Hepatobiliary and Pancreatic Disease
The Team Approach to Management

Hepatobiliary and Pancreatic Disease
The Team Approach to Management

Henry A. Pitt, M.D.

Professor and Vice Chairman, Department of Surgery,
Johns Hopkins University School of Medicine;
Deputy Director, Section of Surgical Sciences,
Johns Hopkins Hospital, Baltimore

David L. Carr-Locke, M.D.

Associate Professor of Medicine, Harvard Medical School;
Director of Endoscopy, Department of Gastroenterology,
Brigham and Women's Hospital, Boston

Joseph T. Ferrucci, M.D.

Chairman, Department of Radiology,
Boston University School of Medicine, Boston

Foreword by
William P. Longmire, Jr., M.D.
Professor Emeritus of Surgery,
University of California, Los Angeles,
UCLA School of Medicine;
Honorary Staff, Department of Surgery,
UCLA Medical Center, Los Angeles

Little, Brown and Company
Boston   New York   Toronto   London

Library of Congress Cataloging-in-Publication Data

Hepatobiliary and pancreatic disease: the team approach to management / [edited by] Henry A. Pitt, David L. Carr-Locke, Joseph T. Ferruci.
    p.   cm.
    Includes bibliographical references and index.
    ISBN 0-316-70915-8
    1. Liver—Diseases—Treatment. 2. Biliary tract—Diseases—Treatment. 3. Pancreas—Diseases—Treatment. 4. Health care teams. I. Pitt, Henry A. II. Carr-Locke, David L. III. Ferrucci, Joseph T., 1937-
    [DNLM: 1. Liver Diseases—therapy. 2. Pancreatic Diseases—therapy. 3. Patient Care Team. WI 700 H5252 1995]
    RC845.H42 1995
    616.3'6—dc20
    DNLM/DLC
    for Library of Congress   94-46416
                                       CIP

Printed in the United States of America

MV-NY

Sponsoring Editor: Nancy E. Chorpenning
Production Services: Textbook Writers Associates
Cover Designer: Ethan Thomas

Contents

Foreword

Over the last several years, significant changes have occurred in the management of many of the diseases of the hepatobiliary and pancreatic systems, and there are now a variety of diagnostic and treatment methods available. The editors, aware of these changes, have drawn together experts from the fields of surgery, gastroenterology, and radiology to collaborate in an authoritative discussion of the frequently complex problems that arise in these closely related systems. In the past, management of a particular patient's problem often depended on the discipline of the original physician to whom the patient had been referred. Historically, these specialists, being particularly familiar with the management literature in their own field, may have overlooked other, possibly more suitable, management options involving related disciplines.

To obviate this difficulty, the editors have selected experts from pertinent fields to present the various options available for the management of 42 complex hepatobiliary and pancreatic diseases. Thus, there is presented in each chapter a balanced discussion of management options from which a preferred course of action is developed.

Gone are the days of the unquestioned authority, knowledge, and judgment of a single specialist—whether surgeon, internist, or radiologist—in the management of the often complex problems presented in this field, problems often requiring multiple diagnostic procedures as well as combined treatment modalities that one specialist is rarely properly prepared to carry out. Surgeons, particularly those of some years' standing, may find it a bit trying at times to give up the time-honored belief that the surgeon is the unquestioned "captain of the team." Instead, we must realize that for optimum results, there must be a collegial attitude of shared input and responsibility, even though only one colleague continues to serve as the patient's doctor.

The multidisciplinary approach of this book is unique. It will undoubtedly prove useful to the physician and ultimately will benefit the patient.

William P. Longmire, Jr., M.D.

Preface

In recent years, hepatobiliary and pancreatic disease has become a recognized subspecialty. This evolution has occurred as our knowledge of the etiology and pathogenesis of, as well as our ability to diagnose and treat, diseases of the liver, biliary tract, and pancreas have expanded dramatically. Interestingly, this subspecialization has taken place simultaneously in the broad fields of surgery, gastroenterology, and radiology. A similar phenomenon is also occurring in oncology and pathology. As a result, multiple diagnostic and therapeutic options have become available for patients with hepatobiliary and pancreatic problems.

As an increasing number of management options have been developed, considerable controversy has arisen among subspecialists as to the optimal approach. In general, the surgical, gastroenterologic, and radiologic literature has tended to be biased in favor of the particular subspecialist's technique. The editors believe, on the other hand, that our patients are best served by a multidisciplinary approach to management. This book is a reflection of the editors' philosophy and should present a unique contribution to the literature.

The editors have identified 42 hepatobiliary and pancreatic problems that require a team approach to management. A national and international group of experts were invited to discuss these patient problems. For each chapter, a surgeon, a gastroenterologist, or a radiologist was identified as the lead author. However, these specialists were then asked to include at least one, and usually two or three, coauthors from different subspecialties.

The result is a fascinating blending of ideas, which represents the state-of-the-art team approach to management of hepatobiliary and pancreatic disease in the mid-1990s.

One hundred and thirty-two authors have contributed to this book. These experts include 57 surgeons, 37 gastroenterologists, 30 radiologists, and 8 individuals in the fields of medical and radiation oncology, pathology, parasitology, and pharmacology. The surgeons include specialists in hepatobiliary and pancreatic surgery, laparoscopy, liver transplantation, pediatric surgery, and trauma surgery. The gastroenterologists include experts in endoscopy as well as adult and pediatric hepatology. The radiologists include subspecialists in the fields of interventional and diagnostic radiology. These experts have provided views from 29 institutions in five countries and five continents.

The authors were asked to discuss etiology, pathogenesis, and diagnosis but to focus on management and results. Management options and controversies were to be covered, and a preferred approach was to emerge. Rather than an exhaustive bibliography, the authors have provided a maximum of ten recent or classic selected readings. The editors believe that this unique formula has resulted in a balanced view of the present management of hepatobiliary and pancreatic disease.

H.A.P.
D.L.C.-L.
J.T.F.

Contributing Authors

Stanley G. Alexander, M.D.
Assistant Professor of Radiology, Indiana University Hospital; General Radiologist, Wishard Memorial Hospital, Indianapolis
23. Sclerosing Cholangitis

Giuseppe Aliperti, M.D.
Assistant Professor of Medicine, Washington University School of Medicine; Director, Section of Interventional and Pancreaticobiliary Endoscopy, Barnes Hospital, St. Louis
17. Gallbladder Stones

Emil J. Balthazar, M.D.
Professor of Radiology, New York University School of Medicine; Attending Radiologist, and Co-Director of Abdominal Imaging, Tisch Hospital and Bellevue Hospital Center, New York
33. Pancreatic Necrosis

Peter A. Banks, M.D.
Associate Professor of Medicine, Harvard Medical School; Director of Clinical Gastroenterology Service, Brigham and Women's Hospital, Boston
29. Acute Pancreatitis

James M. Becker, M.D.
James Utley Professor of Surgery, Boston University School of Medicine; Surgeon-in-Chief, Boston University Medical Center, Boston
29. Acute Pancreatitis

Steven J. Beningfield, FF Rad(D) S.A.
Professor of Radiology, University of Cape Town Medical School; Chairman, Department of Radiology, Groote Schuur Hospital, Cape Town, South Africa
38. Pancreatic Trauma

Martin M. Berman, M.D.
Associate Professor of Pathology, University of Connecticut School of Medicine, Farmington, Connecticut; Attending Pathologist, Hartford Hospital, Hartford, Connecticut
12. Benign Hepatic Tumors

Desmond H. Birkett, M.D.
Associate Professor of Surgery, Boston University School of Medicine; Chief of General and Gastrointestinal Surgery and Surgical Endoscopy, Boston University Medical Center, Boston
20. Acute Cholecystitis

Philippus C. Bornman, M.D.
Professor of Surgery, University of Cape Town Medical School; Chief Specialist, Department of Surgery, Groote Schuur Hospital, Cape Town, South Africa
38. Pancreatic Trauma

Edward L. Bradley III, M.D.
Professor and Vice Chairman, Department of Surgery, State University of New York at Buffalo School of Medicine; Head, Department of Surgery, Buffalo General Hospital, Buffalo, New York
33. Pancreatic Necrosis

David C. Brooks, M.D.
Assistant Professor of Surgery, Harvard Medical School; Assistant Surgeon, Brigham and Women's Hospital, Boston
18. Choledocholithiasis

John L. Cameron, M.D.
Professor and Chairman, Department of Surgery, Johns Hopkins University School of Medicine; Surgeon-in-Chief, Johns Hopkins Hospital, Baltimore
42. Pancreatic Cancer

Paolo Caraceni, M.D.
Clinical and Research Fellow, Oklahoma Transplant Institute, Baptist Medical Center of Oklahoma, Oklahoma City
1. Hepatitis

William D. Carey, M.D.
Head, Section of Hepatology, Department of Gastroenterology, Cleveland Clinic Foundation, Cleveland
2. Hepatic Failure

David L. Carr-Locke, M.D.
Associate Professor of Medicine, Harvard Medical School; Director of Endoscopy, Department of Gastroenterology, Brigham and Women's Hospital, Boston
18. Choledocholithiasis

Lin Chang, M.D.
Assistant Professor of Internal Medicine, University of California, Los Angeles, UCLA School of Medicine, Los Angeles; Staff Gastroenterologist, Harbor-UCLA Medical Center, Torrance, California
39. Islet Cell Tumors

Chang-Yi Chen, M.D.
Professor of Medicine, Kaohsiung Medical College; Former Director, Division of Gastroenterology, Kaohsiung Medical College Hospital, Kaohsiung, Taiwan
22. Biliary Parasites

Eng-Rin Chen, M.D.
Professor of Parasitology, Kaohsiung Medical College, Kaohsiung, Taiwan
22. Biliary Parasites

Kent-Man Chu, MBBS (HK), FRCS (Ed), FCS (HK)
Department of Surgery, The University of Hong Kong, Queen Mary Hospital, Hong Kong
21. Acute Cholangitis

Francisco G. Cigarroa, M.D.
Instructor in Surgery, Johns Hopkins University School of Medicine and Johns Hopkins Hospital, Baltimore
15. Biliary Atresia

Lisa M. Colletti, M.D.
Assistant Professor of Surgery, University of Michigan Medical School; Attending Surgeon, University of Michigan Hospital, Ann Arbor, Michigan
36. Chronic Pancreatitis

Paul M. Colombani, M.D.
Professor of Surgery, Pediatrics, and Oncology, Johns Hopkins University School of Medicine; Children's Surgeon-in-Charge, Department of Pediatric Surgery, Johns Hopkins Hospital, Baltimore
15. Biliary Atresia

Robert D'Agostino, M.D.
Assistant Professor of Radiology, Boston University Medical School; Attending Radiologist, Boston University Medical Center, Boston
10. Hemobilia

Daniel J. Deziel, M.D.
Associate Professor of General Surgery, Rush Medical College of Rush University; Associate Attending Surgeon, Rush-Presbyterian-St. Luke's Medical Center, Chicago
31. Pseudocysts

Anna Mae Diehl, M.D.
Associate Professor of Medicine, Johns Hopkins University School of Medicine; Staff Physician, Division of Gastroenterology/Hepatology, Johns Hopkins Hospital, Baltimore
6. Budd-Chiari Syndrome

Frederic E. Eckhauser, M.D.
Professor of Surgery, University of Michigan Medical School; Chief of Gastrointestinal Surgery, and Director of Multidisciplinary Gastrointestinal Tumor Clinic, University of Michigan Hospital, Ann Arbor, Michigan
36. Chronic Pancreatitis

Steven A. Edmundowicz, M.D.
Associate Professor of Medicine, Department of Gastroenterology and Hepatology, Jefferson Medical College of Thomas Jefferson University; Chief of Endoscopy, and Director of Clinical Gastrointestinal Services, Thomas Jefferson University Hospital, Philadelphia
17. Gallbladder Stones

Peter J. Eisenberg, M.D.
Clinical Assistant, Department of Radiology, Harvard Medical School and Massachusetts General Hospital, Boston
8. Hepatic Abscesses

Grace H. Elta, M.D.
Associate Professor of Internal Medicine, University of Michigan Medical School; Staff Physician, Departments of Internal Medicine and Gastroenterology, University of Michigan Hospital, Ann Arbor, Michigan
36. Chronic Pancreatitis

Stefano Fagiuoli, M.D.
Senior Fellow, Oklahoma Transplantation Institute, Baptist Medical Center of Oklahoma, Oklahoma City
1. Hepatitis

Sheung-Tat Fan, MS, FRCS (Glasgow), FACS
Professor of Surgery, The University of Hong Kong; Honorary Consultant, Department of Surgery, Queen Mary Hospital, Hong Kong
13. Hepatocellular Carcinoma

David V. Feliciano, M.D.
Professor of Surgery, Emory University School of Medicine; Chief of Surgery, Grady Memorial Hospital, Atlanta
11. Hepatic Trauma

Carlos Fernandez-Del Castillo, M.D.
Assistant Professor of Surgery, Harvard Medical School; Assistant Surgeon, Massachusetts General Hospital, Boston
34. Pancreatic Hemorrhage

Joseph T. Ferrucci, M.D.
Chairman, Department of Radiology, Boston University School of Medicine, Boston
20. Acute Cholecystitis

Elliot K. Fishman, M.D.
Professor of Radiology and Oncology, Johns Hopkins University School of Medicine and Johns Hopkins Hospital, Baltimore
40. Cystic Neoplasms

James H. Foster, M.D.
Professor Emeritus of Surgery, University of Connecticut School of Medicine, Farmington, Connecticut
12. Benign Hepatic Tumors

Ivor C. Funnell, FCS (SA)
Consultant Surgeon, Department of Gastroenterology, University of Cape Town Medical School and Groote Schuur Hospital, Cape Town, South Africa
38. Pancreatic Trauma

Steven Goldschmid, M.D.
Associate Professor of Medicine, Emory University School of Medicine; Chief of Gastroenterology and Endoscopy, Veterans Administration Medical Center, Atlanta
25. Biliary Fistulas

Gregory J. Gores, M.D.
Associate Professor of Medicine, Mayo Medical School, Rochester, Minnesota
7. Noninflammatory Cysts

Louise B. Grochow, M.D.
Associate Professor of Oncology, Johns Hopkins University School of Medicine, Baltimore
42. Pancreatic Cancer

Ziv J. Haskal, M.D.
Assistant Professor of Radiology, University of Pennsylvania School of Medicine and Hospital of the University of Pennsylvania, Philadelphia
4. Portal Hypertension

Glenn A. Healey, M.D.
Staff Physician, Department of Radiation Oncology, Lahey Clinic, Burlington, Massachusetts
27. Gallbladder Cancer

J. Michael Henderson, M.B., Ch.B.
Chairman, Department of General Surgery, The Cleveland Clinic Foundation, Cleveland
2. Hepatic Failure

H. Franklin Herlong, M.D.
Associate Professor of Medicine, and Associate Dean for Student Affairs, Johns Hopkins University School of Medicine; Active Staff, Department of Medicine, Johns Hopkins Hospital, Baltimore
3. Cirrhosis

Thomas J. Howard, M.D.
Assistant Professor of Surgery, Indiana University School of Medicine and Indiana University Medical Center, Indianapolis
23. Sclerosing Cholangitis

Ralph H. Hruban, M.D.
Associate Professor of Pathology, Johns Hopkins University School of Medicine; Director of Cardiovascular-Respiratory Pathology, Johns Hopkins Hospital, Baltimore
40. Cystic Neoplasms

Kevin S. Hughes, M.D.
Staff Surgeon, Department of General Surgery, Lahey Clinic, Burlington, Massachusetts
14. Hepatic Metastases

John G. Hunter, M.D.
Associate Professor of Surgery, Emory University School of Medicine; Chief of Gastrointestinal Surgery, Emory University Hospital, Atlanta
25. Biliary Fistulas

Leon G. Josephs, M.D.
Assistant Professor of Surgery, Boston University School of Medicine; Staff Surgeon, Sections of Gastrointestinal and Vascular Surgery, Boston University Medical Center, Boston
10. Hemobilia

Anthony N. Kalloo, M.D.
Assistant Professor of Medicine, Johns Hopkins University School of Medicine; Director of Therapeutic Endoscopy, Johns Hopkins Hospital, Baltimore
16. Biliary Cysts
24. Benign Strictures

Marshall M. Kaplan, M.D.
Professor of Medicine, Tufts University School of Medicine; Chief, Division of Gastroenterology, New England Medical Center, Boston
5. Primary Biliary Cirrhosis

John A. Kaufman, M.D.
Instructor in Radiology, Harvard Medical School; Vascular Radiologist, Massachusetts General Hospital, Boston
34. Pancreatic Hemorrhage

Stephen L. Kaufman, M.D.
Professor of Radiology, Emory University School of Medicine; Director of Interventional Radiology, Emory University Hospital, Atlanta
25. Biliary Fistulas

Chen-Guo Ker, M.D., Ph.D.
Professor of Surgery, Kaohsiung Medical College; Chief of Hepatobiliary and Pancreatic Surgery, Kaohsiung Medical College Hospital, Kaohsiung, Taiwan
22. Biliary Parasites

Michael B. Kimmey, M.D.
Associate Professor of Medicine, University of Washington School of Medicine; Director of Gastrointestinal Endoscopy, University Hospital Medical Center, Seattle
30. Gallstone Pancreatitis

Andrew S. Klein, M.D.
Associate Professor of Surgery, Johns Hopkins University School of Medicine; Director of Liver Transplantation, Johns Hopkins Hospital, Baltimore
3. Cirrhosis
6. Budd-Chiari Syndrome

James A. Knol, M.D.
Associate Professor of Surgery, University of Michigan Medical School; Staff Surgeon, University of Michigan Hospital, Ann Arbor, Michigan
36. Chronic Pancreatitis

Kenyon K. Kopecky, M.D.
Professor of Radiology, Indiana University School of Medicine; Staff Radiologist, Indiana University Hospital, Indianapolis
23. Sclerosing Cholangitis

Richard A. Kozarek, M.D.
Clinical Professor of Medicine, University of Washington School of Medicine; Chief of Gastroenterology, Virginia Mason Clinic, Seattle
37. Pancreatic Fistulas

Jake Krige, M.D.
Associate Professor of Surgery, University of Cape Town Medical School; Senior Consultant, Department of Surgery, Groote Schuur Hospital, Cape Town, South Africa
38. Pancreatic Trauma

Ewa Kuligowska, M.D.
Professor of Radiology, Boston University School of Medicine; Director of Body Imaging, Department of Radiology, Boston University Medical Center, Boston
20. Acute Cholecystitis

Edward C. S. Lai, MBBS (HK), FRCS (Ed), FRACS, FACS, MS
Reader and Director of Endoscopy Unit, Department of Surgery, The University of Hong Kong; Honorary Consultant, Department of Surgery, Queen Mary Hospital, Hong Kong
21. Acute Cholangitis

Sum P. Lee, M.D., Ph.D.
Professor of Medicine, University of Washington School of Medicine; Chief of Gastroenterology, Veterans Affairs Medical Center, Seattle
30. Gallstone Pancreatitis

Glen A. Lehman, M.D.
Professor of Medicine, Division of Gastroenterology/Hepatology, Indiana University Medical Center, Indianapolis
23. Sclerosing Cholangitis

Curtis A. Lewis, M.D.
Assistant Professor of Radiology, Emory University School of Medicine; Director of Vascular-Interventional Radiology, Grady Memorial Hospital, Atlanta
11. Hepatic Trauma

David R. Lichtenstein, M.D.
Instructor in Medicine, Harvard Medical School; Associate Physician, Division of Gastroenterology, Brigham and Women's Hospital, Boston
18. Choledocholithiasis

Christopher Liddle, BSc (Med.), MBBS, Ph.D., FRACP
Senior Lecturer in Pharmacology, University of Sydney; Head of Clinical Pharmacology, Westmead Hospital, Sydney, Australia
9. Hydatid Disease

Keith D. Lillemoe, M.D.
Associate Professor of Surgery, Johns Hopkins University School of Medicine; Active Staff, Department of Surgery, Johns Hopkins Hospital, Baltimore
24. Benign Strictures

Pamela A. Lipsett, M.D.
Assistant Professor of Surgery, Johns Hopkins University School of Medicine; Attending Physician, Department of Surgery, Johns Hopkins Hospital, Baltimore
16. Biliary Cysts

J. Miles Little, M.D.
Professor of Surgery, University of Sydney; Surgeon, Westmead Hospital, Sydney, Australia
9. Hydatid Disease

Lawrence Lumeng, M.D.
Professor of Medicine, Indiana University School of Medicine; Director of Gastroenterology and Hepatology, Indiana University Medical Center and Veterans Administration Medical Center, Indianapolis
23. Sclerosing Cholangitis

Rene Male, M.D.
Gastroenterology Fellow, Department of Medicine, Indiana University School of Medicine and Indiana University Medical Center, Indianapolis
23. Sclerosing Cholangitis

Terence A. S. Matalon, M.D.
Associate Professor of Radiology, Department of Diagnostic Radiology/Nuclear Medicine, Rush Medical College of Rush University; Director of Interventional Radiology, Rush-Presbyterian-St. Luke's Medical Center, Chicago
31. Pseudocysts

Francis D. Milligan, M.D.
Associate Professor of Medicine, Johns Hopkins University School of Medicine; Active Staff, Part-Time Faculty, Department of Medicine, Johns Hopkins Hospital, Baltimore
42. Pancreatic Cancer

Christopher P. Molgaard, M.D.
Staff Radiologist, Lahey Clinic Medical Center, Burlington, Massachusetts
14. Hepatic Metastases

Peter R. Mueller, M.D.
Associate Professor of Radiology, Harvard Medical School; Head of Abdominal Imaging and Interventional Radiology, Massachusetts General Hospital, Boston
8. Hepatic Abscesses
32. Pancreatic Abscesses

Michel M. Murr, M.D.
Research Fellow, Department of Surgery, Mayo Medical School, Rochester, Minnesota
41. Ampullary Carcinoma

Abdul Nadir, M.D.
Liver Transplant Fellow, Oklahoma Transplant Institute; Baptist Medical Center of Oklahoma, Oklahoma City
1. Hepatitis

David M. Nagorney, M.D.
Professor of Surgery, Mayo Medical School and Mayo Clinic, Rochester, Minnesota
7. Noninflammatory Cysts

Ali Naji, M.D., Ph.D.
Professor of Surgery, University of Pennsylvania School of Medicine and Hospital of the University of Pennsylvania, Philadelphia
4. Portal Hypertension

William H. Nealon, M.D.
Professor of Surgery, University of Texas Medical Branch, University of Texas Medical School at Galveston, Galveston, Texas
19. Hepatolithiasis

Henry Ngan, FRCP, FRCPE, FRCR
Professor and Head, Department of Diagnostic Radiology, The University of Hong Kong; Honorary Consultant, Department of Diagnostic Radiology, Queen Mary Hospital, Hong Kong
13. Hepatocellular Carcinoma
21. Acute Cholangitis

Richard A. Oberfield, M.D.
Clinical Instructor in Medicine, Harvard Medical School; Staff Medical Oncologist, Lahey Clinic, Burlington, Massachusetts
27. Gallbladder Cancer

Andrew J. Oishi, M.D.
Resident in General Surgery, Mayo Medical School, Rochester, Minnesota
41. Ampullary Carcinoma

Carlos A. Pellegrini, M.D.
Professor and Chairman, Department of Surgery, University of Washington School of Medicine; Chief of Surgery, University Hospital Medical Center, Seattle
30. Gallstone Pancreatitis

Bret T. Petersen, M.D.
Consultant in Gastroenterology, Mayo Clinic, Rochester, Minnesota
41. Ampullary Carcinoma

Daniel Picus, M.D.
Associate Professor of Radiology, Washington University School of Medicine; Chief of Vascular and Interventional Radiology, Edward Mallinckrodt Institute of Radiology, Barnes Hospital, St. Louis
17. Gallbladder Stones

Henry A. Pitt, M.D.
Professor and Vice Chairman, Department of Surgery, Johns Hopkins University School of Medicine; Deputy Director, Section of Surgical Sciences, Johns Hopkins Hospital, Baltimore
16. Biliary Cysts
40. Cystic Neoplasms

Richard A. Prinz, M.D.
Helen Shedd Keith Professor and Chairman, Department of General Surgery, Rush Medical College of Rush University; Chairman, Department of Surgery, Rush-Presbyterian-St. Luke's Medical Center, Chicago
31. Pseudocysts

Florecia G. Que, M.D.
Instructor in Surgery, Mayo Medical School; Department of Surgery, Mayo Clinic, Rochester, Minnesota
7. Noninflammatory Cysts

David W. Rattner, M.D.
Associate Professor of Surgery, Harvard Medical School; Associate Visiting Surgeon, Massachusetts General Hospital, Boston
8. Hepatic Abscesses
32. Pancreatic Abscesses

Ernest J. Ring, M.D.
Professor of Radiology, University of California, San Francisco, School of Medicine; Chief of Radiology, Mount Zion Medical Center, San Francisco
4. Portal Hypertension

Ian C. Roberts-Thomson, M.D.
Associate Professor of Medicine, University of Adelaide; Director, Department of Gastoenterology, The Queen Elizabeth Hospital, Adelaide, S.A. Australia
26. Motility Disorders

Richard J. Rohrer, M.D.
Associate Professor of Surgery, Tufts University School of Medicine; Chief of Transplant Surgery, New England Medical Center, Boston
5. Primary Biliary Cirrhosis

Ricardo L. Rossi, M.D.
Associate Professor of Surgery, Harvard Medical School; Chairman, Department of General Surgery, Lahey Clinic, Burlington, Massachusetts
27. Gallbladder Cancer

Alfred D. Roston, M.D.
Advanced Therapeutic Endoscopy Fellow, Department of Medicine, Harvard Medical School, and Division of Gastroenterology, Brigham and Women's Hospital, Boston
18. Choledocholithiasis

Raymond A. Rubin, M.D.
Assistant Professor of Medicine, Jefferson Medical College of Thomas Jefferson University, Philadelphia
4. Portal Hypertension

Michael G. Sarr, M.D.
Associate Professor of Surgery, Mayo Medical School; Chair, Division of Gastroenterology and General Surgery, Mayo Clinic and Mayo Foundation, Rochester, Minnesota
41. Ampullary Carcinoma

Scott J. Savader, M.D.
Assistant Professor of Radiology, Johns Hopkins University School of Medicine; Interventional Radiologist, Johns Hopkins Hospital, Baltimore
6. Budd-Chiari Syndrome
16. Biliary Cysts

Robert H. Schapiro, M.D.
Associate Clinical Professor of Medicine, Harvard Medical School; Director of Endoscopy Unit, Massachusetts General Hospital, Boston
35. Pancreas Divisum

Kathleen B. Schwarz, M.D.
Associate Professor of Pediatrics, Division of Pediatric Gastroenterology and Nutrition, Johns Hopkins University School of Medicine, and Johns Hopkins Hospital, Baltimore
15. Biliary Atresia

John Sekijima, M.D.
Assistant Professor of Medicine, University of Washington School of Medicine; Staff Gastroenterologist, Veterans Affairs Medical Center, Seattle
30. Gallstone Pancreatitis

Pai-Ching Sheen, M.D., Ph.D.
Professor of Surgery, Division of Hepatobiliary and Pancreatic Surgery, Kaohsiung Medical College, and Kaohsiung Medical College Hospital, Kaohsiung, Taiwan
22. Biliary Parasites

Stuart Sherman, M.D.
Assistant Professor of Medicine, Indiana University School of Medicine, and Indiana University Medical Center, Indianapolis
23. Sclerosing Cholangitis

Gregory T. Sica, M.D.
Instructor in Radiology, Harvard Medical School; Associate Radiologist, Brigham and Women's Hospital, Boston
29. Acute Pancreatitis

Gregory J. Slater, M.D.
Clinical Fellow, Department of Radiology, Harvard Medical School; Clinical Fellow, Section of Abdominal Imaging and Intervention, Massachusetts General Hospital, Boston
32. Pancreatic Abscesses

Nathaniel J. Soper, M.D.
Associate Professor of Surgery, Washington University School of Medicine; Staff Surgeon, Barnes Hospital, St. Louis
17. Gallbladder Stones

Bruce E. Stabile, M.D.
Professor of Surgery, University of California, Los Angeles, UCLA School of Medicine, Los Angeles; Chairman, Department of Surgery, Harbor-UCLA Medical Center, Torrance, California
39. Islet Cell Tumors

Steven M. Strasberg, M.D.
Professor of Surgery, Washington University School of Medicine; Head, Division of Gastrointestinal Surgery, Barnes Hospital, St. Louis
17. Gallbladder Stones

Mark A. Talamini, M.D.
Assistant Professor of Surgery, Johns Hopkins University School of Medicine; Attending Surgeon, Johns Hopkins Hospital, Baltimore
40. Cystic Neoplasms

Paul J. Thuluvath, M.D.
Assistant Professor of Medicine, Johns Hopkins University School of Medicine, Baltimore
28. Cholangiocarcinoma

James Toouli, MBBS, FRACS
Professor of Surgery, Flinders University of South Australia; Senior Director of Gastrointestinal Surgical and Liver Transplant Unit, Flinders Medical Center, Bedford Park, Adelaide, S.A. Australia
26. Motility Disorders

L. William Traverso, M.D.
Associate Clinical Professor of Surgery, University of Washington School of Medicine; Attending Surgeon, Virginia Mason Medical Center, Seattle
37. Pancreatic Fistulas

Jane I. Tsao, M.D.
Staff Surgeon, Lahey Clinic, Burlington, Massachusetts
14. Hepatic Metastases

Xabier de Aretxabala Urquiza, M.D.
Associate Professor of Surgery, Universidad de la Frontera; Vice Chairman, Biliary-Pancreas Team, Temuco Regional Hospital, Temuco, Chile
27. Gallbladder Cancer

Michael F. Uzer, M.D.
Assistant Professor of Medicine, Section of Digestive Diseases, Rush Medical College of Rush University; Director of Therapeutic Endoscopy, Rush-Presbyterian-St. Luke's Medical Center, Chicago
31. Pseudocysts

Eric vanSonnenberg, M.D.
Professor of Internal Medicine and Surgery, and Professor and Chairman of Radiology, University of Texas Medical Branch, University of Texas Medical School at Galveston, Galveston, Texas
19. Hepatolithiasis

David H. Van Thiel, M.D.
Medical Director of Liver and Digestive Disease Center, and Transplantation Medicine, Baptist Medical Center of Oklahoma, Oklahoma City
1. Hepatitis

Anthony C. Venbrux, M.D.
Associate Professor of Radiology, Johns Hopkins University School of Medicine; Associate Director, Cardiovascular and Interventional Radiology, Johns Hopkins Hospital, Baltimore
28. Cholangiocarcinoma
42. Pancreatic Cancer

David P. Vogt, M.D.
Staff Surgeon, General Surgery/Transplant Center, The Cleveland Clinic Foundation, Cleveland
2. Hepatic Failure

David T. Walden, M.D.
Assistant Professor of Medicine, and Director of Endoscopy, Department of Internal Medicine, University of Texas Medical Branch, University of Texas Medical School at Galveston, Galveston, Texas
19. Hepatolithiasis

Arthur C. Waltman, M.D.
Associate Professor of Radiology, Harvard Medical School; Director of Vascular Radiology, Massachusetts General Hospital, Boston
34. Pancreatic Hemorrhage

Andrew L. Warshaw, M.D.
Harold and Ellen Danser Professor of Surgery, Harvard Medical School; Chief of General Surgery, and Associate Chief of Surgical Services, Massachusetts General Hospital, Boston
35. Pancreas Divisum

Timothy J. Welch, M.D.
Assistant Professor of Diagnostic Radiology, Mayo Medical School; Consultant, Department of Diagnostic Radiology, Mayo Clinic, Rochester, Minnesota
7. Noninflammatory Cysts

Charles F. White, M.D.
Clinical Assistant Professor of Medicine, Harvard Medical School; Staff Physician, Department of Medical Oncology, Lahey Clinic, Burlington, Massachusetts
14. Hepatic Metastases

Adam B. Winick, M.D.
Instructor in Radiology, Johns Hopkins University School of Medicine; Instructor in Cardiovascular and Interventional Radiology, Johns Hopkins Hospital, Baltimore
24. Benign Strictures

Gerhard R. Wittich, M.D.
Professor and Vice Chairman of Radiology, University of Texas Medical Branch, University of Texas Medical School at Galveston, Galveston, Texas
19. Hepatolithiasis

John Wong, Ph.D.
Professor and Head, Department of Surgery, The University of Hong Kong; Chief of Service, Department of Surgery, Queen Mary Hospital, Hong Kong
13. Hepatocelluar Carcinoma

Harlan I. Wright, M.D.
Fellow, Oklahoma Transplant Institute, Baptist Medical Center of Oklahoma, Oklahoma City
1. Hepatitis

Allan G. Wycherley, FRACR
Clinical Lecturer, Department of Radiology, Flinders University School of Medicine; Head of Nuclear Medicine Section, Department of Radiology, Flinders Medical Centre, Adelaide, S.A. Australia
26. Motility Disorders

Charles J. Yeo, M.D.
Associate Professor of Surgery, Johns Hopkins University School of Medicine; Attending Surgeon, Johns Hopkins Hospital, Baltimore
28. Cholangiocarcinoma

Alan M. Zuckerman, M.D.
Assistant Professor of Radiology, Emory University School of Medicine; Attending Radiologist, Emory Clinic, Atlanta
25. Biliary Fistulas

Hepatobiliary and Pancreatic Disease
The Team Approach to Management

1

Hepatitis

David H. Van Thiel
Stefano Fagiuoli
Paolo Caraceni
Harlan I. Wright
Abdul Nadir

The word *hepatitis* is a generic term identifying an inflammatory condition of the liver. Clinically, hepatitis is defined as an elevation of the serum aminotransferase levels. It occurs in two principal clinical situations: as acute and chronic hepatitis. Acute hepatitis is of recent onset ($\leq$ 3–6 months); chronic hepatitis is characterized either by a documentable history of abnormal liver enzymes for more than 6 months or by overt evidence of disease chronicity, such as biopsy evidence of disease, often occurring in association with hepatic fibrosis or cirrhosis; splenomegaly with hypersplenism; ascites; or some other complication of portal hypertension.

Etiology and Pathogenesis

Acute Hepatitis

Acute hepatitis is characterized by hepatocellular injury (increased aminotransferase levels) with or without associated jaundice of recent onset. Because the clinical outcome differs markedly depending on the severity and the rapidity of clinical onset of identifiable hepatic injury, acute hepatitis is most often divided into four distinct clinical syndromes (Fig. 1-1): fulminant hepatitis, subfulminant hepatitis, subacute hepatic failure, and classical hepatitis. In general, fulminant hepatitis follows a very rapid course, with the time from clinical onset to hepatic coma being 2 weeks or less. In subfulminant hepatitis, the clinical onset is less rapid but hepatic coma

develops within 2 to 6 weeks. Subacute hepatic failure is characterized by a disease process that persists beyond 6 weeks and often progresses directly to chronic hepatitis and cirrhosis within 3 to 6 weeks without any evidence of a clinical remission. Overt hepatic coma may or may not occur in subacute hepatic failure, but some degree of hepatic encephalopathy is always present (grades 1–3). Routine or classical hepatitis is the most common syndrome of acute hepatitis. Classical hepatitis is characterized by hepatic injury of short duration (3–6 weeks of illness or less) that does not lead to either hepatic coma or progress to disease chronicity.

The more common causes of acute hepatitis are shown in Table 1-1. The vast majority of acute hepatitis cases are caused by a handful of common hepatotropic viruses. The second most frequent broad class of cases of acute hepatitis are those that occur as a consequence of a drug exposure, usually as a therapeutic misadventure but occasionally as an intentional overdose or poisoning (Table 1-2).

A common form of acute hepatitis that is rarely recognized as such is that caused by hepatic injury occurring as a consequence of anoxia/ischemia. The usual courses for this condition are hepatic hypoperfusion or venous congestion associated with diseases or with dysfunction of an organ other than the liver, such as occurs with low-output cardiac failure, congestive heart failure, major pulmonary embolism, shock, or sepsis. The other forms of

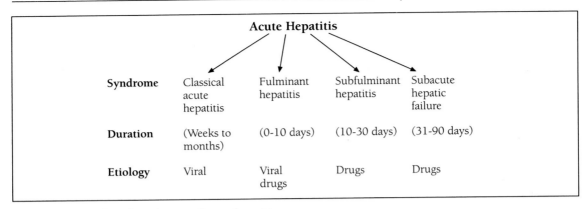

Figure 1-1. Four clinical syndromes of acute hepatitis.

Table 1-1. Acute Hepatitis

Hepatitis due to infection
  Viruses
    Common viral hepatitides
      Hepatitis A
      Hepatitis B
      Hepatitis C
      Hepatitis D + B
      Hepatitis E
    Opportunistic hepatitides
      CMV
      EBV
      Herpes
      Adenovirus
    Unusual geographically restricted forms of acute hepatitis
      Dengue
      Yellow fever
      Ebola
  Bacteria
  Rickettsia
  Other agents
Drug-induced hepatitis
  Therapeutic misadventures
  Overdoses
Toxin-induced hepatitis
  Amanita phalloides
Physical injury
  Anoxia/ischemia (hypoperfusion)
  Congestion/stasis
  Granuloma
  Heat
  Systemic disease
  Infection
  Lipidosis
  Amyloid
  Metastatic cancer

Table 1-2. Common Causes of Drug- or Toxin-Induced Toxicity

Acetaminophen
Diclofenac
Diphenylhydantoin
Disulfiram
Fipexide
Gold injections
Halothane
Isoniazid
Ketoconazole
Nicotinic acid (sustained release)
Valproic acid

acute hepatitis are seen much less often and are identified as a result of either a high index of suspicion or unique clinical circumstances.

Chronic Hepatitis

Chronic hepatitis is defined as liver cell injury that continues for at least 6 months and usually much longer. Chronic hepatitis is most effectively divided into two main types: chronic cholestatic and chronic hepatocellular liver disease. The more common chronic cholestatic liver diseases of adults and children which are included in the overall rubric of chronic hepatitis differ markedly (see Fig. 1-1). Adults, particularly women, are likely to have

Table 1-3. Chronic Hepatocellular Diseases and Their Therapies

Disease Type	Characteristics	Therapy
Autoimmune		
Type 1	Ana+; HLA B_8Dr_3+	Immunosuppressants
Type 2	Anti-LKM+	Antiviral agents
Type 3	SLA+; HLA B_8Dr_3+	Immunosuppressants
Viral		
Hepatitis B	HBsAg+ HBV-DNA+	Antiviral agents
Hepatitis C	HCV-RNA+	Antiviral agents
Cryptogenic		Unknown
Drug-induced (see Table 1-2)		Drug withdrawal
Ethanol-induced		Alcohol abstinence
Familial		
Hemochromatosis		Iron removal
Wilson's disease		Copper elimination
Alpha$_1$-antitrypsin deficiency		Gene therapy
Tyrosinemia		Tyrosine-restricted diet; gene therapy
Others		Variable, depending upon the specific pathogenetic mechanisms of the disease process

primary biliary cirrhosis (PBC). Nearly equal numbers of men and women, with only a slight predominance of men, have primary sclerosing cholangitis (PSC), which often occurs in association with inflammatory bowel disease, particularly, but not exclusively, ulcerative colitis. In contrast, the most common cholestatic disease in children is biliary atresia followed by one or another of the multitude of chronic cholestatic syndromes that have been either described or identified in children.

Despite the preceding, the term *chronic hepatitis* generally is used to refer to a chronic hepatocellular disease process. The multitude of chronic hepatocellular diseases are most easily distinguished from each other on the basis of their presumed etiology (Fig. 1-1; Table 1-3). Such a classification of chronic hepatocellular disease not only enables the physician to distinguish between the various liver diseases but also directs the clinician to the appropriate type of therapy for each (see Table 1-3).

Diagnosis and Management

The many skills required to diagnose, treat, and manage an individual with either acute or chronic hepatitis necessitate a team of professionals working through a single clinician, the hepatologist, who must have a working knowledge of all the skills required.

Hepatologist

The team starts with and principally serves the patient through the hepatologist and primary care physician. The hepatologist orchestrates the involvement of the larger team of professionals who are working with the primary care physician. The hepatologist's task is to identify the specific disease process, characterize its severity, define the prognosis, and select and manage the appropriate therapy (Fig. 1-2). As a result, the clinical skill of the hepatologist merges with that of each of the other team members.

Pathologist

The clinical pathologist performs the numerous biochemical, serologic, and histopathologic examinations requested by the hepatologist that relate to the patient's disease process, its diagnosis, and its management. The pathologist must be able to perform and analyze laboratory tests and recognize patterns of histopathology.

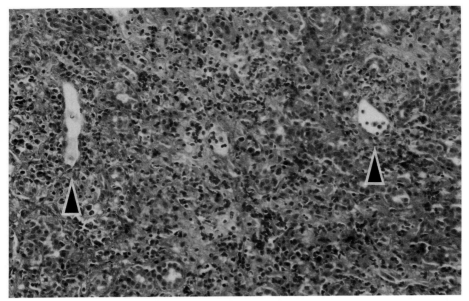

Figure 1-2. Severe Acute Viral Hepatitis: Extensive destruction of the liver parenchyma has occurred, and no normal lobular architecture is apparent. Two central veins (arrowheads) are present. These structures are in closer approximation than normal, reflecting collapse of the intervening parenchyma, which now contains only cellular debris, inflammatory cells, and regenerating hepatocytes. (Courtesy of Dr. James M. Crawford, Brigham and Women's Hospital, Boston). (H&E stain, original magnification 150×.)

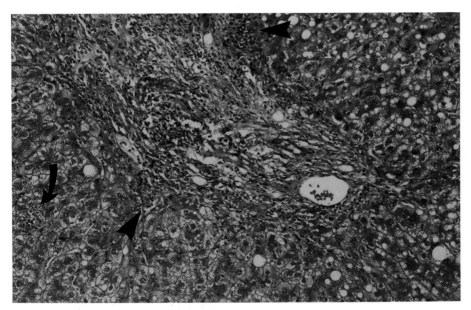

Figure 1-3. Chronic Viral Hepatitis: A portal tract is markedly enlarged by fibrous tissue scarring, and a moderate number of mononuclear inflammatory cells are present. Necroinflammatory activity is present at the interface between the portal tract and the parenchyma (arrowheads). Clusters of inflammatory cells are evidence for focal destruction of lobular hepatocytes (arrow). (Courtesy of Dr. James M. Crawford, Brigham and Women's Hospital, Boston.) (H&E stain, original magnification 150×.)

The ultimate basis for a diagnosis of a chronic liver disease is a liver biopsy (Fig. 1-3). The pathologist must be aware of the subtle histologic features of viral hepatitis (particularly of the more unusual forms) to avoid underdiagnosis. The distinction between fibrotic changes and early cirrhosis can be very difficult to make but is of paramount importance because fibrosis is somewhat reversible. The histopathologic examination of a liver biopsy should include special staining for appropriate viral antigens (HBV, HDV, and CMV in particular), alpha$_1$-antitrypsin globules, iron, copper-associated proteins, reticulin, and a collagen stain (Trichrome). The direct measurement of iron and copper content in the liver (μg/dry weight) should also be determined.

Epidemiologist

The clinical epidemiologist investigates individual patients identified as having viral hepatitis for behaviors that may have contributed to their condition. The epidemiologist may develop plans for behavioral change to prevent the spread of the viral infection. In addition, the epidemiologist attempts to identify common source outbreaks and to identify others at risk for viral hepatitis as a result of their association with or contact with the individual patient.

Immunologist

The clinical immunologist is responsible for performing the many immunologic assays required to identify and characterize the different forms of chronic hepatitis. In addition, the immunologist monitors the clinical response of the patient to the various antiviral or the many biological response modifiers that are used to either treat viral hepatitis or to modify the aberrant immunologic response that characterizes the specific form of hepatitis the patient may have. This often necessitates close interaction not only with the hepatologist but also with the pathologist and virologist.

Virologist

The virology laboratory is essential for identifying the specific viral agent responsible for an individual case of viral hepatitis (see Table 1-1). The laboratory must be able to identify not only the usual forms of viral hepatitis seen most often in practice, but also the many unusual causes of opportunistic or geographically restricted forms of viral hepatitis that can occur (Table 1-4). The latter skill is essential in an age when jet travel enables an individual to change hemispheres or circle the globe within a day. The virology laboratory also must be able to detect mutant viruses that have either greater virulence or resistance to available antiviral treatments. Finally, the virologist should be able to detect the development of mutants that occur as a consequence of active treatment.

Surgeon

The hepatologic surgeon is responsible for treating the complications of portal hypertension or hepatic cancer that occur in patients with advanced chronic hepatitis. In addition, the surgeon plays a critical role when medical therapy is no longer possible or indicated, and the patient requires liver transplantation for either acute or chronic hepatic failure.

The functional reserve of the liver must be carefully assessed prior to any surgical procedure in patients with chronic hepatitis if untoward postoperative complications are to be avoided. Either the magnetoencephalograph (MEGx) test or the caffeine-antipirine test can be used to provide a quantitative measure of residual hepatic function.

Oncologist

The oncologist is required to manage and direct the treatment of hepatic cancer when it develops in individuals with advanced chronic liver disease. Usually, this is a hepatocellular carcinoma (HCC); however, in patients with PSC, cholangiocarcinomas are more likely. Several new drugs are now available which are effective either alone or in combination for the treatment of HCC. Before using any one of these agents, it is essential to determine its actions and potential toxicity, as well as to completely evaluate the function of the tumor-free liver. In patients with viral hepatitis, these agents can, like steroids, promote viral replication, either exacerbating latent viral disease or, upon withdrawal (between cycles of therapy), precipitating fulminant hepatic failure.

Table 1-4. Specific Tests Useful in the Diagnosis and Management of Viral Hepatitis

HAV		Anti-HAV IgM
		Anti-HAV IgG
HBV		
	Serum	HBsAg
		Anti-HBsAg
		Anti-HBc IgM
		Anti-HBc IgG
		HBeAg
		Anti-HBe IgG
		HBV-DNA
		DNA polymerase
		HBV-DNA by PCR
	Tissue	HBsAg (extracytoplasmatic/intracytoplasmatic/nuclear)
		HBcAg (nuclear/cytoplasmatic) (focal/diffuse)
		HBsAg, HBcAg
		HBV-DNA
HCV		
	Serum	Anti-HCV
		RIBA II
		HCV-RNA by PCR
	Tissue	HCV-RNA (in situ hybridization)
HDV		
	Serum	Anti-HDV IgM
		Anti-HDV IgG
		HDV-RNA
		HDV-RNA by PCR
	Tissue	HDVAg (immunofluorescence/immunostaining)
		HDV-RNA (in situ hybridization)
HEV		
	Serum	Anti-HEV IgM
		Anti-HEV IgG

Radiologist

The radiologist is less often identified as a member of the team than are the others identified so far. Yet the radiologist has much to contribute in complicated cases of hepatitis. In cases of acute hepatic failure, CT measurements of hepatic size (Fig. 1-4) and quantitative HIDA scanning can provide valuable information as to when and if liver transplantation will be necessary. In cases of chronic disease, serial ultrasound imaging of patients with cirrhosis is useful in detecting hepatocellular carcinomas when they are still treatable either medically (percutaneous ethanol injections, chemotherapy, or chemoembolization) or surgically. In addition, the recent development of the transjugular intrahepatic portosystem shunt (TIPS) procedure has been helpful in cases of advanced chronic hepatitis with a variety of complications associated with portal hypertension.

Dietician

The clinical dietician is needed to advise the patient and the patient's family on how to optimize the nutritional status and fluid and electrolyte requirements of the patient. The dietician's role is most crucial in cases of acute hepatic failure and end-stage liver disease, when the nitrogen load and sodium intake of the patient may have to be highly regulated and managed, as well as tailored to the individual patient's needs or tolerance. Protein calorie malnutrition is a common and difficult condition to diagnose and manage in patients with chronic hepatitis. Malnutrition is a major prognostic indicator in chronic liver disease. Insulin resistance is ubiquitous in individuals with chronic liver disease. Frequent feedings with moderate-carbohydrate, high-fiber, low-fat diets rich in branched-chain amino acids may improve both insulin resistance and nitrogen balance.

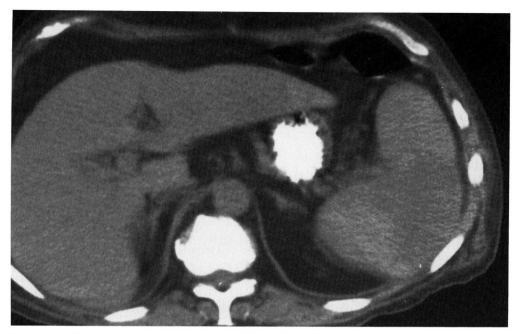

Figure 1-4. CT scan demonstrating a small, nodular cirrhotic liver.

Pharmacologist

Because the liver is central to the biotransformation and excretion of xenobiotics, the clinical pharmacologist plays an important role in advising the hepatologist on which drugs are available for clinical use in patients with liver disease, which should be used with caution or avoided altogether, and which should be monitored, as well as how and when to do so. In addition, the clinical pharmacologist is responsible for identifying any potential drug interactions that might occur in a given patient as a consequence of the various medical treatments being utilized for other organ system disease processes. This typically requires a working knowledge of the metabolism, interactions, and indications for drugs utilized by a given patient for both hepatic disease and the numerous nonhepatic confounding disease processes that may exist in the patient.

Intensive Care Specialists

The patient with acute or chronic hepatitis can be admitted to the intensive care unit for a variety of

Table 1-5. Situations Requiring Intensive Care Unit Hospitalization for Hepatitis

Acute Hepatitis	Chronic Hepatitis
Fulminant hepatic failure	Advanced-stage hepatic encephalopathy
Subfulminant hepatic failure	Variceal bleeding
Subacute hepatic failure	Bleeding from portal hypertensive gastropathy
	Hepatorenal syndrome
	Spontaneous bacterial peritonitis
	Bacteremia (sepsis)

reasons (Table 1-5). In each case, the assistance of an intensive care specialist is often crucial to the optimal management of the patient. This statement is particularly true if the patient is a potential liver transplant candidate. Often other services, such as pulmonary medicine, cardiology, and particularly nephrology, are consulted at the same time.

Results

The outcome of patients with acute and chronic hepatitis varies considerably depending upon the specific cause and treatment. Even the common viral hepatitides differ significantly in their tendency to resolve or progress to chronic hepatitis. For example, hepatitis A is usually self-limited, whereas hepatitis B is much more likely to develop into chronic hepatitis, cirrhosis, and hepatocellular carcinoma. Similarly, drug-induced hepatitis may be subclinical or life-threatening, depending on the agent and the dose. Toxin-induced hepatitis from *Amanita phalloides,* on the other hand, is almost always severe, leading to hepatic failure and the need for liver transplantation.

The outcome of treatment for some of the chronic hepatitides, such as primary biliary cirrhosis (Chap. 5) and primary sclerosing cholangitis (Chap. 23), will be outlined in more detail later in this book. Similarly, the results of treatment for end-stage viral, cryptogenic, drug-induced, and alcohol-induced hepatocellular diseases will be discussed in more detail in the chapters on hepatic failure (Chap. 2), cirrhosis (Chap. 3), and portal hypertension (Chap. 4). Of these causes for chronic hepatitis, alcohol is the most common in this country. Clearly, the results of all treatments for patients with alcohol-induced liver disease are directly related to the patient's ability to remain abstinent from this drug.

Conclusions

As must be evident, the various hepatitides, whether acute or chronic, are complex diseases that require a multitude of clinical and laboratory talents if they are to be diagnosed and treated correctly. This typically necessitates the interaction of a team of professionals rather than the skill of a single physician. Nonetheless, the many skills and services required by a given patient with hepatitis are best orchestrated by a single individual—the hepatologist.

Selected Readings

Balistreri WF, et al. New methods for assessing liver function in infants and children. *Ann Clin Lab Sci* 1992; 22(3):162–174.

Ellis LM, Demers ML, Roh MS. Current strategies for the treatment of hepatocellular carcinoma. *Curr Opin Oncol* 1992; 4(4):741–751.

Gitlin N, Serio KM. Ischemic hepatitis: Widening horizons. *Am J Gastroenterol* 1992; 87(7):831–836.

Kurosaki M, et al. Rapid sequence variation of the hypervariable region of hepatitis C virus during the course of chronic infection. *Hepatology* 1993; 18:1293–1299.

Riely CA, Vera SR. Liver biopsy in the long-term follow-up of liver transplant patients: Still the gold standard. *Gastroenterology* 1990; 99(4):1182–1183.

Sanyal AJ, Zfass AM. MEGX: From bench to bedside. *American J Gastroenterol* 1992; 87(7):919–921.

Sherlock S, Dick R, VanLeeuwen DJ. Liver biopsy today: The royal free hospital experience. *J Hepatol* 1985; 1(1):75–85.

Tank KC, Howard ER. Biliary atresia. *Baillieres Clin Gastroenterol* 1989; 3(1):211–229.

Weiner AJ, et al. Evidence for immune selection of hepatitis C virus (HCV) putative envelope glycoprotein variants: Potential role in chronic HCV infections. *Proc Natl Acad Sci USA* 1992; 89:3468–3472.

Yoshiba M, Sekiyama K, Sugata F, et al. Activation of hepatitis C virus following immuno-suppression treatment. *Dig Dis Sci* 1992; 37:478.

2

Hepatic Failure

WILLIAM D. CAREY
DAVID P. VOGT
J. MICHAEL HENDERSON

Acute liver failure is a syndrome characterized by the rapid onset of severe liver dysfunction in a patient who has no prior history of liver disease. Jaundice, coagulopathy, and encephalopathy are the major clinical manifestations. Acute liver failure occurs because of either massive or submassive hepatic necrosis. In the former, the disease runs its course within 8 weeks of onset; in the latter up to 26 weeks may elapse. Improvement in mortality rates has accompanied improved understanding of the nature of complications for some but not all causes of acute liver failure. With intensive supportive measures, survival rates for established acute liver failure range from 10% to 25% for most causes. Surgical issues in these desperately ill patients are the placement and management of intracranial pressure measurement devices and orthotopic liver transplantation. Liver transplantation appears to improve survival rates from 50% to 85%. Early transfer to a center with expertise in managing this syndrome, particularly to a center which offers liver transplantation, is necessary for optimal salvage.

Etiology

Common causes of acute liver failure are severe viral hepatitis (A, B, [sometimes complicated by delta virus], or C), drug intoxication (especially acetaminophen taken in a suicide attempt), and occasionally mushroom poisoning (usually *Amanita* sp.). Table 2-1 indicates the etiology of acute liver failure in one North American liver unit. Other possible causes include ischemia, acute Budd-Chiari disease, Wilson's disease, and fatty liver of pregnancy. An excellent overview has recently been published. Medications must always be considered as a possible cause in acute liver failure. Sometimes this is difficult to prove; nevertheless, all medications which are nonessential should be discontinued. Table 2-2 indicates some drugs associated with acute liver failure.

Pathogenesis

The pathogenesis of acute liver failure very much depends on the etiology. Drugs may cause liver cell failure by disrupting essential intracellular processes or by causing accumulation of toxic metabolic products. Only occasionally do hepatotrophic viruses (hepatitis A, B, C, delta, E) cause massive cell death. Severe disease is unlikely to be due to the virulence of the virus but instead is probably caused by deficiencies in host response. The injury caused by hepatitis B, for example, is felt to be due mainly to the immunological response to the virus. Hepatitis C, on the other hand, is directly cytopathic. These differences are not absolute and may not directly explain why each virus only occasionally results in massive hepatic injury.

In idiosyncratic drug reactions a variety of mechanisms are apparent as well. Although direct membrane injury may occur, many drugs exhibit a histologic response which does not suggest membrane injury. For example, marked microvesicular fatty changes are seen with valproic acid–induced liver injury. Alpha methyldopa (Aldomet) and iso-

Table 2-1. Diagnosis of Acute Liver Failure in 61 Patients

Diagnosis	Percent	Survival Rate
Non-A, non-B hepatitis	28%	24%
Acetaminophen	25%	67%
Hepatitis B	16%	10%
Drug reaction	10%	17%
Ischemic hepatitis	8%	40%
Delta hepatitis	5%	67%
Wilson's disease	3%	0%
Hepatitis A	2%	0%
Reye's syndrome	2%	0%
Amanita mushroom	2%	0%

Source: Modified from Donaldson BW, et al. The role of transjugular biopsy in fulminant liver failure: Relationship to other prognostic indicators. *Hepatology* 1993; 18:1370–1376.

Table 2-2. Drugs Which May Cause Acute Liver Failure

Infrequent	Rare	Synergistic Toxicity
Amiodarone	Carbamazepine	Acetaminophen/
Dapsone	Etoposide	isoniazid
Disulfiram	(VP-16)	Alcohol/
Halothane	Flutamide	acetaminophen
Isoniazid	Imipramine	Rifampin/
Phenytoin	Interferon	isoniazid
Propylthiouracil	alpha	Trimethoprim/
Valproate	Ketaconazole	sulfamethoxazole
	Labetalol	
	Lisinopril	
	Ofloxacin	

Source: Lee WM. Acute liver failure. *N Engl J Med* 1993; 329:1862–1970. Reprinted by permission of the *New England Journal of Medicine.*

niazid liver injury have similar manifestations as autoimmune chronic active hepatitis.

The basis for acetaminophen liver injury is particularly well understood. Metabolism of acetaminophen ordinarily results in a small amount of toxic metabolite production (*N*-acetyl-*p*-benzoquinonimine [NAPQI]) via a cytochrome P-450 enzyme system (Fig. 2-1). Ninety percent or more is metabolized, forming glucuronide or sulfate conjugates which are excreted in bile. The small amount of toxic NAPQI formed is rapidly transformed to form mercapturic acid metabolites of acetaminophen. This reaction requires glutathione. When normal pharmacologic doses of acetaminophen are consumed, there is sufficient glutathione, and NAPQI does not accumulate. However, glutathione can easily be depleted by large amounts of acetaminophen, resulting in the accumulation of NAPQI, which

causes cell death by covalently binding to intracellular proteins. Chronic alcoholism and certain medications increase cytochrome P-450 enzyme levels and so make acetaminophen toxic at a daily dosage much lower than that usually considered to be toxic.

Diagnosis

Acute liver failure usually results in change in mental state. It often progresses to death with or without treatment within 3 weeks, often much sooner. Those with submassive liver injury may live for up to 6 months before succumbing. Diagnosis is usually not difficult. In a previously well person, the rapid emergence of jaundice, an altered mental state, and markedly abnormal liver tests and coagulation factors make consideration of this syndrome likely. Occasionally sepsis with disseminated intravascular coagulation, thrombotic thrombocytopenic purpura, and leptospirosis may mimic acute liver failure, but the distinctive clinical features of each of these illnesses or syndromes make the differential diagnosis easy in most cases. Also, an acute exacerbation of chronic liver disease (e.g., acute alcoholic hepatitis superimposed upon Laënnec's cirrhosis) may cause confusion. On rare occasions, a patient may present with features of massive hepatic necrosis who has unsuspected metastatic cancer replacing most of the liver.

Typically, laboratory tests confirm the clinical suspicion of acute liver failure. The direct-reacting bilirubin level is almost always elevated, and the prothrombin time is prolonged. Transaminase levels are usually markedly elevated, often dramatically. It is also noteworthy that the level of transaminase elevation is a poor predictor of the level of liver necrosis and of outcome. The patient with a rapidly shrinking liver size because of hepatic necrosis may have a falling level of transaminase, with the decreasing number of hepatocytes available to necrose, indicating, paradoxically, that the liver disease is worsening rather than improving.

More difficult than establishing that acute liver failure is present is discerning the etiology. However, etiology is important because therapy and prognosis are dependent, in part, upon the specific cause. It is important to question the patient (if alert) and family about possible exposures to viral

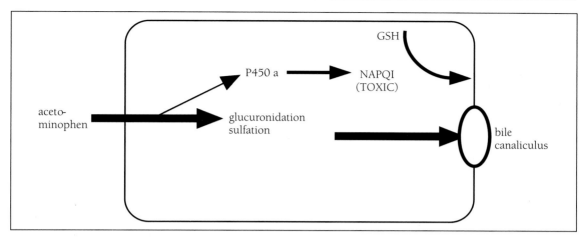

Figure 2-1. Schematic of events in acetaminophen metabolism. Ten percent forms a toxic metabolite, *N*-acetyl-*p*-benzoquinonimine (NAPQI). Glutathione (GSH) detoxifies this metabolite but is present in limited quantities. Large doses of acetaminophen, or moderate doses in the setting of an upregulated cytochrome P-450 system, overwhelms the capacity of glutathione to handle NAPQI.

hepatitis, about medication use, and about psychosocial instability which might point to acetaminophen overdose. If overdose is suspected or established, the time of ingestion is of critical value in planning treatment.

Laboratory studies are of value in the diagnosis both of the syndrome and of the specific cause. Viral markers are important, as is an acetaminophen drug level test and a toxicology screen to look for coingestions. One must keep in mind that antibodies to hepatitis C (the commonest cause of non-A, non-B hepatitis) take months to develop, so this test will almost always be negative in the setting of acute liver failure from hepatitis C. The increasing availability of HCV-RNA levels using the polymerase chain reaction or the branched DNA method represents a real advance in the early detection of acute hepatitis C. In most laboratories, however, this assay is run only occasionally, so results are often delayed considerably. Acute hepatitis B may be presumptively diagnosed in the presence of hepatitis B surface antigen or IgM antibody to the hepatitis B core antigen. The presence of anti-HBs rules out acute hepatitis B. Acute hepatitis A is diagnosed when IgM anti-hepatitis A is present. Autoantibodies are frequently present in acute liver injury, but their presence in this setting does not necessarily establish the diagnosis of autoimmune chronic hepatitis.

Wilson's disease may be hard to diagnose with confidence in the setting of advanced acute liver failure unless Kayser-Fleischer rings are present in the cornea of the eyes. In 95% of cases of Wilson's disease the serum ceruloplasmin will be reduced. In almost all other liver conditions this protein is present in either normal or increased amounts. However, in many cases of advanced liver failure of any cause, ceruloplasmin levels are diminished. Since nearly all cases of Wilson's disease can be excluded by demonstrating a normal or elevated ceruloplasmin level, this test should be part of the battery of screening tests in acute liver failure. A slit lamp examination to demonstrate Kayser-Fleischer rings around the cornea is also essential. Urinary copper levels, elevated in Wilson's disease, are often hard to interpret in acute liver failure. Wilson's disease is especially suspected in the young patient (under 40). Other clues to the possibility include the presence of a Coombs' test negative hemolytic anemia.

Recent interest in transjugular liver biopsy as a safe alternative to percutaneous biopsy in the patient with coagulopathy has emerged. In expert hands it is possible to obtain adequate liver tissue in almost all cases. Although general anesthesia is usually required in children, most adults can be biopsied using only local anesthesia and intravenous sedation. In about one in six cases the diagnosis will be altered after liver biopsy results are known. Since this technique is not without potential complications, and since therapy in established acute liver failure is not usually altered in the short run by knowledge of etiology, the authors have reserved transjugular biopsy for special or confusing cases.

Management

Formerly, acute liver failure was treated exclusively by medical staff, for there were no substantial surgical issues. Two factors have made this a disease best treated by a team of medically and surgically trained specialists (Fig. 2-2). Increased understanding that cerebral edema may be the proximate cause of death (through cerebellar herniation and consequent brain stem compression) has led to the involvement of neurosurgeons. With timely placement of devices for directly monitoring intracranial pressure, and with treatment directed at lowering such pressure, this complication often can be prevented or delayed. Despite an absence of controlled clinical trials, there is widespread agreement that liver transplantation may salvage 50% to 85% of those with acute liver failure. Thus the transplant team needs to be involved in a timely way for those patients deemed to be candidates. Figure 2-2 indicates the clinical course of the hospitalized patient with acute liver failure and the approximate time each specialist is called upon to contribute to patient care.

Care of the patient with acute liver failure presents two major challenges: (1) prevention and treatment of complications and (2) early selection of patients who should undergo urgent liver transplantation. The management required for acute liver failure rapidly intensifies once a change in mental state becomes apparent, for it is in this group of patients that fatalities occur. As a matter of routine, intensive nursing services need to be available to monitor the rapidly changing status of the patient. Liver tests, white blood cell count, and prothrombin time are assessed daily. Blood sugars should be monitored several times daily (discussed below). Estimation of liver cell mass and of the patency of hepatic arterial and venous supply is needed when liver transplantation is considered a possibility. For this reason, ultrasound and computerized tomography are helpful diagnostic tools. They provide information about liver size and contour, the presence of ascites, intrahepatic parenchymal masses, and vascular patency. Serial studies, obtained over the course of several days, which demonstrate significant loss in liver volume and the emergence of ascites help select those patients who will need transplantation.

Figure 2-2. The time course of acute liver failure and the integration of medical and surgical specialists required for optimal patient management. (PSE, portosystemic encephalopathy.)

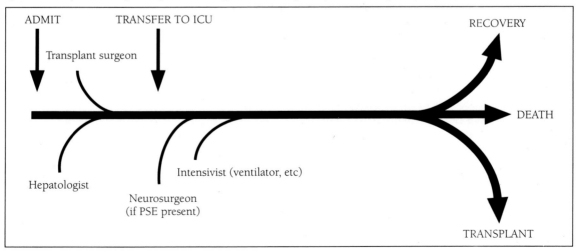

The problems posed by established acute liver failure include the following:

- Sepsis
- Coagulopathy
- Renal failure
- Encephalopathy
- Acute cerebral edema
- Metabolic disorders

Each time a patient is admitted to the intensive care unit with acute liver failure, an inventory of these items (SCREAM) should be made and systematically addressed.

Sepsis

Sepsis is likely, in part, because the acute liver failure patient is immunocompromised. Contributing factors are impaired Kuppfer's cell phagocytosis, depressed cellular and humoral immunity, and decreased complement levels. The median time to onset of sepsis is 5 days after admission. Bacterial infection occurs in more than 80%. *Staphylococcus aureus,* streptococci, and enteric coliform bacteria are the most common infecting organisms. Many of the infections seen in patients with acute liver failure are gut-derived. Because of the high risk of infection, frequent surveillance cultures of blood, urine, and sputum are mandatory. If ascites is present, it, too, should be tested by cell count, differential, and culture. A low threshold for beginning empiric antibiotic therapy (as opposed to prophylaxis) is necessary.

A recent report of selective gut decontamination in a group of patients with acute liver failure suggests that the incidence of enterobacterial infections can be nearly eliminated through the use of such a program (Table 2-3). Forty-seven percent of patients developed infection with enterobacteria (*Escherichia coli, Klebsiella* spp., *Proteus* spp., *Enterobacter* and *Serratia*) prior to the introduction of selective gut decontamination, whereas only 3% developed such infections when given selective decontamination. Norfloxacin 400 mg q24h and 1 × 10^6 nystatin (Mycostatin) q6h was the regimen most often used. The incidence of other gram-negative and gram-positive infections was not decreased. Effect on mortality was hard to compare directly since

patients treated before selective decontamination was used were also treated in an era when transplantation was never employed.

In patients who survive for more than a few days, invasive fungal infections (typically *Candida* or *Aspergillus*) may occur in up to one third, but may be hard to diagnose with certainty antemortem. Indwelling vascular catheters and the lungs are common sources. A patient who appears to get better and then relapses may well have developed invasive fungal infection. Those with renal insufficiency are at particularly high risk. An unexplained temperature elevation (or one that persists after all identified bacterial infections are being treated appropriately), particularly if the white blood cell count is elevated, should raise the index of suspicion for a fungal coinfection. The authors' approach in all acute liver failure patients is to administer norfloxacin and nystatin to achieve selective gut decontamination even in the absence of established infection. Daily chest x-rays and pan culture for bacteria and fungi are done. The threshold to begin broad-spectrum antibiotics is quite low. In a patient not responding, a further search for fungal infection is considered on a case-by-case basis.

Table 2-3. Bacteria Causing Infection in Acute Liver Failure Patients Who Did (Group I) and Did Not (Group II) Receive Poorly Absorbable Antibiotics

	Group I (n=34)	Group II (n=57)
Enterobacteria	1	27 (p < .001)
Escherichia coli	1	17
Klebseilla spp.	0	4
Proteus spp.	0	4
Enterobacter-Serratia	0	2
Other gram-negative bacilli	2	5
Pseudomonas aeruginosa	0	3
Acinetobacter calcoaceticus	1	2
Capnofitophaga ochracea	1	0
Gram-positive cocci	12	16
Streptococcus pneumoniae	0	3
Streptococcus faecalis (enterococcus)	3	5
Other *Streptococcus*	0	5
Staphylococcus epidermidis	7	1
Staphylococcus aureus	2	2

Source: Adapted from Salmeron JM, et al. Selective intestinal decontamination in the prevention of bacterial infection in patients with acute liver failure. *J Hepatol* 1992; 14:280–285.

Coagulopathy

Coagulation disorders occur because all coagulation proteins except factor VIII are produced in the liver. Failure of the liver to produce these factors results in abnormal coagulation. Factors V and VII have the shortest half-lives. Some have advocated repeated factor V determination as a dynamic measure of synthetic function. This recommendation seems unnecessary, however. Superimposed infection may lead to disseminated intravascular coagulation. Prophylactic administration of fresh-frozen plasma is not necessary or desirable, although the plasma is usually given at least to cover invasive procedures, such as the neurosurgical placement of an intracranial pressure measuring device (see below). Gastrointestinal bleeding may be due either to coagulation abnormalities or to erosive gastritis. The incidence of upper gastrointestinal bleeding in acute hepatic failure has been reduced by the administration of H_2 receptor antagonists. When intravenous omeprazole is available, this drug will likely be the agent of choice.

Renal Failure

Renal failure occurs in 50% to 60% of patients. Hepatorenal syndrome, acute tubular necrosis, and glomerulonephritis are among the causes. The degree of renal dysfunction is underestimated by measurement of BUN and creatinine levels because the liver is the site of urea synthesis, and creatinine may be excreted in higher than normal amounts by the renal tubule.

Most often the renal failure is functional, that is, reversible. It frequently is oliguric, and the urine sediment is bland unless there is deep jaundice, in which case "dirty brown casts" may be seen. Avid sodium retention (urine sodium < 10 mEq/liter) is the rule. Renal failure can just as easily develop in those with normal or even high intravascular volume, and does not respond to either further volume challenge or to diuretics. Renal failure in the intensive care unit may also develop from the administration of nephrotoxic drugs or from acute volume loss from gastrointestinal bleeding. Acetaminophen overdose may result in direct renal toxicity which will usually be nonoliguric.

When renal failure is recognized, the first step is to ensure that intravascular volume is adequate.

Hydration may be guided by the central venous pressure, or by a challenge with albumin. If oliguria is a feature, an attempt to increase urine volume with loop diuretics (e.g., furosemide) is appropriate. Rigorous studies demonstrating the value of "renal dose" dopamine (2–4 µg/kg/hr) are lacking. Nevertheless, this agent is frequently employed in the authors' unit. Ultrafiltration is effective in patients who are threatened by fluid overload (although fluid overload characterized principally by ascites does not require ultrafiltration). Hemodialysis may be required in severe cases, which are characterized by hyperkalemia or severe acidosis, and should not be withheld in this setting. The patient should not, of course, be heparinized during dialysis.

Encephalopathy

The patient with acute liver failure has some degree of hepatic encephalopathy. By the time stage III encephalopathy is present, the patient should be transferred to an intensive care unit. The differential diagnosis of neurologic deterioration in a liver failure patient includes cerebral edema, hypoglycemia, and intracerebral bleeding. Of these, cerebral edema is the most lethal and frequent. It occurs in 60% to 70% of patients who succumb. The pathophysiology of cerebral edema is poorly understood. A combination of cytotoxic and vasogenic mechanisms is probably responsible for impaired neuronal Na+/K+ ATPase activity, a disrupted blood-brain barrier, and accumulation of osmotically active amino acids in the brain cells. Progressive cerebral edema results in intracerebral hypertension, brain stem herniation, and brain death.

Acute Cerebral Edema

Encephalopathy in acute liver failure has, at least in part, a different basis from that occurring in the cirrhotic. In acute liver failure there frequently is no association with aromatic amino acids; gut cleansing is generally ineffective. However, recent studies indicate an association between the level of plasma ammonia in experimental acute liver failure and decreases in brain function, suggesting that ammonia is of key importance in the encephalopathy which develops after both acute and chronic liver injury. In addition, a substantial risk of acute cerebral edema exists and frequently produces tonsillar herniation and death of the patient from brain stem compression. The frequency of cerebral edema occurring in fulminant hepatic failure may be as high as 85%. The pathophysiology of cerebral edema in acute liver failure has recently been reviewed. This complication needs to be prevented whenever possible.

Significant cerebral edema is difficult to recognize on clinical grounds. Headache, projectile vomiting, bradycardia, and papilledema are usually absent. Noninvasive measures such as CT scanning are also relatively insensitive in identifying this rapidly progressive complication. In one center in which an epidural pressure transducer was routinely placed in 15 patients with fulminant hepatic failure, elevated intracranial pressure (> 15 mm Hg) was identified in 11 patients (73%). Routine CT scans showed evidence of effacement or flattening of cortical sulci, reduction in size, or narrowing or obliteration of the cerebral ventricles or cisterns. In addition, generalized decreased attenuation of the hemispheres was observed in only 27% of cases where increased intracranial pressure had been identified by pressure measurement. Although head CT scanning cannot be counted on to identify increased intracranial pressure, it can identify structural intracranial changes, such as intracranial bleeding. This information is important, and a routine head CT scan forms part of the initial assessment of the patient with acute liver failure and progressing neurological deterioration.

Two types of intracranial pressure (ICP) monitors are currently in use, epidural and intraparenchymal. The former has a lower incidence of intracerebral bleeding, but is not as sensitive as the latter. Even with severe coagulopathy, these devices can be used safely, either in the intensive care unit or in the operating room after the administration of fresh-frozen plasma. The authors rely on direct measurement of intracranial pressure in the setting of acute liver failure.

Intracranial pressure should be kept at less than 25 mm Hg if possible. Fever, systemic hypertension, and psychomotor agitation may all raise the ICP. Measures useful in lowering the ICP include elevation of the head of the bed 30 degrees, hyperventilation of the intubated patient to a P_{CO_2} of 30 mm Hg, mannitol administration, and barbiturate-induced coma. If mannitol is required, it is given in a bolus of 0.5 to 1.0 g/kg to keep the serum osmolality in the range of 310 to 320 mOsm/liter. Mannitol cannot be used in oliguric patients who do not exhibit a diuretic response to mannitol. Barbiturate coma lowers the ICP by causing cerebral vasoconstriction and decreasing both cerebral oxygen demand and neuronal metabolic activity. Neither lactulose nor neomycin improves encephalopathy from acute liver failure, and both cause gas formation within the gastrointestinal tract, which increases the difficulty of the transplant operation. Therefore, they should be avoided.

Severe cerebral edema is defined as an ICP of greater than 30 mm Hg for 60 minutes or longer. Patients who suffer severe cerebral edema have a 60% to 70% incidence of significant neurological injury if they survive at all. In addition to monitoring the ICP, one must calculate the cerebral perfusion pressure (CPP) by subtracting the ICP from the mean arterial pressure (MAP):

$$CPP = MAP - ICP$$

Patients whose CPP falls below 40 mm Hg for more than 2 hours should not be considered for transplantation because of the very high likelihood of severe irreversible brain injury. Corticosteroids such as dexamethasone are uniformly of no help in preventing or treating the cerebral edema seen in acute liver failure.

Metabolic Disorders

A variety of metabolic disorders may also be seen. A centrally mediated respiratory alkalosis is common and should not be corrected. Metabolic acidosis, particularly in the patient with acetaminophen liver failure, is an ominous finding with a 90% mortality rate if the arterial pH is less than 7.30. Hypoglycemia due to impaired gluconeogenesis and depleted glycogen stores may have disastrous consequences when severe. Daily glucose requirements are always at least 300 g. Blood sugars must be monitored frequently (several times daily and whenever there is a deterioration in mental function), and hypoglycemia should be treated aggressively. Ordinarily, intravenous fluids containing 10% dextrose should be administered to acute liver failure patients. If central vascular access is available, a 20% dextrose solution should be administered. Rapid correction of hypoglycemia (blood sugars less than 40 mg/dl) should be treated by means of bolus infusions of 50% dextrose.

Over the course of their illness, 60% to 70% of patients need ventilatory support, usually because of encephalopathy. The authors intubate electively all patients with grade III and IV encephalopathy, both to prevent aspiration and to allow hyperventilation in those patients with cerebral edema.

The patient with acetaminophen overdose presents special challenges and opportunities. If the condition is recognized early, intervention has a high probability of preventing liver failure. Special criteria, as noted above, need to be borne in mind when deciding if liver transplantation is needed. Therapy is directed toward preventing the buildup of NAPQI or hastening its metabolism. When initially seen, an acetaminophen overdose patient should have vomiting induced by ipecac, if the patient is seen within 4 hours of the ingestion. If this is given within 1 hour, acetaminophen blood levels may be decreased by more than three quarters. Administration of charcoal (6 g/g acetaminophen) will decrease absorption of acetaminophen. Of course, charcoal will also decrease absorption of the antidote, acetylcysteine (see below), but the beneficial effects more than compensate for this effect.

Acetylcysteine (Mucomyst) given orally or via nasogastric tube is a source of glutathione. It may also be given intravenously if the patient is comatose or if gastrointestinal absorption cannot be counted upon. Acetylcysteine is especially helpful if given within 16 hours of acetaminophen ingestion. Some evidence suggests that it may have a small beneficial effect if treatment is initiated as much as 36 hours after ingestion, but the authors believe that the value of treatment is substantially lost if not started within 16 hours. Therapy should be initiated empirically if it is likely that an adult has taken more than 7.5 g. Children who have taken more than 140 mg/kg should also be treated.

Orally the drug is given as a 10% or 20% solution in a soft drink or in water. The initial dose is 140 mg/kg. Then 70 mg/kg is given every 4 hours for total of 17 doses (1330 mg/kg over 68 hours).

One must remember to give the dose an hour after oral charcoal is given because of the decreased absorption of acetylcysteine with charcoal. When intravenous acetylcysteine is required, the following schedule is suggested:

- 150 mg/kg in 200 ml dextrose 5% in water (D5W) over 15 minutes
- 50 mg/kg in 500 ml D5W over 4 hours
- 100 mg/kg in 1 liter D5W over 16 hours
     Total dose 300 mg/kg

Blood levels may help to determine if a full course of therapy needs to be given. They will also help to predict the likelihood of severe liver injury. However, since predictions are based on groups, an individual's sensitivity to the toxic effects of acetaminophen will vary; therefore, one must err on the side of overtreatment. The following nomogram may be helpful (Fig. 2-3). Blood levels earlier than 4 hours after ingestion may underestimate the risk because of incomplete absorption. Alcohol, coingestions, and other factors must be taken into account as well.

Finally, the use of cimetidine intravenously prior to acetaminophen overdose has been shown in experimental animals to protect the liver. Cimetidine occupies binding sites on the cytochrome P-450 enzyme and thereby partially blocks the formation of NAPQI. However, the use of this agent in humans many hours after ingestion has not been shown to reduce substantially the toxicity of acetaminophen overdoses.

Results

The prognosis of a patient with acute liver failure is important to determine. Those with a good prognosis need continued optimal medical therapy; but when the likelihood of survival is low, those who have no contraindication for liver transplantation should be evaluated and listed for an organ search as soon as possible. No controlled trials have been performed comparing liver transplantation with continued medical therapy. A key to selecting patients for liver transplantation in acute liver failure is judging the relative risk of dying with and without a transplant. As discussed below, patients with acute liver failure from hepatitis A have a much different prognosis than those with non-A non-B hepatitis, and need to be considered separately. The decision to proceed with liver transplantation without benefit of randomized controlled trials is much easier to make for the patient with a very bleak outcome than for those whose likelihood of survival without surgery is much greater.

Identification of early indicators of prognosis in acute liver failure is essential. Many retrospective analyses of this disorder highlight the poor prognostic features which may evolve during hospitalization. But late-occurring clinical or laboratory features are frequently the least helpful, because they may presage an irretrievable situation. More helpful are easily monitored aspects of a case at the outset. Of the variables most helpful, the etiology of the

acute liver failure is the most powerful. Those whose acute liver failure is due to hepatitis A, for example, have a 45% survival rate. Acetaminophen-induced liver failure, hepatitis B, and idiosyncratic drug reactions have a survival rate of 34%, 23%, and 14%, respectively. The worst prognosis, as noted, is from non-A, non-B hepatitis–induced acute liver failure, which has a meager 9% survival rate.

Age is also an important determinant of survival, especially for acute liver failure caused by factors other than acetaminophen. Those under age 10 or over 40 are particularly likely to do poorly. The grade of encephalopathy on admission plays a role in the early prediction of outcome, although the relationship is complicated and apparently paradoxical. For example, in one study of nonacetaminophen acute liver failure, survival was lowest (12%) in those admitted with grades 0 to II coma, compared with those with grades III to IV coma (20%

Figure 2-3. Plasma levels of acetaminophen can serve as a useful guide to risk of liver toxicity during the first 16 hours after ingestion. (From Rumack et al. Acetaminophen overdose. *Arch Int Med* 1981; 141:380–385. Used with permission.)

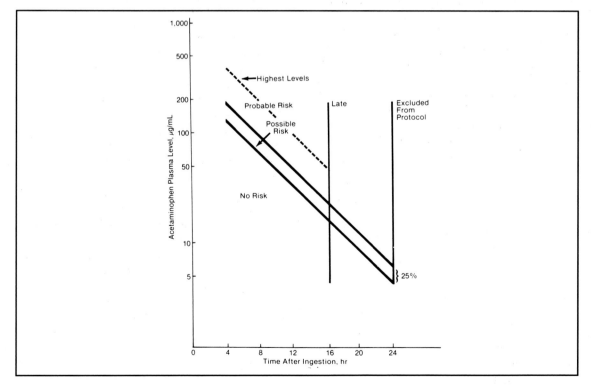

survival). Finally, duration of jaundice prior to encephalopathy plays a prognostic role. When this interval is 7 days or less, the survival rate is 34%, but when greater than 7 days is only 7%. For acetaminophen-induced acute liver failure, an initial arterial blood pH less than 7.30 is also associated with a poorer outcome.

Traditionally, histology has not played much of a role in the evaluation and management of acute liver failure. In part this is due to the fairly rapid progression to coagulation defects, which makes conventional percutaneous biopsy unsafe. A larger reason is that the treatment of liver failure usually does not change as a result of the biopsy. Exceptions to this rule may exist. For example, the patient with acetaminophen overdose usually is obvious because of personal or family recognition of the overdose. In an occasional patient this history may be withheld. If a biopsy were done immediately, therapy might be initiated. These situations are unusual, however.

When transjugular biopsy has been used, the finding of extensive (> 70%) cellular necrosis correlated with nonsurvival, although this feature was neither as sensitive nor as specific as the Kings College criteria, a system which does not require biopsy. Therapy was not apparently altered in any case as a result of the biopsy. In short, although liver biopsy is technically feasible and relatively informative and safe, its value in the management of acute liver failure seemed marginal.

On the basis of a great deal of experience, the Kings College Hospital has developed useful guidelines for determining which patients ought to be given early consideration for a liver transplant rather than continued medical management. It is clear that acetaminophen acute liver failure requires a different set of conditions before medical failure is likely. Obviously, finding a suitable donor requires time and luck. Continued aggressive medical measures are needed until a donor can be identified. Table 2-4 indicates criteria mandating a consideration for liver transplantation.

Unproven Therapies

Other treatment measures have been advocated, often with great enthusiasm based on scant information. Case reports and small series of novel treat-

Table 2-4. Criteria Mandating Consideration for Liver Transplantation

Acetaminophen	Other Causes

1. pH < 7.30
   OR
	1. Prothrombin time > 100 sec
	   OR

2. a) Prothrombin time
      > 100 sec
      AND
   b) Creatinine > 300
      μmol/liter
      AND
   c) PSE[a] grade III
      or IV
	2. Any three of the following:
	   a) Age < 10 or > 40
	   b) Etiology NANB[b] hepatitis,
	      halothane, drug reaction
	   c) Jaundice preceded PSE >
	      7 days
	   d) Prothrombin time > 50 sec
	   e) Bilirubin > 300 μmol/liter

[a]PSE = portosystemic encephalopathy.
[b]NANB = non-A, non-B.
Source: Adapted from O'Grady JG, et al. Early indicators of prognosis in fulminant hepatic failure. *Gastroenterology* 1989; 97:439–445.

ments for acute liver failure abound. To date, none have been shown in controlled clinical trials to be of benefit. Toxin removal by apheresis or plasma perfusion over sorbents such as charcoal or resins is based on the model of the failing liver as one unable to metabolize and excrete toxins. In this regard, comparisons to renal failure are often made. Such comparisons are conceptually flawed. The liver is much more important than the kidney as a synthetic organ. Novel attempts to encapsulate porcine or human hepatocytes within fibers and to utilize the synthetic as well as detoxifying properties of living cells overcome many of the conceptual limitations mentioned above. Although only anecdotal information is currently available, this approach deserves careful evaluation as a bridge to liver transplantation.

Glucagon and insulin have been shown in animal models to be essential for liver regeneration after subtotal hepatectomy. Infusion of these hormones in acute liver failure has not resulted in improved survival, however. Prostaglandin infusions (e.g., alprostadil [Prostin VR]) have received recent attention, but controlled trials are just now under way. One recent uncontrolled trial of 17 patients who received continuous infusion of prostaglandin E_2 reported a 76% survival rate. Other uncontrolled trials showed no effect of prostaglandin E_1. Corticosteroids have no role to play in the treatment of acute liver failure.

Liver Transplantation

The survival rate for emergency liver transplantation for acute liver failure ranges from 50% to 85%. Formidable hurdles to more extensive use of liver transplantation include a rapidly deteriorating patient and the general unavailability of donor organs. Often a less than ideal liver donor is used because of the urgency of the situation. Blood type ABO-incompatible grafts may be used as a stopgap, but up to 60% of such recipients will require retransplantation with a compatible graft. Reduced-size grafts may also be employed.

Although orthotopic replacement liver transplantation is currently the preferred surgical treatment of acute liver failure, auxiliary orthotopic and heterotopic transplants have been performed. The premise of this approach is that, with time, the native liver will recover, and the transplanted liver will be needed to sustain life for only a relatively brief period. This procedure involves removing a portion of the diseased liver, thus allowing either a reduced or whole graft to be placed in an orthotopic position. In a heterotopic transplant, none of the diseased liver is removed, and a reduced or whole graft is placed in a nonanatomic location, usually the right lower quadrant. The majority of these procedures in recent years have been performed in children and teenagers. A potentially attractive aspect of these procedures is the need for only short-term immunosuppression. As the native liver regenerates, one permits the donor organ to atrophy by withdrawing antirejection therapy.

Conclusions

Acute liver failure is a complex disorder with diverse etiologies. Proper management requires a team approach (Table 2-5). Recognition and treatment of the myriad complications will allow many of these patients to survive long enough to undergo liver transplantation. Optimal management requires a hepatology team, a sophisticated intensive care unit, neurosurgical expertise, and liver transplant capabilities. Early referral for evaluation and treatment will give the patient the greatest opportunity for survival.

Table 2-5. Highpoints in Management of the Acute Liver Failure Patient

Transfer to intensive care unit if stage III or IV coma develops.

Obtain emergent CT scan of the head.

STAT neurosurgery consult for evaluation and placement of ICP monitor.

Treat cerebral edema aggressively.

Perform elective endotracheal intubation in stage III coma to protect airway.

Make frequent surveillance cultures.

Follow selective gut decontamination protocol; noroxin, nystatin, (and oral antibiotic paste while intubated).

Low threshold to use of empiric antibiotics if infection suspected.

Use dialysis support for either fluid removal or hemodialysis.

Use Swan-Ganz catheter placement for hemodynamic monitoring and resuscitation.

Follow gastrointestinal bleeding prophylaxis with H_2 blocker +/− sucralfate.

Selected Readings

Blei AT. Cerebral edema and intracranial hypertension in acute liver failure: Distinct aspects of the same problem. *Hepatology* 1991; 13:376.

Bosman DK, et al. Changes in brain metabolism during hyperammonemia and acute liver failure: Results of a comparative 1H-NMR spectroscopy and biochemical investigation. *Hepatology* 1990; 12:281.

Donaldson BW, et al. The role of transjugular biopsy in fulminant liver failure: Relationship to other prognostic indicators. *Hepatology* 1993; 18:1370–1376.

Lee WM. Acute liver failure. *N Engl J Med* 1993; 329: 1862–1870.

Munoz S, et al. Elevated intracranial pressure and computed tomography of the brain in fulminant hepatocellular failure. *Hepatology* 1991; 13:209.

O'Grady JG, et al. Early indicators of prognosis in fulminant hepatic failure. *Gastroenterology* 1989; 97: 439–445.

Rolando N, et al. Fungal infection: A common unrecognized complication of acute liver failure. *J Hepatol* 1991; 12:1–9.

Rumack BH, et al. Acetaminophen overdose. *Arch Int Med* 1981; 141:380–385.

Salmeron JM, Tito L, Rimola A, et al. Selective intestinal decontamination in the prevention of bacterial infection in patients with acute liver failure. *J Hepatol* 1992; 14:280–285.

Williams R, Gimson AES. Intensive liver care and management of acute hepatic failure. *Dig Dis Sci* 1991; 36:820–826.

3

Cirrhosis

H. FRANKLIN HERLONG
ANDREW S. KLEIN

Etiology and Pathogenesis

Cirrhosis is caused by chronic necroinflammatory diseases of the liver resulting in fibrosis and nodular regeneration. The clinical sequelae of cirrhosis result from a combination of impaired hepatocellular function, obstruction to the flow of bile, and alterations in hepatic blood flow caused by disruption of the normal hepatic architecture. A variety of hepatic diseases can cause cirrhosis (Table 3-1). Some of these disorders affect predominantly hepatocytes (e.g., viral hepatitis, alpha$_1$-antitrypsin deficiency, drug-induced liver disease), whereas others injure the biliary system (e.g., sclerosing cholangitis, primary biliary cirrhosis, graft versus host disease). Finally, diseases of the hepatic circulation may result in cirrhosis (Budd-Chiari syndrome, chronic congestive heart failure, veno-occlusive disease).

Diagnosis

The most reliable diagnosis of cirrhosis is made when fibrosis and nodular regeneration are seen on a liver biopsy specimen. A needle biopsy can accurately diagnose micronodular cirrhoses caused by alcohol, jejunoileal bypass, methotrexate, and alpha$_1$-antitrypsin deficiency. Long-standing viral or autoimmune hepatitis can result in a macronodular cirrhosis with large regenerating nodules. On occasion, the percutaneous liver biopsy needle may sample the contents of a nodule and the histologic specimen may look remarkably normal except for distorted architecture.

Ultrasonography is not a reliable modality for diagnosing cirrhosis; CT scan and MRI may show an irregular hepatic contour with distinct nodularity (Fig. 3-1). Finding large collateral portal vessels can help confirm the diagnosis of cirrhosis. If imaging studies are equivocal and percutaneous biopsy cannot be performed safely because of a coagulopathy or other contraindications, measuring the wedged hepatic venous pressure can identify portal hypertension with a presumptive diagnosis of cirrhosis. A technetium Tc 99m scan can show patchy hepatic uptake and shift of tracer to the bone marrow and spleen, suggesting an underlying cirrhosis.

Management

When possible, therapy should always be directed toward the underlying cause of the hepatic injury. Immunosuppressive agents are useful in patients with autoimmune liver disease but not in those with viral hepatitis. In patients with hemochromatosis, mobilization of iron with phlebotomy or desferoxamine retards fibrosis, and penicillamine is useful in eliminating hepatic copper in Wilson's disease. Some patients with hepatitis B and C may benefit from interferon alpha. Other drugs used to slow the progression of cirrhosis in certain diseases include colchicine, ursodeoxycholic acid, and methotrexate. Unfortunately, for many patients with chronic liver disease, no effective treatment for the underlying disease has been established and progression to cirrhosis is inevitable. Since no therapy has been

Table 3-1. Causes of Cirrhosis

Viral
    Hepatitis B, hepatitis C, hepatitis D
Drugs and toxins
    Alcohol, carbon tetrachloride, methotrexate, phenothiazines
Inherited disorders
    Hemochromatosis, Wilson's disease, alpha$_1$-antitrypsin
    deficiency
Vascular disorders
    Budd-Chiari syndrome, chronic congestive heart failure,
    venoocclusive disease
Biliary tract disorders
    Primary biliary cirrhosis, sclerosing cholangitis, graft vs. host
    disease, bile duct strictures
Miscellaneous
    Granulomous liver disease, schistosomiasis, autoimmune
    liver disease

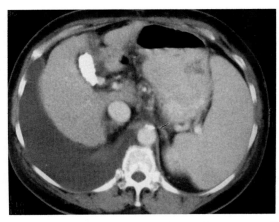

Figure 3-1. A CT scan of the abdomen showing a small nodular liver, enlarged spleen, and ascites. This patient has cirrhosis from chronic hepatitis C.

shown to reverse hepatic fibrosis in established cirrhosis, hepatic transplantation is at present the only definitive therapy for cirrhosis. Criteria for transplantation vary among transplant centers; but for the most part, transplantation is recommended in suitable candidates when life expectancy is less than 1 year. For those patients with cirrhosis who are not candidates for transplant or those patients awaiting transplantation, therapy consists predominantly of managing the complications of portal hypertension and impaired hepatic synthetic function. The complications discussed here include (1) impaired nutrition, (2) ascites, (3) spontaneous bacterial peritonitis, (4) the hepatorenal syndrome, (5)

hepatic encephalopathy, and (6) alterations in drug metabolism.

Impaired Nutrition

Signs of malnutrition are common in patients with cirrhosis, and most common in hospitalized patients with alcoholic liver disease. It has been hard to define the exact relationship between malnutrition and survival in patients with cirrhosis because many adverse physiologic processes are present at the same time. The nutritional status of a patient with cirrhosis, however, can be used to predict operative mortality and to assess the prognosis for liver transplantation.

Malnutrition develops in patients with cirrhosis because of poor dietary intake, malabsorption, maldigestion, and increased energy requirements. Nutritional therapy in patients with cirrhosis should correct protein calorie malnutrition while providing an adequate substrate for hepatic regeneration. The results of controlled trials using various amino acid formulations remain inconclusive. This, combined with the heterogeneity among cirrhotic patients, makes it difficult to provide specific recommendations for nutritional supplementation. However, even in patients with a history of hepatic encephalopathy, adequate daily protein (1.5 g/kg) and calorie (40 kcal/kg) intake should be attempted.

Alterations in the plasma amino acid profile in patients with cirrhosis (decreased branched-chain amino acids and elevated aromatic amino acids) have led to several trials of branched-chain amino acid (BCAA) supplementation in patients with cirrhosis. Controlled and uncontrolled data indicate that BCAA therapy provides no proven benefit over standard amino acid supplementation in most patients with cirrhosis. In a very select population of patients who develop encephalopathy with protein supplementation, BCAA preparations are better tolerated. Because these preparations are very expensive and efficacy has not been clearly established, BCAA formulations are not used in most patients with cirrhosis.

Ascites

Ascites is a frequent complication in patients with cirrhosis and usually implies a poor prognosis. Fewer than half of patients with cirrhosis who develop ascites live more than 2 years. A diagnostic paracentesis should be performed in all patients when ascites is first detected and when there is unexplained deterioration in an otherwise well-compensated cirrhotic patient with ascites. If there is any doubt about the presence of ascites, a blind paracentesis should not be attempted because of the risk of inadvertent puncture of the bowel. Ultrasonography can reliably detect even small amounts of ascites and can determine the location where a safe paracentesis can be performed. The risk of hemorrhage from a diagnostic paracentesis is low and does not require coagulation factor support even when the prothrombin time is prolonged. Using a Z-track will prevent a postparacentesis leak.

Complete laboratory analysis of ascitic fluid should include cell count with differential, culture for bacteria, and determination of total protein and albumin concentration. Measurement of ascitic fluid amylase, culture for AFB, and cytopathologic examination should be included if there is clinical evidence of pancreatic ascites, tuberculosis, or tumor, respectively. Determining the serum/ascitic fluid albumin gradient is helpful in establishing the etiology of ascites. A gradient between the serum and ascitic fluid albumin concentration of greater than 1.1 g/dl is suggestive of portal hypertension, whereas a smaller gradient indicates nonhepatic etiologies such as peritoneal malignancy, tuberculous peritonitis, or the nephrotic syndrome where the portal pressure is normal.

About 10% of patients with ascites develop a right pleural effusion which can be disabling (Fig. 3-2). Such effusions are often quite large and do not respond to diuretic therapy. Pleurodesis rarely reduces fluid accumulation. Portal decompression or hepatic transplantation is required to control this complication in most patients.

Dietary salt restriction and diuretic therapy are the mainstays of the management of ascites. Diuretic therapy leads to mobilization of ascites primarily because of a decrease in the rate of formation rather than an increase in the rate of reabsorption. A diuretic regimen which achieves a weight loss of 0.5 to 1.0 kg/d should be instituted. Fluid restriction is unnecessary unless the serum sodium concentration falls below 130 meq/liter.

Measuring the urinary sodium concentration is a useful adjunct to assess the efficacy of diuretic

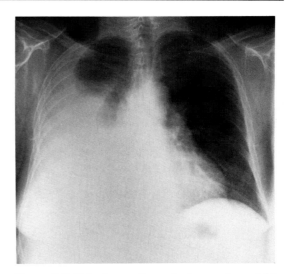

Figure 3-2. This chest radiograph shows a large right pleural effusion (hepatic hydrothorax). The analysis of the pleural fluid is identical to ascites. The left lung is clear and the cardiac silhouette normal.

therapy. A random urine sample is usually sufficient. A diuretic regimen which induces negative sodium balance (urinary sodium excretion greater than dietary sodium intake) will control ascites accumulation in most patients with cirrhosis. Urinary sodium concentration is also helpful in determining the potency of a diuretic regimen needed to mobilize ascites. Patients who excrete more than 50 meq/24 hr of sodium on a 1-g sodium diet can be treated with salt restriction alone. When the sodium excretion is between 25 and 50 meq/24 hr, spironolactone should be added. If sodium excretion is less than 25 meq/24 hr, a combination of a loop diuretic (furosemide, bumetanide) and spironolactone should be used.

Patients who fail to excrete more than 10 meq/24 hr of sodium on a combination of salt restriction and a potent diuretic regimen have refractory ascites. Therapies used in these patients include therapeutic paracentesis, portal systemic shunts, peritoneovenous shunts, or liver transplantation (Table 3-2). Therapeutic paracentesis is effective in controlling tense ascites and is well tolerated in most patients. Removal of 5 to 10 liters of ascitic fluid can be done safely without causing symptomatic electrolyte disturbances. Whether plasma volume expansion with albumin after therapeutic paracen-

Table 3-2. Options for Refractory Ascites

Therapeutic paracenteses
Peritoneovenous shunt (LeVeen, Denver shunts)
Transjugular intrahepatic portosystemic stent (TIPS)
Surgical side-to-side portal systemic shunt
Liver transplantation

tesis reduces electrolyte abnormalities and azotemia remains controversial.

In the past peritoneovenous shunts (LeVeen or Denver) were used to treat ascites refractory to medical therapy. A number of potential complications limit the usefulness of these shunts. In about 30% of patients the shunt fails for mechanical reasons. In some of these patients, repositioning the distal end of the shunt may restore function. In others the valve becomes clogged and needs to be replaced. Some patients with underlying heart disease fail to increase their cardiac output in response to the increased delivery of fluid into the right heart. Unless left ventricular function improves, the shunt will fail. The most serious complication of peritoneovenous shunts is coagulopathy with hemorrhage.

Portal decompression by a surgical side-to-side shunt will control ascites, but the morbidity and mortality from shunt surgery prevent the use of this form of therapy in the majority of patients with cirrhosis and ascites. Recently, transjugular intrahepatic portal systemic shunts (TIPSs) have been used in a limited number of patients as an alternative to surgically created shunts. Uncontrolled reports suggest that this therapy may be efficacious in patients with refractory ascites. The long-term effectiveness of this therapy is yet to be determined, but early reports suggest that maintaining shunt patency is a problem in many patients. Liver transplant is the most effective therapy for the control of refractory ascites and should be considered in all patients with refractory ascites who are otherwise good candidates for transplant.

Spontaneous Bacterial Peritonitis

Bacterial infection of ascitic fluid in patients with cirrhosis is common. Secondary bacterial peritonitis develops with perforation of the bowel or when bacteria leak into the ascitic fluid from localized pockets of infection such as subhepatic or perinephric abscesses. In the vast majority of patients with cirrhosis, bacterial infection of the ascites occurs with no obvious "inoculation" site and is called spontaneous bacterial peritonitis (SBP). In about a third of patients with SBP no signs or symptoms of infection are detected. It is not possible to distinguish secondary peritonitis from spontaneous bacterial peritonitis on the basis of clinical signs and symptoms. Analysis of the ascitic fluid is essential in diagnosing bacterial infection and determining whether it is secondary or primary (Fig. 3-3).

An ascitic fluid polymorphonuclear leukocyte (PMN) count greater than 250 cells/mm^3 should lead to empiric antibiotic therapy. Direct inoculation of the ascitic fluid into blood culture bottles at the bedside can increase the yield of confirmatory culture data. Since the Gram stain is positive in fewer than 10% of specimens, empiric antibiotic therapy is based on the epidemiology of SBP infection. The most commonly encountered organisms include *Escherichia coli*, streptococci, and *Klebsiella* species. Anaerobic infections account for fewer than 1% of all cases of SBP. Cefotaxime, a third-generation cephalosporin, is the drug of choice in the treatment of suspected SBP. Aminoglycosides should be avoided because of the high rate of nephrotoxicity in cirrhotic patients. Two grams of cefotaxime administered intravenously every 8 hours for 7 days should be sufficient. Antibiotic coverage can be altered if culture results identify resistant organisms. In some asymptomatic patients a positive ascitic fluid culture will be obtained when fewer than 250 PMNs are detected in the fluid. In these patients with asymptomatic monomicrobial ascites a repeat paracentesis with cell count and culture should be performed. If the cell count remains low and a repeat culture is negative, no treatment is required.

It is crucial to distinguish spontaneous bacterial peritonitis from secondary peritonitis because secondary peritonitis usually requires surgical intervention. Secondary peritonitis should be suspected in patients with a total ascitic fluid protein greater than 1 g/dl, glucose less than 50 mg/dl, or multiple organisms cultured from the ascitic fluid. When secondary peritonitis is suspected, metronidazole plus cefotaxime should constitute the initial empirical antibiotic regimen. An aggressive search is insti-

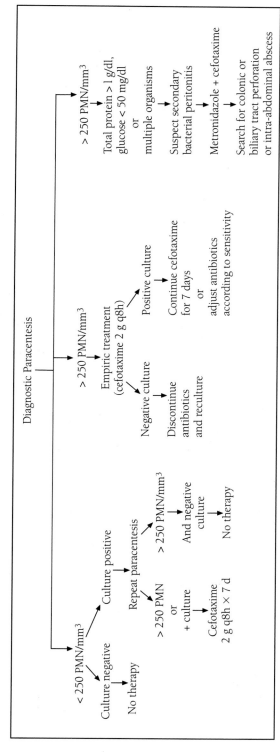

Figure 3-3. Diagnosis of bacterial peritonitis. PMN = polymorphonuclear leukocyte count.

tuted for evidence of colonic or biliary tract perforation or loculated infections such as a perinephric or subhepatic abscess.

Patients with cirrhosis in whom the ascitic fluid contains less than 1 g/dl of protein are particularly susceptible to recurrent episodes of bacterial peritonitis. This increased susceptibility is related to decreased antimicrobial activity of ascitic fluid. The probability of an episode of spontaneous bacterial peritonitis developing in cirrhotic patients with less than 1 g/dl of protein is 20% within 6 months. The prevalence of bacterial peritonitis and other gram-negative bacterial infections in these patients can be reduced by prophylactically administering norfloxacin (400 mg bid).

The Hepatorenal Syndrome

In patients with cirrhosis, renal failure may occur in the absence of clinical, biochemical, or histologic evidence of underlying renal disease (hepatorenal syndrome). The development of the hepatorenal syndrome is a grave prognostic sign with a mortality around 90%. Recovery is dependent on improvement in hepatic function. Rarely is renal failure the cause of death in these patients, since creatinine and blood urea nitrogen levels are only moderately elevated. Instead, the hepatorenal syndrome is but one of many complicating factors in a patient with advanced liver disease. Although the hepatorenal syndrome is most commonly seen in patients with cirrhosis, it can complicate fulminant hepatic failure or hepatic malignancy. Ascites and signs of hepatic encephalopathy frequently accompany the hepatorenal syndrome. Moderate hypotension secondary to peripheral vasodilation is common.

Laboratory abnormalities in the hepatorenal syndrome include increases in the serum creatinine and blood urea nitrogen concentrations, frequently in the setting of oliguria and hyponatremia (Table 3-3). Avid proximal reabsorption of sodium leads to urinary serum concentrations less than 10 meq/liter. The fractional excretion of sodium is less than 1% with a urine-plasma creatinine ratio greater than 30. These findings help distinguish the hepatorenal syndrome from acute tubular necrosis, where urinary sodium excretion is often greater than 20 meq/liter and the urine-plasma creatinine ratio is less than 20.

It may be difficult to distinguish the hepatorenal syndrome from intravascular volume depletion, since both are characterized by low urinary sodium concentrations. In this setting measuring the central venous pressure (CVP) is the most accurate way to reliably assess intravascular volume. A trial of intravascular volume expansion is indicated if the CVP is less than 5 cm of saline; one gradually increases the CVP to 12 cm of saline and observes for a natriuresis or increase in urine volume. Overexpansion of the intravascular volume should be avoided since it may lead to congestive heart failure or esophageal variceal hemorrhage.

No therapies directed at renal hemodynamic changes in patients with the hepatorenal syndrome have been successful. Dopamine, vasodilatory prostaglandins, lysine vasopressin, peritoneovenous shunts, and therapeutic paracentesis with intravascular volume expansion have not improved the prognosis in patients with the hepatorenal syndrome. The prognosis of hepatorenal syndrome reflects the severity of the underlying liver disease. In most patients with cirrhosis little can be done to improve hepatic function; therefore, it is obvious why the prognosis is so poor. In the majority of patients with cirrhosis who develop the hepatorenal syndrome, hepatic transplantation provides the only chance for survival.

Table 3-3. Differential Diagnosis of Renal Failure in Patient with Cirrhosis

	Acute Tubular Necrosis (antibiotics, ischemia)	Prerenal Azotemia (dehydration, over diuresis)	Hepatorenal Syndrome
Urine volume	Variable, usually < 1000 ml/d	< 1000 ml/d	< 500 ml/d
Urinary sodium excretion	> 20 meq/liter	< 10 meq/liter	< 10 meq/liter
Urine-plasma creatinine ratio	< 20	> 30	> 30
Central venous pressure	Normal	< 3 cm H_2O	Normal

Hepatic Encephalopathy

Hepatic encephalopathy is a complex neuropsychiatric syndrome which complicates both acute and chronic liver disease. The clinical spectrum of hepatic encephalopathy is wide, ranging from minor changes in personality to frank coma. Alterations in neuromuscular transmission, typified by asterixis, are frequently seen. No single laboratory test is diagnostic of hepatic encephalopathy, although the diagnosis should be suspect in patients with a normal plasma ammonia level. Psychomotor tests and electroencephalographic readings are useful in diagnosing early encephalopathy and in assessing response to treatment.

Hepatic encephalopathy develops when portal blood is shunted around a poorly functioning liver. Toxic substances, presumably caused by the action of bacterial flora on a nitrogenous load, accumulate in the blood and subsequently in the central nervous system. Certain factors can precipitate encephalopathy by increasing toxin production or increasing cerebral sensitivity to toxic agents. These factors include azotemia, gastrointestinal bleeding, hypoglycemia, alkalosis, systemic infections, and sedative drugs. The prognosis for recovery from an encephalopathic episode is better when a precipitating factor can be identified than when the onset of encephalopathy is caused by worsening hepatic function.

After precipitating causes have been eliminated or treated, empiric therapy for hepatic encephalopathy is initiated (Table 3-4). A very low protein diet should be prescribed (< 20 g/d). As encephalopa-

Table 3-4. Therapy for Hepatic Encephalopathy

Treat precipitating causes.
  Hypokalemia, GI bleeding, infection
Decrease toxin production.
  Low-protein diet
Administer antibiotics.
  Neomycin, metronidazole, ampicillin, vancomycin
Increased toxin elimination and decreased absorption.
  Lactulose, lactose, Lactilol, vegetable diet
"Inactivate" toxins.
  Sodium benzoate, ketoacids
Correct plasma abnormalities which increase effect of toxins.
  Branched-chain amino acids, zinc supplementation
Inhibit CNS effects of toxins.
  Benzodiazepine receptor antagonists, bromocriptine, L-dopa

thy improves, dietary protein can be increased to 1.5 g/kg/d. Intravenous protein administered as protein hydrolysates or mixtures of synthetic amino acids does not cause hepatic encephalopathy. Diets consisting of primarily vegetable rather than animal protein are often better tolerated by patients susceptible to hepatic encephalopathy. The extra fiber in vegetable diets rather than their amino acid composition is likely responsible for their beneficial effects. As previously discussed, branched-chain amino acid enriched mixtures are not useful in the vast majority of patients with hepatic encephalopathy.

Lactulose remains the drug of choice for hepatic encephalopathy. Thirty milliliters tid PO will result in a satisfactory response. Lactulose enemas can be given initially to comatose patients. Suppression of gut bacteria through orally administered antibiotics is effective treatment for hepatic encephalopathy in many patients. Neomycin has been largely replaced by metronidazole because of concerns about neomycin's ototoxicity, nephrotoxicity, and antibiotic-associated diarrhea. Initially, 250 mg of metronidazole is given three times a day. If symptoms improve, the dose is tapered to the lowest dosage required to control encephalopathic symptoms.

Recent data suggest that benzodiazepinelike compounds acting at the benzodiazepine receptor complex in the central nervous system play a role in the pathogenesis of hepatic encephalopathy. As a result several reports using benzodiazepine antagonists have suggested improvement in patients with hepatic encephalopathy. Since no controlled trials have been reported to assess the efficacy of benzodiazepine antagonists, this treatment must be considered, at present, experimental. As with other complications of cirrhosis, hepatic encephalopathy refractory to medical management is considered an indication for hepatic transplantation.

Alterations in Drug Metabolism

Since the liver is the site of biotransformation and excretion of many drugs, cirrhosis can affect drug disposition. Other factors, such as age, nutritional status, and simultaneous use of other medications, may also affect hepatic drug metabolism. Although there is a large volume of information about drug metabolism in patients with cirrhosis, a few practical recommendations can assist the clinician in the use of drugs in patients with cirrhosis.

Patients with cirrhosis are susceptible to infections and frequently require antibiotic therapy. Fortunately, most antibiotics can be used safely and effectively. Exceptions include cephalosporins that contain a methyltetrazole thiol group (cefamandole, cefoperazone, and cefotetan) which can interfere with the synthesis of vitamin K–dependent coagulation factors and lead to significant bleeding. Alternative cephalosporins, such as cefotaxime or cefoxitin, should be used. Aminoglycoside antibiotics should be avoided when possible in patients with cirrhosis because of their enhanced susceptibility to aminoglycoside nephrotoxicity.

Aspirin and nonsteroidal inflammatory agents (NSAIDs) should be used cautiously in patients with cirrhosis. Since aspirin is metabolized in the liver, when it is used, a reduced dosage is advisable. The effect of both aspirin and NSAIDs on platelets, combined with their tendency to cause gastritis, enhances the risk of bleeding in patients with cirrhosis. NSAIDs inhibit the synthesis of vasodilatory prostaglandins and can lead to impaired renal function. Since patients with cirrhosis are particularly susceptible to alterations in renal function (hepatorenal syndrome), it is best to avoid these agents entirely in patients with cirrhosis. Acetaminophen in therapeutic doses can be used safely in patients with cirrhosis. In the absence of phase I enzyme systems induction by alcohol or other drugs, acetaminophen hepatoxicity does not occur when used at usual doses.

Sedatives, particularly benzodiazepines, should be used cautiously in patients with cirrhosis. Precipitation or exacerbation of hepatic encephalopathy by these agents is common. The benzodiazepines, chlordiazepoxide (Librium), and diazepam (Valium), which require several metabolic steps in the liver, should be replaced, when possible, by oxazepam (Serax) and lorazepam (Ativan), which require fewer metabolic steps.

Occasionally, patients with cirrhosis require antihypertensive therapy. Two classes of antihypertensive medications should be used with caution in patients with cirrhosis. Angiotensin-converting enzyme inhibitors (captopril, enalapril) can precipitate renal insufficiency. In addition, alpha-adrenergic receptor antagonists, like prazosin, lead to hypotension in patients with cirrhosis.

Specific guidelines for drug use in patients with

cirrhosis are difficult to provide since there is great heterogeneity among these patients. In general, however, only essential medications should be given to patients with cirrhosis. The clinician should be aware of changes in hepatic clearance and protein binding that can affect the bioavailability of medications. Whenever possible, serum blood levels should be monitored in patients to assess for evidence of toxicity.

Results

The treatment of end-stage cirrhosis is liver transplantation. The results of hepatic transplantation are affected by multiple factors, including age, patient status, and underlying disease. The overall results of transplantation in the United States from 1985 through 1992 are presented in Fig. 3-4. The results for adults and children were almost identical (see Fig. 3-4A), with 1-, 3-, and 5-year survivals being approximately 80%, 72%, and 65%, respectively. Among adults over 50 years of age, however, survivals are approximately 10% lower at each time point. Patient status at the time of transplantation is also crucial to outcome. Results are best for patients who are working or attending school full-time, approximately 5% worse for homebound adults or infants who are failing to thrive, 15% to 20% worse for patients in intensive care units, and 25% to 30% worse for patients on life support.

Significant differences in outcome may also occur as the result of the patient's underlying disease process. However, the overall results of transplantation are the same when patients with alcoholic cirrhosis are compared to all other adults (see Fig. 3-4B). On the other hand, patients with primary biliary cirrhosis and primary sclerosing cholangitis fare significantly better than those who undergo transplantation for fulminant hepatic failure or malignancy (Fig. 3-5A). Similarly, results of transplantation for children are best for metabolic disorders, intermediate for biliary atresia, and worst for fulminant hepatic failure and neonatal hepatitis (see Fig. 3-5B).

Conclusions

Cirrhosis is the end stage of many liver diseases. When possible, therapy should be instituted at a

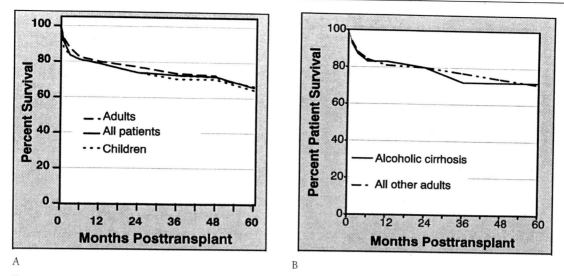

Figure 3-4. A. Five-year actuarial survival of all patients transplanted in the United States between 1985 and 1992. B. Five-year actuarial survival of patients transplanted for alcohol-related liver disease compared to all other adults.

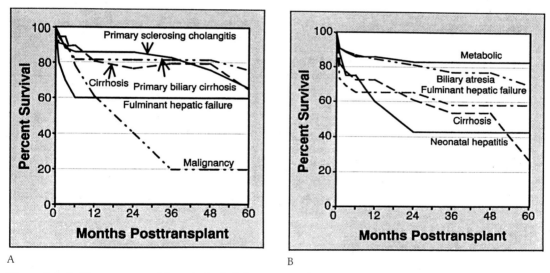

Figure 3-5. A. Five-year actuarial survival of adult recipients segregated by liver disease. B. Five-year actuarial survival of pediatric recipients segregated by liver disease.

precirrhotic stage to prevent this complication. However, for many liver diseases no effective therapy has been established to prevent the progression to cirrhosis. Therapy in these patients is directed primarily at controlling the complications of portal hypertension. These complications include ascites with an inherent risk for spontaneous bacterial peri-tonitis, hepatic encephalopathy, and, in patients with very advanced disease, the hepatorenal syndrome. With the exception of the hepatorenal syndrome, these complications can be controlled in most patients with medical therapy. When medical therapy fails to control the complications, then a liver transplantation is the preferred modality of therapy in patients who are suitable candidates for this procedure.

Selected Readings

Akriviadis EA, Runyon BA. The value of an algorithm in differentiating spontaneous from secondary bacterial peritonitis. *Gastroenterology* 1990; 98:127–133.

Conn HO. Complications of portal hypertension. In Gary Gitnick (ed), *Current Hepatology,* vol. 13. St. Louis: Mosby, 1993. Pp. 223–267.

Epstein M. Functional renal abnormalities in cirrhosis: Pathophysiology and management. In Zakim D, Boyer TD (eds), *Hepatology: A Textbook of Liver Diseases.* Philadelphia: Saunders, 1990. Pp. 493–512.

Epstein M. The hepatorenal syndrome: New perspectives. *N Engl J Med* 1992; 327:1810–1811.

Ferenci P, Grimm G, Meryn S, et al. Successful long-term treatment of portal-systemic encephalopathy by the benzodiazepine antagonist flumazenil. *Gastroenterology* 1989; 96:240–243.

Gonwa TA, Poplawski S, Paulsen W, et al. Pathogenesis and outcome of hepatorenal syndrome in patients undergoing orthotopic liver transplant. *Transplantation* 1989; 47:395–397.

McCullough AJ. Disorders of nutrition and intermediary metabolism. In Rector WG (ed), *Complications of Chronic Liver Disease.* St. Louis: Mosby, 1992. Pp. 182–211.

Raiford DS, Mitchell MC. Disorders of drug disposition. In Rector WG (ed), *Complications of Chronic Liver Disease.* St. Louis: Mosby, 1992. Pp. 238–252.

Rector WG Jr, Reynolds TB. The serum-ascites albumin gradient is superior to the ascites total protein concentration in the separation of "transudative" and "exudative" ascites. *Am J Med* 1986; 77:83–86.

Runyon BA. Care of patients with ascites. *N Eng J Med* 1994; 330:337–342.

4

Portal Hypertension

Ziv J. Haskal
Raymond A. Rubin
Ali Naji
Ernest J. Ring

Although significant advances have been made in the understanding of the pathophysiology of portal hypertension, the treatment of its complications still presents a formidable clinical challenge. The appropriate and effective application of medical, percutaneous, and surgical therapies requires close cooperation between hepatologists, interventional radiologists, and surgeons. This chapter will review the pathogenesis and management of one of the major complications of portal hypertension, i.e., variceal bleeding, and will suggest a multidisciplinary approach to this difficult clinical problem.

Etiology and Pathogenesis

The portal vein is a high-volume, low-pressure conduit formed by the confluence of the splenic, superior mesenteric, and inferior mesenteric veins. Additional tributaries include the left gastric/coronary and short gastric veins, which drain the distal esophagus and gastric cardia, respectively. Portal blood mixes with hepatic arterial blood in the hepatic sinusoids. Sinusoidal blood drains through central veins into the hepatic veins, which return the blood to the heart through the inferior vena cava.

The pressure in the portal vein normally exceeds hepatic vein pressure by 3 to 6 mm Hg. In patients with cirrhosis the effects of increased intrahepatic sinusoidal resistance are transmitted back through the valveless portal circulation. This resistance increases the pressure gradient between the portal and systemic circulation. An increased portosystemic gradient (PSG) is also seen in cases of prehepatic and posthepatic portal hypertension (Table 4-1).

As the PSG increases, the splanchnic venous outflow is redirected through native portosystemic collaterals, including submucosal varices. Although these portosystemic communications have been described in nearly every segment of the alimentary tract, the great majority of varices occur at the cardioesophageal junction. The risk of bleeding from these esophageal varices has been related to the patient's modified Childs-Pugh class, the size of the varices, and the presence of red wales on the varices. Several investigators have corroborated that a PSG exceeding 12 mm Hg is a necessary, but insufficient, condition for spontaneous esophageal variceal hemorrhage.

Approximately one quarter to one third of patients with cirrhosis and quiescent esophageal varices will suffer variceal hemorrhage. The probability of 1-year survival following this index variceal hemorrhage is approximately 30% to 50%, with a high proportion of deaths occurring during the initial hospitalization and the following 2 to 3 months. The mortality is highest for patients with advanced cirrhosis, that is, those with Childs' class B and C cirrhosis. Management of esophageal variceal hemorrhage, therefore, focuses on treatment of acute bleeding, secondary prevention of recurrent hemor-

31

Table 4-1. Causes of Portal Hypertension

Prehepatic
  Idiopathic portal hypertension
  Portal vein thrombosis
  Schistosomiasis
  Extrahepatic portal hypertension caused by toxins
  Extrahepatic arteriovenous fistula
Sinusoidal
  Alcoholic liver disease
  Viral hepatitis
    Autoimmune hepatitis
    Primary biliary cirrhosis
    Sclerosing cholangitis
    Hemochromatosis
    Wilson's disease
    Acute liver failure
  Congenital hepatic fibrosis
  Intrahepatic arteriovenous fistulae
  Alpha$_1$-antitrypsin deficiency
Posthepatic
  Veno-occlusive disease
  Budd-Chiari syndrome
  Constrictive pericarditis
  Right-sided congestive heart failure

rhage, and primary prophylaxis of the initial bleeding episode.

Diagnosis

Portal hypertension is usually manifested by its complications, including variceal bleeding, jaundice, ascites, encephalopathy, and splenomegaly. Diagnostic evaluation can include laboratory, endoscopic, histologic, and radiographic evaluation to assess for ongoing hepatic inflammation, cholestasis, and synthetic dysfunction.

Esophagogastroduodenoscopy (EGD) is the primary diagnostic tool for detecting esophageal varices. Typically, these appear as blue serpiginous engorged submucosal lesions within the lower esophagus. EGD may also identify certain stigmata indicating an increased risk of esophageal variceal bleeding, such as overlying clots and red wales. Gastric endoscopy may reveal mucosal edema and hyperemia or the characteristic mosaic mucosal pattern of "portal hypertensive gastropathy." Gastric fundal varices can be very difficult to distinguish from edematous proximal gastric folds. This discrepancy may account for the highly variable reports of the prevalence of gastric varices in patients with known esophageal varices. In patients with lower gastrointestinal bleeding, anorectal varices may be mistaken for hemorrhoids. Notably, unlike hemorrhoids, anorectal varices can extend above the dentate line, are easily compressible, and rapidly refill upon release. Finally, diagnostic endoscopy is crucial in excluding nonvariceal sources of hemorrhage, which can coexist with gastroesophageal varices in up to one half of cases.

Angiographic evaluation may be indicated when the diagnosis of portal hypertension is in question, when ectopic intestinal varices are suspected, or when percutaneous or surgical shunt placement or liver transplantation is anticipated. Angiography is also valuable in excluding nonvariceal, arterial sources of acute gastrointestinal bleeding.

Selective arteriography of the visceral arterial axis is performed with particular attention to the venous phase (arterial portography). Splenic arteriography can demonstrate retardation or reversal of splenic vein flow, fugal filling of the coronary and/or short gastric veins, venous occlusions, and spontaneous splenorenal shunts. The venous phase of the superior mesenteric arteriogram will opacify the portal vein or demonstrate periportal collaterals in cases of portal vein thrombosis. Superior mesenteric arteriography will also outline enteric varices in most cases. Hepatic arteriography may show arterial findings suggestive of cirrhosis and hepatofugal flow in the portal vein, confirming the presence of significant portal hypertension. Small hepatocellular carcinomas may be an incidental finding in approximately 6% of patients with cirrhosis annually. Finally, arteriovenous fistulae causing portal hypertension can be identified and occluded with transcatheter embolization.

Hepatic venography and inferior venacavography are useful in suspected cases of portal hypertension due to Budd-Chiari syndrome and hepatic veno-occlusive disease. Wedged hepatic venous pressure measurements can estimate portal pressure and allow calculation of the PSG. The technique of transsplenic portography has been largely replaced by direct transhepatic portal catheterization. Finally, in patients with advanced coagulopathies or ascites, transvenous liver biopsy can provide histologic confirmation of cirrhosis while obviating the risk of intraperitoneal hemorrhage following transhepatic biopsy.

Management

Options

The treatment of variceal hemorrhage in portal hypertensive patients is a complex issue. Several options exist for management of acute variceal hemorrhage, primary prophylaxis of initial bleeding, and secondary prevention of recurrent hemorrhage. Options include medical therapy, endoscopic sclerotherapy and variceal band ligation, surgical portosystemic shunts, transjugular intrahepatic portosystemic shunts (TIPSs), and liver transplantation.

Several pharmacologic agents are used to halt acute esophageal variceal hemorrhage. Continuous intravenous vasopressin infusion lowers portal pressure and PSG primarily by constricting splanchnic arterioles and venules and reducing splanchnic venous outflow into the liver. Vasopressin may also mechanically diminish flow to esophageal varices by increasing lower esophageal sphincter pressure. Importantly, concomitant vasoconstriction at other sites may result in adverse effects, such as cardiac and cerebrovascular ischemia. The simultaneous administration of nitrates by intravenous, topical, or sublingual routes not only effectively prevents these adverse effects but also further decreases the PSG. Intravenous somatostatin infusion and synthetic somatostatin analogue infusion reduce azygos blood flow (an indicator of collateral circulation) and PSG without systemic vasoconstrictive effects. The mechanism by which somatostatin accomplishes these hemodynamic effects is not well understood.

Pharmacologic therapy also plays an important role in the primary and secondary prevention of esophageal variceal hemorrhage. Chronic administration of nonselective beta blockers, such as propranolol, has been the mainstay of medical therapy. Propranolol decreases PSG but has a less reliable effect on portal pressure. Nonselective beta blockers reduce splanchnic blood flow both by blocking vasodilatory beta$_2$ receptors and by decreasing cardiac output (perhaps leading to reflex alpha-adrenergic mediated splanchnic vasoconstriction). Beta blockers may be used alone or in combination with other obliterative or decompressive techniques for prophylaxis of variceal bleeding.

Acute endoscopic management focuses upon rapid control of bleeding varices and exclusion of other peptic sources of concomitant bleeding. Chemical irritants are injected directly into or adjacent to actively bleeding varices or those with stigmata indicating a high likelihood of rebleeding (e.g., red wales or clots overlying varices). Alternatively, the varices may be suctioned toward the channel of the endoscope and encircled by "O"-shaped rubber bands deployed from within the instrument. Both sclerotherapy and banding ligation result in varix thrombosis, with subsequent superficial ulceration and re-epithelialization of the overlying mucosa. Although endoscopic does not affect PSG, obliteration of esophageal varices does redirect flow through other collateral pathways which are less likely to bleed, such as the splenic to renal vein network. In some cases, however, obliteration of esophageal varices results in enlarging gastric varices.

Sclerotherapy and banding ligation have also been used for treatment of anorectal, peristomial, and proximal gastric fundal varices. Butyl cyanoacrylate and other "glues" are currently being investigated for treatment of gastric varices. Large and small intestinal varices typically lie beyond the reach of the endoscope and are thus best treated by percutaneous or surgical means.

If endoscopic means successfully control the initial episode of bleeding, then serial endoscopic therapy is performed until variceal obliteration is achieved or procedural complications warrant other intervention. Typically, these outpatient sessions are performed at 1- to 2-week intervals to allow interval healing of mucosal ulcerations.

Reduction of the portosystemic gradient and variceal decompression can be achieved by the creation of surgical or percutaneous portosystemic shunts. Operative shunts can be divided into total, partial, and selective. Totally diverting portacaval shunts are rarely performed today except in cases of uncontrolled variceal bleeding because of their association with accelerated liver failure and unacceptable rates of hepatic encephalopathy. Small stoma portacaval and small-bore prosthetic mesocaval "H" grafts allow partial decompression of the portal system, resulting in lower rates of portosystemic encephalopathy (PSE) and liver failure. The distal splenorenal (Warren) shunt selectively diverts flow from the short gastric and coronary veins filling esophageal and gastric varices into the systemic circulation while preserving mesenteric to portal flow and thus portal perfusion. The Warren shunt

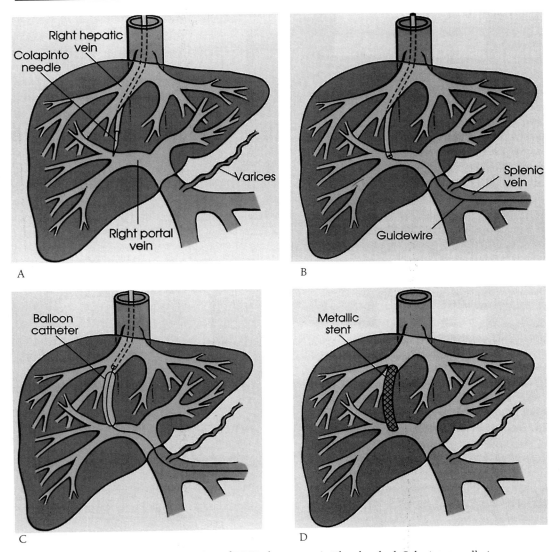

Figure 4-1. Diagrammatic representation of TIPS placement. A. The sheathed Colapinto needle is advanced out of a hepatic vein into a portal vein branch. Varices are present. B. A guidewire is advanced through the needle into splenic vein. C. The parenchymal liver tract is dilated using a balloon angioplasty catheter. D. The metallic stent is deployed within the shunt tract. E. If numerous varices remain after the shunt is dilated to 10 mm diameter and the portosystemic gradient remains elevated, then a second TIPS is constructed. (From Haskal ZJ, Ring EJ. Technique and results of transjugular intrahepatic portosystemic shunts (TIPS). In Cope C (ed), *Current Techniques in Interventional Radiology*. Philadelphia: Current Medicine, 1994; 1:2–2.10. Used with permission.)

is usually reserved for elective cases because its creation is more technically demanding and time-consuming than other surgical shunts. Finally, esophageal transection and gastric devascularization (Sugiura procedure) can be used to prevent recurrent variceal hemorrhage, particularly in cases of splenic vein thrombosis. This option is not widely practiced in the United States.

The transjugular intrahepatic portosystemic shunt (TIPS) offers a percutaneous method of par-

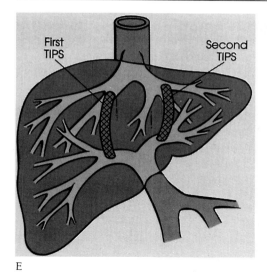

E

Figure 4-1. (continued).

tial portal decompression. A TIPS is created with fluoroscopic guidance under intravenous conscious sedation. In brief, an internal jugular approach is used to pass a long curved needle from within a hepatic vein through the hepatic parenchyma into a branch of the portal vein. The portal vein is thus catheterized, its pressure measured, and its flow imaged angiographically. The bridging liver tract is dilated using an angioplasty balloon and lined with a metallic stent to prevent recoil of the surrounding hepatic parenchyma from collapsing the conduit. The stent is progressively enlarged with balloon catheters until portal venography and pressure measurements indicate that adequate decompression has been achieved (Fig. 4-1). Typical endpoints include reduction of the PSG below 12 mm Hg and disappearance of variceal flow during splenic venography. Coil or alcohol embolization of varices can also be performed as part of the procedure. In experienced hands, the average procedure time is approximately 1.5 hours.

Finally, liver transplantation has been successfully performed in the setting of variceal hemorrhage. Although transplantation can provide definitive therapy, few patients warrant this treatment on the basis of bleeding alone. In addition, the shortage of donor organs often precludes emergent transplant.

Controversies

Most experts agree that the initial treatment of acute esophageal hemorrhage is vigorous resuscitation, vasoconstrictive medication (vasopressin plus nitrates or somatostatin), and diagnostic and therapeutic endoscopy. Since beta blockers may blunt an adequate chronotropic response to hemorrhage, most clinicians do not suggest their use during active bleeding. There are few advocates of shunt surgery or TIPS as first-line therapy during the first episode of esophageal variceal hemorrhage. This situation stems, in part, from the proven ability of sclerotherapy to control bleeding in most cases. In addition, encephalopathy and possible decompensation of hepatic function are real risks after portosystemic shunting.

The appropriate salvage treatment of patients who fail endoscopic treatment of acute bleeding is, however, quite controversial. Balloon tamponade may be used as a temporizing measure, but patients with advanced cirrhosis who fail consecutive endoscopic treatments have an overwhelming high mortality without other therapy. In this situation, TIPSs or surgical portosystemic shunts are the two main options. The type of surgical shunt performed often depends on the patient's acute medical condition and whether he or she is a transplantation candidate. For suitable patients, emergent liver transplantation may be performed depending on organ availability.

Few data are available regarding the appropriate management of acute variceal bleeding from a nonesophageal origin. Although some reports of successful endoscopic treatment of gastric and anorectal variceal hemorrhage have been published, these varices and intestinal varices that lie beyond the endoscope are best treated by surgical shunts or TIPSs.

The proper management of nonbleeding esophageal varices for prevention of recurrent hemorrhage is a highly charged issue. Given the high mortality of patients with cirrhosis after an index bleed, significant debate exists regarding proper management after a patient survives an acute esophageal variceal hemorrhage. Beta blockers offer an inexpensive therapy with few adverse effects. Their use may, however, be contraindicated in patients with obstructive pulmonary disease, diabetes mellitus, and congestive heart failure due to systolic dysfunction. Furthermore, prescription drug therapy in potentially noncompliant patients with active substance abuse may have little impact on the course of variceal bleeding.

Serial endoscopic treatment is labor-intensive and requires frequent physician visits in the first few months after a variceal bleed. Complications of sclerotherapy include dysphagia, esophageal stricture formation, and perforation. Portosystemic shunts can improve other complications of portal hypertension such as ascites and portal hypertensive gastropathy, but may accelerate hepatic failure by diverting significant portal flow. TIPSs are prone to stenosis and occlusion because of excessive intraluminal pseudointimal hyperplasia. Since this problem can lead to recurrent bleeding, periodic surveillance shunt sonography, and possibly reintervention, are necessary. This requirement may be untenable in poorly compliant patients. The uncertain long-term patency of TIPSs compared with surgical shunts may make them less appropriate in patients with early stages of cirrhosis (e.g., Childs' class A) who have an anticipated long survival. In alcoholic patients with Childs' A disease, TIPSs and surgical shunts might be postponed because simple abstinence from alcohol may improve their liver disease. For patients awaiting liver transplantation, however, a TIPS, in particular, can serve as a bridge to transplantation by effectively reducing the risk of recurrent bleeding and potentially controlling refractory ascites.

Given that only one quarter to one third of patients with cirrhosis and varices will ultimately bleed from their varices, the benefits of a primary preventative therapy clearly need to outweigh its potential disadvantages. Propranolol provides a relatively inexpensive prophylactic therapy which is fairly well tolerated. Whereas results of endoscopic sclerosis for primary prevention of esophageal variceal bleeding have been disappointing, the role of serial endoscopic band ligation is indeterminate. Surgical shunts are not advocated for primary prevention. Comparative studies of TIPSs in this setting have not been performed.

Most of the literature on the bleeding complications of portal hypertension focuses on esophageal variceal bleeding and gives little attention to nonesophageal sources. Moreover, most of these trials

are heavily weighted toward patients with alcohol-related cirrhosis. Few studies concentrate on other causes of portal hypertension, such as veno-occlusive disease, Budd-Chiari syndrome, and idiopathic extrahepatic portal hypertension.

Preferred Approach

The initial management of acute variceal bleeding focuses on the usual principles of successful resuscitation and stabilization, including securing an adequate airway, restoring intravascular volume, correcting coagulopathies, and employing vasopressors, when necessary. Practically, the infusion of vasopressin and nitrates or of somatostatin is often initiated prior to diagnostic endoscopy in patients with suspected variceal bleeding. If other sources of hemorrhage are identified at endoscopy, these medications can be promptly discontinued with little untoward effect. If esophageal varices are actively bleeding or bear stigmata of rebleeding, endoscopic sclerotherapy or possibly band ligation should be performed.

For patients who fail endoscopic therapy, balloon tamponade may temporarily control bleeding while treatment decisions are organized and the patient is stabilized. Portal decompression becomes particularly important in this setting. The ability of an experienced interventional radiologist to create a TIPS within 2 hours in almost all patients has, in many institutions, eliminated the role of surgery in the emergent setting. The efficacy of TIPS at arresting acute variceal bleeding is proven. Not surprisingly, the best predictors for early survival after TIPS include the absence of pre-existing or incipient multisystem failure and pneumonia. This fact emphasizes the need to promptly assess the effect of endoscopic therapy during an acute bleeding episode and to perform TIPS, if indicated, before the multiorgan failure ensues and significantly worsens survival. Acute gastric or intestinal variceal hemorrhage and continued oozing from portal hypertensive gastropathy are generally not amenable to endoscopic intervention and should be promptly treated with the portal decompression provided by TIPSs or surgical shunts.

Once a patient survives an acute variceal bleed, the authors recommend elective serial endoscopic sclerotherapy until varices are eradicated or the patient becomes refractory or intolerant. Adjunct therapy with beta blockers has not been shown to augment the effect of endoscopic treatment on rebleeding or mortality. At the present time, TIPS cannot be considered primary therapy for prevention of recurrent bleeding. TIPS is best applied in patients with cirrhosis who fail sclerotherapy. Surgical portosystemic shunts can be used in lieu of TIPS for patients with well-preserved hepatic function (i.e., Childs' class A cirrhosis) in whom liver transplantation is unlikely and long-term survival is anticipated. The decision to offer elective TIPSs, distal splenorenal, or mesocaval shunts to a patient must depend, in part, on the local expertise of the interventional radiologists and surgeons, and on the ability of the patient to comply in a follow-up program. It is important to emphasize that once the decision has been made to decompress the portal system, the chosen approach should be performed promptly and electively when procedural morbidity is at its nadir.

Finally, for patients with medium to large esophageal varices which have never bled, primary prophylaxis with nonselective beta blockers (e.g., propranolol or nadolol) has the best therapeutic risk-benefit ratio when compared to the other treatment options. Although most clinicians titrate the dose of beta blockers to achieve a decrease in pulse rate by 25%, this guideline does not accurately predict the actual reduction of the portosystemic gradient. Actual measurement of wedged hepatic venous pressures can reflect the effect on PSG, but this measurement requires that the patient undergo an invasive venous catheterization. Promising research with sonography and magnetic resonance angiography may allow noninvasive determination of portal pressure and allow accurate titration of these medications.

Results

Acute Treatment

With aggressive resuscitation and supportive management, acute esophageal variceal bleeding will cease in about 50% of cases. Although intravenous somatostatin or vasopressin plus nitroglycerin has been shown to effectively control hemorrhage in 50% to 65% of patients, it has been difficult to prove that these medications decrease mortality compared with placebo infusion. The in-hospital survival for Childs' class C patients treated for acute esophageal variceal bleeding with these drugs is only 35% to 40%.

Endoscopic sclerotherapy or banding ligation (with or without vasopressin) will stop acute esophageal variceal bleeding in 80% to 90% of patients. The success rate is significantly lower for bleeding gastric varices. Creation of partial or totally diverting surgical portosystemic shunts effectively halts esophageal, gastric, and intestinal variceal bleeding in over 90% of cases. Emergent surgery and advanced Childs' class C disease are associated with a surgical mortality rate of up to 50%.

A TIPS functions most like a side-to-side portacaval shunt and is thus as effective as surgical shunts at arresting acute bleeding. If the PSG is reduced to below 12 mm Hg and variceal flow is eliminated, then variceal bleeding stops in virtually all cases. Advantages of TIPS include its ability to be performed rapidly with a technical success rate of over 95%. The risk of general anesthesia in a hemodynamically unstable patient with potentially limited hepatic reserve is obviated by the ability to create a TIPS under conscious sedation (Fig. 4-2).

The contraindications to TIPS are few, including polycystic liver disease and pre-existing right heart failure. The latter is important because the sudden inflow of high-pressure portal blood into the right atrium can lead to further cardiac decompensation in such patients. Portal vein occlusion does not preclude TIPS placement, although it makes the procedure lengthier and more difficult to perform (Fig. 4-3).

Although many procedural complications from TIPS have been described, severe complications occur in less than 1% of cases. Reported complications include contrast reactions, transient renal failure, hemobilia, myocardial ischemia, hepatic infarction, and pulmonary edema. Thirty-day survival after TIPS is highly correlated with the condition of the patient prior to TIPS. At the Hospital of the University of Pennsylvania, active variceal hemorrhage promptly arrested in 43 out of 45 patients who underwent TIPS placement. Nearly all of the patients who expired within 30 days of TIPS placement died from pre-existing multiorgan failure, aspiration pneumonia and/or adult respiratory distress syndrome. Advanced cirrhosis, as reflected

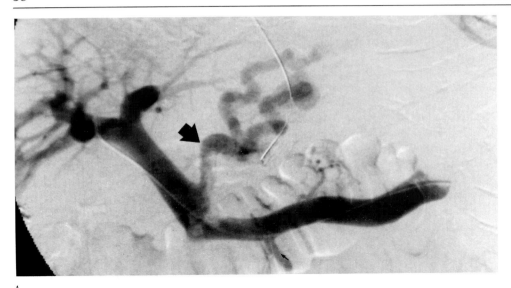

A

B

Figure 4-2. Case 1: Placement of TIPS in a patient with a patent portal vein. A 43-year-old woman presents with acute esophageal variceal bleeding refractory to emergent sclerotherapy. A. Initial transjugular venogram demonstrates hepatopedal portal flow with fugal flow into the coronary vein (arrow). A nasogastric tube is faintly seen. The portosystemic gradient is 23 mm Hg. B. Transjugular portogram after placement of a 10-mm right hepatic to right portal vein TIPS (arrow) demonstrates flow through the shunt into the hepatic vein. No significant variceal flow remains. The portosystemic gradient is now 10 mm Hg.

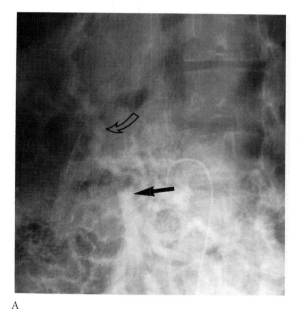

A

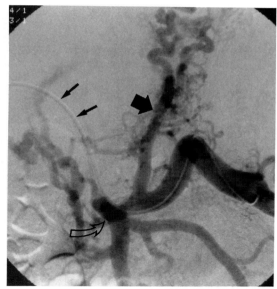

B

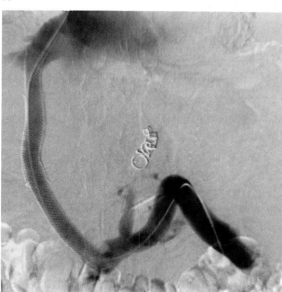

C

Figure 4-3. Case 2: Placement of a TIPS in a patient with a chronically occluded portal vein. A 61-year-old male with Childs' class C Laënnec's cirrhosis presents for TIPS 2 weeks after his seventh episode of recurrent gastric and esophageal variceal hemorrhage. He had undergone seven prior episodes of sclerotherapy. A. Venous phase of a superior mesenteric arteriogram demonstrates distal thrombosis of the superior mesenteric vein (arrow). A large periportal collateral vessel (curved arrow) is seen near the site of the thrombosed portal vein.
B. Transhepatic splenic venogram demonstrates occlusion of the superior mesenteric (curved arrow) and splenic veins at their confluence with the thrombosed portal vein. There is fugal flow into a large coronary vein (arrow). The transhepatic catheter, coursing through the occluded main portal vein, is faintly seen (small arrows). The portosystemic gradient is 42 mm Hg. C. Splenic venogram obtained after portal thrombectomy, transjugular shunt placement, and coil embolization of the coronary vein. There is no residual variceal flow. The portosystemic gradient is 12 mm Hg.

by Childs' class, was associated with diminished survival. Notably, a pre-TIPS APACHE II score (Acute Physiology and Chronic Health Evaluation) exceeding 20 was associated with an over twelvefold increased risk of early demise independent of Childs' class (author's data, ZJH).

The most significant adverse effect of portal diversion by any means is portosystemic encephalopathy (PSE). Precise comparisons of PSE rates for TIPSs and surgical shunts are difficult to perform because of varying methods of assessing and reporting. For example, some investigators prescribe prophylactic oral lactulose therapy for all patients, whereas others reserve it for those who develop spontaneous PSE. Despite these caveats, the rate of PSE after TIPS appears similar to that reported in surgical shunt series, ranging between 18% to 25%. Between 4% and 7% of patients with new or worsened encephalopathy after TIPS do not respond to protein restriction and oral lactulose therapy. Associated risk factors for PSE include pre-existing encephalopathy and patient age exceeding 60 years. In cases of severe encephalopathy after shunting, the TIPS can be thrombosed with the temporary placement of a balloon occlusion catheter within the shunt. Alternatively, the shunt lumen can be reduced in diameter by deployment of a flow-limiting stenotic stent (Table 4-2A–F).

In most cases, however, encephalopathy after TIPS diminishes with time as the shunt lumen is incorporated within a layer of pseudointima and collagen tissue. This natural process usually reduces the shunt lumen diameter by 1 to 2 mm and thus lessens the amount of portal diversion (Fig. 4-4).

Secondary Prevention

Serial endoscopic therapy is complicated by rebleeding in 20% to 50% of patients treated for prevention of recurrent hemorrhage. Rebleeding often occurs in the first 2 months after initiating treatment, before the varices have been obliterated. Varices can be completely eradicated in 60% to 80% of patients, although they may recur 1 to 2 years later. The eradication of varices requires fewer sessions with banding ligation compared with sclerotherapy. The rate of complications (such as esophageal strictures and infections), however, is significantly higher with sclerotherapy than with ligation. A meta-analysis performed by Infante-Rivard and colleagues concluded that serial sclerotherapy reduced the number of deaths by 25% compared with placebo after patients survived an index variceal bleed. Conflicting data have been reported regarding possible long-term survival benefits for patients treated with serial banding ligation as opposed to sclerotherapy.

Trials comparing serial sclerotherapy to beta blockers have shown either no difference or a modest advantage of sclerotherapy with respect to rebleeding and survival. The combination of elective sclerotherapy and beta blockade does not appear to decrease recurrent bleeding or death compared to treatment with beta blockers alone in patients with advanced cirrhosis.

No consistent difference has been reported in rebleeding rate or mortality in secondary prevention studies comparing selective to nonselective surgical shunts, although up to 30% occlusion rates have been described for mesocaval "H" graft procedures. Several studies have corroborated the expected lower prevalence of encephalopathy after selective shunts, although these differences appear to diminish somewhat over time. The major randomized trials comparing serial sclerotherapy to surgical shunts have differed with respect to the percentage of patients with alcohol-related liver disease, proportion of patients in each Childs' class, and the intervals between the index bleed and treatment. Although the frequency of rebleeding has been consistently higher in patients treated with sclerotherapy (requiring surgical rescue in 30% to 40% of patients), survival was either the same or slightly better with endoscopic therapy.

The initial results for gastric variceal sclerotherapy were extremely disappointing, involving frequent rebleeding and ulcerations. Although randomized, blinded trials have not been performed, these results have been improved by using either a combination of paravariceal preceding intravariceal injections of sclerosant or intravariceal injections of butyl cyanoacrylate. In the most enthusiastic reports, combination sclerotherapy has been demonstrated to control bleeding in up to 75% of cases; most reports indicate significantly less success. Recurrent bleeding complicates both strategies in at least 15% to 35% of cases. The use of nonselective beta blockers for prevention of nonesophageal variceal bleeding has not been adequately studied.

The role of transplantation in portal hypertensive patients was addressed in 1988 by Iwatsuki et al., who reported a group of 302 Childs' class C patients with variceal bleeding who underwent transplantation. Ninety-five percent of patients had nonalcoholic cirrhosis. Seventy-three percent of patients had undergone prior sclerotherapy, and 15% had prior surgery for variceal bleeding. One-year survival in this group was 79%, and 5-year actuarial

Table 4-2. Multicenter Clinical Results of TIPS Placement

	Univ. of Penn. ($n = 87$)	Freiburg ($n = 100$)	UCSF ($n = 250$)
A. INDICATIONS			
Bleeding	81 (93%)	100 (100%)	203 (81%)
Acute	45	10	75
Chronic	36	83	130
Ascites	4	NA	31
Preoperative	2	NA	8
B. CLINICAL INFORMATION			
Gender (M/F)	53/34	67/33	161/89
Age			
Mean	53.8	57	51.6
Range	20–84	18–84	5–84
Childs-Pugh class			
A	8%	27%	12%
B	44%	51%	42%
C	48%	22%	46%
C. ETIOLOGY OF LIVER DISEASE			
Alcoholic	49	68	125
Postnecrotic	21	19	51
Cryptogenic	11	9	34
Primary biliary cirrhosis	4	3	9
Budd-Chiari	2	—	5
Other	—	1	24
D. OUTCOME			
Technical success	100%	93%	97%
Dead < 30 days	30%	3%	13%
Dead > 30 days	6.9%	6%	17%
Transplanted	6.9%	NA	20%
E. HEMODYNAMIC RESULTS (mm Hg)			
Portosystemic gradient			
Preshunt	24	21.5	23
Postshunt	11	9.2	10
F. COMPLICATIONS			
Bleeding			
Intra-abdominal	3	6	4
Hemobilia	0	4	2
Fever	23	—	24
Renal failure	—	—	2
Encephalopathy			
New or worse	23%	25%	25%
Uncontrolled	5%	7%	5%

survival was 71%, with a median follow-up of just over 2 years. Clearly, transplantation is impractical as a widespread salvage procedure for uncontrolled variceal hemorrhage. Nevertheless, this report does emphasize that in appropriately selected patients with variceal bleeding and Childs' class C cirrhosis, survival after transplantation is markedly improved compared with that achieved with other therapeutic options.

At present, the long-term efficacy of TIPS in preventing recurrent bleeding is related to maintenance of shunt patency. Shunt stenosis resulting in

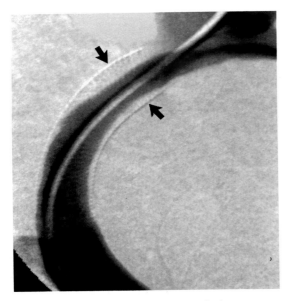

Figure 4-4. Case 3: Follow-up 18-month shunt venography in an asymptomatic 64-year-old male. Magnified view of the TIPS demonstrates a patent shunt with pseudointimal hyperplasia lining the stent (arrows). The appearance is unchanged from that seen 10 months after shunt placement.The portosystemic gradient was 13 mm Hg.

recurrent elevation of portal pressures has been seen in one third to one half of patients at one year after TIPS. This problem is almost exclusively due to excessive pseudointimal proliferation within the shunt lumen or the outflow hepatic vein. This significant rate of early shunt narrowing warrants sonographic, venographic, or endoscopic follow-up every 6 months in all TIPS patients. Once pseudointimal hyperplasia has been shown to stabilize in a given patient, annual studies may be adequate to assess shunt function. In the majority of cases, shunt stenosis or occlusion can be managed in a short outpatient visit by balloon angioplasty or placement of additional metallic stents. Several centers have reported assisted shunt patencies 85% to 92%. Finally, several centers are currently investigating the role of coated stents and other modifications which may blunt the pseudointimal hyperplasia within the shunt and prolong primary shunt patency.

Primary Prophylaxis

Pagliaro and colleagues compiled a meta-analysis to assess the effectiveness of beta blockers and endoscopic sclerotherapy in preventing first bleeding and reducing mortality in patients with cirrhosis and esophageal varices. The incidence of bleeding in trials of beta blockers was significantly reduced (pooled odds ratio, 0.54), particularly in patients with large or medium-sized varices or those with varices and a PSG exceeding 12 mm Hg; however, only a trend toward reduced mortality was detected. The trials examining sclerotherapy for primary prevention have been of variable quality. The favorable results noted in some reports were obtained mainly in early studies of lesser quality. Adequately controlled studies evaluating TIPS or surgical shunts in primary prevention have not been performed. Presently, these options should not be utilized in patients without prior variceal bleeding.

Conclusions

Initial management of acute esophageal variceal hemorrhage should focus upon diagnostic and therapeutic endoscopy. In cases of acute bleeding where patients are intolerant of or have become refractory to sclerotherapy, TIPS placement provides a rapid and reliable nonoperative method of lowering portal pressure and halting bleeding. TIPSs and smallbore or selective surgical shunts both provide viable options in the prevention of recurrent bleeding in patients with esophageal, gastric, or ectopic varices. Large-scale randomized, controlled trials comparing TIPS with endoscopic and surgical intervention are necessary to compare the effects of these treatments upon survival, quality of life, and cost. The promising role of TIPS in treating other complications of portal hypertension such as refractory ascites must also be studied in prospective controlled trials.

The role of portosystemic shunting for primary prophylaxis against variceal hemorrhage is indeterminate. Thus, neither TIPS nor surgical shunts should be applied in this setting. Patients with asymptomatic varices are best managed with drug therapy.

Clearly, management of patients with cirrhosis and variceal hemorrhage remains a complex and demanding endeavor. The multitude of available therapies requires a multidisciplinary collaboration between hepatologists, general and transplant surgeons, and interventional radiologists. The appropriate choice of therapy must be based on the local expertise of the treatment team and their consensus opinion in each individual case.

Selected Readings

Greig JD, Garden OJ, Carter DC. Prophylactic treatment of patients with esophageal varices: Is it ever indicated? *World J Surg* 1994; 18:176–184.

Haskal ZJ, et al. Intestinal varices: Treatment with the transjugular intrahepatic portosystemic shunt. *Radiology* 1994; 191:183–187.

Henderson JM. Role of distal splenorenal shunt for long-term management of variceal bleeding: *World J Surg* 1994; 18:205–210.

Infante-Rivard, C, Esnaola S, Villeneuve JP. Role of endoscopic sclerotherapy in the long-term management of variceal bleeding: A meta analysis. *Gastroenterology* 1989; 96:1594–1600.

Iwatsuki S, et al. Liver transplantation in the treatment of bleeding esophageal varices. *Surgery* 1988; 104: 697–705.

LaBerge JM, et al. Creation of transjugular intrahepatic portosystemic shunt (TIPS) with the Wallstent endoprosthesis: results in 100 patients. *Radiology* 1993; 187:413–420.

Pagliaro L, et al. Prevention of first bleeding in cirrhosis. A meta-analysis of randomized trials of nonsurgical treatment. *Ann Intern Med* 1992; 117:59–70.

Rodriguez-Perez F, Groszmann RJ. Pharmacologic treatment of portal hypertension. *Gastroenterol Clin North Am* 1992; 21:15–39.

Rossle M, et al. The transjugular intrahepatic portosystemic stent-shunt procedure for variceal bleeding. *N Engl J Med* 1994; 330:165–171.

Rypins EB, Sarfeh IJ. Small-diameter portacaval H-graft for variceal hemorrhage. *Surg Clin North Am* 1990; 70:395–404.

5

Primary Biliary Cirrhosis

Marshall M. Kaplan
Richard J. Rohrer

Primary biliary cirrhosis (PBC), a chronic, progressive, liver disease that occurs predominantly in middle-aged women, is characterized by the destruction and subsequent disappearance of small intralobular bile ducts. The gradual decrease in the number of intrahepatic bile ducts leads to worsening cholestasis, portal inflammation, and scarring, and eventually to cirrhosis and liver failure.

Etiology and Pathogenesis

Although the etiology of PBC is still unknown, most data suggest that it is due to some inherited abnormality of immunoregulation. The precise nature of the defect is unknown. Likewise, it is unclear whether all who inherit this presumed abnormality are destined to develop PBC or whether an additional factor, such as a triggering event, is also required in genetically susceptible individuals. Numerous abnormalities of humoral and cell-mediated immunity occur in PBC. Increased serum levels of IgM are found in most patients, and most have high titers of various autoantibodies. These include antinuclear antibodies antimitochondrial antibodies, antithyroid antibodies, antiacetylcholine-receptor antibodies, and antiplatelet antibodies. An association exists between PBC and other autoimmune diseases, such as autoimmune thyroiditis, rheumatoid arthritis, and scleroderma. In one study, 84% of PBC patients had one other "autoimmune" disease, and 41% had two or more. The complement system is in a chronically activated state via the classical pathway in PBC, and complement turnover is increased.

Antimitochondrial antibody (AMA) is detected in 90% to 95% of patients with PBC. The major autoantibody found in PBC patients has been called anti-M2. This antibody is directed principally against the dihydrolipoamide acetyltransferase component (E2) and branched ketoacid dehydrogenase-E2 of the pyruvate dehydrogenase complex on the inner mitochondrial membrane. The relationship between the antimitochondrial antibodies and immunologic bile duct injury is not clear, since the M2 antigen is not tissue-specific, and its intracellular location should reduce its immunogenicity. However, a recent report demonstrates that a molecule that shares some antigenic determinants with the E2 subunit of pyruvate dehydrogenase is expressed on the luminal surface of biliary epithelial cells from PBC patients but not in primary sclerosing cholangitis patients or control subjects. Expression of this autoantigen on the luminal surface of biliary epithelial cells might lead to antibody-mediated attack by IgA antibodies, the antibody present in bile. On the other hand, repeated studies have shown that there is no correlation between the presence or titer of AMA and the severity or course of PBC.

Cellular immunity is also disordered in PBC. The immunologic injury to bile ducts in PBC appears to be mediated by activated T cells. A recent study has shown that the E2 antigens stimulate interleukin-2 production by cloned T cells isolated from liver tissue in PBC patients. The predominant cell type found in portal areas of the liver in late-stage PBC is the CD3$^+$, CD4$^+$, and CD8$^-$. CD8$^+$ cells appear to be the predominant cell type directly attacking the bile ductular cells. These lymphocytes express class II human leukocyte antigens (HLAs) and interleukin-2 receptors and produce tumor necrosis factor and interferon gamma, cytokines that can cause bile duct injury. Bile ductular cells in PBC demonstrate increased expression of class I major histocompatibility complex (MHC) antigens, HLA-A, HLA-B, and HLA-C. In addition, bile duct cells in PBC patients also express certain class II HLAs that are not expressed in normal persons, such as DR, DP, and DQ. That PBC is histologically similar to hepatic graft-versus-host disease and liver allograft rejection, two disorders mediated by activated T cells, also suggest an immunologic T-lymphocyte–mediated process.

In addition to immunologic destruction of small bile ducts, secondary damage to hepatocytes occurs in PBC from the accumulation in the hepatic lobule of toxic concentrations of bile acids such as taurocholate and chenodeoxycholate (Fig. 5-1). Some histologic features of PBC, such as "foamy degeneration" of hepatocytes, may be attributed to the noxious effects of bile acids. Cholestasis, per se, causes increased expression of Class I HLAs on hepatocytes and renders them better targets for an immunologically mediated attack. Treatment with ursodeoxycholic acid (UDCA) reduces expression of class I HLAs by hepatocytes, in addition to mitigating the toxicity of naturally occurring bile acids such as cholic acid and chenodeoxycholic acid.

Diagnosis

Clinically, primary biliary cirrhosis mimics extrahepatic bile duct obstruction. Now that PBC is diagnosed at early stages, approximately 50% of patients are asymptomatic at the time of diagnosis. They are recognized because of abnormal blood tests or, less often, because of physical findings such as unexplained hepatomegaly or splenomegaly. This form of presentation is a distinct difference from earlier experience, in which most patients were symptomatic (Tables 5-1, 5-2). The most common initial symptoms are fatigue and itching. Many patients note darkening of the skin due to the increased deposition of melanin. Jaundice is usually a later symptom. Other manifestations of PBC include osteoporosis with bone pain and spontaneous fractures of vertebrae and ribs, hypercholesterolemia with xanthomas and xanthelasmas, and an increased in-

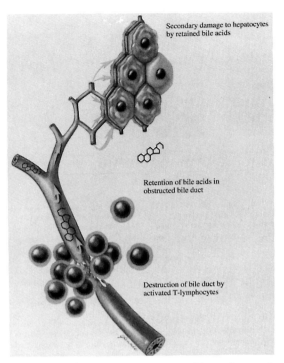

Figure 5-1. Schematic representation of the pathogenesis of primary biliary cirrhosis. A small bile duct is surrounded by T lymphocytes. Secretion into bile of subtances such as bile acids is blocked because of bile duct damage and obliteration, and these substances accumulate in and around hepatocytes. This situation causes a secondary injury to hepatocytes. (From Kaplan MM, Primary biliary cirrhosis. *Resid Staff Physician*, 1993; 39:65. Used with permission.)

cidence of other autoimmune disorders such as sicca syndrome, hypothyroidism, the CREST syndrome, and arthritis.

The diagnosis of primary biliary cirrhosis should be considered in all patients with unexplained cholestatic liver disease so that appropriate diagnostic tests can be done and unnecessary invasive tests and/or surgery can be avoided. The diagnosis is based on characteristic liver function tests: that is, greatly elevated serum alkaline phosphatase and gamma glutamyl transpeptidase levels and only moderately elevated serum aminotransferase levels, usually less than 300 IU. Ninety-five percent of patients with primary biliary cirrhosis will have a positive antimitochondrial antibody test. Most will have elevations of serum IgM. It is essential that mechanical bile duct obstruction be excluded.

Table 5-1. Symptoms of Primary Biliary Cirrhosis at Presentation[a]

Symptom	% Affected, Yale[b] (1955–1979)	% Affected, Mayo[c] (1974–1984)	% Affected, Combined[d] (1955–1984)
None	13	17[e]	16[f]
Pruritus	58	70	64
Fatigue, malaise	24	73	50
Dark urine	NS[g]	44	44
Light-colored stool	NS	34	34
Jaundice	23	41	32
Weight loss	13	27	20
Abdominal pain	12	21	17
Bone pain	NS	15	15
Gastrointestinal hemorrhage	1	9	5
Fever	NS	3	3

[a]Symptoms at time of diagnosis or referral in 592 patients with primary biliary cirrhosis. Data compiled from 280 patients at Yale and 312 patients at Mayo Clinic. At Mayo Clinic 424 patients were used to calculate the percentage of asymtomatic patients.
[b]Data from Roll J, et al. The prognostic importance of clinical and histological features in asymptomatic and symptomatic primary biliary cirrhosis. *N Engl J Med* 1983; 308:1.
[c]Data from Dickson ER, Fleming CR, Ludwig J. Primary biliary cirrhosis. In Popper H, Schaffner F (eds), *Progress in Liver Diseases,* vol. 6. New York, Grune & Stratton, 1978. P. 487. By permission.
[d]Reprinted by permission of the publisher from Diminished survival in asymptomatic primary biliary cirrhosis. A prospective study, by Balasubramaniam K, et al, *Gastroenterology,* vol. 98, p. 1567. Copyright 1990 by the American Gastroenterological Association.
[e]n = 424.
[f]n = 704.
[g]NS = not stated.

Table 5-2. Physical Findings in Patients with Primary Biliary Cirrhosis at Presentation[a]

Physical Finding	% Affected, Yale[b] (1955–1979)	% Affected, Mayo[c] (1974–1984)	% Affected, Combined[d] (1955–1984)
Hepatomegaly	70	51	60
Jaundice	52	41	46
Hyperpigmentation	37	53	45
Splenomegaly	43	28	35
Spider nevi	NS[e]	29	29
Excoriations	NS	27	27
Xanthelasmas, xanthomas	28	18	22
Esophageal varices	NS	14	14
Edema	NS	12	12
Clubbing	NS	4	4

[a]Physical findings in 592 patients with primary biliary cirrhosis at time of diagnosis or referral. Data compiled from same patients as in Table 5-1.
[b]Data from Roll J, et al. The prognostic importance of clinical and histological features in asymptomatic and symptomatic primary biliary cirrhosis. *N Engl J Med* 1983; 308:1.
[c]Data from Dickson ER, Fleming CR, Ludwig J. Primary biliary cirrhosis. In Popper H, Schaffner F (eds), *Progress in Liver Diseases,* vol. 6. New York, Grune & Stratton, 1978. P. 487. By permission.
[d]Reprinted by permission of the publisher from Diminished survival in asymptomatic primary biliary cirrhosis: A prospective study, by Balasubramaniam K, et al, *Gastroenterology,* vol. 98, p. 1567. Copyright 1990 by the American Gastroenterological Association.
[e]NS = not stated.

Techniques such as ultrasound and CT imaging are adequate except in patients with negative antimitochondrial antibody tests. Endoscopic cholangiography should be done in this group to rule out primary sclerosing cholangitis or other disorders. Diagnosis should be confirmed by percutaneous liver biopsy. The biopsy will also allow histologic staging and aid in prognosis.

Histologically, PBC has been divided into four stages. In stage I, there are so-called florid bile duct lesions, characterized by the infiltration and destruction of small bile ducts by mononuclear cells, predominantly T lymphocytes (Fig. 5-2). Stage II is characterized by ongoing bile duct destruction, the absence of bile ducts in some portal triads, and atypical bile duct proliferations in others (Fig. 5-3). The inflammation extends beyond the portal triads. In stage III, there is more extensive fibrosis and linkage of adjacent portal triads by bands of scar tissue. Stage IV is characterized by cirrhosis. These patients are often distinguishable from those with other types of cirrhosis by a striking diminution in the number of bile ducts seen.

Management

The treatment of primary biliary cirrhosis has three goals: (1) management of the symptoms and complications that result from chronic cholestasis; (2) suppression or reversal of the underlying pathogenetic process, destruction of small intralobular hepatic bile ducts; and (3) assessment of the severity of PBC in order to optimize the timing of liver transplantation. Currently, no proven medical treatment for PBC clearly prevents the slow progression to liver failure. Although several drugs look promising in patients with histologically early disease, patients with cirrhosis, portal hypertension, and serum bilirubin levels chronically above 3 mg/dl almost all have medically untreatable disease. They will ultimately require liver transplantation. Thus

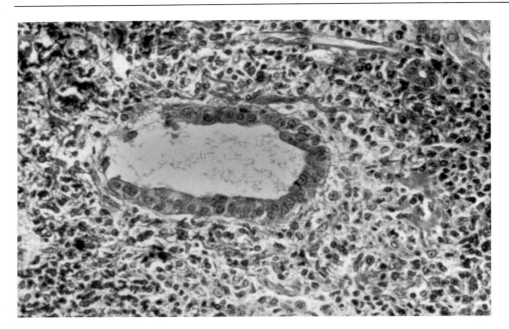

Figure 5-2. Florid bile duct lesion in PBC. A bile duct is surrounded by lymphocytes. Some bile duct cells are vacuolated, and epithelial cells have been dislodged from one quadrant of a bile duct (Masson trichrome, ×310).

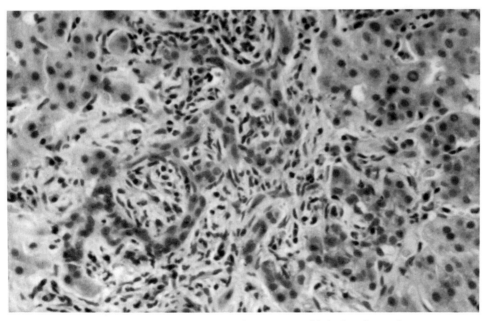

Figure 5-3. Stage II lesion in primary biliary cirrhosis. Atypical bile duct hyperplasia is present. Bile ducts are tortuous, and few are cut in cross section. The inflammatory cell infiltrate is primarily lymphocytes with occasional neutrophils (H & E, ×310).

management is directed at symptoms, such as pruritis, and complications, such as bone disease.

Pruritus

The earliest and most disconcerting symptom in primary biliary cirrhosis is pruritus. The itching is worse at bedtime and may cause insomnia and extensive excoriations because of the overwhelming urge to scratch. The pruritus is caused by the inability of the liver to excrete certain substances into bile. These presumably accumulate in the skin and produce the itching. The pruritogenic substance is not known but binds to cholestyramine, a nonabsorbed quaternary ammonium resin. Cholestyramine taken orally will relieve the itching of primary biliary cirrhosis as long as there is adequate bile flow: that is, stools are not acholic (clay-colored). The usual dosage of cholestyramine is 4 g tid, taken just before or with meals. Cholestyramine takes 2 to 4 days to relieve itching from the time it is started. If itching fails to respond to the usual dose of cholestyramine within 4 days, the dose should be increased in 4-g increments up to 24 g/d. Doses above 24 g/d are rarely more effective, although doses as high as 36 g/d have been tolerated. However, some patients have difficulty taking cholestyramine because of its taste and consistency. Its palatability can be improved by mixing it with fruit juice or applesauce, or by pureeing it with fruits in a food processor.

Cholestyramine may cause severe constipation. This problem can be treated with laxatives or bulking agents. Many drugs will bind to cholestyramine and be poorly absorbed. Hence, medications should be taken as far apart from the cholestyramine as possible, at least 2 hours before or after cholestyramine is taken. Blood levels of fat-soluble vitamins A, D, E, and K should be periodically monitored or replacement therapy given, since patients requiring cholestyramine may malabsorb fat-soluble vitamins. Cholestyramine usage has also been associated with folic acid deficiency. Concomitant treatment with folic acid, 1 mg/d, is recommended, or serum folate should be monitored. For patients who cannot tolerate cholestyramine, colestipol hydrochloride, another nonabsorbed anion exchange resin, may be used. This agent is as effective as cholestyramine

and has the same side effects. The starting dose is 5 mg tid orally.

Rarely, the pruritus in primary biliary cirrhosis will not respond to cholestyramine. In such instances, large-volume plasmapheresis may be effective. Unfortunately, plasmapheresis is expensive and impractical if used chronically. Its beneficial effects usually last for 2 to 4 weeks, at which time the plasmapheresis must be repeated. Antihistamines and other related anti-itch medicines are rarely effective as treatment for severe pruritus but may help in mild pruritus if given before bedtime. Recent data suggest that the itching in some patients may be related to stimulation of opioid receptors within the brain. Such patients have responded to the short-term administration of opioid antagonists such as naloxone.

A number of patients with pruritus note that their itching worsens if they eat rich, fatty meals. Conversely, some have reported that their itching improves if they eat a low-fat diet. Diet treatment has not been critically evaluated but is innocuous. If these measures fail to relieve the itching, rifampin may be tried. The dose is 150 mg PO bid if the serum bilirubin is greater than 3 mg/dl and 150 mg tid, if the serum bilirubin level is lower. If all of these fail, there are anecdotal reports of patients whose itching has responded to phototherapy with UVB light, methyl testosterone, corticosteroids, and cimetidine.

Malabsorption

Some patients with primary biliary cirrhosis who are clinically jaundiced have steatorrhea, which may cause diarrhea, including troublesome nocturnal diarrhea. The steatorrhea is due primarily to inadequate concentrations of bile acids within the small intestinal lumen, below the critical micellar concentration. Patients with concomitant sicca syndrome may also have pancreatic insufficiency. This problem may be treated with replacement pancreatic extract. Symptomatic steatorrhea can be partially corrected by restricting dietary fat. Medium-chain triglyceride (MCT) may be added if caloric supplementation is required to maintain body weight. Each milliliter of MCT oil contains 7.5 calories. Most patients can tolerate 60 ml/d without difficulty. The MCT oil may either be taken directly by the teaspoon or be used in cooking as a substitute for shortening and salad oil.

Patients with primary biliary cirrhosis may malabsorb the fat-soluble vitamins A, D, and K (Figs. 5-4, 5-5). Deficiencies of vitamin E are uncommon except in patients with advanced disease awaiting liver transplantation. Vitamin A deficiency occurs in approximately 30% of patients but is rarely symptomatic. It is as practical to prevent vitamin A deficiency with dietary supplements of vitamin A, 15,000 U/d (three times the recommended daily allowance), as it is to measure serum levels on a regular basis. Vitamin K deficiency rarely occurs in primary biliary cirrhosis unless the patient takes cholestyramine on a regular basis and is deeply jaundiced. The prothrombin time is normal in most patients until late in the course of disease, when there are signs of liver failure. Vitamin K rarely has to be given except to these patients.

Bone Disease

Osteopenia with spontaneous bone fractures is a serious problem that occurs in approximately 20% of patients with primary biliary cirrhosis. The metabolic bone disease most commonly associated with primary biliary cirrhosis is osteoporosis, not osteomalacia. Osteomalacia occurs rarely and only in patients with far-advanced disease. The osteoporosis is manifested by bone pain and spontaneous fractures, usually of the vertebral bodies and ribs. Neither the cause nor the treatment of the osteoporosis is known. Patients with primary biliary cirrhosis may have low serum levels of 25-hydroxy vitamin D, but serum levels of the most active vitamin D metabolite, 1,25(OH)$_2$ vitamin D, are normal.

The following treatment regimen is suggested, more in the belief that it will not hurt and may have placebo effect than in the conviction that it will stabilize or reverse the bone loss. First, oral calcium supplements may be given, 1.0 to 1.5 g calcium/d. The safety of calcium can be easily monitored by measuring serum calcium levels and 24-hour urinary calcium excretion. Twenty-four-hour urinary calcium excretion should be less than 200 mg/d. Because of the low serum levels of 25-hydroxy vitamin D, supplementation with low doses of vitamin D, 50,000 U biw, or 25-hydroxy vitamin D$_3$, 20 mcg/d, may be given. The goal is to maintain the serum 25-hydroxy vitamin D level in the high or normal range. Treatment with 25-hydroxy vitamin D will correct or prevent the osteomalacia that occurs in patients with advanced disease. No information is available about the efficacy or safety of medications used to treat postmenopausal osteoporosis, such as calcitonin, etidronate, or sodium fluoride. They are best not used. Only liver transplantation has been shown to improve the osteoporosis seen in PBC. Bone thinning actually worsens for up to 6 months after transplantation because of physical inactivity and corticosteroids but then improves, even on low-dose corticosteroids.

Xanthomas

Less than 10% of patients with primary biliary cirrhosis develop xanthomas. Planar xanthomas may

Figure 5-4. Serum vitamin A levels in 52 patients with primary biliary cirrhosis. Serum levels are normal in patients with stages I and II disease (hatched area). Many are low in patients with stages III and IV disease. (Reprinted by permission of the publisher from Fat soluble vitamin nutriture in primary biliary cirrhosis, by Kaplan MM, et al, *Gastroenterology*, vol. 95, p. 787. Copyright 1988 by the American Gastroenterological Association.)

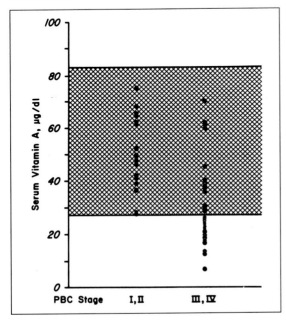

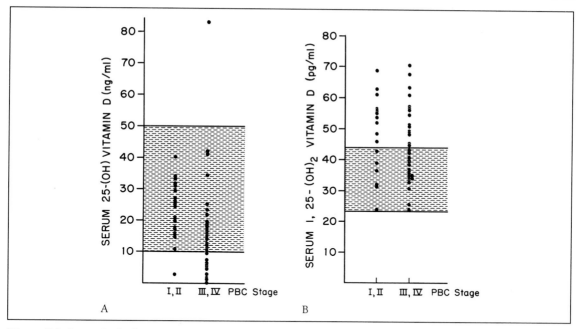

Figure 5-5. Serum 25-hydroxy vitamin D (A) and 1,25-dihydroxy vitamin D (B) levels in patients with primary biliary cirrhosis. The hatched area indicates the normal range. (Reprinted by permission of the publisher from Fat soluble vitamin nurture in primary biliary cirrhosis, by Kaplan MM, et al, *Gastroenterology,* vol. 95, p. 787. Copyright 1988 by the American Gastroenterological Association.)

occur on the palms of the hands, become painful, and interfere with manual dexterity. Xanthomas on the soles of the feet may also cause pain and make walking difficult. If xanthomas become truly symptomatic, they can be treated with large-volume plasmapheresis done at 1- to 2-week intervals. The goal is to remove cholesterol from the body. Each plasmapheresis will lower the serum cholesterol level by approximately 50%. Once the serum cholesterol level approaches normal, xanthomas will gradually resolve.

Anemia

Iron deficiency anemia may occur in primary biliary cirrhosis, often in patients without obviously advanced disease. A thorough search for a site of gastrointestinal blood loss should be done, even in the absence of overt GI blood loss. Some patients may have unexpectedly severe portal hypertension. Chronic intermittent blood loss from congestive gastropathy or esophageal varices is a possible

cause. If treatment with oral iron is not adequate, the usual modalities to treat bleeding from portal hypertension should be considered: beta blockers, endoscopic ligation of varices, and transjugular intrahepatic portosystemic stent shunt (TIPS), in that order.

Autoimmune Disorders

Other autoimmune disorders, such as Sjögren's syndrome and the CREST syndrome, may occur in patients with primary biliary cirrhosis. Treatment is symptomatic. More importantly, as many as 25% of primary biliary cirrhosis patients may be (or become) hypothyroid. Routine tests for thyroid function, such as the total T_4 or free T_4 index, may be misleading, because these patients have increased serum concentrations of thyroid-binding globulin. Hypothyroidism is best evaluated by measuring the thyroid-stimulating hormone (TSH). Hypothyroid biliary cirrhosis patients respond normally to replacement thyroid hormone.

Liver Failure and Portal Hypertension

Patients with advanced primary biliary cirrhosis develop symptoms of liver failure, such as ascites and bleeding esophageal varices, similar to patients with other types of liver disease. Liver transplantation is the treatment of choice in patients with impending liver failure and in those who have bled from esophageal varices and have cirrhosis or jaundice. They should all be referred to a liver transplant surgeon to prepare for liver transplantation. The treatment of hemorrhage from portal hypertension is similar to that in patients with other types of cirrhosis and is typically a temporizing action until liver transplantation can be done. Most patients with large varices, whether or not they have bled, should be placed on a nonspecific beta-adrenergic blocker such as propranolol in a dose that lowers the resting pulse by 25%. Large varices are best ablated with endoscopic banding therapy. Sclerotherapy is reserved for the unusual patient in whom banding cannot be done. If bleeding recurs despite the above treatment, transjugular intrahepatic portosystemic stent shunts (TIPSs) should be placed. TIPS has largely replaced the distal splenorenal shunt in PBC patients.

Results

The management of patients with primary biliary cirrhosis is rapidly changing, for two reasons. First, colchicine and ursodiol have been shown to combine efficacy and safety. Methotrexate may be even more effective, but its toxicity in PBC limits its use to clinical trials, Second, agreement how exists that primary biliary cirrhosis is a progressive disease in virtually all patients. PBC eventually becomes irreversible, usually at the time that cirrhosis develops. The risk-benefit ratio of drugs such as colchicine and ursodiol is clearly better than that of no treatment and awaiting liver failure with the need for liver transplantation. In addition to undergoing the risk of major surgery, patients who survive liver transplantation face a lifetime of treatment with cyclosporine, corticosteroids, azathioprine, and antihypertensive agents. Because specific therapy is a rapidly evolving and still controversial area, relevant clinical data will be reviewed.

Ineffective or Toxic Drugs

Drugs used to treat many autoimmune diseases have been disappointing. Results of controlled trials of D-penicillamine, corticosteroids, chlorambucil, azathioprine, and cyclosporine have been disappointing. These drugs will not be discussed further. They are rarely, if ever, used to treat PBC currently, except in clinical trials.

Promising Drugs

COLCHICINE

The authors and others have studied the effects of colchicine, 0.6 mg bid, versus placebo in primary biliary cirrhosis during the past 14 years. Colchicine-treated patients had small but significant improvement in levels of serum albumin, bilirubin, alkaline phosphatase, aminotransferases, and cholesterol after 2 years compared to those on placebo (Fig. 5-6). Of greater importance, colchicine decreased the risk of dying of liver failure (Fig. 5-7). Four years after entry, the cumulative mortality from liver disease in the authors' study was 21% in colchicine-treated patients and 47% in patients taking placebo. However, no improvement was noted in the histologic progression of the disease, nor were symptoms or physical findings benefited (see Fig. 5-6). Little toxicity was observed, but 10% of patients developed diarrhea which disappeared when the dose was lowered to 0.6 mg every day. Two other studies have similar but less significant results. With meta-analysis, colchicine significantly decreased the risk of dying of liver failure. Current data suggest that colchicine may slow the progression of primary biliary cirrhosis but does not stop it. Colchicine is safe, inexpensive, and well tolerated.

URSODIOL

The results of four studies employing ursodiol, 10 to 15 mg/kg/d, are even more encouraging. Ursodiol produced striking reductions in serum alkaline phosphatase, gamma-glutamyl transpeptidase, alanine aminotransferase, and aspartate aminotransferase, and stabilization of serum bilirubin (Fig. 5-8). Histologic improvement was less impressive. These studies were short-term, up to 2 years. Ursodiol also lessened the need for cholestyramine in some patients with pruritus and decreased manifes-

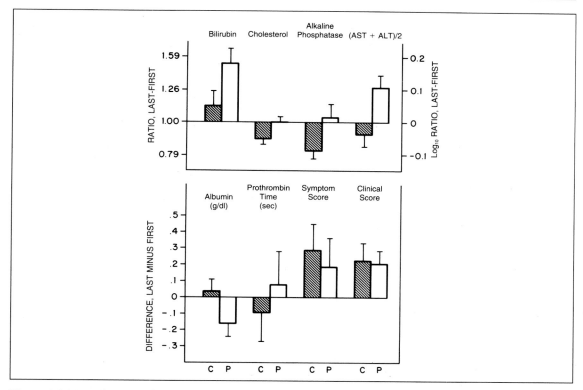

Figure 5-6. Mean changes in biochemical tests and clinical evaluations during a 2-year period after entry among patients receiving colchicine (C, hatched bars) or placebo (P). Top panel: geometric mean relative changes in serum bilirubin, cholesterol, alkaline phosphatase, and aminotransferase. (Relative change is ratio of last observed value to initial value.) Lower panel: arithmetic mean changes in serum albumin, prothrombin time, symptom score, and clinical score. (Change is difference between last observed value and initial value.) (From Kaplan MM, et al. A prospective trial of colchicine for primary biliary cirrhosis. *N Engl J Med* 1986; 315:1448–1454. Reprinted by permission of the *New England Journal of Medicine*.)

tations of autoimmunity. Little toxicity, other than diarrhea, has been reported. Preliminary results of two of these multicenter studies have recently been reported after 4 years of follow-up. The biochemical improvement noted at 2 years has been sustained for 4 years. Of greater importance, referral for liver transplantation was significantly decreased in patients treated with ursodiol (Fig. 5-9).

These results suggest that ursodiol is safe and may be effective in slowing the rate of progression. Preliminary data suggest that even larger doses of ursodiol, 15 to 17 mg/kg body weight/d, may increase efficacy. Of note, most of the beneficial biochemical effects of ursodiol occur within 2 to 3 months of initiating therapy. However, efficacy is usually lost after 2 years in patients with advanced disease, those with cirrhosis and jaundice.

METHOTREXATE

The authors have recently reported their experience with low-dose oral pulse methotrexate in 14 patients with precirrhotic primary biliary cirrhosis and are currently conducting a prospective, double-blind trial of methotrexate versus colchicine. The dose of methotrexate is 15 mg/week PO, given as 5 mg q12h for three doses each week. In the open-label trial, a striking improvement in biochemical tests was observed in response to methotrexate. In addition, debilitating fatigue and itching disappeared in symptomatic patients. There was also an

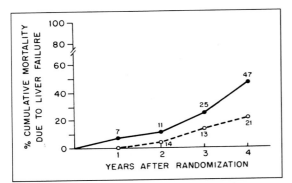

Figure 5-7. Cumulative mortality due to liver failure of patients assigned colchicine (dashed line) or placebo (solid line) during 4-year period after entry. Patients assigned placebo at entry crossed over to colchicine treatment at 2 years. At 4 years cumulative mortality among colchicine-treated patients was significantly lower than among patients who received placebo during the first 2 years of study ($P = 0.05$, one-tailed test; $P = 0.10$, two-tailed test). (From Kaplan MM, et al. A prospective trial of colchicine for primary biliary cirrhosis. *N Engl J Med* 1986; 315:1448–1454. Reprinted by permission of the *New England Journal of Medicine*.)

encouraging improvement in liver histology, much less inflammation after 1 and 2 years of methotrexate, and an apparent decrease in fibrosis in several patients treated for 2 years or longer. Of note, most patients had a striking but transient increase in aminotransferase levels, up to fivefold elevations, 1 to 8 months after beginning methotrexate. Aminotransferase levels then improved in all of these patients and became normal in some. Paradoxically, a transient increase of aminotransferase levels appears to be a marker for an ultimately good response to methotrexate. No hepatotoxicity has been seen.

However, with methotrexate therapy bone marrow suppression and particularly allergic pneumonitis are potential risks that must be watched for. A reversible but worrisome interstitial pneumonitis is more common in PBC than in other diseases and limits its use to controlled trials in which patients are closely monitored. In contrast to the ursodiol response, which occurs within 2 to 3 months of initiating therapy, the response to methotrexate occurs slowly and is often not obvious until 6 to 10 months after starting methotrexate. A sustained biochemical and histological improvement then appears and continues for many years. Patients with advanced primary biliary cirrhosis, i.e., those with

cirrhosis and jaundice and/or portal hypertension, do not respond to methotrexate, nor to any drug studied so far. These patients should be referred for liver transplantation.

Liver Transplantation

At present, successful medical treatment of PBC is defined in terms of temporization rather than outright cure, implying that progression to end-stage liver disease will be universal in the majority of patients who live long enough (Fig. 5-10). Provided no contraindications are present, most such patients, particularly those who already have histologic stage III or IV at time of diagnosis will therefore require liver transplantation, since no other remedy for entrenched liver failure exists. Fortunately, enough intrinsic uniformity in advancing PBC is available to allow a measure of predictability not enjoyed by most other causes of end-stage liver disease. It would be appropriate to allude briefly to ultimate transplant options in a conversation at the time histologically advanced PBC is diagnosed; but for the vast majority of patients, actual transplant evaluation should await the development of worrisome trends in symptoms, signs, or laboratory data.

Mild fatigue is often related more to psychosocial factors than to liver disease and, by itself, need not trigger major concern. Progressive debilitating fatigue in patients with stage III and IV disease which cannot be ascribed to any other cause should, however, prompt a transplant inquiry, even in the face of relatively preserved synthetic function. Muscle wasting, fluid retention, bone disease (occasionally severe), and infection may follow; since liver donors are everywhere in short supply and "seniority" is a significant factor in organ distribution schemes, early registration on a transplant list is desirable. This fact is particularly so for small-stature women, since finding a size-matched donor may be difficult. When the serum bilirubin level has worsened past 6 mg/dl (100 µmol/liter), 2-year survival is very unlikely, and 1-year survival with transplantation already exceeds that expected with maximal medical therapy (Fig. 5-11). Varying degrees of difficulty controlling ascites, hypoalbuminemia, and prolongation of the prothrombin time worsen the picture. By the time any degree of func-

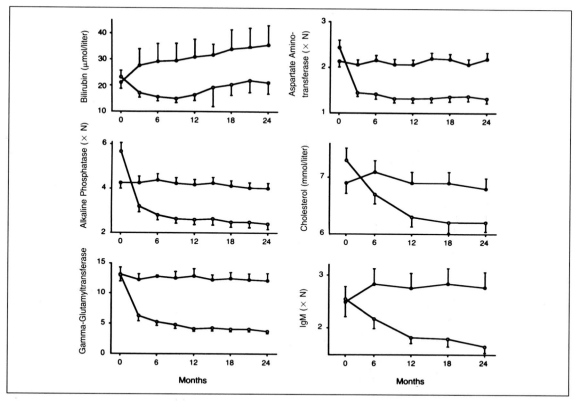

Figure 5-8. Mean (±SEM) changes in serum bilirubin, alanine aminotransferase (ALT), and alkaline phosphatase levels. Open circles indicate values in the ursodiol group, and closed circles indicate values in the placebo group. (From RE Poupon et al. A multicenter controlled trial of ursodiol for the treatment of primary biliary cirrhosis. N Engl J Med 1991; 324:1548. Reprinted by permission of the New England Journal of Medicine.)

Figure 5-9. Probability of responding to treatment with ursodiol (solid line) or placebo (dashed line). Kaplan-Meier estimates were used. The rates of treatment failure in the two groups were significantly different ($P < 0.01$ by Cox regression model). (From RE Poupon et al. A multicenter controlled trial of ursodiol for the treatment of primary biliary cirrhosis. N Engl J Med 1991; 324:1548. Reprinted by permission of the New England Journal of Medicine.)

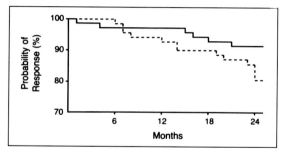

tional debility is present despite optimal medical attention, all PBC patients should have been evaluated by a liver transplant team.

Variceal hemorrhage is not uncommon. Although it may be severe, variceal hemorrhage generally responds well to medical measures and aggressive sclerotherapy or banding. Rebleeding is less common than when cirrhosis is due to alcoholic liver disease or chronic active hepatitis, and progression in hemorrhage from portal gastropathy is unusual. Recourse to transjugular intrahepatic portosystemic shunting (TIPS) for control of hemorrhage is less necessary than in these other types of cirrhosis. For the rare patient with recurrent hemorrhage who is otherwise asymptomatic and has preserved hepatic synthetic function, surgical shunting may be appropriate and afford years of

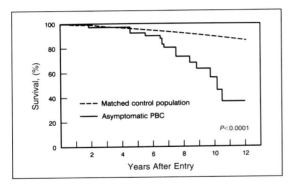

Figure 5-10. Survival (Kaplan-Meier estimate) of 73 asymptomatic primary biliary cirrhosis patients (solid line) and age-, sex-, and race-matched controls (dashed line). Asymptomatic primary biliary cirrhosis patients had a fourfold increase in the mortality rate (P < 0.001). (Reprinted by permission of the publisher from Diminished survival in asymptomatic primary biliary cirrhosis: A prospective study, by Balasubramaniam K, et al, *Gastroenterology*, vol. 98, p. 1567. Copyright 1990 by the American Gastroenterological Association.)

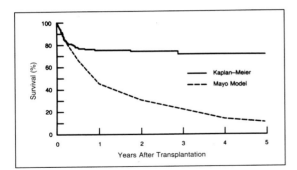

Figure 5-11. Actual (Kaplan-Meier) survival after transplantation in 161 patients with primary biliary cirrhosis and estimated survival without transplantation as predicted by a survival model (stimulated control). (From Markus BH, et al. Efficacy of liver transplantation in patients with primary biliary cirrhosis. *N Engl J Med* 1989; 320:1709. Reprinted by permission of the *New England Journal of Medicine*.)

good-quality life. The distal splenorenal shunt is preferred, but if this is anatomically inappropriate, a mesocaval shunt can be used in order to spare the portal vein. Encephalopathy usually occurs rather late in the course of PBC. Malignant transformation of either hepatocytes or biliary epithelial cells is rare.

Patients with PBC have traditionally fared better than other adults undergoing liver transplantation. In the United States, the PBC population now accounts for 8% of liver transplants performed annually. The lead time afforded by relatively early diagnosis and slow progression of disease allow for better pretransplant medical management than with many other causes of end-stage liver disease. Paradoxically, improved medical therapy may soon push back typical age at transplantation from the 50s to the 60s and may worsen outcome due to the intercurrent development of other medical conditions. A hard, enlarged native liver and bulky peripheral adenopathy may be nuisances, but the surgery is usually technically unremarkable. Posttransplant management is the same as for any other patient. Immunosuppression generally consists of cyclosporine or tacrolimus and low-dose corticosteroids with or without azathioprine. Recurrent disease in the first decade after transplant, if it occurs at all, must be very uncommon. In this circumstance most practitioners suspect that maintenance immunosuppression is preventative. One- and five-year survival after transplantation are typically 10% better than for other adults undergoing transplantation, with figures approaching 90% and 75%, respectively, being reported by selective centers. Though immunosuppression is lifelong, the quality of posttransplant life is quite uniformly good, as measured by both objective and subjective standards.

Conclusions

Virtually all patients with primary biliary cirrhosis have a progressive and potentially serious disease. If one waits too long to treat, patients may develop cirrhosis and irreversible disease. Hence, all patients without clinically advanced disease should be treated. Ideally, each should be enrolled in a prospective, randomized treatment trial. However, this possibility is not practical for most patients with primary biliary cirrhosis. For those patients not enrolled in randomized trials, treatment should be initiated with ursodiol cholic acid, 14 to 17 mg/kg body weight/d. If all liver function tests return to normal after 4 months of therapy, the drug should be maintained. If after 4 months liver function tests are improved but not normal, or are not improved, colchicine, 0.6 mg bid, should be added. Each drug acts differently and the efficacy of both drugs may be additive. A percutaneous liver biopsy should be performed 12 to 18 months after starting treatment. If there is no worsening of histology, the same treatment should be continued indefinitely, and liver biopsies should be done every 2 to 3 years. If there is definite histologic worsening on ursodiol and colchicine, methotrexate might be added.

Methotrexate may be more effective treatment than either ursodiol acid or colchicine. However, methotrexate is more toxic. Patients must be warned about the risk of pneumonitis and instructed to call a physician if there is any hint of this complication: namely, unexplained fever, cough, or dyspnea. If methotrexate is to be used outside a treatment trial, a percutaneous liver biopsy should be done at baseline and after 1 and 2 years of treatment. A complete blood count and platelet count should be done monthly, and biochemical tests of liver function should be done every 2 months. Patients should be seen every 2 months.

The next several years should see more results of treatment trials in primary biliary cirrhosis. The hope is that there will be effective treatment for early, precirrhotic PBC. However, it is unlikely that patients who are jaundiced or who have cirrhosis or any manifestation of portal hypertension will respond to medical treatment. These patients should be referred for liver transplantation evaluation.

Selected Readings

Balasubramaniam K, et al. Diminished survival in asymptomatic primary biliary cirrhosis: A prospective study. *Gastroenterology* 1990; 98:1567–1571.

Dickson ER, et al. Prognosis in primary biliary cirrhosis: Model for decision making. *Hepatology* 1989; 10:1–7.

Gershwin ME, Mackay IR. Primary biliary cirrhosis: Paradigm or paradox for autoimmunity? *Gastroenterology* 1991; 100:822–833.

Kaplan MM. Primary biliary cirrhosis. *N Engl J Med* 1987; 316:521–528.

Kaplan MM, et al. A prospective trial of colchicine for primary biliary cirrhosis. *N Engl J Med* 1986; 315:1448–1454.

Kaplan MM, Knox TA. Treatment of primary biliary cirrhosis with low-dose weekly methotrexate. *Gastroenterology* 1991; 101:1332–1338.

Kaplan MM, et al. Fat soluble vitamin nutriture in primary biliary cirrhosis. *Gastroenterology* 1988; 95:787–792.

Lombard M, et al. Cyclosporin A in primary biliary cirrhosis: Results of a long-term placebo controlled trial and effect on survival. *Gastroenterology* 1990; 104:519–526.

Markus BH, et al. Efficacy of liver transplantation in patients with primary biliary cirrhosis. *N Engl J Med* 1989; 320:1709–1713.

Poupon RE, et al. A multicenter controlled trial of ursodiol for the treatment of primary biliary cirrhosis. *N Engl J Med* 1991; 324:1548–1554.

6

Budd-Chiari Syndrome

ANDREW S. KLEIN
ANNA MAE DIEHL
SCOTT J. SAVADER

Etiology and Pathogenesis

The Budd-Chiari syndrome (BCS) is a rare, often fatal disease which results from hepatic venous outflow obstruction. Two anatomically distinct forms of the BCS are recognized: (1) membranous occlusion of the suprahepatic inferior vena cava (IVC) and (2) thrombosis of the major hepatic veins. IVC occlusion due to membranous webs, the most common form worldwide, is most prevalent in Eastern countries and is unusual in the United States except in regions with a large population of Asian descent. The remainder of this chapter will focus primarily upon the thrombotic form of the BCS. Despite recent diagnostic advances, the etiology of the thrombotic process is uncertain in approximately one third of patients. In the remainder, hepatic vein thrombosis is the consequence of hypercoagulability induced by certain hematologic conditions, hyperestrogenic states, locally invasive malignancies, perihepatic infections, or abdominal trauma (Table 6-1).

Clinical Features

Patients with the BCS develop progressive ascites, abdominal discomfort, and variable biochemical evidence of liver dysfunction. Typically, symptoms prompt medical evaluation within weeks of hepatic vein thrombosis. However, in some patients florid clinical features of portal hypertension and hepatic parenchymal failure develop over only a few days.

Profound encephalopathy and jaundice consistent with fulminant hepatic failure may result. In a small number of patients, the course is much more protracted, and the clinical picture is reminiscent of the gradual deterioration that occurs with other causes of cirrhosis. The chronic form of the BCS may only be correctly diagnosed at the time of anatomic imaging during an evaluation for liver transplantation.

The clinical and histopathological features of the BCS reflect the consequences of obstructed hepatic venous flow (Tables 6-2, 6-3). Hepatic vein obstruction produces congestion of blood within the terminal hepatic venules and hepatic sinusoids, as well as the clinical finding of hepatomegaly. Abdominal tenderness is most likely related to acute hepatic capsular distention, compounded by the generalized abdominal distention which accompanies the rapid accumulation of ascites. Congestion also increases sinusoidal pressure, which in turn compromises portal venous perfusion of the liver. Splenic venous drainage is subsequently impeded, resulting in secondary splenic engorgement and splenomegaly. Since portal venous perfusion supplies the bulk of nutrients to the liver, hepatocyte viability may be compromised. Indeed, zone 3 hepatocytes which are most distant from the portal venous inflow may suffer necrosis. Consequent reductions in the functioning hepatocyte mass are manifest by hepatic synthetic and excretory dysfunction, leading to jaundice. Chronic increases in sinusoidal pressure eventually cause generalized hepatocyte atrophy and fibrosis.

Table 6-1. Conditions Associated
with Hepatic Vein Thrombosis

Condition	Prevalence (%)
Idiopathic	25–30
Hematologic disorders	20–30
Polycythemia rubra vera	
Paroxysmal nocturnal hemoglobinuria	
Myeloproliferative disorders	
Tumors	10
Hepatocellular carcinoma	
Renal cell carcinoma	
Adrenal carcinoma	
Other	
Infections	10
Amebic abscess	
Aspergillosis	
Hydatid cysts	
Oral contraceptives	10
Pregnancy	10
Trauma	2

Source: Modified from Mitchell MC, et al. Budd-Chiari syndrome:
etiology, diagnosis and management. *Medicine* 1982; 61:199.

Table 6-2. Clinical Features of
the Budd-Chiari Syndrome

Signs	Prevalence (%)
Ascites	80–90
Hepatomegaly	75–80
Splenomegaly	40–50
Right upper quadrant tenderness	40–50
Jaundice	< 50
Variceal bleeding	Rare, late event
Hepatic encephalopathy	Rare, late event

Table 6-3. Histologic Features of
the Budd-Chiari Syndrome

Congestion in terminal hepatic veins and hepatic sinusoids
Zone 3 hepatocyte necrosis
Fibrosis, particularly in zone 3

Increased sinusoidal pressure also triggers compensatory renal mechanisms which attempt to restore hepatocyte perfusion by restricting renal sodium excretion to increase plasma volume. Unfortunately, the expanded plasma volume only exacerbates sinusoidal pressure elevations, and fluid is forced out of the vascular compartment and into hepatic interstitial spaces. Increased interstitial fluid prompts compensatory increases in lymphatic flow. However, eventually the ability of the lymphatic system to return this fluid to the intravascular compartment is overwhelmed, and ascites begins to form.

Meanwhile, collateral vessels begin to open within the splanchnic bed in an effort to decompress the engorged hepatic sinusoids. These collateral vessels provide a low-resistance pathway for blood flow, and portal venous shunting begins. Increased pressure in portosystemic collaterals can result in variceal hemorrhage and contributes to the development of hepatic encephalopathy. Expansion of the vascular bed and losses of intravascular fluid into the ascitic compartment eventually jeopardize perfusion of other vital organs. This situation, in turn, triggers hormonal and autonomic reflexes to maintain blood flow to these tissues, but at the price of heightened renal salt and water retention. The latter, of course, only exacerbates ascites formation.

Diagnosis

The BCS should be suspected in patients with sudden onset of ascites, especially if they have associated conditions which increase the risk of hepatic vein thrombosis (see Table 6-1). Important initial diagnostic tests include blood cell counts and chemistries and an evaluation of the ascitic fluid. Elevations in the hematocrit and/or platelet count suggest underlying myeloproliferative disorders, which are associated with hepatic vein thrombosis in at least one third of patients. Typically, the serum bilirubin level is only mildly elevated. Liver enzymes are usually slightly increased but may be dramatically elevated in patients with abrupt total obstruction of hepatic venous outflow. Hypertransaminemia may be overshadowed by alkaline phosphatase elevations in patients with chronic hepatic vein obstruction and long-standing hepatic congestion. High ascitic fluid protein concentrations (> 3 g/dl) are suggestive of BCS, but are documented in only a minority of patients. Hypoalbuminemia reflects the substantial protein loss into ascitic fluid and should not be misinterpreted as an indication of synthetic dysfunction.

Ultimately, the diagnosis of the BCS rests on demonstration of hepatic vein obstruction. Initial evaluation of patients with suspected BCS is usually noninvasive in nature. A nuclear medicine liver-spleen scan may be performed with technetium Tc 99m sulphur colloid. Early in the disease, the study may be normal or demonstrate only minimal hepatocyte dysfunction. An abnormal scan will show an enlarged liver with inhomogeneous up-take. As the disease progresses, the right and left lobe congestion increases and function decreases, with a subsequent increase in the size and activity of the caudate lobe. The caudate lobe "hot spot" is explained by the independent venous drainage into the inferior vena cava (IVC), which is typically spared from thrombotic occlusion even when the three main hepatic veins are involved. Unfortunately, this classic appearance is seen in only 17% of patients. Single-photon-emission computerized tomography (SPECT) is a process in which axial, sagittal, or coronal images are obtained during a liver-spleen scan utilizing computer reconstruction. This technique can in some cases provide enhanced functional detail, which may improve the overall sensitivity of nuclear medicine imaging.

Many authors have reported that color flow and duplex-Doppler ultrasound provide an accurate means of diagnosing the BCS. Sonographically the hepatic veins may demonstrate thickening, stenoses, irregularities, obstruction, and intrahepatic collateralization. The IVC may be narrowed, may be shifted to the right secondary to caudate lobe hypertrophy, or may demonstrate intraluminal thrombus. Color flow duplex ultrasound may be used to evaluate flow characteristics and direction. In the Budd-Chiari patient, blood flow signals may be absent, reversed, turbulent, or contiguous. Some of the limitations of sonography include the inability to consistently image webs, underestimation of thrombus or tumor extent, overlying bowel gas artifacts, and the operator dependency in determination of Doppler blood flow analysis. Advantages include its noninvasive nature, multiplanar imaging capabilities, availability, and relatively low cost.

Magnetic resonance imaging (MRI) has proven to be valuable in the evaluation of patients with suspected BCS due to its ability to detect blood flow and provide multiplanar imaging of the abdomen and liver. MRI can depict the hepatomegaly, inhomogeneous liver enhancement (particularly on T_2-weighted images), varices, and ascites typically seen in this group of patients. The asymmetric compression of the IVC common to the Budd-Chiari syndrome is also clearly visualized, as is the extrahepatic splanchnic venous circulation.

The classic computerized tomographic findings of the Budd-Chiari syndrome include hepatomegaly and ascites. On a contrast-enhanced image, two important additional findings are noted: (1) a patchy inhomogeneous contrast enhancement pattern of the liver with a central fan-shaped area of greatest enhancement decreasing toward the periphery, and (2) nonvisualization of the hepatic veins. IVC compression by an enlarged caudate lobe and gastroesophageal and splenic hilar varices may be seen.

The noninvasive studies are most helpful in confirming the diagnosis of the Budd-Chiari syndrome when the findings from multiple modalities are combined. Nonetheless, despite advances in noninvasive imaging, hepatic venography is still the gold standard for the diagnosis of the Budd-Chiari syndrome. During venographic evaluation, inferior venacavography should initially be performed. The inferior venacavogram classically shows the intrahepatic IVC to be "pointed" or to have a "steeple"-shaped configuration (Fig. 6-1A). Complete occlusion with retroperitoneal collaterals may be seen. Sixty-five percent of patients with the BCS are found to have significant compression or total occlusion of their IVC. Right atrial and IVC pressures (infrahepatic, intrahepatic, and suprahepatic levels) should be obtained to further evaluate and assess objectively the degree of caval compression. This information is vital in selecting the most appropriate form of therapy for each patient.

Following venacavography, a transjugular or basilic vein cannulation is performed in an attempt to image the hepatic veins directly. Angiography may demonstrate thrombus in the hepatic vein(s) with occlusion in the most acute phase of the disease or the more typical "spider web" appearance of partially recanalized and collateralized vessels in the chronic phase (Fig. 6-1B). If the hepatic veins cannot be selectively catheterized, a percutaneous transhepatic injection into the liver with a 22-gauge Chiba needle will demonstrate the spider web collateral venous pattern.

Liver biopsy results are helpful in guiding the management of patients with the BCS. By distin-

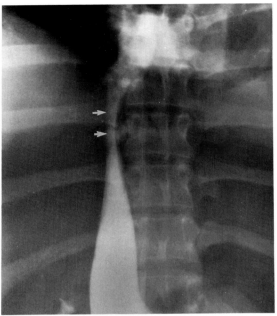
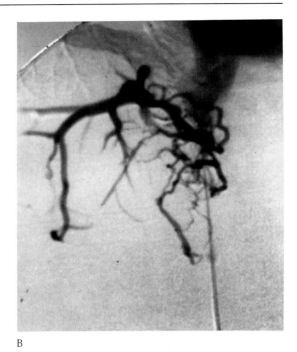

A   B

Figure 6-1. A 33-year-old female who developed the BCS 4 months postpartum. A. Classic "steeple"-shaped suprarenal IVC (arrows) secondary to caudate lobe hypertrophy. B. "Spider web" appearance of the hepatic veins, which occurs secondary to collateralization and recanalization. (From Society of Cardiovascular and Intentional Radiology Videodisc II, Portal Hypertension. Used with permission.)

guishing patients with predominant liver congestion and necrosis from others who have progressed to a more advanced stage of established fibrosis/cirrhosis, histology identifies subgroups likely to benefit from portal decompressive procedures and liver transplantation, respectively. Biopsy findings also distinguish liver congestion that results from obstruction of the large hepatic veins (e.g., Budd-Chiari syndrome) from that which follows obliteration of the terminal hepatic venules in veno-occlusive disease. When severe coagulopathy or massive ascites jeopardizes the safety of percutaneous liver biopsy, tissue can be obtained via a transjugular approach.

Management and Results

Medical

Optimal treatment of hepatic vein thrombosis requires surgical or invasive radiologic intervention.

Spontaneous resolution of the thrombotic form of the BCS has occurred but is a rare event. Nonetheless, medical management of patients with BCS should not be neglected. Patients with associated myeloproliferative disorders require therapy for those conditions. Phlebotomy often is necessary to normalize the hematocrit in patients with polycythemia rubra vera. Patients with essential thrombocytosis may benefit from treatment with hydroxyurea. Oral contraceptives and other synthetic estrogens should be discontinued. When hepatic vein thrombosis results from perihepatic infection, aggressive antibiotic therapy is crucial. Although there is little evidence that anticoagulant therapy can dissolve established thrombi, patients with documented hypercoagulability are typically treated with systemic anticoagulant therapy to minimize the risk of de novo thrombosis. Diuretic therapy is usually necessary to control ascites accumulation, but may need to be supplemented with large-volume paracentesis. Hepatic encephalopathy is treated with lactulose and, if necessary, dietary protein restriction.

A number of case reports have appeared in the literature in which thrombolytic therapy utilizing either urokinase or streptokinase has been used to treat the IVC thrombosis which can occur as a primary or secondary event in patients with the BCS. Multi-side-hole infusion catheters can be placed from a common femoral venous approach, either unilaterally or bilaterally, for direct infusion of the thrombolytic agent into the caval thrombus. At the authors' institution, three patients have been effectively treated with IVC thrombosis, all of whom presented with severe lower extremity edema rather than the BCS. The principle, however, is the same. Direct infusion of the thrombolytic agent into the clot is preferable to systemic intravenous administration, in which the activity and concentration of the agent is reduced substantially during first passage through the liver. For direct infusion, the authors recommend a loading dose of 240,000 to 360,000 IU urokinase followed by 100,000 to 260,000 IU/hr for 55 to 96 hours. If, for some reason, systemic delivery is preferred, urokinase (4400 IU/kg loading dose followed by 4400 IU/kg/hr) or streptokinase (250,000 IU loading dose over 30 minutes followed by 100,000 IU/hr) may be given for a duration of 72 to 96 hours.

When hepatic vein thrombosis occurs, the clot typically extends out to the fifth-order hepatic vein radicals and into the hepatic venules. Thus, even if the major hepatic veins can be catheterized, which is uncommon, effective delivery of the agent to the entire hepatic venous system is unlikely, not to mention that the normal direction of blood flow in the hepatic veins is counterproductive to successful thrombolysis at all levels. In addition to the risk of hemorrhage, pulmonary embolism has been reported with venous thrombolysis. Critics of thrombolytic therapy argue that in most cases of the BCS diagnosed in the United States, the hepatic veins are clotted; thus attempts at thrombolysis are generally ineffective and only result in delayed institution of appropriate therapy.

No reports have been published describing successful hepatic vein thrombolysis with intra-arterial delivery of urokinase or streptokinase via the hepatic artery. In addition to the immediate loss of some of the agent due to first-pass metabolism within the liver, alterations in venous outflow most likely result in a shunting of the agent away from the clotted vessels within the liver.

Surgical

Surgical therapy for the BCS falls into one of four general categories: (1) excision or ablation of the obstructing lesion, (2) peritoneovenous shunt, (3) portosystemic shunt, or (4) orthotopic liver transplantation (OLT). For patients with membranous occlusion of the vena cava, it may be possible to excise or surgically dilate the caval web, or to perform cavoplasty or venoplasty. However, thrombotic occlusion of the hepatic vein(s) is not correctable by a direct surgical approach such as this. Since a minority of patients in this country suffer from the membranous form of the BCS, these methods are used infrequently. Peritoneovenous shunts (LeVeen or Denver shunts) also have a very limited role in the management of the BCS. Although the insertion of these devices may temporarily palliate the patient's ascites, the unrelieved hepatic congestion and portal hypertension invariably progresses with the development of hepatic cirrhosis and end-stage liver failure. Transient symptomatic improvement may accompany the placement of a peritoneovenous shunt, which should be reserved for high-risk patients who are not candidates for more definitive therapy. If necessary, these devices can be inserted using local anesthetics and intravenous sedation.

PORTOSYSTEMIC SHUNTS

The most frequently used form of therapy for the BCS is portosystemic shunting. A variety of portosystemic shunt operations have been designed to convert the portal vein from an inflow vessel to an outflow vessel, thus decompressing the congested liver. Relief of the elevated sinusoidal pressure eliminates the pathophysiologic state thought to be responsible for the hepatic deterioration which inevitably develops in untreated patients. Success of portosystemic shunting is limited by the inability of these procedures to reverse established cirrhosis. A preoperative liver biopsy is essential in determining the presence of cirrhosis, which is a relative contraindication for a shunt and an indication for liver transplantation.

Although there is general agreement that portosystemic shunting is the treatment of choice for most noncirrhotic patients with the BCS, considerable debate exists regarding which shunt procedure is best. Orloff has championed the use of portacaval shunts, which in his reported experience are associated with excellent long-term patency and patient survival (85% at 3–16 years). Others who have attempted to construct portacaval shunts in patients with the BCS have been less enthusiastic. The caudate lobe hypertrophy which usually accompanies the BCS has been found to render this particular shunt operation difficult or occasionally impossible. The authors prefer to use the superior mesenteric vein (SMV) for access to the portal venous circulation. For patients with no evidence of IVC obstruction, a mesocaval "C" shunt is preferred. A 14- to 16-mm Dacron tube graft is sewn end to side to the infrarenal IVC. The graft is navigated in a gentle C-shaped curve to the SMV where this vessel passes over the third portion of the duodenum and behind the neck of the pancreas. At this location the SMV is usually more than 1 cm in diameter and of sufficient caliber to construct a widely patent end-to-side anastomosis with the Dacron graft.

In the presence of significant IVC obstruction (as evidenced by a reduction in IVC diameter by more than 75% or a pressure gradient between the right atrium and infrahepatic IVC which exceeds 20 mm Hg) splanchnic blood must be diverted directly into the right atrium by a mesoatrial shunt. For the mesoatrial shunt, a 16-mm ring-reinforced polytetrafluoroethylene (PTFE) prosthesis is sewn end to side to the SMV in a fashion similar to that used for the mesocaval shunt. The graft is then passed into the lesser sac, over the liver, substernally into the mediastinum, and finally into the right chest. The pericardium is opened, and the graft is then sewn to the side of the right atrium. To prevent extrinsic compression, the long (60-cm) prosthesis is supported by a noncompressible silicone rubber sleeve at the level of the sternum.

Both the mesocaval and mesoatrial shunts can be performed well away from the congested liver and porta hepatis, which does not then become a reoperative field if liver transplantation should be required at some point in the future. The 5-year survival rate for patients undergoing mesocaval or mesoatrial shunts is 75% to 85%.

LIVER TRANSPLANTATION

Orthotopic liver transplantation (OLT) is a well-accepted form of therapy for selected cases of end-stage liver failure. Initial enthusiasm for the use of total liver replacement to treat BCS patients was tempered with concerns over recurrence of disease in the transplanted liver. The potential for patients with hypercoagulable disorders to experience other vascular thrombotic events after transplantation was realized in several Budd-Chiari patients who developed portal vein and/or hepatic artery occlusion in the early postoperative period. Anticoagulation, instituted within 24 to 48 hours of the transplant, was found to substantially reduce the risk of arterial or venous thrombosis. Patients are initially heparinized to a target APTT of 1.5 to 2.0 times control. Long-term anticoagulation is maintained with daily sodium warfarin (Coumadin) titrated to a prothrombin time of 1.5 to 1.8 times control. Alternatively, antithrombotic regimens employing hydroxyurea (500–2000 mg/d titrated to a platelet count of 100,000–200,000) and aspirin (325 mg/d) have been suggested by one group as equally effective in preventing clot formation in the transplanted organ, and do not subject the patient to the risk of the hemorrhagic complications which accompany long-term anticoagulation. Using lifelong anticoagulation or antithrombotic medication, transplant centers in both the United States and Europe have recently reported 3-year survival rates of 76% to 88% among patients transplanted for the BCS. Perhaps more important than patient survival statistics is the finding that rehabilitation and quality of life following OLT for the BCS are generally excellent.

Radiological

Interventional radiological procedures have a role both as primary therapy for the BCS and as an adjunct to surgically constructed portosystemic shunts.

PRIMARY THERAPY

Percutaneous transluminal angioplasty (PTA) can be utilized for the treatment of the Budd-Chiari syndrome in the following settings: (1) focal stenosis of the hepatic vein(s) or IVC due to either a congenital or postinflammatory web(s); (2) segmental stenosis of the intrahepatic segment of the IVC; and (3) occlusion of the suprahepatic segment of the IVC. PTA is ideally suited for treating focal stenoses, and the high success rate can obviate the need for more invasive surgery. In cases of recurrent stenosis, obstruction, or web(s), PTA can be repeated on a per-need basis with minimal risk and short-term hospitalization, and without precluding future use of other therapies such as thrombolysis, vascular stenting, portosystemic shunting, or liver transplantation.

PTA for hepatic vein or IVC stenosis is performed in an analogous fashion to that used for peripheral PTA. For an IVC stenosis, techniques are used to place one or more guidewires across the obstruction and into the right atrium or superior vena cava. Balloon catheters, appropriately chosen after proper sizing from a cut film inferior venacavogram, are passed over the guidewire(s) and positioned across the obstruction. The balloon(s) are inflated until the waist resolves and are kept inflated for 60 to 120 seconds.

If the obstruction is located within a hepatic vein or at the hepatic vein–IVC confluence, balloon dilatation can be performed from a transfemoral approach (Fig. 6-2). However, the anatomy of these lesions is often such that a transjugular approach will provide better access to the lesion. Stenoses or obstruction involving the hepatic veins is treated as described for the IVC. Following completion of an angioplasty procedure, anticoagulation with heparin should be continued for a minimum of 24 hours, and conversion to sodium warfarin or aspirin and dipyridamole is recommended for a minimum of 3 months to allow for adequate healing of the angioplasty site with minimal risk of postprocedure thrombosis. In summarizing multiple small series of patients with the BCS treated with PTA alone, a total of 15 patients underwent a mean of 1.5 dilatations per patient during a period ranging from 6 to 37 months. The mean patency rate following PTA was 12 months.

PTA of the IVC or hepatic veins, although proven to be extremely beneficial in providing at least short-term (12-month) patency of treated stenoses and obstructions, will often require repeated procedures because of restenosis. The stenoses and obstructions commonly seen in patients with the Budd-Chiari syndrome tend to be extremely fibrotic

in nature, with a significant degree of elastic recoil. Percutaneously placed intraluminal vascular stents are designed to maintain luminal patency across a persistent or recurrent region of vascular stenosis following balloon dilatation. In addition, stents may be used for lesions which are extremely difficult or impossible to approach surgically. Vascular stents can be used in both the hepatic vein and the IVC; however, proper and adequate sizing of the stents is necessary to prevent embolization to the heart or pulmonary circulation. In addition, the stents must not extend superiorly from the hepatic vein or IVC into the right atrium, or inferiorly into the infrahepatic IVC, or they can interfere with surgical removal of the liver if OLT is required. These stents typically undergo incorporation into the wall of the vessel secondary to neointima formation.

Budd-Chiari patients may not only present with IVC narrowing as the primary etiology of their disease, but may also develop this problem as a secondary complication of congestive hepatomegaly. Although adequate flow across the area of narrowing is usually sufficient to prevent IVC thrombosis, this situation may not always be the case. In addition, if there is greater than 75% luminal narrowing or the right-atrial–IVC pressure gradient is greater than 20 mm Hg, the flow across the obstruction will be insufficient to maintain patency of a mesocaval shunt (Fig. 6-3). In these situations, placement of intravascular stents within the intrahepatic IVC to support luminal patency will not only prevent IVC thrombosis but will allow for selection of a mesocaval shunt in place of the more extensive mesoatrial shunt.

Creation of a transjugular intrahepatic portosystemic shunt (TIPS) has been used to treat a small number of patients with the BCS in the United States and Japan. TIPS has been shown to effectively reduce postsinusoidal portal hypertension in patients with the BCS. Although early reports are encouraging, additional studies are necessary to evaluate the risk-benefit ratio and long-term patency rates in this particular group of patients.

SECONDARY INTERVENTION

The most common technical complication of portosystemic shunting is stricture formation at the surgical anastomosis. This problem has been reported in

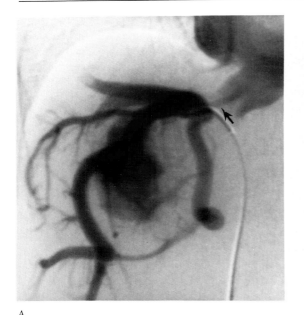

A

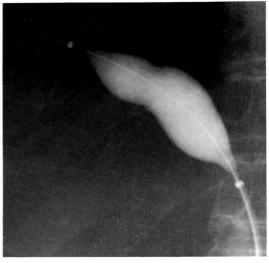

B

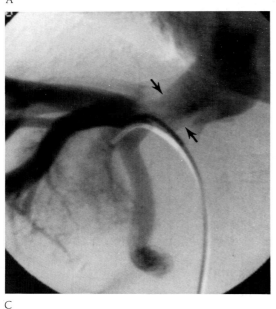

C

Figure 6-2. A 70-year-old female with the BCS secondary to stenosis of the hepatic vein confluence. A. Pre-PTA hepatic venogram demonstrates an extremely tight stenosis (arrow) at the confluence of the hepatic veins, with a 20-mm Hg gradient. B. The hepatic vein confluence is dilated with a 20-mm × 4-cm balloon catheter. C. Following PTA, the confluence appears significantly improved (arrows) and the gradient is reduced to 2 mm Hg post-PTA. (From Society of Cardiovascular and Intentional Radiology, Videodisc II, Portal Hypertension. Used with permission.)

up to 44% of shunted patients despite the relatively large diameter (14–16 mm) of the Dacron or PTFE grafts used to construct the shunt. As the stricture increases in severity, a progressive decrease in flow through the graft occurs. Patients experience weight gain, increasing abdominal girth, and pain second-ary to reaccumulation of ascites and hepatomegaly. Some evidence suggests that incomplete decompression of the liver (i.e., patent shunt but elevated portal venous pressure) is associated with persistent hepatic injury, resulting in fibrosis and cirrhosis. Eventually, shunt thrombosis, the end result and

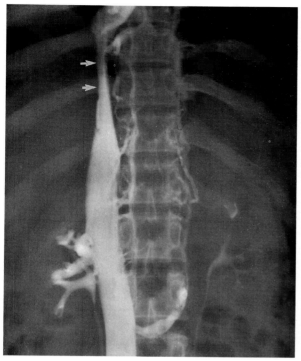
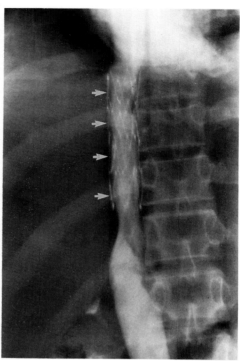

A   B

Figure 6-3. A 28-year-old female with the BCS secondary to polycythemia rubra vera. A. High-grade stenosis of the intrahepatic portion of the IVC (arrows) with an 18-mm Hg gradient noted 17 months after PTA of the shunt anastomosis. B. Following failure of PTA to significantly reduce the gradient, four modified Rosch-Z stents (arrows) were placed within the IVC to prevent mesocaval shunt thrombosis. The gradient was subsequently reduced to 1 mm Hg.

most devastating complication of anastomotic stricturing, can occur.

The authors have noted that a rather fragile relationship exists between the pressure gradient across the shunt anastomosis and the development of symptoms, which is quite variable from patient to patient. Small pressure gradients (< 10 mm Hg) across the shunt anastomosis in some patients can result in significant symptomatology with return of abdominal pain and ascites. Thus, any gradient greater than 3 mm Hg in the symptomatic patient should be treated if no other etiology for shunt malfunction or patient symptomatology can be determined. Angioplasty of a strictured shunt or surgical anastomosis can be performed in the standard fashion. Minor improvements in the pressure gradient have been shown to result in dramatic clinical improvement, obviating the need for surgical intervention (Fig. 6-4). For patients who do require repeat PTA procedures, or for those in whom the initial PTA yields poor results due to the elasticity of the lesion, vascular stents may be used to protect and maintain patency across the treated region.

Thrombosed shunts may be treated with urokinase or streptokinase in order to re-establish patency (Fig. 6-5). Placement of an infusion catheter or catheters directly into the shunt as distal as possible is recommended to expose the thrombus to the maximum amount of thrombolytic agent. Creation of a channel through the thrombus with the catheter and guidewire, and subsequent direct infiltration of the clot with 250,000 to 500,000 units of urokinase, may promote a complete and rapid result.

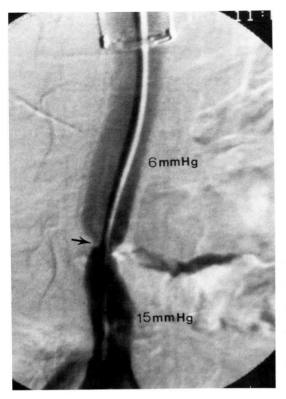

A

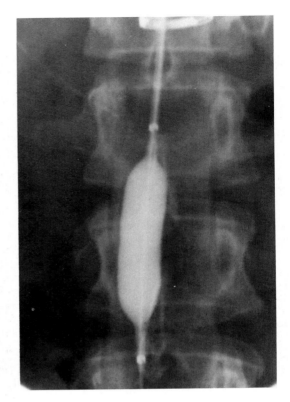

B

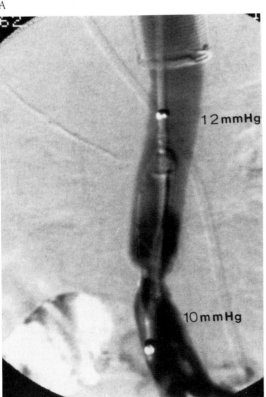

C

Figure 6-4. A 48-year-old female status post mesoatrial shunt for the BCS. A. Mesoatrial shunt evaluation following representation with symptoms demonstrated a stenosis (arrow) at the shunt–superior mesenteric vein anastomosis with a 9-mm Hg gradient. B. The stricture was dilated with an 18-mm × 3-cm balloon catheter. C. Following dilatation, the stenosis did not appear significantly changed; however, the gradient was reduced to 2 mm Hg. The patient's symptoms subsequently resolved.

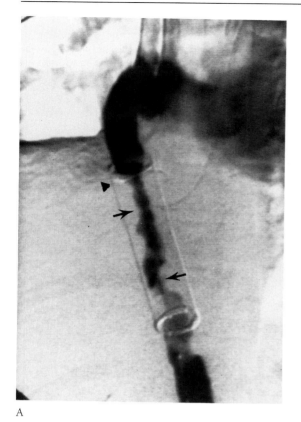

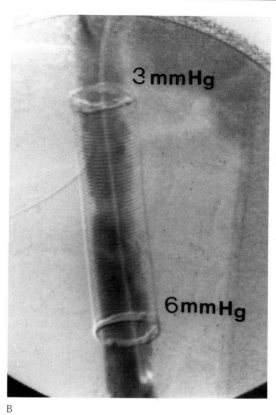

A

B

Figure 6-5. A 19-year-old female with the BCS secondary to oral contraceptives. A. The mesoatrial shuntogram demonstrates significant narrowing of the lumen (arrows), primarily within the substernal support tube (arrow heads) of the shunt. B. Following 36 hours of urokinase therapy, there was marked improvement in the intraluminal appearance of the shunt. The gradient across the support tube was reduced to 3 mm Hg. (From Savader SJ, et al. Percutaneous intervention in portosystemic shunts in Budd-Chiari syndrome. *JVIR* 1991; 2:489–495. Used with permission.)

Conclusions

The BCS should be suspected in patients who present with a rapid onset of ascites and abdominal discomfort, especially in the setting of a known hypercoagulable disorder. Screening for hepatic vein occlusion is best accomplished initially with MRI. If the hepatic veins appear patent by MRI, a second noninvasive procedure such as color flow Doppler imaging should be performed to confirm this observation. However, hepatic venography supplemented by inferior cavography and hemodynamic pressure measurements remains the gold standard for establishing a diagnosis of the BCS. The liver biopsy then provides essential information for therapeutic planning. The presence of fibrosis or cirrhosis is a contraindication to surgical or radiological decompressive procedures and should alert the clinician to consider OLT as definitive therapy for the BCS. The noncirrhotic patient is best served by initial attempts at portosystemic decompression. Until long-term follow-up is available for the recently introduced TIPS procedure, surgically constructed portosystemic shunts (mesocaval or mesoatrial) should be considered the procedures of choice. Nonetheless, interventional radiologic procedures—PTA, thrombolytic therapy, and insertion of intravascular stents—play a crucial role in the primary and secondary therapy of the Budd-Chiari syndrome.

In light of the excellent results anticipated after OLT, some have suggested that liver replacement should be the procedure of choice for *most* patients with the BCS. The authors would recommend a more selective approach because of (1) the unpredictable availability of donor organs, (2) the ever-widening gap between the number of patients awaiting transplantation and the number of organ donors, (3) the need for and consequences of life-long immunosuppression therapy after OLT, and (4) the substantial difference in cost between OLT and standard surgical or radiological treatment. In addition to histologic findings of fibrosis or cirrhosis, indications for OLT in Budd-Chiari patients include fulminant hepatic failure and anatomic contraindications to shunting (i.e., portal vein thrombosis with SMV patency), or as salvage for patients with failed surgical shunts. Implementation of a multimodality therapeutic approach should result in an excellent prognosis for the majority of patients with the Budd-Chiari syndrome.

Selected Readings

Bismuth H, Sherlock DJ. Portosystemic shunting versus liver transplantation for the Budd-Chiari syndrome. *Ann Surg* 1991; 214(5):581–589.

Klein AS, et al. Current management of the Budd-Chiari syndrome. *Ann Surg* 1990; 212(2):144–149.

Orloff MJ, Girard B. Long term results of treatment of Budd-Chiari syndrome by side to side portocaval shunt. *Surg Gynecol Obstet* 1989; 168:33–41.

Peltzer MY, et al. Treatment of Budd-Chiari syndrome with a transjugular intrahepatic portosystemic shunt. *JVIR* 1993; 4:363–367.

Savader SJ, et al. Percutaneous intervention in portosystemic shunts in Budd-Chiari syndrome. *JVIR* 1991; 2:489–495.

Shaked A, et al. Portosystemic shunt versus orthotopic liver transplantation for the Budd-Chiari syndrome. *Surg Gynecol Obstet* 1992; 174(6):453–459.

Wang Z, et al. Recognition and management of Budd-Chiari syndrome: Report of one hundred cases. *J Vasc Surg* 1989; 10(2):149–156.

7

Noninflammatory Cysts

FLORENCIA G. QUE
GREGORY J. GORES
TIMOTHY J. WELCH
DAVID M. NAGORNEY

Cystic lesions of the liver are encountered commonly in clinical practice as a result of the advent of modern imaging techniques. The vast majority of these lesions are asymptomatic simple cysts. Most simple cysts can be diagnosed reliably on the basis of radiographic imaging features and do not require therapeutic intervention. Occasionally, symptoms may be associated with liver cysts. When symptomatic, patients with cystic lesions usually present with abdominal pain or an abdominal mass. The clinician must determine whether symptoms are related to the cyst and, if so, which intervention is preferable. Indeed, the treatment of liver cysts depends on the type of cyst and the presentation. This chapter describes the etiology, pathology, diagnosis, and management of noninflammatory cystic lesions of the liver, emphasizing a team approach by gastroenterologists, radiologists, and surgeons.

Cystic lesions of the liver can be broadly divided into four groups: congenital, inflammatory, neoplastic, and traumatic. Congenital cysts of the liver are most common and include simple cysts and polycystic liver disease (PLD). Inflammatory cysts are discussed in Chapter 8. Primary cystic neoplastic lesions are the rare cystadenomas and the rarer cystadenocarcinomas. Traumatic cysts arise from an injury to the liver which causes either a subcapsular hematoma or a transected biliary duct.

Congenital Cysts

Congenital cysts of the liver are dilatations of the biliary tree which are lined with biliary epithelium. Simple cysts usually lack continuity with the biliary ductal system. Patients with symptoms associated with these cysts can present in a variety of ways. The treatment, which should be determined by the presentation and imaging studies, includes percutaneous aspiration, percutaneous sclerotherapy, cyst fenestration, combined liver resection and cyst fenestration, and liver transplantation.

Etiology and Pathogenesis

Simple cysts and PLD reputedly arise from an aberration of the normal development of the intrahepatic bile ducts. Around the third week of fetal development, the hepatobiliary system arises from a solid proximal endodermal anlage that gives rise to the hepatocytes and small intralobar ductal cells. The distal anlage is the origin of the gallbladder and the main biliary ductal cells. Moschowitz in 1906 postulated that aberrant ducts are formed during embryogenesis and result in cysts. Later, VonMeyenburg postulated the excess development of intralobular bile ducts which over time became dilated. The biliary epithelium secretes fluid which accumulates and forms cysts. These cysts enlarge over time because they lack biliary drainage. Recent work in mice has challenged the previously postu-lated etiologies. Alternatively, defective production of the basement membrane in bile ducts has been hypothesized. The basement membrane of the bile duct heaps up on itself and causes dilatation of the proximal bile ducts. The enlarged bile ducts eventually compress the communication with other bile ducts. Fluid rapidly accumulates within the obstructed biliary segment and macroscopic cysts arise. Finally, an additional etiologic factor may be cystic dilatations of biliary microhamartomas in the development of liver cysts in PLD.

Histologically, simple cysts are lined by cuboi-dal epithelia. These lesions are small clusters of bile ducts surrounded by fibrous tissue which are not connected to the portal tracts. As the cysts enlarge, the epithelium flattens and becomes fibrotic. Figure 7-1 is a histologic photograph of the lining of a cyst from a patient with PLD. The tissue has been treated with cytokeratin 19, a stain specific for bile duct epithelium, which confirms biliary origin.

Diagnosis

PRESENTATION

Simple cysts are the most commonly encountered cystic lesions of the liver. These are usually solitary but can be multiple. They are distributed randomly throughout the liver and vary widely in size, from a few millimeters to greater than 20 cm. Although simple cysts are usually discovered incidentally dur-ing imaging studies, approximately 10% of patients will have symptoms. Usually, symptoms develop insidiously as a consequence of cyst expansion and adjacent organ compression. Complications of cysts are uncommon but include hemorrhage, infection, and biliary obstruction. Hemorrhage, the most fre-quent complication, is usually heralded by sudden acute abdominal pain. Hypotension is unusual un-less the cyst is huge or hemorrhage is uncontained by cyst rupture. Signs and symptoms of sepsis will accompany cyst infection and jaundice with bile duct obstruction.

Figure 7-1. A photomicrograph of the cyst wall from a patient with polycystic liver disease. The tissue has been treated with cytokeratin 19, a stain specific for bile epithelium. The dark lining of the cyst demonstrates biliary epithelial lining of the cyst. (From Dr. Douglas Jefferson, Tufts University, Medford, Massachusetts. Used with permission.)

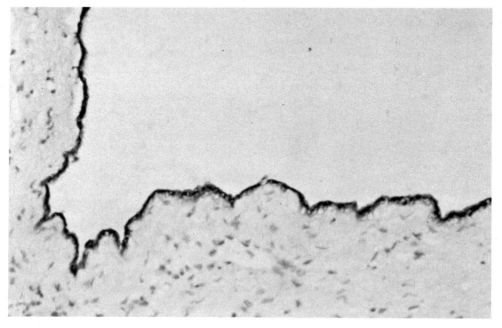

Percutaneous catheter drainage may also represent an effective therapy for rupture of hepatic amebic abscesses, which is seen as a complication in approximately 2% of patients overall and is associated with a mortality of 6% to 42% with rupture into the peritoneal cavity. With the use of multiple catheters, large sump systems, and copious irrigation, surgery may be avoided. However, if the patient has diffuse peritoneal signs or does not respond to percutaneous drainage, surgery should be undertaken.

Conclusions

Pyogenic hepatic abscesses are now seen most commonly in patients with underlying biliary tract disease and especially in those with malignant obstruction. CT is the diagnostic procedure of choice. Management options include medical treatment with antibiotics, open surgical drainage, and radiologic percutaneous drainage. Percutaneous drainage has become the method of choice for most patients, but surgery should be considered when an intra-abdominal source requires therapy and when percutaneous drainage fails. Amebic abscesses are caused by the parasite *Entamoeba histolytica* and are usually diagnosed with ultrasound and serology. The vast majority of these patients respond to metronidazole alone. Percutaneous drainage is reserved for patients who do not respond to medical therapy

and for large abscesses in the left lobe that are prone to rupture. Surgery is required in a small percentage of patients whose abscesses have ruptured or do not respond to percutaneous drainage.

Selected Readings

Bernardino ME, et al. Percutaneous drainage of multiseptated hepatic abscess. *J Comp Assist Tomogr* 1984; 8(1):38–41.

Bertel CK, van Heerden JA, Sheedy PF. Treatment of pyogenic hepatic abscesses: Surgical vs percutaneous drainage. *Arch Surg* 1986; 121:554–558.

Do H, et al. Percutaneous drainage of hepatic abscesses: Comparison of results in abscesses with and without intrahepatic biliary communication. *AJR* 1991; 157:1209–1212.

Gerzof SG, et al. Intrahepatic pyogenic abscesses: Treatment by percutaneous drainage. *Am J Surg* 1985; 149:487–493.

Halvorsen RA, et al. The variable CT appearance of hepatic abscesses. *AJR* 1984; 141:941–946.

Johnson RD, et al. Percutaneous drainage of pyogenic liver abscesses. *AJR* 1985; 144:463–467.

Pitt HA, Zuidema GD. Factors influencing mortality in the treatment of pyogenic hepatic abscess. *Surg Gynecol Obstet* 1975; 140:228–234.

Ralls PW, et al. Medical treatment of hepatic amebic abscess: Rare need for percutaneous drainage. *Radiology* 1987; 165:805–807.

Thompson JE, Forlenza S, Verma R. Amebic liver abscess: A therapeutic approach. *Rev Infec Dis* 1985; 7:171–179.

vanSonnenberg E, et al. Percutaneous abscess drainage: Current concepts. *Radiology* 1991; 181:617–626.

9

Hydatid Disease

Christopher Liddle
J. Miles Little

Etiology and Pathogenesis

Hydatid disease occurs in regions of the world where sheep are plentiful and eradication programs are absent or underfunded. In South America and the countries around the Mediterranean, the incidence is high. In parts of South America, for example, the incidence varies between 13 and 76 new cases for every 100,000 of population each year. In the United States of America, Great Britain, and northern Europe, the disease is rare, appearing in immigrants or travelers. Approximately 200 new cases per year are diagnosed in the United States. Eastern Australia, where the disease remains endemic in Victoria and New South Wales, has an intermediate incidence. Given the frequency of international travel, internists and surgeons in most parts of the world need to know something about the pathology, natural history, diagnosis, and treatment of clinical hydatid disease.

Types of Parasites

The commonest form of hydatid disease is caused by *Echinococcus granulosus*. *E. granulosus* infection in humans is a localized cystic disease, found most commonly in the liver (about 70%) or lung (about 25%). *E. multiocularis* infection is uncommon. The main endemic areas are in the Northern Hemisphere, specifically central Europe, Siberia, Japan, Alaska, and northern Canada. *E. multilocularis* causes alveolar echinococcosis of the liver, an invasive disease which does not have the well-demarcated, cystic structure of *E. granulosus* infection. *E. multilocularis* behaves more like a hepatic malig-

nancy and may spread by way of blood vessels. The prognosis in this condition is grave if the disease is extensive.

Two rare forms, *E. vogleri* and *E. oligarthrus*, behave like *E. multilocularis* in humans. They are found only in South America and are not further considered in this chapter.

Life Cycle

The hydatid is a dimorphic parasite. It exists exclusively as a short flat worm in the primary (definitive) host, which is usually a member of the dog family. The cestode lives in the small bowel of the primary host, is some 4 to 6 mm in length, and has three to five segments below the head. The terminal segment of the worm is the gravid segment, which contains between 300 and 500 ova. The gravid segment is periodically shed, and the ova (oncospheres) are passed in the dog's feces. The ova are resistant to drying; they may remain viable for weeks after being passed. A grazing animal, the intermediate host, swallows the ova. This animal is typically the sheep, though cattle, pigs, and camels may also become infected. The outer covering of each ovum is digested by gastric acid, allowing the hexacanth embryo to hatch in the upper bowel, to penetrate the bowel wall and gain access to the portal circulation or the lymphatic system. Although most embryos are trapped in the liver, some pass through to the lungs or beyond to any other part of the body. The life cycle is completed when the dog eats contaminated offal (Fig. 9-1).

Humans usually contract the disease in childhood or adolescence when ova are swallowed after

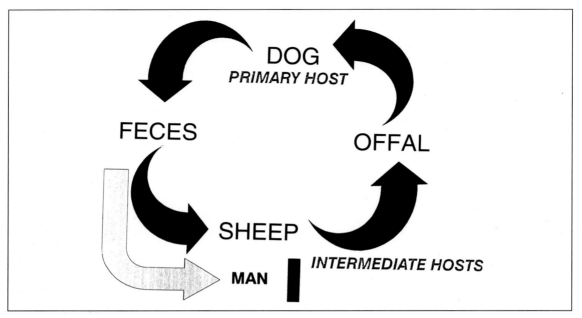

Figure 9-1. The life cycle of *Echinococcus granulosus*.

contact with an infected dog. The ova adhere to the dog's coat, and simple handling of the animal may lead to infection. Ova may also contaminate vegetables and grass in the vicinity of the dog. Man is an accidental intermediate host, representing a dead end for the parasite, since dogs seldom have access to human viscera. The life cycle of *E. multilocularis* is a little different. The primary host is usually a fox, and the intermediate host a microtine rodent such as the vole or the lemming.

An understanding of this life cycle is important. Preventative campaigns based upon prevention and eradication of infection in dogs have been demonstrated to markedly reduce the incidence of human hydatid disease. For instance, the incidence of hydatid disease in Tasmania decreased from 15 cases per 100,000 to less than 2 cases per 100,000 between 1965 and 1978. Simple advice to a patient and family also depends on a good comprehension of the life cycle. A tendency exists for families to segregate those who are known to be infected, but humans are not infective to other humans.

Structure in the Intermediate Host

The mature cyst of *E. granulosus* characteristically contains three layers, regardless of the organ in which it grows.

1. The adventitia, a layer of scar tissue and compressed host organ tissue
2. The laminated membrane, a gelatinous acellular layer manufactured by the parasite, loosely adherent to the adventitia, making a natural cleavage plane through which the infective part of the parasite can be removed
3. The germinal epithelium, from which the brood capsules bud, and containing protoscoleces or potential worm heads.

The fluid within the cyst may contain minute daughter cysts and viable fragments of germinal epithelium. Spillage of fluid into a body cavity can cause further hydatids to develop.

The intermediate phase of *E. multilocularis* has a different structure. The adventitial layer does not confine the parasite, nor is there a major cystic cavity within the mass of parasitic tissue. Instead, the parasite infiltrates like a malignancy and forms microcysts, which make up a honeycomblike structure. Because no natural cleavage plane exists between the parasite and the host organ, the surgical approach to *E. multilocularis* involves principles similar to those used in cancer surgery.

Development of Hydatid Cysts

Infestation usually occurs in childhood; growth is slow, about 0.3 cm per year. As hydatid cysts grow, they tend to make their way toward regions of low pressure. In the liver, for example, they make their way from the depths of the liver toward the peritoneal surface, particularly beneath the diaphragm. Cysts may also make their way into nearby bile ducts and, less frequently, into the hepatic veins. In the lung, cysts tend to present themselves on the pleural surface of the lung and to rupture into the bronchi. Compression of surrounding tissue occurs, but so slowly that there are usually no symptoms associated with even large cysts.

As the cyst grows, the attachment of the laminated membrane to the adventitia becomes more tenuous, and the laminated membrane tends to break away from the adventitia. This shearing stimulates the parasite to form daughter cysts (Fig. 9-2). Daughter cysts are most commonly contained within the cavity of the main cyst as endogenous daughter cysts. Exogenous daughter cysts form outside the cavity of the main cyst when the adventitia splits as it stretches. For reasons that remain unclear, hydatid cysts most often involve the right lobe of the liver. In approximately one third of patients a single cyst is present, with the remainder having multiple cysts.

Diagnosis

Clinical Features

Because a hydatid cyst grows slowly, the patient may be completely unaware of the parasite, even when it reaches a large size. Abdominal pain, hepatomegaly, palpable tumor, nonspecific dyspeptic symptoms, fevers, and jaundice were the most common presenting features in a large series. Symptoms

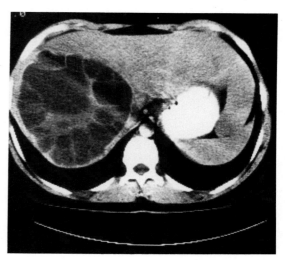

Figure 9-2. CT scan demonstrating hydatid cyst of the liver with multiple daughter cysts.

tend to occur in association with complications. As the cyst dies, leakage of fluid produces pericystitis, which causes pain and low-grade fever. When bacterial infection occurs, the patient presents with the clinical picture of an abscess. A growing hydatid may erode the tubular structures within the parenchyma of the host organ. Extrusion of hydatid membrane may occur into the bile ducts, the bronchi (Fig. 9-3), or the blood vessels. Obstructive jaundice, the coughing up of hydatid fluid and membrane (resembling grape skins), and multiple pulmonary emboli can all occur. Leakage of bile into a hydatid cyst usually results in death of the main cyst, although not necessarily of daughter cysts, and may be accompanied by severe pain. Hydatids can cause allergic phenomena. Urticaria, pruritus, asthma, and even anaphylaxis may occur.

At times, a roentgenogram obtained for other purposes will show a densely calcified cyst in an elderly person who has never been aware of hydatid infection. Calcification does not mean that the cyst is dead, and even a heavily calcified cyst may contain viable elements. Similarly, the widespread use of abdominal CT scanning and ultrasound will often diagnose unsuspected disease, particularly in endemic areas.

Physical findings are often unimpressive. Hydatid cysts in the liver usually occur in the dome

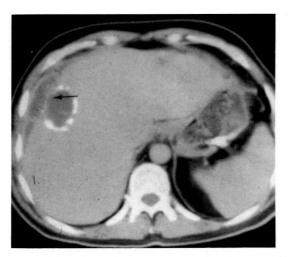

Figure 9-3. CT scan demonstrating rupture of a hydatid cyst through the diaphragm into a bronchus.

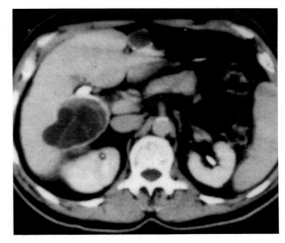

Figure 9-4. CT scan demonstrating calcified hydatid cysts in both the right and left lobes of the liver.

of the right liver in segments VII and VIII, and push the liver downward as they grow. The commonest physical finding, therefore, is diffuse hepatomegaly rather than identification of a mass in the liver. Pulmonary signs may depend on the degree of pressure exerted on the bronchi, on consolidation surrounding the cyst, and on rupture of the cyst into the bronchi.

Serological Tests

Serological tests have a long history in the investigation and management of hydatid disease. A large number of tests are available, but those most commonly used are the complement fixation test (CFT), indirect fluorescent antibody test, enzyme-linked immunosorbent assay (ELISA), radioallergosorbent test (RAST), and specific immunoelectrophoretogram (IEPG or arc-5 test).

Usually, at least two of these tests should be performed. Even so, false-positive and false-negative results will occur. The complement fixation test is useful because it becomes negative after cure of a hydatid cyst and can therefore be used to assess the efficacy of treatment. Complement fixation is not, however, particularly sensitive, and many false negatives occur. The IEPG or arc-5 test is the most specific test so far devised.

Imaging

The diagnosis of hepatic hydatid disease is most often made following imaging of the liver, either by ultrasound or radiological techniques. Although a laminated structure or the presence of calcification is highly suggestive of hydatid disease, it may sometimes be difficult to differentiate from other space-occupying lesions of the liver, particularly if the cyst is small. Although ultrasound is the preferred modality, other modalities may be required to confirm the diagnosis or to determine the full extent of hepatic involvement (Fig. 9-4). Heavy plaques of calcification are seen in the walls of dead cysts, although live daughter cysts may survive within the main cyst. Ultrasound and CT scans can establish the diagnosis of hydatid disease when daughter cysts are identified within a mother cyst (see Fig. 9-2). CT scanning is more sensitive in detecting extrahepatic abdominal disease and probably should be performed if surgery is planned. It is particularly important to define the relationship between the cyst and adjacent structures, such as the inferior vena cava. These considerations may modify the extent of planned surgery.

Large and recurrent hydatid cysts may require additional investigation. Endoscopic retrograde cholangiopancreatography (ERCP) or bronchogra-

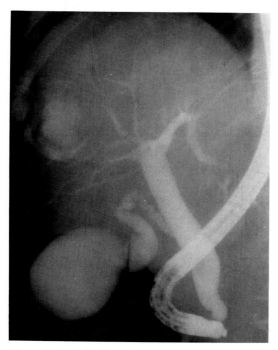

Figure 9-5. ERCP demonstrating communication of a hydatid cyst in the right lobe with the biliary tree.

phy may be helpful when previous surgery has distorted local anatomy or the surgeon suspects a communication between a cyst and the biliary (Fig. 9-5) or bronchial tree. Angiography is seldom indicated. Magnetic resonance imaging produces clear and detailed pictures, but its place in diagnosis is not yet established. Radioisotope scanning has no place in diagnosis.

Management and Results

Options

Several approaches to the treatment of hepatic hydatid disease have been tried, but open surgical evacuation of cysts with obliteration of the cavity remains the treatment to which other therapies must be compared in terms of both safety and efficacy. The recent proliferation of surgical procedures that can be accomplished using the video laparoscope suggests that this technique may be useful in managing some hepatic hydatid cysts. However, published series are still small and are restricted to cysts that are visible and easily accessible. Rapid developments in interventional radiology and ultrasound have generated a number of studies utilizing percutaneous aspiration of cysts followed by injection of scolecidal agents. This latter approach should be used with caution because the risk of peritoneal contamination with scoleces exists and, as mentioned below, scolecidal agents have been associated with significant complications. In patients with recurrent or complicated disease, or in whom coexistent medical problems contraindicate surgery, systemic administration of antihelminthic agents is another possibility.

In the treatment of *E. multilocularis* infection hepatic resection is usually required because there is no clear margin for pericystectomy to be performed. Indeed, in extensive disease, liver transplantation may be the only hope of cure.

Surgical Treatment

Although the simplest treatment is evacuation and drainage, this form of management is not a good one unless the cyst is infected with bacteria. The old operation of marsupialization, in which the open cyst is sutured to the parietal peritoneum so that a drainage track is formed at this site, is also outdated, since the morbidity is high.

The standard procedure for treating most cysts in soft tissue is cystectomy or pericystectomy with evacuation of the cyst and obliteration of the residual cavity. This operation can be used in almost any organ affected by echinococcosis. Adequate exposure is important, since evacuation of the cyst must be carried out under complete control to avoid spilling its contents. Rarely is it necessary to open the chest, even when the cyst occurs in the dome of the right liver. Exploration should be carried out to search for previously undetected cysts. It is important to examine the retroperitoneum, since hepatic hydatids sometimes extrude laminated membrane and germinal epithelium into the bare area. Infective material may track downward as far as the pelvis in the extraperitoneal tissue. Cysts may be found in the lesser omentum around the pancreas, in the spleen, and in the kidneys in association with hepatic hydatids. The use of operative ultrasound is most helpful in determining the extent of disease and in detecting the presence of exoge-nous daughter cysts that might otherwise be missed.

Once the disease has been adequately assessed, the area around the cyst should be packed with sponges soaked with hypertonic saline solution. Three percent saline solution appears to be less irritating to tissues than alternative scolecides. Once the packing is complete, it is traditional to attempt to aspirate as much as possible of the contents of the cyst, and to replace the aspirate with a scolecide. Silver nitrate (0.5%), hypertonic saline (3% or 20%), 2% formalin, and cetrimide have been used, but there is little evidence of their effectiveness in the clinical setting. All of them depend on reaching an adequate concentration within the cyst; it is impossible, however, to predict the degree of dilu-tion caused by residual cyst contents. In addition, both formalin and hypertonic saline have been as-sociated with a progressive sclerosing cholangitis when injected accidentally into the biliary tree. It is rarely possible to evacuate a cyst completely; and indeed, if there are many daughter cysts and if the laminated membrane is detached from the wall of the main cyst, it may be impossible to remove more than a few milliliters of fluid.

A useful device to assist in maintaining control is an evacuation cone. The suction cone devised by Aarons has a grooved inferior rim connected to a side arm. The side arm is connected to suction, sealing the cone to the surface of the cyst. An inci-sion is then made through the center of the cone, and the large-bore evacuation tubing is used to clear away the material that pours out and to suck away fluid and laminated membrane from the inside of the cyst. Evacuation takes place in the plane be-tween laminated membrane and adventitia. Using the sucker tubing as the source of vacuum is the most effective way to remove the laminated mem-brane as it falls away from the adventitia.

Once the cyst has been evacuated, the incision in the adventitia is enlarged, and the depths of the cyst are inspected. In a large hepatic cyst, unsus-pected daughter cysts may be found in the depths of the main cavity. These daughter cysts should be extracted with the suction tubing. The inner lin-ing of the adventitia is then swabbed with 3% saline solution, and the cyst is partly filled with 3% saline solution to kill any residual viable ele-ments.

The saline solution is aspirated, and all redun-dant adventitia is removed. In the liver, this excision is taken back to the surrounding viable liver tissue, and the liver edge is oversewn to secure hemostasis. This procedure usually leaves a saucer-shaped cav-ity in the liver, which must now be inspected for bile leaks. The most effective way to detect bile is to pack the residual cavity with a clean, dry sponge and to compress the adjacent liver between the hands. After a minute the sponge is removed and inspected for bile staining. Bile leaks are closed. Cholangiography should be carried out, and the common duct explored if there is evidence of lami-nated membrane within it.

In the lung, closure of dead space by suture may be possible. In the liver, various techniques of closure have been reported, but the most effective is omentoplasty. The greater omentum is mobilized from the transverse colon, preferably maintaining the blood supply from both the right and left gas-troepiploic arteries. The omentum is laid into the cavity (Fig. 9-6). Bile leakage is common for several days after removal of a hepatic hydatid, but gener-ally stops spontaneously.

Calcified cysts in the liver measuring up to about 12 cm and situated well away from the infe-rior vena cava can be treated by cystopericystectomy (Fig. 9-7). A dissection plane is developed between the adventitia and the liver. This plane is not clearly defined, and is crossed by bile ducts and vessels. The advantage of the operation is that calcified tis-sue is removed, and the dead space is easier to close. More blood is lost during cystopericystectomy than is usual during the standard operation of evacuation and omentoplasty. Complete excision of cysts in other areas, such as the retroperitoneum, can be achieved with the same technique. Hepatic, pulmo-nary, or renal resection may be necessary for the treatment of complex cysts with multiple exoge-nous daughter cysts and for recurrences.

Cysts superinfected with bacteria are consid-ered to be abscesses and are treated as such by drainage and antibiotics. Infection in a calcified cyst often persists until all the calcified material has been removed. Persistent biliary fistulas may be found in heavily calcified cysts. An asymptomatic, heavily calcified cyst in an elderly person should be left alone, since the potential morbidity of surgical re-moval outweighs the benefit.

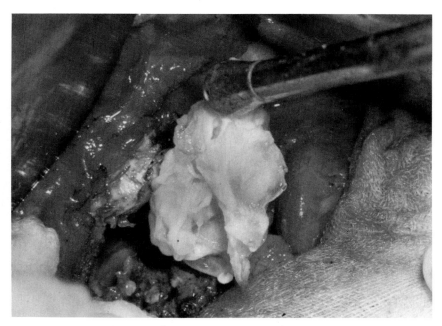

Figure 9-6. Operative picture demonstrating removal of a daughter cyst from a thick-walled cyst that was packed with omentum.

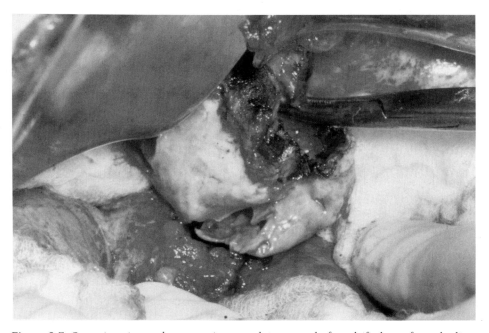

Figure 9-7. Operative picture demonstrating complete removal of a calcified cyst from the liver.

The mortality of surgical treatment should be lower than 5%. Reported recurrence rates in the literature vary widely and are usually proportional to the intensity of postoperative follow-up and ultrasound examination. In the authors' experience, a recurrence rate of 22% was found, with all recurrences occurring within the first 3 years. Recurrence is much more common among patients who have evidence of spread of the disease at the time of the primary operation. Recurrence can also occur because of spillage of cyst fluid during an operation.

Drug Treatment

The benzimidazoles can be used for the drug treatment of echinococcosis. Albendazole in particular appears to be effective in some cases. Albendazole is metabolized by the liver to albendazole sulfoxide. This metabolite is able to penetrate the hydatid cyst and probably explains the superior efficacy of albendazole as compared to earlier benzimidazoles, such as mebendazole. The benzimidazoles interfere with glucose absorption by the parasite. Albendazole is usually given in a dose of 10 mg/kg/d in two divided doses for 28 days. The drug is then suspended for 14 days, and liver function tests and full blood counts are checked. An ultrasonic or radiological measurement of cyst size is carried out. After 14 days without drug treatment, the cycle is repeated and continued until cyst measurements are stable for two successive examinations.

The results of albendazole treatment for *E. multilocularis* infection have been disappointing. Although drug treatment may retard disease progression, it does not eliminate the parasite in animal models or in humans.

Hepatic toxicity is common during albendazole therapy, with up to 85% of patients exhibiting abnormalities of liver enzymes. In some patients a severe hepatic reaction has been noted which has recurred on rechallenge. Neutropenia, proteinuria, febrile reactions, and alopecia have also been reported.

In Australia, albendazole is available only for clinical trials, and its use is restricted to patients with recurrent disease, with multiple body cavities affected, with surgically inaccessible disease, or with serious associated medical conditions. Albendazole seems particularly effective treatment for recurrent *E. granulosus* detected on routine follow-up examination after primary hydatid surgery.

Guided Aspiration and Injection

Over the last several years, some authors have described the use of ultrasound- or CT-guided needle aspiration of hepatic hydatid cysts followed by injection of a scolecidal agent. Generally, 95% sterile alcohol has been used as the scolecide and appears to be reasonably safe. Most series have reported a decrease in cyst size on serial imaging, and in one study a decrease in antibody titers to *E. granulosus* was also noted. Authors have acknowledged the risk of peritoneal contamination with viable scoleces, but this complication appears to be rare. Unfortunately, these studies have been on small numbers of patients, and a randomized study comparing aspiration and injection to surgery has not been performed.

Controversies

Overall, little controversy exists regarding the need for surgery in hydatid disease of the liver. The place for laparoscopic and percutaneous procedures remains to be defined, and these techniques should be restricted to clinical trials at present.

A more difficult area is the use of albendazole, either as monotherapy or in combination with surgery. Treatment with albendazole for at least 1 month prior to surgery, at a dose of 10 mg/kg/d, has been shown to eliminate viable protoscoleces in some patients. Advocates suggest that such treatment may reduce the recurrence rate after surgery. However, this hypothesis has not been subjected to a controlled trial. As monotherapy, the efficacy of albendazole has been examined in several studies utilizing serial ultrasound or CT examinations. Generally, these studies have involved small numbers of patients and have reported widely differing results. Overall, in about 50% of patients some change in cyst appearance has been documented, with a lesser number having virtual disappearance of disease. Thus dispute about the value of treatment with albendazole for patients first presenting with hydatid disease still exists. Clearly, a large-scale trial of albendazole monotherapy is required, preferably compared to surgery in a randomized fashion.

With regard to the use of guided aspiration and scolecidal injection of cysts, again, randomized studies in comparison to surgery are required. This therapeutic approach is potentially attractive for less complex hepatic disease, and the possibility for combination with systemic albendazole treatment exists.

Conclusions

Hydatid disease of the liver is a common entity in certain areas of the world. Eradication programs should be the primary focus because they are of proven benefit. Surgery remains the treatment of choice, with cystectomy or pericystectomy being the preferred procedure. Less invasive procedures and drug therapy have been advocated, but their role in the management of this disease remains to be determined.

Selected Readings

Braithwaite PA. Hydatid disease: Epidemiology and pathology. *Aust N Z J Surg* 1983; 53:203–209.

Khuroo MS, et al. Percutaneous drainage versus albendazole therapy in hepatic hydatidosis: A prospective randomized study. *Gastroenterology* 1993; 104: 1452–1459.

Little JM, Deane SA. Hydatid disease. In Blumbart LH (ed), *Surgery of the Liver and Biliary Tract*. Edinburgh: Churchill Livingstone, 1988. Pp. 955–966.

Little JM, Hollands MJ, Ekberg H. Recurrence of hydatid disease. *World J Surg* 1988; 12:700–704.

Morris DL, et al. Albendazole—objective evidence of response in human hydatid disease. *JAMA* 1985; 253: 2053–2057.

Pitt HA, Korzelius J, Tompkins RK. Management of hepatic echinococcosis in Southern California. *Am J Surg* 1986; 152:110–115.

Teres J, et al. Sclerosing cholangitis after surgical treatment of hepatic echinococcal cysts. *Am J Surg* 1983; 53:694–697.

10

Hemobilia

ROBERT D'AGOSTINO
LEON G. JOSEPHS

Hemobilia, once considered a rare condition, is now being reported with increasing frequency. Hemobilia has been described in the setting of traumatic injury of the liver, cholelithiasis, neoplasms and inflammatory disease of the liver and biliary system, and primary vascular disease of the liver. A comparison of three large series reviewing causes of hemobilia (Table 10-1) indicates that trauma is the leading etiology. In comparing Sandblom's 1972 collective series with Curet's 1984 and Yoshida's 1987 series, one sees an overall increase in traumatic causes of hemobilia, with a large jump in percentage of iatrogenic trauma in the 12 to 15 years between these series. This increase most likely reflects the increased use of percutaneous liver biopsy and transhepatic procedures for the diagnosis and treatment of hepatobiliary diseases.

Etiology and Pathogenesis

Percutaneous transhepatic procedures are associated with a high incidence of vascular complications, such as arterial pseudoaneurysm and arterioportal venous fistula. A 4% incidence of hepatic vascular injuries is found following percutaneous transhepatic cholangiography, and a 5% incidence occurs after percutaneous liver biopsy. Following the placement of indwelling transhepatic drainage catheters, the incidence of vascular injuries shown angiographically may reach 25%. With the close anatomic proximity of the branches of the portal vein, the hepatic artery, and the intrahepatic bile ducts, concurrent injury to these structures during these procedures seems unavoidable. The rate and severity of injury increase with large-caliber instruments and more central liver punctures. Long-term indwelling catheter drainage may also cause pressure necrosis of biliary ducts and adjacent vessels. This complication can occur in up to 5% of cases and may take days to months to occur. Delayed rupture of a posttraumatic pseudoaneurysm or an arteriovenous fistula into the biliary system produces the clinical findings of hemobilia. Iatrogenic bleeding can also arise secondary to cholecystectomy and surgical manipulation in the biliary tree. Ductal exploration can also lead to mucosal laceration. Such complications can arise from both open and laparoscopic approaches.

Approximately 15% to 20% of all blunt abdominal injuries and 25% of penetrating wounds of the abdomen involve the liver. Hemobilia may complicate up to 3% of cases and is more likely to occur after blunt injury. Posttraumatic hemobilia usually arises from arteriobiliary fistulae, and intraparenchymal hematoma, biloma, or necrotic tissue will increase the likelihood of formation of fistulae and pseudoaneurysms.

Primary vascular causes of hemobilia include aneurysmal disease of the hepatic artery, vasculitis, or, very rarely, portal vein aneurysm. Portal hypertension leading to hemobilia is rare and is usually related to a large periportal or gallbladder wall varix that ruptures. Nevertheless, in patients with portal hypertension, trauma is still the most common cause of hemobilia.

Hemobilia from gallstone-related disease is usually occult. Cases of cystic artery erosion by gallstones and hemorrhagic necrosis complicating

Table 10-1. Hemobilia Cases: Number (Percentage) by Cause

	Sandblom (1972) (n = 355)	Curet (1984) (n = 86)	Yoshida (1987) (n = 103)
Trauma (iatrogenic)	59 (17)	50 (58)	42 (41)
(accidental)	137 (38)	23 (27)	20 (19)
Gallstone-related	53 (15)	—	9 (9)
Inflammatory	46 (13)	—	10 (10)
Primary vascular	38 (11)	—	15 (14)
Neoplastic	22 (6)	—	7 (7)
Other	—	13 (15)	—

cholangitis and cholecystitis have been reported. Inflammatory lesions causing hemobilia are mostly related to gallstones except in the Far East, where *Ascaris* infestation is prevalent. Cases of hemobilia with amebic and hydatid infection of the liver have also been reported.

Diagnosis

Hemobilia has been classically described as presenting with a triad of pain, jaundice, and gastrointestinal bleeding, but larger series have shown this to be the case in less than 50% of patients. In these series 70% of patients presented with biliary colic, and 60% with jaundice, in addition to the constant feature of gastrointestinal bleeding. The bleeding may range from scant to profuse and intermittent to continuous, and may arise from communication to the biliary tree at any level. Severe large-volume hemorrhage is more likely to occur in patients undergoing percutaneous biliary drainage procedures for malignant biliary obstruction as a result of abnormal liver function or biliary infection. Blood clots in the biliary system may cause acute biliary obstruction which leads to the development of cholangitis, cholecystitis, or pancreatitis, or the clots may serve as a nidus for biliary calculi.

The age distribution of patients with hemobilia tends to peak in the sixth decade of life, representing the amount of iatrogenic trauma in people in this age group undergoing invasive testing and treatment. A second concentration of patients occurs in the first four decades of life, representing the higher likelihood of accidental trauma in this age group. Hemobilia from trauma is seen more often in men, whereas gallstone-related bleeding is

more common in women. In Yosida's large series the initial diagnosis of hemobilia was made by endoscopy in 12% of cases, by angiography in 28%, intraoperatively in 34%, and by identifying bleeding via a biliary drainage catheter in 12%.

The authors' team approach to the diagnosis of hemobilia involves initial resuscitation and evaluation, including laboratory analysis of hematocrit, coagulation, and renal and liver function. Endoscopy is performed to exclude other sources of upper gastrointestinal tract bleeding. Although the bleeding of hemobilia can be intermittent, endoscopy is useful in diagnosing 50% of cases, with extended observation of the papilla of Vater recommended. Endoscopic retrograde cholangiopancreatography (ERCP) may also be utilized, with the retrograde cholangiogram identifying intrabiliary filling defects. Although usually not definitive, this finding may suggest the diagnosis. With the diagnosis confirmed, papillotomy and nasobiliary drainage can be performed during ERCP. This maneuver is a useful approach to managing biliary obstruction due to clots.

CT scanning is useful in cases of hemobilia from traumatic origin. CT can identify parenchymal disruptions, hematomas, and bilomas that may be associated with hemobilia (Fig. 10-1A). CT can also identify high-density blood clots in the gallbladder or biliary tree and aid in the diagnosis (see Fig. 10-1B). Tumors of the liver and biliary system, gallstones, and common bile duct stones can also be identified. Ultrasound can also serve a similar role to CT, and may better evaluate gallbladder- and stone-related pathology (see Fig. 10-1C).

Angiography is the most helpful diagnostic modality. With the success of transcatheter therapy,

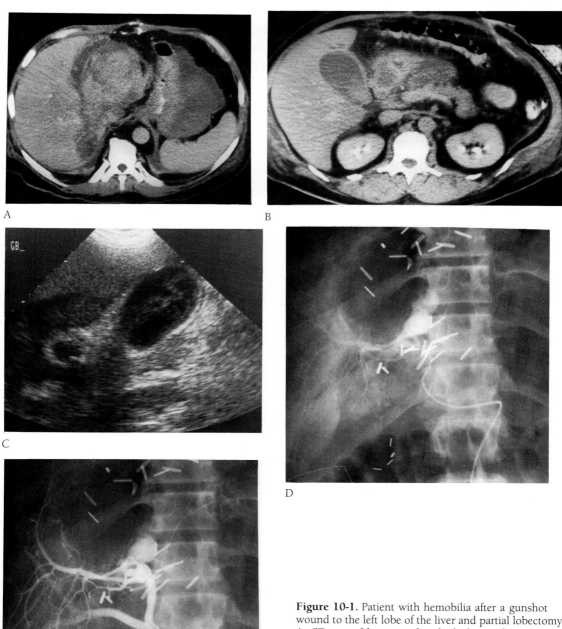

Figure 10-1. Patient with hemobilia after a gunshot wound to the left lobe of the liver and partial lobectomy. A. CT scan of liver revealing high-density hematoma in areas of left lobe. B. Caudal image showing high-density clot in the gallbladder. C. Gallbladder ultrasound image disclosing nonshadowing homogeneous clot. D. Hepatic angiogram demonstrating left hepatic artery pseudoaneurysm. E. Late film from angiogram showing continued filling of pseudoaneurysm and surrounding avascular hematoma.

angiography has become a necessary step in the diagnosis of hemobilia. The identification of a source of bleeding with angiography will dictate a further treatment plan. Angiograms of both the celiac and superior mesenteric arteries are mandatory to evaluate all structures related to the biliary system, including vascular anatomical variants. It is important to examine related structures, including the duodenum for ulcer disease and to be alert for the neovascularity of tumors. In hemobilia related to indwelling biliary drainage catheters, the catheters may need to be removed temporarily during filming to avoid a tamponade effect, which will give a falsely negative evaluation. Subselective angiography should also be performed to identify the exact causative vessel and to help plan transcatheter therapy if indicated. Patency of the portal venous system should also be determined if transcatheter embolization or surgical ligation is planned.

The lesion most often identified in patients with hepatic or biliary bleeding is an arterial pseudoaneurysm (see Fig. 10-1D,E). Hepatic arterioportal vein fistulas are also common. Fistulas from the hepatic artery to the hepatic veins and venobiliary fistulas are rare. Only a fourth of cases will show direct extravasation into the biliary tree. It should be remembered, moreover, that angiography carries a 10% false negative rate.

In patients with a negative diagnostic workup, surgical exploration may be performed without a preoperative diagnosis. Active bleeding from the duodenum may be identified via intraoperative endoscopy or duodenotomy, or may be localized as proximal filling using small bowel Penrose "tourniquets." By performing a lateral duodenotomy, one may observe bleeding directly from the ampulla. An intraoperative cholangiogram may also show the filling defects of clot and confirm the diagnosis.

Treatment and Results

Treatment decisions for hemobilia should be based on the anatomical source of bleeding. In the past the treatment for intrahepatic causes of hemobilia was ligation of the main hepatic arterial branch. Ligation of the hepatic artery is made possible by the dual hepatic blood supply and the extensive collateral blood flow to the liver. The portal vein supplies 75% to 80% of the oxygen and metabolic needs of the liver. Dual hepatic supply also allows highly selective angiographic transcatheter embolization as the treatment of choice in intrahepatic causes of hemobilia. The overall success of embolization is high, providing control of bleeding in over 95% of patients.

The ability to perform subselective embolization has been improved greatly with the development of 0.018-in. and 0.025-in. catheter and wire systems and platinum microcoils. The goal of ligation or embolization is to decrease the pressure head to the lesion without devitalizing the hepatic tissue. This goal is best achieved with highly selective embolization. To prevent recanalization of the feeding vessel, permanent occluding agents, such as spring coils, are recommended. The coils should be packed in and placed both proximal and distal to a pseudoaneurysm and arteriovenous fistula to occlude antegrade and retrograde flow to the lesion (Fig. 10-2A,B,C). The complication rates of transcatheter embolization are low. Since 20% of patients develop minor liver damage manifested as transient elevation in serum liver enzymes levels, these values should be monitored after the procedure.

If highly selective embolization is unsuccessful, embolization of the main hepatic artery or its major branches using spring coils can be performed. Surgical treatment is also very successful if transcatheter therapy fails. However, as initial therapy, surgery does not approach the cure rate and low morbidity of transcatheter embolization. Surgical therapy includes liver suturing, partial hepatic resection, and vessel ligation. When hemobilia accompanies major liver injury, initial surgery with debridement, vessel ligation, and drainage is important, but transcatheter therapy should also be considered as an adjunct to control vascular injuries. Rare portal venous causes of hemobilia should be treated surgically.

Surgical therapy has a reported 77% success rate in extrahepatic causes of hemobilia. Cholecystectomy is the procedure of choice in cases where the gallbladder is the source of bleeding. Subselective embolization has been reported for massive cystic artery hemorrhage, but adjunctive cholecystectomy should be planned. Resectable neoplasms and common bile duct tumors should also be ap-

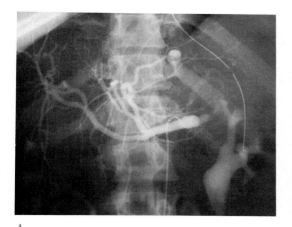

A

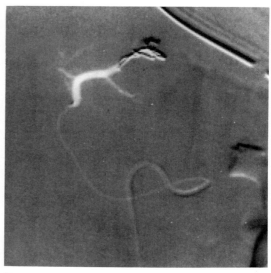

B

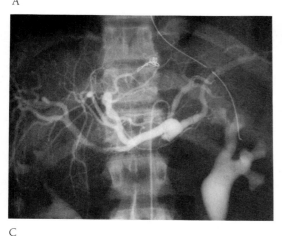

C

Figure 10-2. Hemobilia in a patient after abdominal stab wound. A. Hepatic angiogram with pseudoaneurysm from left hepatic artery branch. B. Subselective catheterization with 0.018-in. guidewire system and placement of microcoils. C. Post embolization microcoils with complete thrombosis of pseudoaneurysm.

proached surgically. Embolization may be considered for unresectable bleeding lesions if it is the safest method and technically possible.

Expectant observation is an option for managing hemobilia in selected cases. Spontaneous cessation of bleeding will occur in one third of patients with hemobilia after percutaneous liver biopsy. Some authors have recommended the placement of clot promoters into percutaneous needle puncture tracts to reduce bleeding complications.

Conclusions

Hemobilia is most often due to trauma, including iatrogenic trauma, and has a 10% overall mortality rate. Successful diagnosis and treatment of hemo-

bilia rely on a high level of clinical suspicion and the joint skills of the endoscopist, radiologist, and surgeon. The identification of biliary bleeding and confirmation of the precise anatomical localization by angiography will help define the therapeutic option. Prompt and definitive intervention is recommended to minimize patient morbidity and mortality.

Selected Readings

Curet P, et al. Hepatic hemobilia if traumatic or iatrogenic origin: Recent advances in diagnosis and therapy, review of the literature 1976 to 1981. *World J Surg* 1984; 8:2–8.

Czerniak A, et al. Hemobilia: A disease in evolution. *Arch Surg* 1988; 123:718–721.

Merrell SW, Schneider PD. Hemobilia: Evolution of current diagnosis and treatment. *West J Med* 1991; 155:621–625.

Sandblom P. Hemobilia: History, pathology, diagnosis, treatment. Springfield, Ill: Thomas, 1972.

Sandblom P, Saegesser F, Mirkovitch V. Hepatic hemobilia: Hemorrhage from the intrahepatic biliary tract, a review. *World J Surg* 1984; 8:41–50.

Schwartz RA, et al. Effectiveness of transcatheter emboli-zation in the control of hepatic vascular injuries. *JVIR* 1993; 4:359–365.

Vajic I. Site and etiology of hemobilia. In *Interventional Radiology* (2nd ed). Baltimore: Williams & Wilkins, 1992.

Yoshida J, Donahue PE, Nyhus LM. Hemobilia: Review of recent experience with a worldwide problem. *Am J Gastroenterol* 1987; 82:448–453.

11

Hepatic Trauma

DAVID V. FELICIANO
CURTIS A. LEWIS

Etiology

The liver is the most commonly injured organ in patients with abdominal trauma. In patients with blunt trauma, 35% to 45% will be noted to have a hepatic injury if laparotomy is necessary. When penetrating trauma has occurred, the incidence ranges from 30% (gunshot wounds) to 40% (stab wounds).

Injuries to the liver during blunt trauma result from strains or physical deformations, including stretching (avulsion of the liver from supporting ligaments), shearing (compression between the lower ribs on the right and the spine), and crushing (direct blows). The majority of such injuries occur in victims of motor vehicle accidents, especially unrestrained drivers and front-seat passengers in frontal collisions. In a patient with contusions of the right lower chest or upper abdominal wall or fractures of the lower six ribs on the right, injury to the liver should be suspected.

As the largest organ in the body, the liver is likely to be injured when a penetrating wound traverses the upper abdomen. Stab, gunshot, or shotgun wounds to the epigastrium, right upper quadrant, or right flank inevitably injure the liver, and most, but not all, of these patients will require a laparotomy.

Diagnosis and Emergency Management

Thoracotomy for Resuscitation

On occasion, a patient with a severe hepatic injury, which often involves the retrohepatic vena cava,

will be in a moribund condition with a massively distended abdomen upon arrival in the emergency department. In older hospitals where the operating room is geographically distant from the emergency department, it may be necessary to perform a left anterolateral thoracotomy with cross-clamping of the descending thoracic aorta prior to transferring the patient to the operating room. This maneuver is the only way to preserve some blood flow to the coronary and carotid arteries during transport, but unfortunately results in a survival rate of only 2% to 7% when applied to victims of abdominal trauma.

Emergency Laparotomy

In many patients with major hepatic injuries from either blunt or penetrating trauma, the location of trauma, profound hypotension temporarily responsive to the infusion of fluids and blood, abdominal distention, and obvious signs of peritonitis mandate an immediate laparotomy without the need for further diagnostic testing. This procedure is indicated even though the surgeon does not have precise knowledge of the presence or extent of a hepatic injury.

Blunt Abdominal Trauma

The diagnosis of intra-abdominal injuries is often difficult even in reasonably stable victims of blunt trauma. Reasons for this include the significant incidence of alcoholic intoxication, associated intracranial injuries, injuries to adjacent structures such as ribs, pelvis, and spine, and multisystem injuries in many of the victims.

If the victim of blunt trauma is hypotensive in the emergency department and the abdomen is one of many potential sites of hemorrhage, then either a diagnostic peritoneal tap and lavage, if necessary, or ultrasonography performed by the surgical team is appropriate. An infraumbilical diagnostic peritoneal tap (supraumbilical if a pelvic fracture is present) is performed with a dialysis catheter or commercially available kit after a nasogastric tube and bladder catheter have been inserted. The return of 10 to 20 ml of gross blood through the lavage catheter in the absence of external bleeding elsewhere, significant intrapleural hemorrhage, or a major pelvic fracture mandates an immediate laparotomy to control hemorrhage, which is most commonly from the liver, spleen, or mesentery.

In a similar fashion, an emergency ultrasound performed with a portable high-resolution real-time unit and a 3.0-MHz transducer is extremely useful in rapidly diagnosing intra-abdominal bleeding as the source of hypotension in a patient with multiple blunt injuries. An experienced surgical ultrasonographer can rule out a pericardial tamponade and rule in intra-abdominal bleeding in less than 3 minutes with a diagnostic accuracy of 90% to 98%. As surgeons gain experience with emergency ultrasound, a precise diagnosis of a hepatic injury will be made before operation in more patients.

Different diagnostic approaches are used in hemodynamically stable victims of blunt trauma. Computerized tomography (CT) has now been used for the evaluation of such patients for approximately 15 years. CT is particularly useful for the detection of hepatic injuries in patients with associated hematuria or pelvic fractures, when a long anesthetic is needed for other injuries, when trauma to the head or spinal cord is present, when there has been delayed presentation of the patient after blunt trauma (Fig. 11-1), and when there are contraindications to diagnostic peritoneal lavage. Except for requiring an injection of contrast, CT is noninvasive and reasonably defines the magnitude of a hepatic injury, along with the amount of intraperitoneal blood that is present. Should the patient with a hepatic injury remain hemodynamically stable during CT evaluation, nonoperative management is likely to be chosen (discussed below).

The other technique used to detect hepatic and other injuries in hemodynamically stable patients

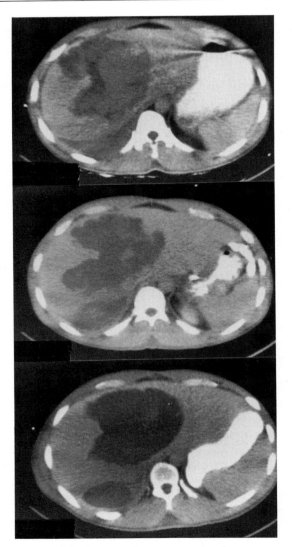

Figure 11-1. Nonoperative management of an intrahepatic hematoma (12/29/86) was chosen for this patient, who presented to the hospital several days after a motor vehicle accident. Sequential CT scans showed liquefaction of the hematoma (1/5/87, 1/16/87). The patient had complete resolution of the hematoma within 6 weeks of the injury. (From Feliciano DV, Pachter HL. Hepatic trauma revisited. *Curr Probl Surg* 1989; 26(7): 453–524. Used with permission.)

has been diagnostic laparoscopy performed under local anesthesia in the emergency center or under general anesthesia in the operating room. The accuracy of laparoscopy in detecting intra-abdominal injuries requiring operation has been comparable to that of diagnostic peritoneal lavage in several series. To date, the ability of diagnostic laparoscopy to significantly lower the incidence of negative or nontherapeutic laparotomies has been no better than that of diagnostic peritoneal lavage or CT. This fact, in addition to the charges for the technique ($430 in emergency department; $3000–$3325 in operating room plus 1-day hospitalization), strongly suggests that laparoscopy should be further studied in experienced trauma centers rather than recommended for widespread usage.

Penetrating Abdominal Trauma

In contrast to patients with blunt multisystem trauma including the abdomen, hypotensive patients or those with peritonitis after suffering penetrating wounds in proximity to the abdomen undergo emergent laparotomy because the area of hemorrhage or reason for peritonitis is obvious.

When a patient with a penetrating (through the peritoneum) anterior (to the anterior axillary line) stab wound is asymptomatic, diagnostic options that have been utilized to detect hepatic and other injuries include serial physical examinations, diagnostic peritoneal tap and lavage, if necessary, and the previously described ultrasonography, diagnostic laparoscopy, and CT. Serial physical examinations result in a 5% to 6% incidence of delayed operations for visceral injuries requiring repair and only a rare unnecessary operation. In a patient with a hepatic injury, such a delay might occur until the volume of blood draining from a small hepatic perforation is significant enough to cause hypotension or peritonitis. Local wound exploration to verify peritoneal penetration followed by a diagnostic peritoneal tap and lavage, if necessary, results in a 1% to 3% incidence of delayed operations for visceral injuries requiring repair. Also, a 5% to 10% incidence of unnecessary operations is caused by intraperitoneal collections of blood originating at the site of the stab wound in the abdominal wall. The role of ultrasonography and diagnostic laparoscopy in patients with possible penetrating anterior stab wounds is still to be determined, though the absence of intraperitoneal blood noted on the former and the absence of peritoneal penetration noted on the latter would clearly be indications for a nonoperative approach. The final approach utilizes

contrast CT to evaluate the magnitude of hepatic and diaphragmatic injuries in stable patients with gunshot wounds to the right upper quadrant and will be discussed under management options in penetrating abdominal trauma, below.

Stable patients who are asymptomatic after suffering flank or back stab or gunshot wounds that might involve the liver may also be evaluated by serial physical examinations. This approach results in a 5% to 8% incidence of delayed operations for visceral injuries requiring repair. An alternative approach is to use triple-contrast CT (intravenous to visualize solid viscera and blood vessels, upper gastrointestinal to visualize the duodenum, rectal to visualize the colon). This technique has a combined false-negative, false-positive incidence of only 2% to 3%, but is both time-consuming and labor-intensive for the radiology department.

Classification

Prior to 1989, no uniformly accepted classification of hepatic injuries existed. This situation was subsequently corrected by the Organ Injury Scaling Committee of the American Association for the Surgery of Trauma (AAST) with the development of the Liver Injury Scale (Table 11-1).

Management

Options in Blunt Trauma

The options for management of patients with blunt hepatic injuries are either nonoperative or operative. Nonoperative management of blunt hepatic injuries in adults was a logical step after the long period of success with nonoperative management of similar injuries in pediatric trauma centers. This approach is recommended only for patients who have been hemodynamically stable since the time of injury or for those with modest hypotension that has responded rapidly to the infusion of crystalloids in the emergency department. Obviously, such patients should have no other indication for laparotomy. The immediate availability of a modern-generation CT scanner, an experienced CT technician, and a radiologist with extensive experience in interpreting abdominal CTs in trauma patients is mandatory.

Table 11-1. Liver Injury Scale, American Association for the Surgery of Trauma

Grade[a]	Injury Description[b]	ICD-9[c]	AIS[d] 85	AIS 90
I. Hematoma	Subcapsular, nonexpanding, < 10% surface area	864.01 864.11	2	2
Laceration	Capsular tear, nonbleeding, < 1-cm parenchymal depth	864.02 864.12	2	2
II. Hematoma	Subcapsular, nonexpanding, 10%–50% surface area Intraparenchymal, nonexpanding, < 2 cm in diameter	864.01 864.11	2	2
Laceration	Capsular tear, active bleeding; 1–3-cm parenchymal depth, < 10 cm in length	864.03 864.13	2	2
III. Hematoma	Subcapsular, > 50% surface area or expanding Ruptured subcapsular hematoma with active bleeding Intraparenchymal hematoma > 2 cm or expanding		3	3
Laceration	> 3-cm parenchymal depth	864.04 864.14	3	3
IV. Hematoma	Ruptured intraparenchymal hematoma with active bleeding		3	4
Laceration	Parenchymal disruption involving 25%–50% of hepatic lobe	864.04 864.14	4	4
V. Laceration	Parenchymal disruption involving > 50% of hepatic lobe		5	5
Vascular	Juxtahepatic venous injuries, i.e., retrohepatic vena cava/major hepatic veins		5	5
VI. Vascular	Hepatic avulsion			6

[a]Advance one grade for multiple injuries to the same organ.
[b]Based on most accurate assessment at autopsy, laparotomy, or radiologic study.
[c]ICD-9 = International Classification of Diseases, Ninth Division.
[d]AIS = Abbreviated Injury Scale, 1990.
Source: Moore EE, et al. Organ injury scaling: Spleen, liver, and kidney. *J Trauma* 29: 1664–1666. © 1989 The Williams & Wilkins Co., Baltimore.

Hepatic lesions that were observed most commonly in the early experience at San Francisco General Hospital were simple parenchymal lacerations, subcapsular hematomas, and intrahepatic hematomas. In addition, there should be no evidence of active bleeding on the CT, no intraperitoneal blood collection over 250 ml, and, again, no other intraperitoneal injury requiring a laparotomy. The majority of such injuries managed nonoperatively in the early experience was AAST grades I to III. With increasing experience in many centers, nonoperative management has been extended to lesions that appear to be AAST grade IV or V on the contrast CT. One reason for this change has been the recognition that CT grading of the magnitude of a blunt hepatic injury is somewhat imprecise. In one recent series by Croce et al., 84% of CT grades of injury were either too high or too low, or a hepatic injury had been missed after the preoperative CT grades were compared to operative findings. Also, hemodynamic stability at the time of admission to the emergency department has been more predictive of the success of nonoperative management than the actual grade of injury in several prospective series.

When nonoperative management of hepatic lacerations or hematomas is chosen, the patient management protocol involves absolute bedrest and monitoring in the surgical intensive care unit, serial examinations, and serial measurements of the hematocrit. The interval for a follow-up abdominal CT varies from center to center, with many centers choosing to perform a repeat CT 2 days after injury to see if there has been substantial worsening (or healing) of the injury during the early period of observation. An alternative approach in the asymptomatic patient is to repeat the abdominal CT 5 to 7 days after the original study in order to plan the remainder of the patient's management. Should the repeat CT show no change in the hepatic injury in the asymptomatic and hemodynamically stable patient, the patient is moved to a stepdown unit or surgical floor for several more days of observation before the next CT. A patient with obvious improvement of the hepatic injury may be discharged home if a family member is available to stay in the house with the patient at all times until an outpatient CT demonstrates substantial healing. A stable patient whose in-hospital follow-up CT demonstrates active hemorrhage is managed with operation or a selective hepatic arteriogram.

It should be obvious that nonoperative management of a significant hepatic injury may not be cost-effective, particularly when repeated outpatient CT scans are performed to document final healing. For this reason, some centers have chosen to observe asymptomatic stable patients without repeat CTs in the outpatient setting. Although Knudson and others have demonstrated persistent intrahepatic defects on CT scans even years after the original period of nonoperative management, these lesions do not appear to cause clinical problems. In general, 90% to 95% of observed hepatic injuries are healed or nearly healed within 8 weeks.

In active patients treated with nonoperative management, the question of return to contact sports such as football, hockey, or rugby is often raised. A safe policy is to forbid a return to any of these activities until near-complete or complete healing of the hepatic injury is observed on the outpatient CT.

Nonoperative management is considered a failure when one of the following is present: (1) repeated episodes of hypotension during observation; (2) continuing need for transfusion; (3) increasing tenderness or signs of peritonitis on physical examination; (4) increase in size of the original injury on CT or clinical evidence of continuing hemorrhage; and (5) an intrahepatic hematoma that is acting as a septic focus. On rare occasions, a hepatic arteriogram with selective therapeutic embolization is preferable to an emergency operation if the patient has other life-threatening injuries mandating continued care in the intensive care unit (increased intracranial pressure, circulatory failure secondary to severe cardiac contusion, respiratory failure requiring jet ventilation, etc.). In all other instances an emergency operation for control of hepatic hemorrhage is appropriate. Operative management of blunt hepatic injuries is currently performed in 75% to 80% of adults, utilizing a wide variety of techniques, to be discussed.

Options in Penetrating Trauma

In asymptomatic patients who have remained hemodynamically stable after suffering penetrating stab wounds directly over the liver in the right thoracoabdominal area or right upper quadrant of the abdomen, nonoperative management is once again appropriate. As previously noted, serial physical examinations in combination with the measurement of serial hematocrits are indicated in such a patient. If a hepatic injury is present, it is presumably small and nonbleeding. On rare occasions bile peritonitis will develop during the period of observation secondary to a perforation of the gallbladder rather than the liver. The period of observation in patients who continue to be asymptomatic is generally 24 hours. The patient is then discharged with specific instructions to return to the emergency department if increasing abdominal pain, nausea and vomiting, or sweating and lightheadedness occur at home. Since late deaths have occurred in rare patients with penetrating wounds involving the colon rather than the liver, the patient is scheduled for an early return to the clinic or the surgeon's office after discharge.

As previously noted, another option in the asymptomatic or mildly symptomatic patient with a stab wound in proximity to the liver is to perform a local wound exploration (for right upper quadrant or epigastric wound) to verify peritoneal penetration. A positive exploration is followed by a diagnostic peritoneal tap and lavage, if necessary. The return of 20 ml of blood on the tap or the presence of 100,000 RBCs/mm^3 on quantitative analysis of the lavage effluent is considered to be a positive study in several trauma centers with extensive experience with the technique. A "negative" exploration of the site of the stab wound should prompt an immediate discharge of the patient from the emergency department, whereas a negative diagnostic peritoneal tap followed by a negative peritoneal lavage mandates 24 hours of in-hospital observation.

A gunshot wound traversing the right thoracoabdominal area has traditionally prompted an emergency operation. Most of these wounds injure the right lower lobe of the lung, the right hemidiaphragm, and the right lobe of the liver. Since the intrapleural hemo- or pneumothorax can be managed by the insertion of a thoracostomy tube and hepatic herniation through a bullet hole in the right hemidiaphragm does not occur, the sole indication for operation would be to repair the injury in the right lobe of the liver. Preliminary evidence from the group at Grady Memorial Hospital suggests that a mildly symptomatic and hemodynamically stable patient who has suffered a right thoracoabdominal gunshot wound should undergo a contrast CT in preference to an emergency operation. If the CT documents that only the liver, hemidiaphragm, and/or right lower lobe of the lung have been injured and minimal intraperitoneal blood is present, nonoperative management is chosen. Nonoperative management has been found to be safe in properly selected patients because healing of transhepatic missile tracks occurs in a fashion similar to that described with blunt hepatic injuries. Further studies from other centers will be necessary to validate this approach. Operative management of penetrating hepatic injuries is currently performed in 90% to 95% of adults, utilizing a wide variety of techniques, to be discussed.

Controversies in Operative Management

Significant changes in the operative management of patients with hepatic injuries have occurred over the past 25 years. In former years limited periods of occlusion of the porta hepatis (Pringle maneuver) coupled with nonselective approaches such as the use of large compressing mattress sutures, frequent lobar resection, and dearterialization of an injured lobe were used. All patients were also managed with open Penrose drainage in the postoperative period. Although these techniques were clearly successful in managing many patients, both postoperative morbidity and mortality were unacceptable in patients with the higher grades of hepatic injury. For example, in the hands of trauma surgeons without extensive experience in elective hepatic resection, the operative mortality for major lobar resection in the trauma patient has been 25% to 50% in several series. This figure decreases to 10% to 15% when an experienced hepatic surgeon performs the resection, but few of these individuals are the primary surgeon in patients with trauma.

In patients with major hepatic injuries treated with the widespread use of compressing mattress sutures to control parenchymal bleeding, prolonged

drainage of bile and necrotic tissue has often been noted in the postoperative period. The early postoperative period has also been characterized by the development of a "liver fever," now thought to be secondary to the necrosis of hepatic tissue under mattress sutures. Finally, perihepatic abscesses often in proximity to the Penrose drain have occurred in 10% to 15% of patients undergoing nonselective management of major hepatic injuries, and all of these have previously been treated with major reoperations.

In addition to the problems described, two other factors have contributed to changes in operative techniques. The first is the large body of data on tolerance of the liver to ischemia that is available from centers with extensive experience in elective hepatic resection and transplantation. The second is the recognition that prolonged complicated operative procedures in patients with major intraabdominal injuries inevitably lead to intraoperative hypothermia, metabolic acidosis, and persistent coagulopathies. These metabolic sequelae, rather than the hemorrhage from the original injury, may cause the demise of the patient.

It is now clear that 60% of patients with blunt hepatic injuries and 90% of patients with penetrating hepatic injuries requiring operation can have areas of hemorrhage controlled with "simple" techniques of hemostasis. The remaining 40% of patients with blunt hepatic injuries and 10% of patients with penetrating wounds will require "advanced" techniques of hepatic hemostasis, including both the nonselective approaches from the past and current selective approaches (Table 11-2).

Preferred Operative Approach

The patient's anterior trunk from the chin to the middle thighs is prepared and draped. This wide draping allows for access to the thorax for an emergency median sternotomy or left anterolateral thoracotomy during laparotomy and for retrieval of the saphenous vein as a vascular conduit for other injuries in the abdomen. Full circumferential preparation and draping of the trunk has been used in a few centers to permit dependent drainage through the bed of the resected twelfth rib after extensive hepatic repairs or resections.

A midline incision from the xyphoid to the pubis is used in any hypotensive patient thought to

Table 11-2. "Advanced" Techniques
for Hepatic Hemostasis

Extensive hepatorrhaphy (mattress sutures)
Hepatotomy with selective vascular ligation (finger fracture or
    cautery to reach vessels and ducts)
Balloon catheter tamponade in track of wound
Resectional debridement with selective vascular ligation
Formal resection (lobectomy)
Selective hepatic artery ligation (SHAL)
Absorbable mesh compressive wrap
Perihepatic packing with laparotomy pads

have significant intra-abdominal injuries. All blood and gastrointestinal contents are manually evacuated with laparotomy pads and a suction device. Blood may also be aspirated with an autotransfusion device even if contamination from the gastrointestinal tract is present, since there is now preliminary evidence that washing and parenteral antibiotics allow for the safe return of such blood to the patient. In patients who have suffered blunt trauma, hemorrhage usually arises from solid organ injuries, whereas injuries to the gastrointestinal tract are less common and injuries to retroperitoneal vascular structures are rare. In patients with penetrating wounds, hemorrhage usually arises from the small bowel, colon, liver, and retroperitoneal or mesenteric vascular structures.

If the source of hemorrhage turns out to be a minor or modest hepatic injury (AAST grade I or II), then only a "simple" technique of hemostasis will be necessary. A capsular avulsion or laceration less than 1 cm in depth with hemorrhage will usually respond to 5 minutes of compression with a laparotomy pad and does not need to be drained. An approved topical agent such as Surgicel (oxidized regenerated cellulose; Johnson & Johnson, New Brunswick, NJ) or Avitene (microfibrillar collagen hemostat; Med Chem Products, Woburn, Mass.) may also be used to control hemorrhage when Glisson's capsule is avulsed. An electrocautery is used to control any remaining bleeders after compression is removed.

Parenchymal lacerations that are 1 to 3 cm deep are AAST grade II injuries and account for more than 50% of all hepatic injuries treated. Such a laceration should be carefully inspected, and any open vessels or bile ducts selectively clipped or suture-ligated. Some centers have approval to use

an experimental topical agent such as Fibrin Sealant (fibrin glue; Immuno AG, Vienna) or even mix their own version using a combination of fibrinogen, thrombin, aprotinin, and calcium chloride. If hemorrhage from the grade II laceration cannot be controlled by a combination of a topical agent and 5 minutes of compression or even use of the electrocautery in a patient with a coagulopathy, then suture hepatorrhaphy is indicated.

Hepatorrhaphy has traditionally been performed using horizontal mattress sutures of No. 0 chromic placed with a large blunt needle. It is easier and just as effective to place a No. 0 or 2–0 chromic suture in a continuous fashion to loosely approximate the edges of the laceration for control of hemorrhage. Hepatic tissue that blanches as the suture is pulled tight will often undergo necrosis in the postoperative period. In the patient without a coagulopathy, the laceration may be left open if selective clipping of bile ducts and vessels has been successful. Although there is no convincing evidence that a grade II laceration needs to be drained in the postoperative period, many surgeons choose to place a closed suction drain beneath the injured lobe for several days.

When preliminary inspection or palpation confirms the presence of a grade III, IV, or V hepatic injury, a vascular clamp is applied to all structures in the hepatoduodenal ligament (Pringle maneuver). This clamp does not need to be removed until hepatic hemostasis is attained, and occlusion times in excess of 60 minutes without postoperative sequelae have been reported from several centers. Either the surgeon or the assistant should then compress the injured lobe with laparotomy pads as the nursing team, anesthesiologist, and blood bank are informed about the magnitude of the hepatic injury. Instruments that should be available in the operating room prior to release of compression include small, medium, and large metallic clips and appliers, a liver clamp, complete vascular surgery tray, sternal saw, and sternotomy retractor. In addition, all of the standard maneuvers used to prevent hypothermia in the injured patient should be instituted (Table 11-3).

The time-honored approach to the control of hemorrhage in deep hepatic lacerations has been the insertion of the previously mentioned horizontal mattress sutures. These sutures compress bleeding vessels in lacerations greater than 3 cm

Table 11-3. Operating Room Maneuvers to Prevent Hypothermia in Patients with Major Hepatic Injuries*

Cover patient's head with turban or "space" hat if this was not done in the emergency department.

Increase temperature level in the operating room, especially if a pediatric patient is the victim.

Place patient on heating blanket in the operating room and turn it on immediately.

Cover patient's lower extremities with plastic garbage bag or "space" blanket in the operating room.

Irrigate nasogastric and thoracostomy tubes with warm saline during laparotomy.

Irrigate open pericardial cavity, pleural cavities, and peritoneal cavity during simultaneous sternotomy-thoracotomy and laparotomy.

Turn up heating cascade on anesthesia machine.

*All fluids and blood products are warmed.

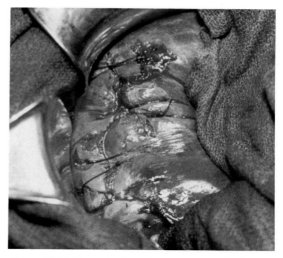

Figure 11-2. Extensive hepatic necrosis resulted when mattress sutures and selective hepatic artery ligation were used to control parenchymal hemorrhage. (Reprinted with permission from Feliciano DV. In Fischer JE, *Common Problems in Gastrointestinal Surgery. Copyright © 1989 by Year Book Medical Publishers, Inc., Chicago.*)

deep or control hemorrhage from the tracks of stab wounds or missiles. As previously noted, this non-selective technique has been used less frequently in recent years because reoperations in patients who have had the adjunct of perihepatic packing have often demonstrated extensive necrosis of hepatic parenchyma under the mattress sutures. This problem may be aggravated by the simultaneous use of selective ligation of the hepatic artery to the injured lobe (SHAL) (Fig. 11-2). Extensive hepatorrhaphies are still appropriate in patients with multiple associated intra-abdominal injuries and an intraoperative coagulopathy that is not controlled by perihepatic packing. The technique is also useful for the surgeon with little or no experience in more selective techniques of hepatic hemostasis. When the technique is used, every attempt should be made to apply only modest tension as the mattress sutures are tied in order to limit the amount of parenchymal necrosis.

In recent years, hepatotomy, or incision into the liver, with selective vascular ligation has been used more frequently to control hemorrhage in deep hepatic lacerations or in the tracks of stab or missile wounds. This technique has been popularized by Pachter and consists of finger fracture or use of the electrocautery in line with a laceration or track of a penetrating wound to allow for visualization of the bleeding vessel. It should be performed early in the operative procedure before multiple transfusions and hypothermia have created a

coagulopathy. Also, unless careful clipping or ligation of vessels in the normal parenchyma is performed, these structures will continue to bleed into the hepatotomy site while the major deep source of hemorrhage is being sought. After the overlying parenchyma is divided, retractors are inserted into the opened laceration or track to help locate the bleeding vessels (Fig. 11-3). Small branches of the hepatic artery are clipped or ligated if they are the source of hemorrhage, and lateral venorrhaphy with No. 5–0 or 6–0 polypropylene suture may occasionally be possible on large intrahepatic branches of the portal vein or hepatic veins. Hepatotomy is extremely valuable as a selective technique, but is best performed by an experienced trauma surgeon who understands the appropriate indications and operative technique.

Diffuse oozing in a deep laceration or hepatotomy site may be treated by the insertion of a viable omental pack mobilized from the stomach and colon. The omental pack is also used as a "filler" in a deep laceration or hepatotomy site, even when there is no active hemorrhage or oozing (Fig. 11-4). The filling of intrahepatic dead space in combination with the introduction of large numbers of mac-

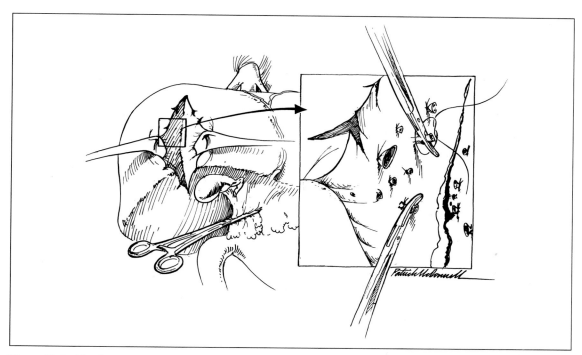

Figure 11-3. After hepatotomy by finger fracture or electrocautery, selective clipping or ligation of disrupted vessels and biliary ducts is performed. (From Feliciano DV. In Schwartz SI, Ellis H, *Maingot's Abdominal Operations,* Norwalk: Appleton & Lange, 1989. P. 492. Used with permission.)

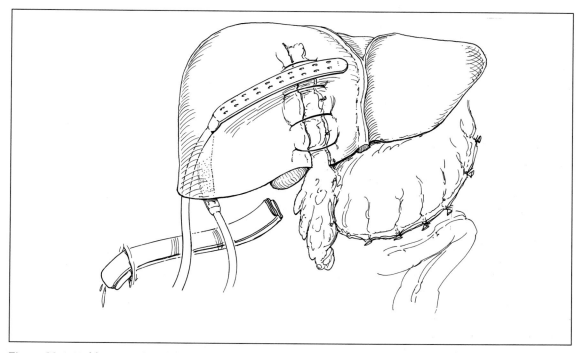

Figure 11-4. Viable omental pack inserted into hepatotomy site. (From Feliciano DV, Pachter HL. Hepatic trauma revisited. *Curr Probl Surg* 1989; 26(7):453–524. Used with permission.)

rophages in the "milky spots" of the omentum may be responsible for the low rate of perihepatic sepsis reported in many recent series. The viable omentum is placed into the deep laceration or hepatotomy site and held in place by chromic sutures that compress the sides of the laceration around the omentum. It is expected that the viable omentum will tamponade capillary oozing, aid in the absorption of local blood and bile, and minimize drainage from the opening in the liver in the postoperative period, but there is no evidence that it will accelerate healing of the hepatic injury. There is, however, much anecdotal evidence that the decreased drainage from the area of injury in the postoperative period lessens the incidence of perihepatic abscesses. With the widespread use of the viable omental pack in the current management of hepatic injuries, it is unlikely that a prospective study to evaluate its benefits will be performed.

Balloon catheter tamponade, a technique used by vascular and cardiac surgeons to control hemorrhage for the past 35 years, has now been applied to a small subset of patients with exsanguinating hemorrhage from complex hepatic injuries. Examples would be patients with penetrating bilobar injuries or those with deep tracks through the middle of a lobe. In either group, deep mattress sutures are unlikely to be effective, and the extensive hepatotomy needed would not appeal to many trauma surgeons. Either a Foley or Fogarty balloon catheter or a combination of a Penrose drain with a preselected length acting as a long balloon over a red rubber catheter is passed into the long track. The balloon catheter is inflated at various depths until hemorrhage from the ends of the track ceases (Fig. 11-5). The Penrose red rubber catheter combination is inflated with a saline and meglumine diatrizoate (Gastrografin) mixture once it fills the whole track.

As a reoperation for removal of the balloon has been performed in patients reported to date, a towel clip or suture closure of the skin only is used once the balloon catheter is in place. After the patient's operative hypothermia and coagulopathy are corrected over the following 24 to 72 hours, the patient is returned to the operating room for evacuation of clot, deflation of the balloon, further techniques of hemostasis as needed, insertion of an omental pack within the track, and a complete examination of all

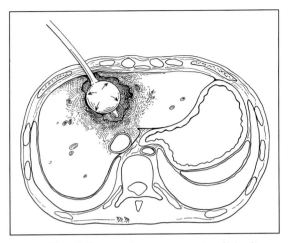

Figure 11-5. Balloon catheter tamponade of bleeding vessels in missile track.

intra-abdominal viscera and vessels if this was not performed at the first procedure. Much as in its use in vascular trauma procedures, rebleeding has not been a problem with deflation of the balloon in a patient without a residual coagulopathy. There will be some patients in whom removal of a balloon catheter passed through the skin at the first operation can be performed by deflation of the balloon in the surgical intensive care unit. A reoperation in order to perform the maneuvers listed above is preferable, however, and should be well tolerated by the hemodynamically stable patient. Balloon catheter tamponade will be necessary in less than 5% of patients with hepatic injuries, but can be life-saving in the complex situations described.

Resectional debridement with selective vascular ligation, a technique similar to hepatotomy, is used to remove devascularized tissue from the edges of the liver or from deep lacerations. In many patients with blunt hepatic injuries, there are areas of disruption containing avulsed vascular structures and biliary ducts. Ligation or clipping of these structures alone is inappropriate because the surrounding hepatic tissue has also been devascularized. Debridement of the entire area is best performed by use of the electrocautery or finger fracture technique in a new line outside the area of injury. This technique allows for the clean division of disrupted vessels and biliary ducts where they are still intact and is followed by formal debridement of all these structure as well as of the devascularized hepatic parenchyma.

Resectional debridement properly performed in a hepatic laceration should leave two flat surfaces in which all vessels and biliary ducts have been ligated or clipped. A viable omental pack is then inserted into the laceration as previously described and fixed in place with absorbable sutures. When resectional debridement is performed on the edge of the liver, an omental pack is not used to cover the raw surface. The reason is that any tamponading effect is lost when only a thin sheet of omentum is wrapped around the raw surface. Moreover, fluid collections may become trapped behind the sheet of omentum and may not be accessible to suction drains placed below the area of debridement.

Formal resection including segmentectomy, lobectomy, or a very extensive resectional debridement used to complete the plane of injury is performed in only 2% to 4% of patients with hepatic injuries. As previously noted, the high mortality associated with resection performed by surgeons without extensive experience in elective hepatic surgery has prompted a shift to nonresectional approaches in most centers. Lobectomy is still indicated (1) when there is total disruption of a segment or lobe, (2) when it is the only technique that will control life-threatening hemorrhage, or (3) when the extent of injury precludes the use of an absorbable mesh compressive wrap or the insertion of perihepatic packs. If a formal hepatic lobectomy is necessary, it may be worthwhile to extend the midline abdominal incision into a median sternotomy. This extension allows for better visualization of the posterior supporting ligaments of the injured lobe and creates less pain, pulmonary complications, and problems with wound healing as compared to an oblique thoracoabdominal incision.

Hepatic lobectomy is performed with a Pringle maneuver in place, but without preliminary hilar dissection and ligation. After division of the posterior supporting ligaments, the dome of the liver is marked with the electrocautery from one side of the gallbladder bed back to the ipsilateral side of the retrohepatic vena cava. This conservative line of resection is indicated to preserve the middle hepatic vein that drains both the medial aspect of the anterior segment of the right lobe and the medial segment of the left lobe. Sacrifice of this vein is

usually not necessary in hepatic lobectomy performed for trauma.

In order to decrease the amount of clipping or ligating as the parenchyma is divided, it may be helpful to place a parenchymal compression clamp (Lin or Longmire) around the lobe to be resected. If the clamp cannot be placed, the surgeon then rapidly and selectively clips or ligates and divides vessels and ducts in the interlobar septum. As the inferior vena cava is approached, the main right hepatic vein can be grasped within the hepatic parenchyma with a Satinsky clamp. On the left side, care must be taken to clamp the left hepatic vein before it joins the middle hepatic vein (in 84% of patients). Selective vascular ligation is then used to control hemorrhage and leakage of bile in the raw edge of the hepatic lobe that remains. As previously noted, a significant incidence of both postoperative perihepatic abscesses and perioperative mortality results when hepatic resection is performed for trauma.

Selective hepatic artery ligation (SHAL) has been used less frequently in recent years as direct transhepatic approaches to parenchymal bleeders have become more common. The primary indication for the technique has been the inability to directly control arterial hemorrhage in a hepatotomy site, blunt laceration, or track of a penetrating wound. If temporary occlusion of the individual artery to the injured lobe causes cessation of arterial bleeding in one of the sites mentioned, then the artery is selectively ligated. Failure of the technique to control hemorrhage indicates ligation of the wrong lobar artery, usually due to an anomalous origin or to injury to an intrahepatic portal vein, hepatic vein, or the retrohepatic vena cava. The safety of the technique arises from the higher oxygen saturation in the portal vein of humans compared to other animals, the absence of portal bacteremia in humans without terminal hypotension, and the extensive collateral arterial flow to each lobe of the liver should its principal artery be ligated. The technique should be used with caution in patients with cirrhosis because flow through the remaining lobar portal vein may already be compromised. Also, some increased necrosis of hepatic parenchyma under tight mattress sutures in the injured lobe usually occurs. The technique of selective hepatic artery ligation is a valuable one but will be necessary in less than 1% of patients with hepatic injuries.

Several reports about the use of absorbable mesh compressive wrapping in controlling hemorrhage from severely disrupted lobes have been published. Much as with its use in patients with major splenic or renal fractures, an absorbable mesh wrap appears to be an effective technique to control oozing. The mesh is applied after selective ligation of disrupted vessels and biliary ducts and debridement of fragmented and devascularized hepatic parenchyma. After the mesh is wrapped around one or both lobes (leaving splits around the suprahepatic vena cava and the portal structures), it is pulled tight so as to compress the remaining hepatic tissue. The mesh is then fixed to itself using a continuous suture line or a TA-90 stapler. The technique is analogous to the use of perihepatic packing for tamponade in patients with coagulopathies or subcapsular hematomas and has the added advantage of avoiding a reoperation in otherwise stable patients. The major disadvantage appears to be the time needed to fully mobilize an injured lobe if this has not been performed previously and then to wrap and fixate the mesh in the patient with hypothermia and a coagulopathy. Absorbable mesh compressure wrapping appears to be a valuable adjunct in managing disrupted lobes that cannot be safely debrided or resected.

Perihepatic packing refers to the insertion of folded dry laparotomy pads between the hemidiaphragm and the injured lobe and, on occasion, under the injured lobe. Packs are placed in approximately 4% to 5% of patients with hepatic injuries, and there is reasonable consensus about the appropriate indications (Table 11-4). The majority of patients who need packing are those with intraoperative coagulopathies associated with metabolic failure—that is, body temperature approaching or less than 32°C and persistent arterial pH less than 7.2. In this group of patients the previously described simple and advanced techniques of hepatic hemostasis will not control diffuse oozing ("nonmechanical bleeding") from exposed hepatic parenchyma or previously placed suture lines. Once a coagulopathy occurs, a nonadherent 30- × 45-cm Steri-Drape (3M, St. Paul, Minn.) is folded on itself and placed over any hepatic parenchyma or suture lines to prevent the dry packs from adhering to

Table 11-4. Indications of Perihepatic Packing

Patient will have to be transferred because of lack of facilities, blood, or experience in dealing with hepatic trauma.

Intraoperative coagulopathy induced by massive transfusion and hypothermia.

Presence of a large nonexpanding subcapsular hematoma.

Failure of routine hemostatic maneuvers in the patient who is not a candidate for a major resectional debridement or lobectomy.

Severe bilobar injury.

Need to terminate operation in a patient with multiple injuries, including the liver and intraoperative hemodynamic or cardiac instability.

these areas as the coagulopathy resolves. Folded dry laparotomy packs are then placed over the Steri-Drape to compress oozing vessels in the injured lobe. If oozing is also occurring on the undersurface of the liver, more laparotomy pads should be inserted beneath the lobe. Only a towel clip or suture closure of the skin is performed because a reoperation will be necessary to remove the packs.

Should there be continued hemorrhage in the early postoperative period, the combination of perihepatic packs and clot may increase intra-abdominal pressure to greater than 25 mm Hg. This pressure will compress the retrohepatic and suprarenal inferior vena cava as well as the renal veins, leading to oliguric renal failure. In the hemodynamically stable patient with oliguria unresponsive to volume replacement, it may be worthwhile to return the patient to the operating room for removal of clot and some laparotomy pads. Perihepatic packs are otherwise removed at 48 to 72 hours in most centers after the patient's hypothermia, coagulopathy, and metabolic acidosis have been corrected.

At the reoperation to remove the perihepatic packs, clots are evacuated, the peritoneal cavity is irrigated clean, and drains are inserted in the right subhepatic and subphrenic areas. The survival rate for patients with perihepatic packing ranged from 43% to 90% (mean 74%) in six series with 10 or more patients reported from 1981 to 1986. In 10% to 15% of survivors, perihepatic fluid collections, infected seromas, or abscesses have occurred, an incidence similar to that reported with other advanced techniques of hepatic hemostasis, emergent or elective hepatic resection for nontrauma indications, or hepatic transplantation. Perihepatic packing continues to be a life-saving maneuver in a highly selected group of patients with hepatic injuries and metabolic or anatomic reasons that preclude continued use of other techniques of hepatic hemostasis.

Several techniques of hepatic hemostasis will usually be used in most patients with grade III, IV, or V hepatic injuries. After control of hemorrhage by hepatotomy, resectional debridement, or chromic sutures, the Pringle maneuver is removed, and selective ligation of residual bleeders is performed. Continued venous oozing in the depths of a hepatotomy site or hepatic laceration can often be controlled by insertion of a viable omental pack, and arterial bleeding may rarely require selective hepatic artery ligation in the porta. An absorbable compressive mesh wrap may then be needed to approximate a disrupted lobe containing viable parenchyma, and perihepatic packs would be the choice if there is diffuse oozing from the injured lobe associated with an intraoperative coagulopathy. A comprehensive knowledge of the techniques described and a flexible operative approach will yield the best results in patients with major hepatic injuries.

Results

In patients with hepatic injuries who survive the perioperative period, the incidence of complications is dependent on the magnitude of the original injury. Injury-related complications such as hyperpyrexia, postoperative bleeding, perihepatic abscess, biliary fistula, and late hemorrhage or hemobilia essentially occur only in patients with grade III, IV, or V injuries (Table 11-5).

Hyperpyrexia

The multicenter report from the Western Trauma Association authored by Cogbill et al. was one of the first to document the significant incidence of postoperative hyperpyrexia in victims of major hepatic injuries. Over 10% of patients had a maximum daily temperature of 39°C or greater for the first 3 consecutive postoperative days, and another 53% were noted to have a maximum daily temperature between 38.0°C and 39.0°C for the same period of time. Although the etiology of this temperature elevation is unclear, the significant incidence in

Table 11-5. Postoperative Complications in Patients with Grade III, IV, or V Hepatic Injuries

	Cogbill et al, 1988[a] (n=129)	Pachter et al, 1992[b] (n=128)
Hyperpyrexia	82 (64%)	Not reported
Coagulopathy/early postoperative bleeding	21 (16%)	2 (1.6%)
Abscess	13 (10%)	11 (8.6%)
Biliary fistula	10 (8%)	9 (7.0%)
Late hemorrhage	9 (7%)	Not reported

[a]Data from Cogbill TH, et al. Severe hepatic trauma: A multi-center experience with 1,335 liver injuries. *J Trauma* 28: 1433–1438. © 1988 The Williams & Wilkins Co., Baltimore.
[b]Data from Pachter HL, et al. Significant trends in the treatment of hepatic trauma: Experience with 411 injuries. *Ann Surg* 1992; 215: 492–502. Used with permission.

patients with blunt disruption strongly suggests that parenchymal necrosis is a contributing factor.

Coagulopathy/Early Postoperative Bleeding

Hemorrhage in the early postoperative period is due to failure to control bleeding vessels in the parenchyma, porta, or retrohepatic area, to a coagulopathy from multiple transfusions and hypothermia, or to a combination of both. The first priority in the surgical intensive care unit is to provide clotting factors through infusions of fresh-frozen plasma. Even in the most experienced trauma centers, actively bleeding trauma patients rarely receive adequate operative replacement of clotting factors in relation to the large volumes of packed red blood cells that are transfused. The second priority is to reverse hypothermia by infusing only warmed fluids and blood, using a warming cascade on the ventilator and covering the entire patient with one of the commercially available warming "cocoons." If repeated episodes of hypotension and increasing abdominal distention occur as clotting factors are being replaced and hypothermia is being reversed, an early reoperation may be necessary. Should only a coagulopathy be present at the early reoperation, the insertion of perihepatic packs as well as intra-abdominal packs and a towel clip closure of only the skin of the incision are appropriate.

An early reoperation is obviously also indicated whenever the coagulopathy and hypothermia have been reversed but persistent bloody drainage or the hypotension-distention combination mentioned above is present. At the reoperation it may be necessary to remove sutures or even the omental pack in order to visualize the source of hemorrhage. Selective hepatic artery ligation or the insertion of perihepatic packs is indicated when the discrete bleeder(s) cannot be controlled by direct clipping or suturing. Continued bleeding in the surgical intensive care unit is best managed by the interventional radiologist (see below).

Perihepatic Abscess

The incidence of perihepatic infected seromas, hematomas, or abscesses depends upon the age of the patient, the magnitude of the hepatic injury, the associated blood loss, the presence of injuries to other organs such as the colon or pancreas, the type of operative repair, and the type of drainage used during the postoperative period. A patient at the highest risk for the development of a postoperative perihepatic abscess is one with a grade III, IV, or V injury, an associated injury to the colon or pancreas, continued bleeding in the postoperative period, and use of open (Penrose) drainage. It is obvious, therefore, that attaining hepatic hemostasis at the first operation and the use of a

closed (Jackson-Pratt) drain in the postoperative period may lower the incidence of postoperative abscesses.

In the patient whose postoperative febrile state persists beyond 5 to 7 days and is associated with a leukocytosis or foul-smelling drainage from either open or closed drains, an emergent CT scan or ultrasound of the abdomen is indicated. A perihepatic fluid collection or abscess detected on the scan is best drained through the flank by the interventional radiologist. First, an 18-gauge Chiba needle is inserted into the collection under CT or ultrasound guidance. The fluid or pus is aspirated to confirm proper placement of the needle as well as to obtain material for Gram's stain and culture. Second, the standard Seldinger technique (guidewire, dilator, drain) is used to insert a van Sonnenberg sump drain with "J" tip (Medi·tech, Watertown, Mass.) into the cavity. When the fluid appears to be viscous, a 14 to 16 French catheter is inserted (Fig. 11-6). The sump catheter may be irrigated on a daily basis with 25 ml of saline containing antibiotics, followed by an injection of 5 ml of the same solution to maintain patency of the catheter. The sump catheter may be replaced with a 10 to 12 French single-lumen catheter over a guidewire as the original cavity is noted to decrease in size on a follow-up

Figure 11-6. A. Right subphrenic abscess demonstrated by sinogram performed through percutaneous catheter on fifty-sixth day after partial right hepatectomy for blunt trauma to the liver. B. Decrease in size of abscess cavity after 8 days of percutaneous drainage. (From Feliciano DV, Pachter HL. Hepatic trauma revisited. *Curr Probl Surg* 1989; 26(7):453–524. Used with permission.)

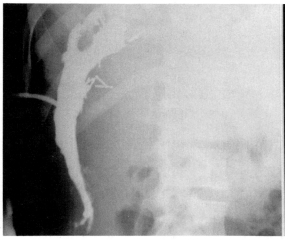 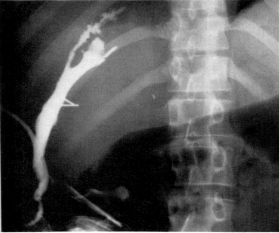

A   B

CT. The percutaneous drain is gradually removed when drainage has ceased, the CT scan demonstrates no residual abscess cavity, and the patient has a normal white blood cell count.

When percutaneous drainage of a perihepatic abscess does not lead to resolution of a septic state in 24 to 48 hours, reoperation is indicated. A first reoperation is performed through a previous drain site or through an extraperitoneal approach such as an anterior subcostal or a posterior incision with resection of the twelfth rib. These directed approaches are based on precise localization of the abscess on abdominal CT or ultrasound. A midline reoperation is indicated in patients who have failed percutaneous drainage or a local extraperitoneal approach and carries the highest morbidity and mortality for the patient.

Biliary Fistula

A postoperative biliary fistula occurs in 8% to 10% of patients with major hepatic injuries. Probable causes include a missed intrahepatic disruption of a biliary duct at operation or dislodgement of a clip or suture on a duct in the postoperative period. Most biliary fistulas are from small ducts, and drainage will be less than 300 ml/d. With drainage of 500 to 750 ml/d, a major duct is obviously leaking. Such a fistula is usually well tolerated if suction drains are in place and fluid and electrolyte status is carefully monitored. In the absence of distal ductal obstruction, a biliary fistula will almost always close within 3 weeks, and most close much sooner. Persistence of a biliary fistula beyond this time should prompt a fistulogram or an endoscopic retrograde cholangiogram. A percutaneous transhepatic cholangiogram may be difficult to perform with the significant distortion that results from a major hepatotomy with omental packing, resectional debridement, or use of an absorbable mesh compressive wrap. A fistulogram that demonstrates major disruption of a large intrahepatic duct 3 weeks after injury should prompt consideration for a reoperation. On rare occasions, resection of the involved residual lobe or an intrahepatic Roux-en-Y hepatodochojejunostomy may be necessary.

A bronchobiliary fistula is a rare complication of a penetrating right thoracoabdominal wound. This fistula has occurred in patients in whom the

original treatment was only a thoracostomy tube inserted for what was presumed to be an isolated intrathoracic wound. A bronchopulmonary fistula has also been seen in patients who drain significant amounts of bile after hepatic repair and have disruption of the diaphragmatic repair performed at the original laparotomy. In either case leaking bile passes through the right hemidiaphragm and enters a bronchial tear in the right lower lobe of the lung. The patient develops a chronic cough productive of bile, usually within 7 to 14 days of the original injury or operation. At a reoperation through the abdomen, the biliary duct should be ligated if it can be found, the perforation in the right hemidiaphragm repaired, and a viable omental pedicle placed between the liver and diaphragm. If significant inflammation and destruction of the right lower lobe of the lung has occurred secondary to the fistula, a right lower lobectomy may need to be performed through a separate right posterolateral thoracotomy.

Late Hemorrhage or Hemobilia

Late hemorrhage into the hepatic parenchyma or hemobilia with gastrointestinal blood originating from the injured liver is essentially always due to a traumatic false aneurysm of one of the intralobar hepatic arteries or a branch. The patient with persistent leukocytosis and right upper quadrant pain in the late postoperative period should undergo a CT scan. If a new large intrahepatic cavity is present, a selective hepatic arteriogram is indicated. In the patient with new-onset gastrointestinal bleeding associated with right upper quadrant pain, the selective hepatic arteriogram is the first study chosen. An arteriogram that demonstrates a ruptured or unruptured traumatic false aneurysm should prompt therapeutic embolization of the involved hepatic artery or branch.

In recent years the Tracker-18 Infusion Catheter (TARGET Therapeutics, Fremont, Calif.) with a distal outer diameter of only 2.7 French has allowed for selective embolization of injured distal branches of the lobar hepatic artery. After precise localization of the bleeding site, a platinum fibered coil for occlusion of vessels is placed into the proximal vessel using a coil pusher. Several coils may need to be inserted to obtain complete occlusion of the

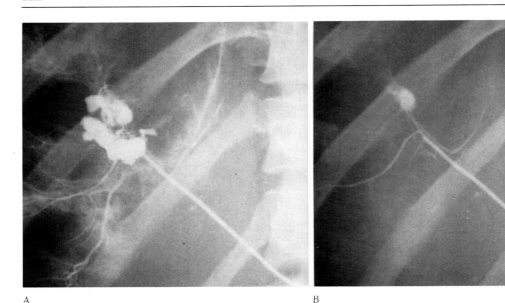

A   B

Figure 11-7. A. Selective right hepatic arteriogram revealed a false aneurysm and hematoma cavity in right lobe of liver in a patient who suffered a gunshot wound previously. B. The responsible artery has been embolized with autologous clot, and the hemorrhage has ceased. (From Feliciano DV, Pachter HL. Hepatic trauma revisited. *Curr Probl Surg* 1989; 26(7):453–524. Used with permission.)

artery at the site of injury. With selective catheterization techniques, the need for injection of autologous clot, absorbable hemostatic material, or larger coil occlusion devices has much diminished in recent years (Fig. 11-7). Even with complete occlusion of a proximal lobar hepatic artery, the ipsilateral lobe should maintain its viability by flow through the portal vein and re-established arterial flow through translobar and subcapsular collaterals within 24 hours.

Mortality

The mean mortality for a large group of patients with hepatic injuries from both blunt and penetrating trauma ranges from 10% to 15% (Table 11-6). Nearly 80% of deaths occur in the perioperative period from shock and transfusion-related coagulopathies. Both the mechanism of injury and the magnitude of the hepatic injury will have a significant impact on survival. For example, the mortality from stab wounds is 5% or less, whereas the operative mortality for major blunt hepatic injuries in tertiary referral centers has been 14% to 31%. The

Table 11-6. Mortality from Hepatic Injuries

Mortality by Etiology

Series	Number of Patients	Blunt Trauma (%)	SW (%)[a]	GSW (%)[b]
Stain et al, 1988[c]	233	25	5	11
Cox et al, 1988[d]	323	31	—	—
Carmona et al, 1982[e]	443	14	2.8	8

Mortality in Grade III, IV, V Injuries[f]

Grade	Number of Patients	Mortality	Hepatic Mortality
III	92 (44%)	23 (25%)	6 (6.5%)
IV	59 (28%)	27 (46%)	18 (30.5%)
V	59 (28%)	47 (80%)	39 (66%)

[a]SW = Stab Wound
[b]GSW = Gunshot Wound
[c]Data from Stain SC, Yellin AE, Donovan AJ. Hepatic trauma. *Arch Surg* 1988; 123: 1251–1255.
[d]Data from Cox EF, et al. Blunt trauma to the liver: Analysis of management and mortality in 323 consecutive patients. *Ann Surg* 1988; 207: 126–134.
[e]Data from Carmona RH, Lim RC Jr, Clark GC. Morbidity and mortality in hepatic trauma: A 5-year study. *Am J Surg* 1982; 144: 88–94.
[f]Source: Cogbill TH, et al. Severe hepatic trauma: A multi-center experience with 1,335 liver injuries. *J Trauma* 28: 1433–1438. © 1988 The Williams & Wilkins Co., Baltimore.

"hepatic" mortality for AAST grade III injuries is only 6.5%, but with grade IV or V injuries, "hepatic" mortality increased to 30.5% and 66%, respectively, in Cogbill's multicenter review.

Conclusions

Injury to the liver occurs in approximately 40% of patients with blunt or penetrating abdominal trauma. Diagnostic peritoneal tap, ultrasonography, computerized tomography, diagnostic laparoscopy, and serial physical examinations may all be indicated in specific circumstances. Similarly, either nonoperative or operative management may be appropriate. Various operative methods to control hemorrhage have been described, and all may be useful for specific injuries. In recent years perihepatic packing, as opposed to major resection, has lowered the mortality of the most severe injuries. The management of postoperative problems such as perihepatic abscess, biliary fistula, and hemobilia often requires a team approach that includes interventional radiologists, endoscopists, and surgeons.

Selected Readings

Beal SL. Fatal hepatic hemorrhage: An unresolved problem in the management of complex liver injuries. *J Trauma* 1990; 30(2):163–169.

Cogbill TH, et al. Severe hepatic trauma: A multi-center experience with 1,335 liver injuries. *J Trauma* 1988; 28(10):1433–1438.

Croce MA, et al. AAST organ injury scale: Correlation of CT-graded liver injuries and operative findings. *J Trauma* 1991; 31(6):806–812.

Feliciano DV, et al. Packing for control of hepatic hemorrhage. *J Trauma* 1986; 26(8):783–743.

Feliciano DV. Diagnostic modalities in abdominal trauma: Peritoneal lavage, ultrasonography, computed tomography scanning, and arteriography. *Surg Clin North Am* 1991; 71(2):241–256.

Feliciano DV, et al. Management of 1000 consecutive cases of hepatic trauma (1979–1984). *Ann Surg* 1986; 204(4):438–445.

Feliciano DV, Pachter HL. Hepatic trauma revisited. *Curr Probl Surg* 1989; 26(7):453–524.

Knudson MM, et al. Nonoperative management of blunt liver injuries in adults: The need for continued surveillance. *J Trauma* 1990; 30(12):1494–1500.

Moore EE, et al. Organ injury scaling: Spleen, liver and kidney. *J Trauma* 1989; 29(12):1664–1666.

Pachter HL, et al. Significant trends in the treatment of hepatic trauma: Experience with 411 injuries. *Ann Surg* 1992; 215(5):492–502.

12

Benign Hepatic Tumors

JAMES H. FOSTER
MARTIN M. BERMAN

In both the laboratory and the clinical situation, the liver exhibits a remarkable ability to grow tumors spontaneously and in response to exogenous stimuli. Most such tumors are benign, and many are innocuous. In patients, these tumors are often discovered incidentally at laparoscopy or open laparotomy done for some other problem. Even more often today, they are found during imaging of the upper abdomen for a wide variety of complaints often unrelated to the tumor. Once discovered, however, such lesions raise several critical questions for the clinician, including whether the tumor is malignant or, if benign, whether it is safer to recommend observation or resection. The answers to those questions require knowledge about the natural history of the several varieties of benign tumor and the morbidity and effectiveness of resection. With appropriate knowledge and experience, the diagnostic workup can be sharply limited and tailored to the individual circumstances of each patient. The predilection of middle-aged females for the more common benign liver tumors and for the most curable of the malignant primary liver tumors sharpens the necessity for accurate diagnosis and clear decision making.

A brief discussion of the various types of benign liver tumors will be followed by recommendations for diagnosis and therapy in three settings: first, when a deliberate approach can be made to the diagnosis and management of an asymptomatic patient with a lesion found on a radiographic image; second, when the tumor is encountered as a surprise finding at laparotomy; and finally, in the unusual situation when some catastrophic event—

usually hemorrhage—has forced emergency laparotomy. Benign cysts and cystadenomas are discussed in Chapter 7 and will only be considered here in relation to differential diagnosis.

Etiology and Diagnosis

Tumors of Vascular Origin

Hemangiomas are said by many to be the most common benign tumor of the liver. Certainly, small capillary hemangiomas are very common and often appear as small, soft, surface lesions which may disappear with manipulation. They have no clinical significance. The larger cavernous hemangiomas are much less common, may be multiple in 10% to 20% of cases, tend to become symptomatic in middle age, particularly in women, and have a natural history that supports an increasingly conservative approach to therapy. Spontaneous rupture is very rare but may follow needle biopsy. However, pain—probably due to acute thrombosis—is suffered by some patients and may become chronic. Thrombocytopenia and hypofibrinogenemia have also been reported, more often in children, in association with these lesions. The fact that most symptoms occur in connection with pregnancy, with multiparity, with the use of birth control medication, and in perimenopausal women suggests that these lesions, which probably have been present since birth, may undergo endocrine-related vascular change. Most giant (greater than 4 cm) cavernous hemangiomas of the liver do not cause symptoms, even when observed for up to 20 years. The author has followed 52 such patients for up to 18 years. Only 2 patients developed symptoms, and in each case those symptoms were not due to the cavernous hemangioma. In one, a rapidly enlarging cyst was found, and in the other, a huge, necrotic liver cell adenoma caused severe symptoms. Others have reported similar associations of cavernous hemangioma with focal nodular hyperplasia, benign cysts, and liver cell adenoma.

The diagnosis of cavernous hemangioma has been remarkably simplified with the use of the technetium Tc 99m–tagged red blood cell scintiscan (Fig. 12-1). That test is quite sensitive and specific, and it is much less expensive and invasive than angiography. Ultrasonography will show an echogenic lesion, and dynamic computerized tomography, magnetic resonance imaging (Fig. 12-2), and angiography also will give characteristic patterns for cavernous hemangiomas, but are necessary only when the clinical suspicion of cavernous hemangioma is strong and the tagged red blood cell scan is not diagnostic. Fine-needle aspiration biopsy is safer than core biopsy but adds little to clinical decision making when the scintiscan is pathognomonic.

Mesenchymal Hamartoma

This lesion is probably the only true hamartoma of the liver. Mesenchymal hamartoma is a rare tumor usually, but not always, found in young children, and more often in males. A hamartoma has a multicystic appearance, produces symptoms by mass effect, and may kill if untreated. Even partial resection has been curative, and malignant degeneration has not been described. Computerized tomography can suggest the diagnosis and define tumor geography well enough to allow safe resection in most cases.

Focal Nodular Hyperplasia and Liver Cell Adenoma

These two solid tumors are discussed together even though most pathologists agree that they are lesions with a differing etiology, histology, presentation, and prognosis. Table 12-1 outlines some of these differences. In the clinical situation, however, these differences are often apparent only by hindsight. Both lesions are usually found in menstruating fe-

males, both are solid, hypervascular tumors often difficult to distinguish from malignancy short of biopsy, and a few tumors will show gross and microscopic features characteristic of both lesions. It may be that they represent different stages of the same process, but this is doubtful.

Focal nodular hyperplasia (FNH) is most often discovered incidentally in adults, but may reach large size and present as a mass lesion in older children around puberty, or during or just after pregnancy. FNH behaves and appears histologically like a reparative lesion, presumably related to a focal injury, perhaps vascular. Malignant degeneration has not been satisfactorily documented. If necrosis and hemorrhage ever occur, these complications must be very rare indeed, perhaps only in those lesions with "mixed" histology. Association of FNH with benign cysts and hemangiomas is well documented. Most importantly, no instance of serious complication is known to have occurred in a patient in whom a definitively diagnosed (biopsy-proven) FNH was left in place.

Even the most modern imaging techniques cannot reliably and consistently distinguish FNH from liver cell adenoma (LCA) or even from certain

Figure 12-1. Technetium Tc 99m–tagged red blood cell scintiscan. Note marked retention of radionuclide in large, right lobe cavernous hemangioma 45 minutes after injection.

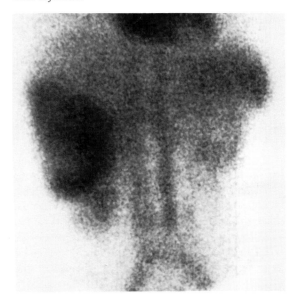

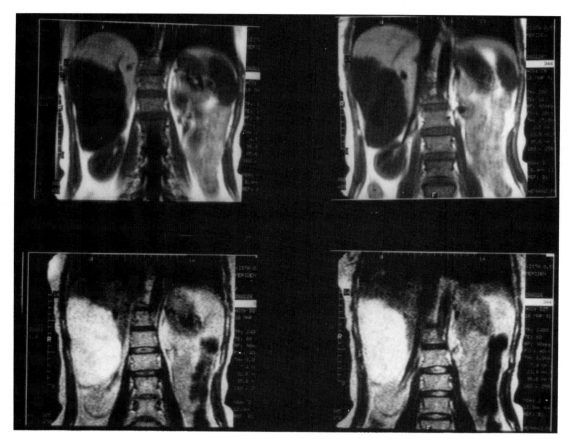

Figure 12-2. MRI of same patient as in Fig. 12-1.

Table 12-1. Clinical Differences Between Focal Nodular Hyperplasia and Liver Cell Adenoma

	Focal Nodular Hyperplasia	Liver Cell Adenoma
Epidemiology	Well described before 1960 10%–20% in males, children, and postmenopausal females OCM association nebulous ? Reparative process	Mostly since 1960 95% in menstrual-aged females, adults only Strong association with dose and duration of OCM ? Neoplastic, hyperplastic
Clinical presentation	Usually asymptomatic Incidental finding Largest with puberty or pregnancy	Mass or pain Rapid growth Hemorrhage and/or necrosis
Gross appearance	Smaller, darker, firmer central scar, nodular Prominent surface vessels 10%–20% multiple	Larger, lighter, softer Necrosis and ecchymosis, and rupture More often multiple
Histologic appearance	Nodular regeneration Bile duct hyperplasia Central scar with dilated blood vessels	No portal triads, zones of necrosis without inflammation Peliosis hepatis Minimal connective tissue
Prognosis if not resected	Benign Involution with time No cancer	May decrease with cessation of OCM Pain and rupture ? Malignant change

OCM = oral contraceptive medication.

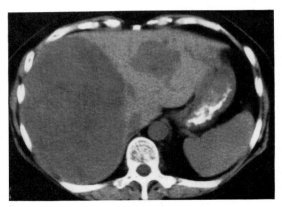

Figure 12-3. CT scan of liver of 54-year-old woman with large liver cell adenoma of right liver observed for 8 years without change in size. Lesion in left lateral segment is a hemangioma.

types of low-grade malignancy (Fig. 12-3). Much has been written about distinguishing LCA from FNH by scintigraphy, because the reticuloendothelial cells in FNH may pick up ^{99m}Tc. Thus, a tumor diagnosed with computerized tomography or ultrasonography that "disappears" with scintigraphy should be FNH, whereas an LCA will persist as a "cold" lesion. Unfortunately, exceptions occur in either direction which mandate biopsy for definitive diagnosis. If a fine-needle aspiration biopsy cannot distinguish FNH from LCA, and if management recommendations will differ for the two lesions, an open wedge biopsy must be done, preferably by a surgeon prepared to resect during the same anesthesia.

In contrast to FNH, 30% to 50% of patients with LCA will present with symptoms, often acute and severe. The large size of the tumor on presentation and the zones of acute necrosis and hemorrhage which are often seen suggest rapid growth, perhaps with a resultant outrunning of required blood supply. Case control investigations have strongly suggested an association between LCA and the dose and duration of oral contraceptive medication. An apparent recent decrease in the instance of LCA may be related to decreased steroid dosage and more careful use of oral contraceptive medication, or may simply be due to the nonreporting of tumors now recognized as fairly common.

Miscellaneous Rare, Benign Tumors

Case reports of a whole variety of epithelial and nonepithelial primary liver tumors document the ability of many of the liver's component cells to form tumors, but most such lesions are too rare to be discussed here. Primary lymphomas, benign teratomas, angiomyolipomas, and bile duct adenomas are among the more common of these rare lesions. Chondromas, leiomyomas, myxomas, schwannomas, and fibromas have also been described. These unusual tumors are usually readily diagnosed and resected in most instances.

Von Meyenberg plexi are small collections of subcapsular bile ducts, usually multiple, which have no clinical significance (unless they are detected and biopsied by an astute clinician suspecting liver metastases and misread by an innocent pathologist as well-differentiated carcinoma). The reader is referred to articles by Craig et al. and Foster for further information about these esoteric lesions.

Management

Clinical Strategies

When a tumor mass is found in the liver of a patient without cirrhosis, the clinician is obliged to find out enough about that mass to allow for decisions about therapy. He must rule out the presence of a resectable primary or secondary cancer and must establish an accurate diagnosis of the specific type of benign tumor, since some will need resection and others will not. Tissue diagnosis becomes very important, but percutaneous needle biopsy should be avoided in patients with possible echinococcal cysts or hemangiomas, and should probably not be done unless the information obtained might be used to avoid general anesthesia or laparotomy.

When a liver mass is found and diagnosed during the workup of an image, repetitive demonstration of the mass by different imaging techniques will seldom be as rewarding as some careful thinking in finding a solution to the problem. Selective angiography, magnetic resonance imaging, and dynamic computerized tomography have not yet added significantly to the usefulness of more conventional measures in the differential diagnosis of mass liver lesions (Fig. 12-4).

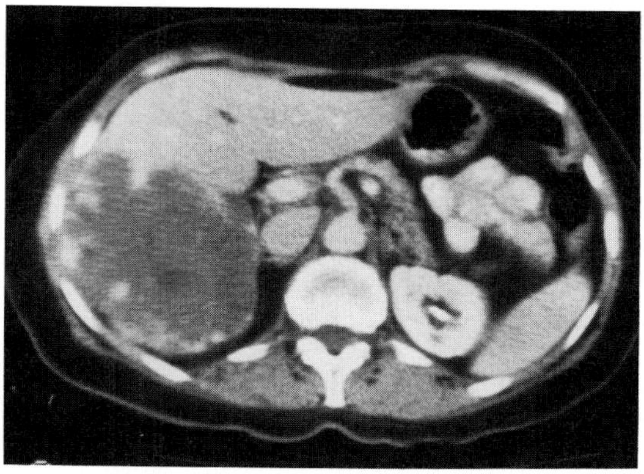

Figure 12-4. Conventional CT scan with contrast of a 38-year-old woman with a symptomatic cavernous hemangioma. Note areas of heterogeneity, suggesting recent thrombosis.

A thorough medical history may reveal a story of previous gastrointestinal malignancy, chronic liver disease, foreign travel, exposure to toxins, chills and fever, sex steroid medications, or even trauma, all of which can point toward a probable diagnosis. Findings within or without the liver on physical examination may provide additional clues to diagnosis. Tumor markers such as carcinoembryonic antigen and alpha-fetoprotein are most helpful in selected instances, but routine tests of liver function almost never assist in the differential diagnosis of a liver mass. Ultrasonography most readily and easily differentiates cystic from solid masses. The management of patients with cystic masses is considered in Chapter 7.

If the mass is greater than 2 cm in diameter, if it is echogenic, and if the patient has no symptoms, the tagged red blood cell scintiscan should be done. If positive, a diagnosis of hemangioma can be made and no therapy recommended (see above). If the lesion does not retain tagged red blood cells and there are no other clues to a specific diagnosis, further workup depends upon the circumstances. If the lesion is peripheral and easily resectable, operation should be recommended to most patients without preoperative tissue sampling. If the lesion is central, and if the patient is a 35-year-old female who has been on birth control pills for several years, a period of a few months (3–6) of observation off

of birth control medication might be chosen *after* fine-needle aspiration biopsy has ruled out cancer. Subsequent failure of a tumor to regress demands accurate tissue diagnosis by core or wedge biopsy by a team prepared to resect almost all lesions except focal nodular hyperplasia. In some circumstances, preoperative percutaneous fine-needle aspiration biopsy is indicated and can be done safely in most patients with normal hemostasis. An experienced cytologist can confidently differentiate cancer, including fibrolamellar carcinoma, from the benign lesions, although he or she cannot be expected to separate LCA, FNH, and hemangioma from each other without a core of tissue sufficient to allow examination of the architecture of the liver cells.

Pathologic Differentiation

During the past 30 years, the pathologist's ability to provide rapid and accurate information has become more critical in the management of patients with liver neoplasia. This need has paralleled the introduction of modern imaging techniques, including computerized tomography, ultrasound, and magnetic resonance imaging. Liver resection is now performed more safely and has been recognized as effective for the treatment of primary and secondary liver neoplasms. Moreover, experience has demonstrated that some benign liver tumors need resection, whereas others do not.

The major area of diagnostic innovation has been the utilization of the image-guided fine-needle aspiration technique (FNA) as a major source of information. This technique has been successfully used in many centers around the world. This method serves as a diagnostic technique which bridges both tissue and cytologic diagnosis.

What should the clinician's expectations be from this technique? The primary task of the pathologist is to separate nonneoplastic hepatocytes from hepatocellular carcinoma, the latter recognizable by an increased nucleus-cytoplasm ratio, atypical large, bare nuclei, and a trabecular grouping of abnormal liver cells surrounded by endothelial cells. If the FNA aspirate is clearly malignant, the pathologist's responsibility is to separate primary hepatocellular carcinoma from metastatic carcinoma, primary cholangiocarcinoma, or even rare mesenchymal neoplasms. To separate hepatocellular carcinoma from metastatic carcinoma, the pathologist depends on criteria of large polygonal cells in the aspirate with central nuclei, malignant cells arranged in a perithelial pattern, and bile pigment. The diagnostic accuracy of both image-guided and non–image-guided FNA is highly accurate for both benign and malignant tumors, showing a sensitivity and specificity of 85.6% and 98.4% and positive and negative predictive values of 99.1% and 76.1% in a study by Edóute et al., with an overall diagnostic accuracy of 89.7%.

The pathologist, after having identified the needle aspiration material to represent benign hepatocytes, must differentiate typical from atypical hepatocytes. Typical hepatocytes are seen with normal liver, focal nodular hyperplasia (FNH) and with liver cell adenoma (LCA), although some adenomas may show enlarged hepatocytes with clear or vacuolated cytoplasm. Distinguishing between LCA and FNH by FNA biopsy alone is often not possible. Even core needle biopsy, particularly for larger tumors, may not be definitive.

Atypical and dysplastic hepatocytes are found with regenerative nodules, with hepatitis B surface antigen positive chronic active hepatitis, and with cirrhosis, as well as adjacent to hepatocellular carcinomas. Differentiation from well-differentiated hepatocellular carcinoma may be difficult. This problem can be minimized by avoiding FNA and choosing instead a core biopsy for patients with diffuse liver disease.

Elective Surgery

Patients with symptomatic primary liver tumors should have them excised whether they are malignant or benign unless tumor geography or the patient's general condition does not allow this procedure. Benign tumors close to major vessels can be excised in most instances because a margin of normal liver tissue is not required to prevent recurrence. Although large tumors may require excision of huge areas beneath Glisson's capsule, the nontumorous residual liver will have already hypertrophied; thus the vast majority of functioning liver tissue can be left in place (Fig. 12-5).

When an unsuspected liver nodule is found at laparotomy or at laparoscopy, the surgeon will be required to make a diagnosis and decision in more urgent circumstances. In general, the purpose for

Figure 12-5. Asymptomatic cavernous hemangioma resected at time of drainage of a huge liver cyst. Note how tumor at lower edge of liver has dragged out a pedicle from near the apex of the gallbladder. The knobby, irregular surface with areas of scarring is typical.

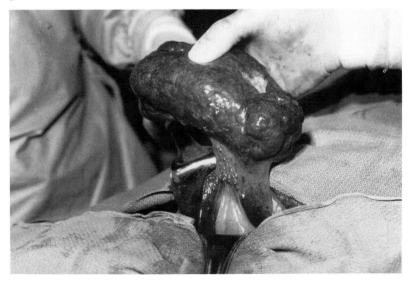

which the operation was undertaken should be completed unless any patient benefit would be negated in the presence of liver metastases. If the liver nodule is on the surface, excision or incision biopsy should be done for noncystic lesions (see Fig. 12-5). If a cyst is suspected, needle aspiration will quickly confirm this diagnosis. Frozen section diagnosis by an experienced pathologist should assist with decisions about further steps. If the gross characteristics of a discrete lesion suggest cavernous hemangioma, operative wedge biopsy can be safely done through the firm areas of the tumor with suture control. Control after biopsy of the softer tissue may prove more difficult.

If the liver lesion is palpable but not visible or near the surface, an attempt should be made to establish the exact geography of the lesion, and a tissue diagnosis by aspiration or core biopsy should be sought. Direct vision is preferable, but a percutaneous-needle core biopsy can be done with digital control alone through almost any abdominal incision. A few moments spent in establishing a diagnosis of the liver lesion, even if there is no thought of resection at this time, will save the patient untold amounts of postoperative time, testing, and cost.

Tumor Hemorrhage

Most surgeons will rarely be called upon to manage a catastrophic complication of benign liver tumor. When this does happen, it usually happens to a young female patient who has had acute abdominal pain and vascular collapse, and who will be found to have hemoperitoneum due to rupture of a benign tumor. The circumstances will usually preclude preoperative investigations. After urgent resuscitation, a large abdominal incision is usually made, and hemorrhage is seen coming from an area of ruptured liver capsule. A discrete tumor mass may be obvious, but sometimes it is difficult to distinguish a ruptured LCA from the spontaneous rupture of the liver (e.g., in pregnancy) or from a ruptured primary or secondary malignant tumor.

The first priority is control of hemorrhage. Many techniques may prove useful, most of which are familiar to trauma surgeons and will not be discussed here. Desperate circumstances may demand more desperate measures. Friable, necrotic, bleeding tumors may be scoped from adjacent liver

with no attention to segmental anatomy or tumor margin to achieve control. The cure of cancer and the niceties of specific tumor diagnosis can be postponed until another day. However, it is usually easy to bluntly debride away a small piece of tissue from the ragged edges of the ruptured crevasse to provide the pathologist with enough material to assist the surgeon with a considered future decision.

Results

Tumors of Vascular Origin

Asymptomatic patients should probably have a repeat image (sonography is probably the least expensive and invasive choice) 6 months after diagnosis to ensure that no change has occurred. On theoretical grounds, violent sports should probably be proscribed and pregnancy should raise concern, but otherwise the patient should be reassured. No catastrophic complication is known to have occurred to a patient in whom a cavernous hemangioma has been left in place in an asymptomatic patient.

Resection in the symptomatic patient may be done more safely than for most tumors. Although anatomic resections are occasionally indicated for geographic reasons, most often enucleation will be a better choice of technique. A definite plane between the cavernous hemangioma and normal liver parenchyma allows blunt dissection with easy separation, even from adjacent major vessels. There are often remarkably few major feeding vessels, which can be ligated as they are encountered.

The value of radiation has never been proven, and the effects of embolization are probably transient at best. If significant pain persists after a period of observation, enucleation should be recommended. It is comforting to know that most patients with cavernous hemangioma will never have symptoms, that life-threatening hemorrhage is very rare, and that episodes of mild pain, probably due to thrombosis, are often transient.

Benign vascular tumors in infants and children may present a more difficult dilemma. Coagulopathies and congestive heart failure (probably due to arteriovenous fistulae) are more common, the lesions are often huge and/or multiple, and there seems to be a spectrum of lesions all the way from tumors resembling mature cavernous hemangiomas of the adult to multifocal endothelial malignancies which can kill quickly. Experience has taught that spontaneous maturation and involution may occur. This situation has prompted a more conservative approach to resection. Whether radiation, steroid therapy, and hepatic artery ligation or embolization aid in promoting involution is debatable, but their use may comfort the parents, the clinician, and the patient in what are sometimes desperate circumstances. Recently, the use of interferon alpha has shown great promise in an anecdotal experience with cavernous hemangiomas in children.

Focal Nodular Hyperplasia and Liver Cell Adenoma

Because most adenomas have been resected, the natural history of these tumors without resection is not well documented. A few patients with multiple lesions have been followed for up to 15 years. Late rupture is quite rare, but at least five instances of histologic cancer have been documented in patients with unresected or only partially resected LCA (Table 12-2). It is unclear whether this is coincidence or progression of benign to malignant disease. Because liver resection can be done quite safely by experienced surgeons, a recommendation for resection of all "resectable" LCA is warranted, even in the asymptomatic patient. The exception is provided by the patient with multiple adenomas whose tumor geography would require total hepatectomy. The risk of transplantation is probably greater than that of malignant change, at least until more is known about this ominous complication. The serial determination of alpha-fetoprotein may be helpful in detecting malignant change if LCA tumors are left in situ, and patients should be monitored for long periods of time.

The question of the relationship of pregnancy to the growth of FNH and LCA remains unresolved. The evidence is scarce, anecdotal, and insufficient to conclude that the risk of tumor complication justifies termination of a wanted pregnancy. Certainly, obstetrician, surgeon, and mother-to-be should all be alert to any sign of trouble and ready to intervene if necessary.

Conclusions

Most benign liver tumors are small and inconsequential. The important larger noncystic lesions include cavernous hemangioma, focal nodular hyperplasia, liver cell adenoma, and a host of very rare, mostly mesenchymal lesions, the most important of which is the mesenchymal hamartoma of children. No therapy is recommended for an asymptomatic patient with a proven diagnosis of cavernous hemangioma or focal nodular hyperplasia, but most other lesions should be resected. An intelligent use of diagnostic measures can sharply limit the number of preoperative tests needed. Perhaps the clinician's most important duty in the management of a patient eventually proven to have a benign liver tumor is to rule out the presence of a resectable malignancy. In spite of rapid improvements in several new imaging techniques, tissue biopsy will usually be required to resolve the important questions.

Selected Readings

Craig JR, Peters RL, Edmondson HA. Tumors of the liver and intrahepatic bile ducts. *AFIP Atlas of Tumor Pathology,* Fascicle 26, Second Series, 1988.
Crawford JM. Pathologic assessment of liver cell dysplasia and benign liver tumors: Differentiation from malignant tumors. *Semin Diagn Pathol* 1990; 7:115–128.

Table 12-2. Transformation from Liver Cell Adenoma to Cancer

Authors	Year	Gender	Age	Interval (yrs)	Alpha-fetoprotein	Resectable	Outcome
Tesluk & Lawrie	1979	Female	34	3	Not done	Yes	Postoperative death
Gordon et al	1986	Female	36	7	Normal	Yes	Disease free, 6 yrs
Leese et al	1988	Male	13	5	High	Transplantation	Disease free, 1 yr
Gyorff et al	1989	Female	53	2	High	No	Died of tumor, 7 mos
Foster & Berman	1994	Female	56	5	Slight increase	No	Died of tumor, 7 mos

Source: Adapted from Foster JH, Berman MM, The malignant transformation of liver cell adenomas, *Arch Surg* 1994; 129:712–717.

Edoute Y, et al. Imaging-guided and nonimaging-guided fine needle aspiration of liver lesions: Experience with 406 patients. *J Surg Oncol* 1991; 48:246–251.

Farlow DC, et al. Investigation of focal hepatic lesions: Is tomographic red blood cell imaging useful? *World Surg* 1990; 14:463–467.

Foster JH. Benign liver tumours. In Blumgart LH (ed), *Surgery of the Liver and Biliary Tract.* London: Churchill Livingstone, 1988. Pp. 1115–1127.

Foster JH, Berman MM. The malignant transformation of liver cell adenomas. *Arch Surg* 1994; 129:712–717.

Ishak KG. Mesenchymal tumors of the liver. In Okuda K, Peters RL (eds), *Hepatocellular Carcinoma.* New York: Wiley, 1976. Pp. 247–308.

Little JM, Kenny J, Hollands MJ. Hepatic incidentaloma: A modern problem. *World J Surg* 1990; 14:448=451.

Rosenberg L. The risk of liver neoplasia in relation to combined oral contraceptive use (review). *Contraception* 1991; 43:643–652.

Tait N, et al. Hepatic cavernous haemangioma: A 10-year review. *Aust N Z J Surg* 1992; 62:521–524.

13

Hepatocellular Carcinoma

Sheung-Tat Fan
Henry Ngan
John Wong

Hepatocellular carcinoma (HCC) is a common malignant disease in Asia and Africa. With immigration of Asians to Western countries, this disease is increasingly seen in other parts of the world. HCC is a highly lethal disease because the tumor usually grows rapidly, the patients often have underlying cirrhosis, and the disease is often diagnosed late. In the majority of cases, HCCs produce few symptoms even when they are huge. Small HCCs are only diagnosed in patients screened by ultrasonography and alpha-fetoprotein monitoring. In recent years, the prognosis is slightly better because an increasing number of small HCCs are being diagnosed. The improvement is also related partly to improved liver resection technique and the availability of effective nonoperative treatment.

Etiology and Pathogenesis

Hepatitis B and C virus infections are the predominant causes of cirrhosis and HCC. The relative risk of patients with hepatitis B virus infection developing HCC is 21.3. The relative risk of patients with hepatitis C cirrhosis developing HCC is 52.3. Dual infections by hepatitis B and C tend to further increase the risk of HCC.

How hepatitis B virus induces hepatocarcinogenesis is not exactly known. It is possible that malignant transformation of hepatocytes is related to the hepatitis B virus X gene protein, which acts as a transcriptional transactivator of many genes, including those associated with cell growth. Heavy cigarette smoking and alcohol consumption are added risk factors in patients with hepatitis infection. Once the viral infection is established, it will take approximately 10 years for patients to develop chronic hepatitis, 21 years to develop cirrhosis, and 29 years to develop HCC.

In areas where HCC is endemic, contamination of food and water by aflatoxin is probably an important factor in hepatocarcinogenesis. Aflatoxin may induce mutation of the tumor-suppressor gene, p53. It is also possible that the hepatitis B virus interacts with p53 protein to provide a growth advantage to cells harboring the mutation. Thus the relative risk of hepatocarcinogenesis on exposure to aflatoxin is 2.4 but is markedly elevated to 60.1 in the presence of hepatitis B virus infection.

In some countries, alcoholic cirrhosis is an important cause of HCC. Hemochromatosis, anabolic steroids, and long-standing primary biliary cirrhosis may occasionally be associated with HCC.

Diagnosis

HCC is usually diagnosed late because the majority of the patients are asymptomatic. Mild symptoms such as distending discomfort are frequently seen in patients who have already harbored a big tumor but are generally well. Sudden sharp pain in the upper abdomen is often due to hemorrhage into the tumor or spontaneous rupture into the peritoneal cavity. When weight loss and cachexia appear, they are often in the preterminal stage. Not infrequently, low-grade fever may be present and is a reaction to central necrosis in a fast-growing tumor. Rare presentations include diarrhea, polycythemia, hypercalcemia, hyperglycemia, acute cholangitis, and acute pancreatitis. In the latter instances, the tumor has eroded into the biliary tract, and tumor fragments are dislodged into the common bile duct or through the ampulla of Vater. When an HCC has eroded into the bile duct, hemobilia may also occur (Fig. 13-1).

Physical examination is often not revealing except in the late stage. Clinical diagnosis of early HCC is therefore impossible, but a high index of suspicion is necessary when interviewing Asian patients for mild upper abdominal symptoms, particularly those who have a history of hepatitis or who are known hepatitis B carriers.

Radiology

Ultrasonography, computerized tomography, hepatic angiography, and portovenography are techniques widely used in the imaging of HCC. Ultrasonography (US) is simple, readily available, and noninvasive. US can detect most HCCs except small ones within a small and cirrhotic liver. The tumor is usually hyperechoic, but it can at times be hypoechoic, especially when it is small in size. US can delineate the extent of the tumor and determine whether daughter nodules are present. Invasion of the main portal vein or its branches, the hepatic

veins, and the inferior vena cava by the tumor can also be detected by US. However, US is often unable to differentiate HCCs from other tumorous lesions in the liver.

Computerized tomography (CT) is the mainstay in the imaging of HCC. The tumor is hypodense in the majority of patients before intravenous contrast, and there is nonhomogeneous enhancement after contrast, with the lesion being still hypodense relative to the normal liver. Necrosis may be seen in the center of the tumor. On rare occasions, the tumor may be hyperdense before intravenous contrast enhancement. The extent of the tumor is usually sharply demarcated by CT (Fig. 13-2), and the presence of daughter nodules in the opposite lobe can be detected (Fig. 13-3). After intravenous injection of contrast, the main portal vein and major intrahepatic branches, the hepatic veins, and the inferior vena cava can normally be visualized. Thus CT is the most helpful modality in showing the surgeon the topographic relationship of the tumor to major vessels and in determining whether the tumor is resectable. However, a small HCC and daughter nodules below 1 cm in diameter can be missed by CT even after contrast enhancement. Moreover, an HCC of the diffuse type may also be difficult to detect on CT. As on US, HCCs are nonspecific in appearance on CT, and cannot be differentiated from other kinds of tumors with certainty. Both US and CT are most helpful in guiding

Figure 13-1. Hepatic angiogram showing a diffuse HCC with contrast leaking into the upper part of the common bile duct (arrow), which was obstructed by tumor fragments.

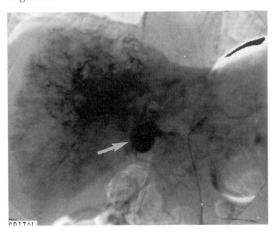

Figure 13-2. CT scan after contrast showing a large HCC in the right lobe extending into segment IV.

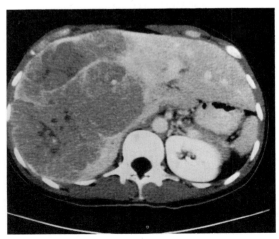

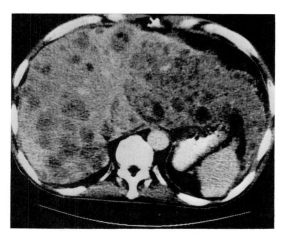

Figure 13-3. CT scan after contrast showing a multicentric HCC in both lobes.

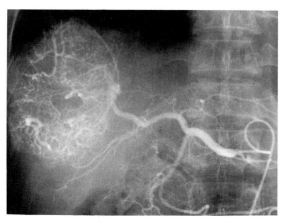

Figure 13-4. Pathological arteries are present in a solitary well-encapsulated HCC in the right lobe during the arterial phase of hepatic angiography.

fine-needle aspiration biopsy or "Trucut" biopsy of the tumor.

Hepatic angiography and portovenography are the most important imaging modalities in the diagnosis of HCCs. The appearance of HCCs on hepatic angiography is relatively diagnostic. HCCs can be solitary, multicentric, or diffuse (Figs. 13-4, 13-5). In the solitary or multicentric type, pathological arteries and sometimes venous lakes may be present within the tumor. Tumor blush can be seen in some HCCs during the capillary phase. Encasement of a branch of the hepatic artery is rare, but occlusion of intrahepatic branches of the portal vein occurs early. In the diffuse type, the pathological vessels are more subtle (Fig. 13-6). Arteriovenous shunting into branches of the portal vein or even into branches of the hepatic vein and thence into the inferior vena cava is not infrequently encountered (Fig. 13-7A, B). Regurgitation of the contrast into the main portal vein may also occur. Hepatic angiography delineates the anatomy of the arterial supply to the liver and will serve as a road map during surgery.

Portovenography is usually performed by injection of the contrast medium into the superior mesenteric artery, with delayed films taken when the contrast medium has reached the portal vein and intrahepatic branches. Tolazoline or papaverine is routinely injected into the superior mesenteric artery immediately prior to the injection of the con-

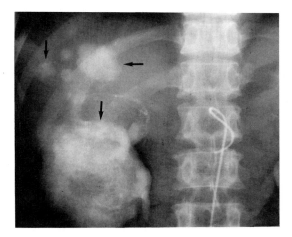

Figure 13-5. Hepatic angiogram showing tumor blush during late capillary phase in a multicentric HCC in the right lobe (arrows).

trast medium to produce transient shunting of blood from the arterial to the venous side so as to improve opacification of the portal vein and branches, unless digital subtraction angiography is used.

Compression, invasion, or complete occlusion of the main portal vein by an HCC is often seen in advanced disease (Fig. 13-8A, B). Invasion of the main portal vein by tumor precludes resection. Transcatheter arterial chemoembolization is contraindicated in the presence of arteriovenous shunting

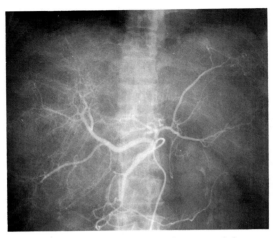

Figure 13-6. Hepatic angiogram showing subtle pathological arteries in a diffuse HCC in both lobes of an enlarged liver.

or complete occlusion of the main portal vein. Extrahepatic peritoneal recurrence of an HCC after a previous hepatic resection occasionally occurs, and this situation may be amenable to further surgical resection. Although CT may demonstrate a nodule adjacent to the hepatic remnant, this finding may be confused with an unopacified loop of bowel. However, angiography will confirm the diagnosis because the recurrent HCC is invariably vascular and receives its blood supply from a branch of the celiac axis or superior mesenteric artery (Fig. 13-9A, B). Thus hepatic angiography and portovenography are not only useful in the diagnosis of an HCC, but are also essential in determining whether the tumor is amenable to surgery or chemoembolization.

Iodized oil computerized tomography (Lipiodol CT) is an imaging technique which is useful in the detection of small HCCs or daughter nodules. In a contracted cirrhotic liver, a small HCC or a daughter nodule may not be diagnosed with certainty by US, CT, or even hepatic angiography. CT performed 7 to 14 days following the injection of 2 to 5 ml of iodized oil into the hepatic artery may be able to detect an HCC in a patient with a strong clinical suspicion of having an HCC because of persistent elevation of serum alpha-fetoprotein but with negative US, CT, and hepatic angiography. The iodized oil accumulates in an HCC and enhances the differentiation of the HCC from normal liver tissue. The uptake of the iodized oil within an HCC is either dense-homogeneous (Fig. 13-10A) or dense-patchy at the periphery and/or in the center of a hypodense area (Fig. 13-10B). A study of the authors demonstrated that when dense-homogeneous and well-circumscribed uptake was present within a lesion, the chance of it being an HCC was high, with the posttest probability being 92.8%. On the other hand, when dense-patchy uptake was present within the lesion, only 76% turned out to be an HCC, since hemangiomas, metastases, and focal nodular hyperplasia could have an identical appearance. It is therefore advisable to perform fine-needle aspiration biopsy of such lesions to clarify the diagnosis, especially when the serum alpha-fetoprotein level is below the diagnostic level.

The authors' study also revealed that the overall sensitivity of iodized oil CT in the detection of small HCCs was as high as 97.1%. Iodized oil CT was superior to hepatic angiography, which could detect HCCs with certainty in only 73.6% of such patients. Unfortunately, the specificity of the technique in the diagnosis of HCC was only 76.9%, since other lesions could also demonstrate a dense-patchy uptake pattern. By virtue of its high sensitivity, iodized oil CT often picks up daughter nodules in the opposite lobe and thus spares the patient a hepatic resection after which the tumor is doomed to recur.

Alpha-Fetoprotein

Alpha-fetoprotein (AFP) is the most important tumor marker of HCCs. AFP is elevated in 80% of patients. The serum level of alpha-fetoprotein is generally proportional to the volume of the tumor. For small HCCs (< 2 cm), alpha-fetoprotein is within normal range in 23% to 55%. Thus the detection of small HCCs in a high-risk population should rely on concomitant ultrasonography and alpha-fetoprotein measurement.

The diagnostic level of serum alpha-fetoprotein for HCC is generally accepted to be 400 to 500 ng/ml, above which a histological confirmation may not be necessary. If the level of alpha-fetoprotein is between 20 and 500 ng/ml, "Trucut" biopsy under ultrasound, CT, or laparoscopic guidance may be necessary. However, the procedure may be dangerous in that it may induce hemoperitoneum or seeding of tumor cells into the peritoneal cavity. In the

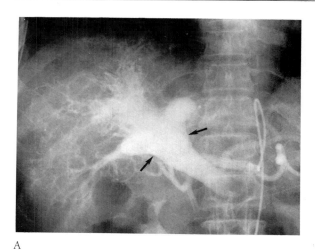
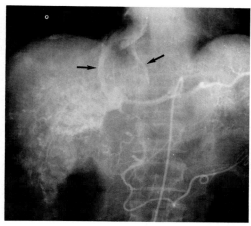

A   B

Figure 13-7. A. Arteriovenous shunting into the portal vein (arrows) during the arterial phase of hepatic angiography in HCC. B. Arteriovenous shunting into hepatic vein and inferior vena cava (arrows) in hepatic angiography in HCC.

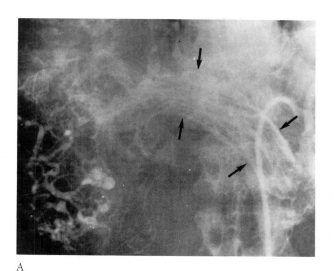
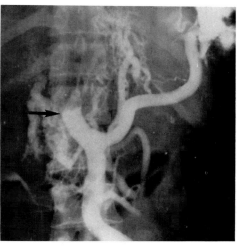

A   B

Figure 13-8. A. Hepatic angiogram showing invasion of lumen of main portal vein (arrows) by HCC, producing the "thread and streak" sign. B. Percutaneous transplenic portovenogram showing complete occlusion of main portal vein (arrow) by HCC with opacification of coronary veins running toward the cardia and lower esophagus.

authors' practice, histological confirmation is only needed when the HCC is considered not resectable and is associated with serum alpha-fetoprotein below the diagnostic level. In this situation, fine-needle aspiration cytology under image guidance is a much safer alternative.

Liver Function

In addition to determining the extent of growth of the HCC, it is mandatory to assess liver function so that one can plan the appropriate treatment. Liver function can be assessed by simple parameters

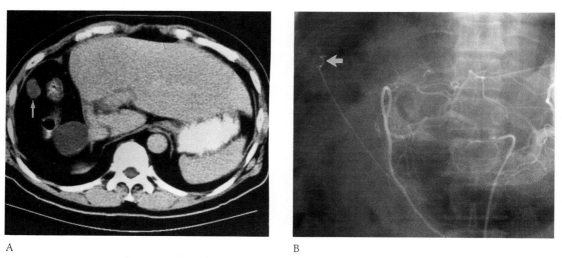

A   B

Figure 13-9. A. A small extrahepatic nodule (arrow) is present in the right upper abdomen on a CT scan of a patient who had a previous right hepatic resection with subsequent elevation of serum alpha-fetoprotein. B. Celiac axis angiogram showing a branch of the inferior epiploic artery supplying a vascular recurrent HCC nodule (arrow) under the diaphragm.

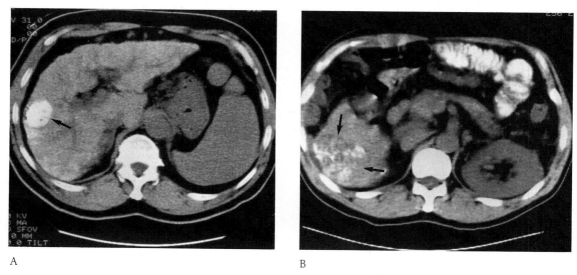

A   B

Figure 13-10. A. A small HCC in the right lobe with dense homogeneous uptake of iodized oil (arrow) on iodized oil CT scan. B. An HCC in the inferior part of the right lobe with dense-patchy uptake of iodized oil (arrows) on iodized oil CT scan.

such as serum bilirubin level, serum albumin level, prothrombin time, and platelet count, or by sophisticated tests such as the sulfobromophthalein sodium (Bromsulphalein) (BSP) retention test, the indocyanine green (ICG) clearance test, the amino-pyrine breath test, the oral glucose tolerance test, and the arterial ketone body ratio. Of all these tests, ICG clearance when combined with volumetric measurement of the liver or CT scan was shown to be superior to the other tests in predicting liver failure. However, the ICG clearance test is not readily available in many hospitals. For practical purposes, selection of a patient with HCC for liver resection would have to be based on visual assessment of the size of the liver that is going to be retained (as seen on US or CT) and a set of normal findings of serum bilirubin level, serum albumin level, prothrombin time, and platelet count. It is important to note that even after careful selection of patients with good liver function for resection, the occurrence of liver failure cannot be prevented if major hemorrhage occurs during the operation or serious intra-abdominal sepsis develops post-operatively.

Management

Surgery

Surgical resection is the treatment of choice when the HCC is confined to one lobe of the liver and the function of the remaining liver is judged to be adequate for supporting the postoperative recovery. Patients with underlying cirrhosis but with nearly normal liver function should not be barred from surgery. Sometimes they can tolerate major hepatectomy well, but meticulous surgical maneuvers and maximum postoperative care are necessary to achieve a satisfactory result.

In planning surgical resection, it is important to achieve a nontumorous margin of at least 0.5 cm on all sides and to preserve as much functioning liver parenchyma as possible. However, for a large tumor, a satisfactory margin may not always be possible, and for small tumors which are encroaching on major vessels near the hilum, a large volume of functioning liver may have to be sacrificed in order to achieve a curative margin and to avoid damage to major vessels. The judgment will be based on preoperative liver function assessment and the confidence of the surgeon in doing a safe operation.

The surgical technique of hepatectomy is well established. Major hepatectomy such as right hepatic lobectomy, left hepatic lobectomy, or extension of the resection to either side of Cantlie's line is usually performed with inflow and outflow vasculature control before parenchymal transection. The portal branch, the hepatic artery, and the hepatic duct of the ipsilateral side are isolated, divided, and sutured at the liver hilum, and then the liver lobe is mobilized by dividing the triangular ligament to expose and control the hepatic vein.

Exposure of the right hepatic vein requires rotation of the right lobe, followed by division of the short venous branches that drain directly from the right lobe of the liver to the inferior vena cava and division of the inferior vena caval ligament that covers the right hepatic vein. If extrahepatic control of the right hepatic vein can be achieved before liver transection, blood loss may be less than in cases without prior control. Clearance of the posterior surface of the liver from the inferior vena cava and rotation of the right lobe will also facilitate transection of the liver in a vertical plane, allow more tumor-free margin, and reduce the hazard of injury to the inferior vena cava. However, forceful rotation of the right lobe, particularly in the presence of a large HCC, is associated with the danger of laceration of the liver; rupture of the tumor; laceration of the right adrenal gland; torsion of the inferior vena cava, leading to reduced venous return to the heart; torsion of the portal vein, leading to relative ischemia of the left lobe; and squeezing of tumor cells into the systemic circulation.

Liver transection can be performed using finger fracture, Kelly clamps, ultrasound aspirators, or water jet dissectors. Liver transection by finger fracture is fast but is less precise and probably is associated with more bleeding. Frequently the plane of transection goes easily into the space between the tumor capsule and the uninvolved liver, resulting in an unsatisfactory tumor-free margin. Transection of the liver using Kelly clamps is a modification of the finger fracture method. Small vessels and ducts are exposed after Kelly clamps are applied at the proposed site of transection. The vessels are then ligated, clipped, or diathermized. This method is efficient but becomes less so when one approaches the deeper position near to the inferior vena cava and hepatic veins, which may be damaged by the clamps.

Ultrasound aspirators and water jet dissectors are as efficient as Kelly clamps in exposing vascular and ductal structures but are much slower, and the equipment is expensive. The water jet dissector is less prone to damage major vessels, but the field is less clear than with the ultrasound aspirator during application. Comparative studies will be required to determine which of the methods or which instrumentation is more efficient than the others, but such a study is difficult to conduct because there will be many variables and differences among surgeons and patients. The final choice is probably dependent on the surgeon's experience with individual methods as well as the availability of equipment.

During liver transection, the necessity of portal inflow occlusion, outflow occlusion, or total vascular isolation is controversial. Normal and cirrhotic liver can tolerate warm ischemia for up to 1 hour, but such a long period of continuous inflow occlusion is definitely not desirable. Thus many surgeons practice intermittent occlusion of 10 to 15 minutes. It is still arguable whether inflow occlusion offers any benefit, particularly in anatomical lobar hepatectomy after ligation and division of appropriate branches of the portal vein, hepatic artery, and hepatic vein. For instance, when liver transection is done on the right side of Cantlie's line in the case of right hepatic lobectomy, the vascular inflow has already been ligated and the right hepatic vein has been controlled; bleeding, if any, will be coming from the middle hepatic vein or its branches. Occlusion of the middle hepatic vein would produce an avascular field, but occlusion of the middle hepatic vein alone is not always possible because the middle hepatic vein is infrequently independent of the left hepatic vein outside the liver.

In a retrospective comparative study, liver transection with or without inflow occlusion did not produce an obvious difference in blood loss or blood transfusion requirement. Total vascular isolation, that is, clamping of portal inflow and of the suprahepatic and infrahepatic inferior vena cava, is advocated, but a completely dry field is not always achieved unless the right adrenal vein is also ligated, a situation that is difficult to achieve when there is an indication for this measure, as in a huge right lobe tumor. To stop blood flow completely, aortic clamping above the celiac axis has been introduced but has not been readily adopted because the ischemic damage to the other viscera cannot be estimated.

Preferred Approach

The authors' preferred method of major hepatectomy is a modification of the standard procedure.

Hilar dissection and division of the appropriate branches of the portal vein and hepatic artery are performed routinely, but dissection for the right or left hepatic duct is avoided so that the bile duct is not thinned out and the arterial supply to the bile duct is not damaged. In the case of a bulky tumor, the liver is not mobilized and rotated, and liver transection is performed at the proposed site by ultrasound aspirator or by water jet dissector without inflow occlusion (Figs. 13-11, 13-12). If the tumor is near the caudate lobe and process, they are separated from the inferior vena cava by division of the short caval branches. Further mobilization of the caudate lobe from the left to right side of the inferior vena cava will expose the middle and right hepatic veins outside the liver, which are divided and sutured. The triangular ligaments are then divided, leading to delivery of the specimen out of the abdominal cavity. For smaller HCCs that necessitate a right hepatectomy, the authors still use the classical approach of mobilization of the right lobe and prior control of inflow and outflow

Figure 13-11. CT scan showing a large HCC in the right lobe. The dotted line shows the direction of the liver transection, going from the anterior surface (arrow) down to the right of the liver hilum, curving to the left to include the caudate lobe, and finally going back to the right side of the inferior vena cava. The inferior vena cava was compressed but not obstructed, a feature often seen in patients who have a large HCC that is still amenable to hepatectomy.

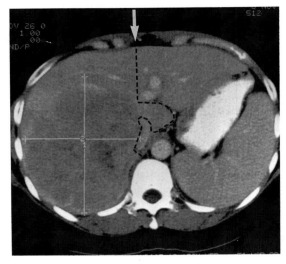

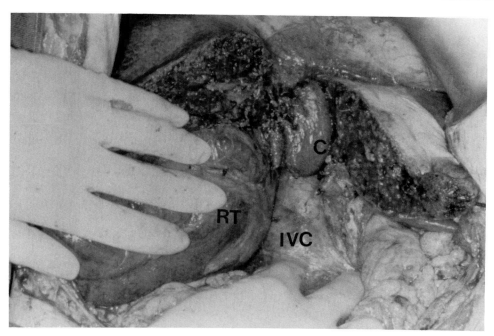

Figure 13-12. Photograph showing the liver transection completed at the right side of the liver hilum, exposing the caudate lobe (C). Further mobilization of the caudate lobe from the inferior vena cava (IVC) will expose the right hepatic vein and complete the mobilization. The surgeon's left hand has displaced the right lobe and tumor (RT).

vasculatures. Parenchymal transection is also performed without the Pringle maneuver.

For small HCCs that can be resected by mono- or bisegmentectomy, it is necessary to mark the boundaries of individual segments by intraoperative ultrasound. Ultrasound-guided puncture and injection of methylene blue into the feeding portal venous branch of the segment harboring the tumor can be used to outline the boundary. In the case of cirrhosis, the mapping may be patchy and unsatisfactory because of arterioportal shunting. The staining can be improved by clamping the hepatic artery. During liver transection, inflow vascular control can be done by the Pringle maneuver, by clamping the unilateral hepatic artery and portal vein, or, after dissection into the hilar plate, by clamping the segmental branch of the portal vein and hepatic artery. Balloon occlusion of the portal venous branch by a cannula placed under ultrasound guidance has also been advocated, but this procedure may cause portal vein thrombosis. The authors' preferred approach is to avoid vascular clamping in the cirrhotic liver. The line of transec-

tion is mapped by intraoperative ultrasound using the landmark of major vasculature. The initial parenchymal transection is made perpendicular to the portal venous branches so as to ligate them as early as possible in order to obtain a relatively dry field.

After hepatectomy, diluted methylene blue solution is injected into the biliary tract via cystic duct cannulation to check for bile leakage. In case of uncertainty about injury to the bile duct, a cholangiogram can also be obtained by the same cannula. The raw area is then covered with greater omentum. In the case of right hepatic lobectomy, the falciform ligament is reconstituted so that the liver remnant will not rotate into the right subphrenic cavity, resulting in twisting of the left and middle hepatic veins.

Transcatheter Arterial Chemoembolization

When an HCC is inoperable because it is very large or there is a daughter nodule in the opposite lobe, transcatheter arterial chemoembolization (TACE) can be offered. TACE is also indicated in some patients with a small solitary HCC in whom surgery is considered too risky because of poor liver function, and in those with recurrence of the HCC after a previous hepatic resection. In TACE, an emulsion of iodized oil and doxorubicin hydrochloride (Adriamycin) or cisplatin is infused slowly into the hepatic artery or a branch supplying the tumor through a catheter inserted via the femoral artery, followed by an absorbable gelatin sponge (Gelfoam) embolization. The authors use cisplatin as the cytotoxic drug of choice. Ten milligrams of cisplatin in 10 ml is mixed with 10 ml of iodized oil by the pumping method into a 20-ml emulsion. The dose of the emulsion infused per treatment session varies from 4 to 40 ml, depending on the size of the tumor. This infusion is followed by "light" absorbable gelatin sponge embolization with absorbable gelatin sponge pellets 1 mm in diameter in a contrast medium. The mixture is injected until the blood flow in the arteries supplying the tumor slows down but before total occlusion occurs.

The infused iodized oil accumulates within the HCC, carrying with it the cytotoxic drug, which is then slowly released and delivered to the tumor at a high concentration, while the concentration delivered to the normal areas of the liver is much lower. Moreover, the amount of the cytotoxic drug reaching the rest of the body is extremely small, thus avoiding the unwanted side effects of systemic chemotherapy. Since an HCC is almost exclusively supplied by branches of the hepatic artery, occlusion of the hepatic artery by embolization will invariably result in some degree of tumor necrosis. The normal areas of the liver will continue to be perfused by branches of the portal vein and will remain viable as long as the main portal vein is patent. Combining the above two modes of therapy, TACE is a safer and more effective procedure than systemic chemotherapy and is well tolerated by the majority of patients.

Chemoembolization is contraindicated under the following conditions:

1. When the main portal vein is completely occluded
2. When arteriovenous shunting either into branches of the portal vein or into branches of the hepatic vein occurs

3. When liver function is severely impaired, as when the serum bilirubin level is above 3.5 mg/dl
4. When extrahepatic metastases are present
5. In HCCs of the diffuse type, which rarely respond to such treatment

After the procedure, two thirds of the patients experience nausea and vomiting, and these symptoms usually last only for a few hours. Upper abdominal pain occurs in just over half of the patients and usually persists for a few days. Pyrexia, which can at times be above 39°C, is present in about half of the patients and can persist for over a week. The levels of serum bilirubin and transaminases (aspartate aminotransferase and alanine aminotransferase) are invariably elevated after TACE but return to the preprocedure level within a week.

More severe complications are sometimes encountered. Perforation of a chronic duodenal ulcer and severe bleeding from peptic ulcers occur occasionally because of the ulcer-producing effect of cisplatin on the gastroduodenal mucosa. The routine administration of an H_2 receptor antagonist or Omeprazole will probably reduce the risk of peptic ulceration. Acute pancreatitis, liver abscess, septicemia, and hepatic encephalopathy have been reported but will respond to conservative therapy.

In the authors' recent study, TACE was administered to 105 patients with inoperable HCC. The treatment sessions were repeated every 1½ to 3 months. The number of treatment sessions each patient underwent varied from 1 to 16, with the mean number being 4.4. The tumor size ranged from 0.5 to 33 cm in maximum diameter, with the median size being 8.5 cm. Overall, the HCC decreased in size, at least initially, in 54% of the patients (Fig. 13-13A, B). In tumors 9 cm or less in size at the commencement of TACE (group 1), 71% responded. In tumors between 9 and 18 cm in size (group 2), only 43% responded. None of the tumors larger than 18 cm in size (group 3) responded. The authors found that the addition of absorbable gelatin sponge embolization enhanced the response of the tumor to treatment in patients in group 2. Occasionally, the extent and number of tumors can be reduced to such a degree that surgical resection becomes possible.

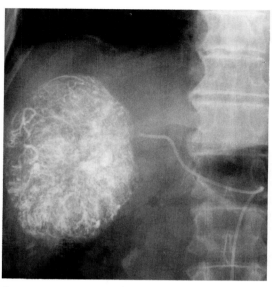
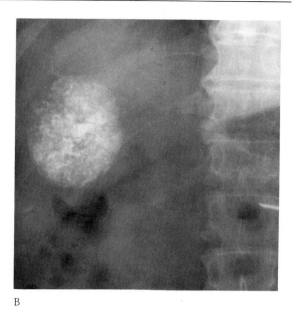

A   B

Figure 13-13. A. Heavy uptake of iodized oil in an HCC 12.5 cm in maximum diameter in the right lobe at the commencement of TACE. B. The HCC has decreased to 8 cm in size after three sessions of TACE.

The overall median survival time in the patients was 12 months. This result compares favorably with the median survival of 3.5 to 7.5 weeks in untreated patients. The median survival time of patients in groups 1, 2, and 3 was 20 months, 8 months, and 1 month, respectively. The median survival time of responders irrespective of tumor size was 36 months, whereas that of nonresponders was only 3 months. Thus the size of the HCC at the commencement of therapy has significant influence not only on the initial response but also on the ultimate survival. Survival was also significantly prolonged in responders.

Alcohol Injection

Ninety-five percent alcohol can be injected directly into a liver tumor under ultrasound guidance. The alcohol exerts its therapeutic effect by desiccation of tumor cells. The treatment is usually limited to small tumors (< 3 cm) and is given when the liver contains no more than three nodules. Alcohol injection is indicated when the liver function is not satisfactory for liver resection. The procedure consists of insertion of a 22-gauge Chiba needle through a puncture probe into the center of the tumor. Two other needles are inserted into the edge of the nodule. After all three needles are in correct position, alcohol is injected slowly while the needle is slowly withdrawn. The alcohol can be seen spreading throughout the tumor on ultrasound screening. After the alcohol injection is completed, the needles are left in situ for 5 minutes so that alcohol spillage into the peritoneal cavity and severe pain will not occur. About 2 to 6 ml of alcohol is given for each treatment session, depending on the size of the tumors, and the treatment is repeated once a week until the whole tumor and about a 5-mm rim of normal liver is covered by alcohol. The treatment is generally considered contraindicated if the patient has ascites, poor liver function, or a bleeding tendency. When the lesion is subcapsular, alcohol injection is also not advisable because spillage of alcohol and tumor cells into the peritoneal cavity is likely.

Systemic Chemotherapy

Systemic chemotherapy is given when there is extrahepatic dissemination of HCC, but the systemic chemotherapy, whether as a single drug, as multiple drugs, or with a potentiating agent (e.g., verapamil), is only occasionally successful. A higher response rate may be observed with heavy doses of multiple drugs, but the side effects are substantial, and the quality of life is very poor. Once the treatment is withdrawn because of side effects, rapid progression of the disease is almost universal. In general, systemic chemotherapy is given only when there is no better treatment option and when the patient's general condition and liver function are still acceptable.

Other Treatment

Other forms of regional or systemic treatment have been reported. Regional therapy utilizing agents that are selectively sequestrated in HCCs, such as I-131, I-131-antihuman HCC isoferritin, yttrium 90, microencapsulated mitomycin and alpha-fetoprotein–adriamycin conjugate, have been shown to be useful, but these studies involved relatively small numbers of patients and none were comparative studies except the study on I-131-isoferritin. In this report, I-131-isoferritin and low-dose chemotherapy led to the same survival rate as full-dose chemotherapy. Since the treatment protocol also involved external irradiation and systemic chemotherapy, it is difficult to determine the role of I-131-isoferritin alone.

In a study carried out in the authors' institution, the administration of intramuscular recombinant interferon alpha-2 induced tumor regression of over 50% in 10% of patients and of 25% to 50% in 12% of patients. Moreover, interferon alpha-2 was superior to doxorubicin. Another randomized controlled trial at the authors' institution has also demonstrated that both tumor regression and survival of patients treated with interferon alpha-2 were significantly better than that of patients who received no antitumor therapy. However, the cost of treatment is prohibitive and therefore not readily available to many patients.

Results

The overall result of the treatment of HCCs is poor because most patients have an advanced stage of the disease or poor liver function. Of all the patients referred to a surgical unit in the authors' institution, only 20% can undergo tumor resection, and another 20% are suitable for TACE. For the others, meaningful treatment cannot be offered because of disseminated disease or poor liver function.

Surgical resection is the only treatment that can offer cure. The 5-year and 8-year survival rates have been 15% and 12%, respectively. However, the hospital mortality rate can be as high as 20% in series that are composed largely of major hepatectomies for large tumors and in the presence of cirrhosis. A lower hospital mortality rate is often seen in series involving patients that have limited resection for small tumors.

The high operative mortality is often due to liver failure and sepsis. Liver failure results from loss of functioning liver mass and injury to the liver remnant during surgery. Sepsis is probably due to enhanced catabolic response, increased proteolysis, and suppression of immunocompetence in patients with underlying chronic liver diseases. In addition to meticulous surgical technique to avoid excessive blood loss and hepatic ischemia, as well as preservation of functioning liver parenchyma, intensive perioperative nutritional therapy may improve the operative result because it can reduce the catabolic response and improve protein synthesis and liver regeneration. In the authors' recent prospective randomized study, perioperative nutritional therapy in the form of intravenous infusion of branched-chain enriched amino acids, dextrose, and medium-chain triglycerides resulted in reduced incidence of postoperative septic complication, reduced requirement of diuretic to control ascites, less weight loss, and higher serum levels of prealbumin, retinol-binding protein, and transferrin. In addition, treated patients had less deterioration of liver function as measured by indocyanine green clearance test, and a slightly lower mortality rate. Such benefits were obvious in cirrhotic patients that had major liver resection but not in patients with minor resection.

After a successful surgical resection, almost 60% of patients manifested recurrence within the first year. Thus the 1-year survival rate was only 65%. The majority (80%) of the recurrences were confined to the liver remnant. These recurrences probably represent undetected or microscopic foci that grow rapidly and concomitantly with liver regeneration. Nevertheless, they are sometimes amenable to further treatments such as TACE, alcohol injection, or even re-resection. In selected cases, solitary extrahepatic recurrences, such as in the lung or omentum, are also amenable to resection. As a result, the postrecurrence survival rate can be significantly prolonged.

However, these treatments are unlikely to be effective unless tumors are relatively small at the time of detection. To detect small recurrences, the authors have adopted a policy of close surveillance using postoperative angiography coupled with ultrasonography and alpha-fetoprotein monitoring. The angiography can be performed via an intra-arterial device ("Implantofix") inserted into the gastroduodenal artery after liver resection. Iodized oil can also be injected via an Implantofix followed by CT to detect early recurrence if the angiography is normal. An alternative approach aiming at deferring postoperative recurrence is adjuvant chemotherapy, which should be administered into the liver itself and into the systemic circulation. In a pilot study, postoperative hepatic artery chemotherapy was found to be effective in prolonging survival in the high-risk group. The validity of such an approach needs to be confirmed in a prospective randomized trial.

The result of TACE has been gratifying, considering the good response in small HCCs and occasionally even in relatively large tumors, as well as the fact that no effective palliative treatments were available in the past. Survival is prolonged and the quality of life is much improved, especially if the tumors decrease in size. There is also usually improvement in well-being, gain in appetite and weight, and reduction in epigastric pain or discomfort. The overall 1-year and 2-year survival rates from the authors' study were 50% and 34%, respectively.

The overall prognosis of HCC with or without treatment is dependent on the size of the lesion. For example, survival rates of 70% and 50% at 5 and 10 years, respectively, after surgical resection of small HCCs have been reported from China. For small HCCs with relatively good liver function selected for alcohol injection, the 1-year survival rate could be as high as 89%. To improve the overall prognosis, it is necessary to screen inhabitants in endemic areas or subjects at risk of developing HCC (known cirrhotics, hepatitis B virus carriers, and family members of patients with HCC). The recommendation for the frequency of screening is 8- to 10-month intervals. Through a combination of ultrasonography and alpha-fetoprotein estimation, 95% of early HCCs can be detected. The cost-effectiveness of screening is, however, debatable. Screening inhabitants in endemic areas or hepatitis B carriers will yield a low discovery rate of early HCCs which are often amenable to resection, but the cost of screening is enormous. However, limiting the screening to cirrhotic patients will be cost effective because it will lead to a high detection rate of tumors which unfortunately are often not suitable for resection or even other forms of treatment because of the multifocal nature of the disease and the underlying cirrhosis. Despite all these controversies, screening programs continue to be carried out in many centers as part of a concerted effort to improve the overall prognosis of HCC.

Conclusions

The future prospect of improving the prognosis of HCC will depend on a concerted effort of physicians to detect small HCCs, of interventional radiologists to provide effective regional treatment, and of surgeons to perform liver resection with a low morbidity and mortality rate. A combination of operative and nonoperative treatment may be necessary in selected patients. The ideal treatment is that which will arrest the progression of chronic liver disease to HCC, but such treatment is unlikely to be available in the foreseeable future.

Selected Readings

Choi TK, et al. Results of surgical resection for hepatocellular carcinoma. *Hepatogastroenterology* 1990; 37: 172–175.

Lai CL, et al. Recombinant interferon-α in inoperable hepatocellular carcinoma: A randomized controlled trial. *Hepatology* 1993; 17:389–394.

Lai ECS, et al. Hepatectomy for large hepatocellular carcinoma: The optimal resection margin. *World J Surg* 1991; 15:141–145.

Lai ECS, et al. Long term results of resection for large hepatocellular carcinoma: A multivariate analysis of clinicopathological features. *Hepatology* 1990; 11: 815–818.

Ngan H. Lipiodol computerized tomography: How sensitive and specific is the technique in the diagnosis of hepatocellular carcinoma? *Br J Radiol* 1990; 63: 771–775.

Ngan H, et al. Treatment of inoperable hepatocellular carcinoma by transcatheter arterial chemoembolization using an emulsion of cisplatin in iodized oil and Gelfoam. *Clin Radiol* 1993; 47:315–320.

Nonami T, et al. The potential role of postoperative hepatic artery chemotherapy in patients with high-risk hepatomas. *Ann Surg* 1991; 213:222–226.

Shiina S, et al. Percutaneous ethanol injection therapy of hepatocellular carcinoma: Analysis of 77 patients. *Am J Roentgenol* 1990; 155:1221–1226.

Taniguchi H, et al. Vascular inflow exclusion and hepatic resection. *Br J Surg* 1992; 79:672–675.

Tjandra JJ, Fan ST, Wong J. Peri-operative mortality in hepatic resection. *Aust N Z J Surg* 1991; 61:201–206.

14

Hepatic Metastases

Jane I. Tsao
Christopher P. Molgaard
Charles F. White
Kevin S. Hughes

Etiology and Incidence

Metastatic neoplasm is the most common malignant disease of the liver in the United States. The majority of hepatic metastases are from primary malignant neoplasms of the colon, pancreas, breast, ovaries, rectum, and stomach (Table 14-1). Metastases reach the liver by four routes: the portal vein, lymphatic channels, the hepatic artery, and direct extension. Primary malignancies from the gastrointestinal tract reach the liver by the portal vein and mesenteric lymphatics; those from the genitourinary tract reach the liver via nearby tributaries of the portal vein; melanoma and lung and breast carcinoma reach the liver by the systemic circulation via the hepatic artery and/or mediastinal lymphatics; primary malignant neoplasms of the biliary tract, pancreas, stomach, and colon may also reach the liver by direct extension.

Hepatic Metastases from Colorectal Carcinoma

Synchronous metastases are instances when both the hepatic metastasis and the primary carcinoma are discovered at the same time. The incidence of synchronous hepatic metastases from colorectal carcinoma is in the range of 15% to 25%.

Metachronous metastasis is the appearance of hepatic metastasis at some time interval following local control of the primary cancer. In 1984 Willett et al. retrospectively reviewed 553 patients who underwent curative resection of colon carcinoma at the Massachusetts General Hospital. They found that 6% of the patients had hepatic metastases alone, and another 11% had peritoneal and/or intra-abdominal lymph nodal metastases concurrent with hepatic metastases. The incidence of hepatic metastases increased in proportion to the stage of the primary colon carcinoma (Table 14-2). The researchers found that the location of the primary colon carcinoma did not affect the incidence or pattern of hepatic metastases. A report from the Memorial Sloan-Kettering Cancer Center in 1984 of 412 patients who underwent curative resection for rectal carcinoma showed that 5% of their patients had metastases involving the liver alone, and another 12% had hepatic metastases concurrent with peritoneal or lymph nodal metastases.

Data from patients with hepatic metastases from colorectal carcinoma treated at St. Mark's Hospital (n = 120), the Memorial Sloan-Kettering Cancer Center (n = 217), and the University of Alabama at Birmingham (n = 147) showed that the distribution of hepatic metastases was bilobar in 50% to 68% of the patients, was limited to the right lobe in 22% to 38%, and was limited to the left lobe in 7% to 13%. The principles of management of patients with hepatic metastases from colon and rectal carcinoma are dictated by the incidence and patterns of metastatic disease.

Table 14-1. Overall Incidence of Hepatic Metastases from Various Primary Neoplasms

Primary Neoplasm	Incidence of Hepatic Metastases (%)
Colon	65
Pancreas	63
Breast	61
Ovary	52
Rectum	47
Stomach	45
Lung	36
Kidney	27

Hepatic Metastases from Noncolorectal Malignant Neoplasms

The incidences and patterns of hepatic metastases from noncolorectal malignant neoplasms have not been as well studied as those from colorectal primaries. Generally, hepatic metastases from noncolorectal primaries occur in the setting of systemic dissemination, and very few patients present with resectable disease limited to the liver. Survival of the majority of patients with unresected hepatic metastases from noncolorectal neoplasms is poor; a mean survival of 6 months for patients with hepatic metastases from carcinoma of the stomach, pancreas (exocrine), breast, and melanoma is generally reported.

In contradistinction, hepatic metastases from carcinoid tumor and pancreatic islet cell tumors are often slow-growing, and prolonged survival is possible despite frequent bilobar and multicentric hepatic involvement. Even without hepatic resection, patients with pancreatic islet cell tumor metastatic to the liver have a median survival of 3.3 years, and patients with carcinoid tumor involving the liver have a 25% 6-year survival rate.

Diagnosis

Laboratory Studies

The carcinoembryonic antigen (CEA) is often elevated in patients who have colorectal carcinoma with hepatic metastases. Often asymptomatic patients will present with elevated CEA levels at interval follow-up after removal of the primary colorectal malignant neoplasm, and diagnostic workup will reveal the presence of hepatic metastases.

The serum alkaline phosphatase level is often elevated in patients with hepatic metastases; frequently, it may be the only abnormally elevated liver enzyme. Other liver enzymes that may be elevated in the face of hepatic metastases are gamma-glutamyl transpeptidase (GGTP), alanine aminotransferase (ALT), aspartate aminotransferase (AST), and lactic dehydrogenase (LDH).

Examination of a 24-hour urine collection for 5-hydroxyindoleacetic acid (5-HIAA) is a relatively sensitive method for detecting metastatic carcinoid tumors within the liver, particularly in symptomatic patients.

Imaging Studies

Ultrasonography (US) and conventional intravenous-contrast–enhanced computerized tomography (CT) have been the main imaging modalities for diagnosing lesions of the liver. Reported sensitivities for detection of hepatic metastases using these imaging studies have been variable, from 41% to 73% for US, and from 48% to 88% for CT; the specificity of both tests is greater than 90%. The appearance of hepatic metastases on CT is quite varied. Lesions are usually less dense than surrounding liver; they may have a thickened ring with mural nodules; on rare occasions they are septated and calcified.

Table 14-2. Incidence of Intra-abdominal Recurrence After Resection of Colon Carcinoma

Duke's Stage	Number of Patients	Liver Alone (%)	Liver and Extrahepatic dz (%)
A	29	0	0
B	335	5	12
C	169	8	28
Total	533	6	17

Source: Willett CG, et al. Failure patterns following curative resection of colonic carcinoma. *Ann Surg* 1984; 200(6):685–690.

Many new developments have occurred in the imaging of the liver during the last 10 years. These have included sequential dynamic bolus CT (DBCT), delayed iodine CT (DICT), CT angiography (CTA), CT arterial portography (CTAP), magnetic resonance imaging (MRI), and intraoperative ultrasound (IOUS).

SEQUENTIAL DYNAMIC BOLUS CT (DBCT)

In this approach, contiguous scans are made through the liver within 3 minutes after and during the rapid injection of 150 ml of 60% iodinated contrast (Fig. 14-1). This is the period of time during which the greatest contrast difference between tumor and normal liver is achieved. Sequential DBCT is now the procedure of choice for surveying or screening hepatic tumors; it has a sensitivity of about 85% to 90% for detecting lesions of the liver.

DELAYED IODINE CT (DICT)

Scans are performed 4 to 6 hours after administration of 60 to 80 g of intravenous iodine. By this time there is increased accumulation of iodine in hepatocytes and thus increased density of the liver parenchyma. This increased density creates an artificial contrast between focal abnormalities that do not take up iodine, such as tumor, and normal liver, which does. DICT has been reported to be more sensitive than DBCT. In one study, DICT detected additional lesions not seen on DBCT in 26% of the patients.

CT ANGIOGRAPHY (CTA) AND CT ARTERIAL PORTOGRAPHY (CTAP)

These studies are invasive, requiring the placement of a catheter in the hepatic artery for CTA and in the superior mesenteric artery for CTAP. The liver is sequentially scanned during the injection of 100 to 150 ml of 60% iodinated contrast at 3 ml/sec (Fig. 14-2). Since the hepatic artery is the sole blood supply of hepatic tumors, hepatic artery injection sharply increases the density of the periphery of tumor nodules when compared to the surrounding normal hepatic parenchyma during CTA. On the other hand, since hepatic tumors are not fed by the portal vein, liver lesions stand out as defects within a field of increased parenchymal density during CTAP (see Fig. 14-2). Both CTA and CTAP boast sensitivities for detecting liver lesions of over 90%. CTA and CTAP are especially sensitive for detecting lesions smaller than 1 cm, which are often missed on intravenous contrast CT. However, the increased sensitivity of CTA and CTAP has not meant increased specificity. Some of the lesions detected may be hepatic cysts or hemangiomas. Several dif-

Figure 14-1. CT scan with IV and PO contrast showing a large metastasis in the right liver.

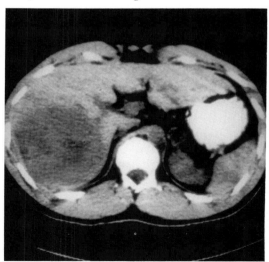

Figure 14-2. Dynamic CT scan showing diffuse liver metastases from colorectal carcinoma.

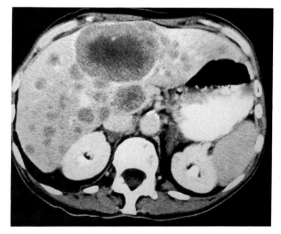

ferent types of perfusion abnormalities can be confused with tumor neovascularization on CTA: therefore, the increased sensitivity may be limited by experience with image interpretation. As experience accumulates with CTA and CTAP, these imaging modalities can provide important additional information in the preoperative evaluation and selection of patients for resection of hepatic metastases.

MAGNETIC RESONANCE IMAGING (MRI)

With MRI, the body is exposed to a magnetic field and gamma radiation is not involved. Depending on the magnetic field used, the intensity of a lesion can be enhanced or that of normal tissue depressed. MRI is ideal for examining blood flow and the presence of clots or tumor in blood vessels. Proper evaluation of the liver with MRI requires considerable technical expertise because a multiplicity of factors may degrade images and cause large lesions to become undetectable. The MRI appearance of hepatic metastasis is usually that of a mass less intense than the surrounding liver on T_1-weighted images, and more intense than the liver on T_2-weighted images. The lesions have irregular borders and thick walls, and may have areas of necrosis and hemorrhage within them. The varied MRI appearance of hepatic metastases overlaps with that of other malignant and benign lesions of the liver. Furthermore, tumors of the same cell type may have varied appearances, depending on their age, size, and degree of hemorrhage and necrosis. MRI and DBCT have similar sensitivities, and both have complementary roles in the survey of liver lesions. The precise role of MRI in the imaging of hepatic metastases remains to be determined.

INTRAOPERATIVE ULTRASOUND (IOUS)

IOUS is performed with a 5.0- or 7.5-MHz transducer which can be gas-sterilized. After the liver is fully exposed and mobilized in the operating room, the ultrasound transducer is placed directly on the liver and the liver is scanned systematically. IOUS depicts the relationship of the tumor to blood vessels and bile ducts. It reveals the confluence of the three hepatic veins as they enter the IVC. The status of resectability or the surgical approach may be altered if tumor involvement or encroachment upon this critical area of vascular confluence is observed on IOUS. IOUS also allows the delineation of portal vein branches to the intrasegmental level. In addition to its diagnostic application, IOUS can be very useful in providing guidance for fine-needle aspiration and core biopsy of deep and nonpalpable hepatic lesions during surgery.

IOUS has resulted in detection of lesions not diagnosed by preoperative imaging or by intraoperative palpation in 3% to 19% of the patients. Most, if not all, of these lesions have been less than 2 cm and not palpable. Several reports have demonstrated IOUS with a sensitivity of 96% to 98% in detecting hepatic metastases and a specificity of 90%. Various clinical reports have claimed that IOUS have affected their surgical approach and management in 19% to 49% of the operations. One study compared the sensitivity of preoperative CTAP with that of IOUS in the detection of hepatic metastases from colorectal carcinoma and found the sensitivities to be 91% and 96%, respectively. This difference was not statistically significant, and the authors concluded that IOUS and CTAP are complementary techniques and that preoperative CTAP does not obviate the potential benefits of IOUS.

The roles of these new imaging modalities in the diagnosis and management of hepatic metastases continue to evolve. Even though many published reports have cited increased sensitivity in the detecton of hepatic lesions with new imaging modalities, data reflecting consistent and reproducible results in large patient samples and across institutional boundaries are still forthcoming.

Laparoscopy

Since 1993 Lahey Clinic has been performing diagnostic laparoscopy prior to laparotomy for patients who are candidates for resection of hepatic metastases based on preoperative imaging studies. Both procedures are done under general anesthesia in the operating room at the same setting. In patients with multiple previous upper abdominal operations, success at laparoscopy may be limited by dense adhesions. In these patients, the authors proceed to laparotomy without unproductive attempts at laparoscopy.

The open method is used for insufflation of a pneumoperitoneum. A 1-cm skin incision is made in the abdominal wall (preferably in the midline) away from previous surgical incisions. Blunt dissection exposes the abdominal wall fascia. The visualized fascia is tented by two anchoring sutures and incised by a scalpel. Often preperitoneal fat is encountered at this point, and a finger is introduced to bluntly enter the peritoneal cavity and ensure clearance of underlying viscera and adhesions. The Hasson trocar (Weck Company, Princeton, NJ) is then placed into the peritoneal cavity via the fascial opening. The pneumoperitoneum is insufflated via the Hasson trocar. The laparoscopic camera and lens system are placed into the distended abdomen via the Hasson trocar. Placement of additional trocars, if needed, is done under direct visualization.

Excellent views of the majority of the liver surfaces are possible via the laparoscope. A 30-degree–angled lens allows good visualization of the dome and posterior surface of the liver, which may be difficult to see well with the standard lens. A five-pronged laparoscopic fan retractor can be used to provide steady retraction of the liver to facilitate mobilization, inspection of the subhepatic space, and biopsy of lymph nodes in the hepatoduodenal ligament if indicated. Furthermore, percutaneous fine-needle aspiration and core biopsies can be obtained with laparoscopic guidance. Appropriate use of diagnostic laparoscopy prior to laparotomy avoids an unnecessary laparotomy in patients with extrahepatic metastases or unresectable hepatic metastases. The morbidity and cost of exploratory laparotomy—incisional pain, postoperative ileus, and hospitalization—are thus avoided. Patients who have had laparoscopy with or without biopsy are usually observed in the hospital for 24 hours; hemoglobin level and hematocrit are checked prior to dismissal.

Management and Results

Woodington and Waugh in 1963 reported a 20% 5-year survival rate and a median survival of 35 months in 20 patients undergoing hepatic resection for metastases from a variety of neoplasms originating from colon, stomach, gallbladder, pancreas (exocrine and endocrine), and cutaneous melanoma. They were among the pioneer hepatic surgeons who first advocated a resective approach to treating patients with metastatic lesions of the liver.

Resection of Hepatic Metastases from Colorectal Carcinoma

Wagner and Adson in 1984 reported an overall 5-year survival rate of 25% among 116 patients with resected hepatic metastases from colorectal neoplasms (Table 14-3). Similar survival rates were found in multi-institutional retrospective and prospective studies.

The Registry of Hepatic Metastases (RHM) is a multi-institutional cooperative effort aimed at

Table 14-3. Survival of Patients with Hepatic Metastases from Colorectal Primaries with and Without Hepatic Resection

	GITSG[a]	Scheele et al.[b]	Wagner and Adson[c]
Unresectable	n = 63	n = 921	—
Median survival (mos)	17	7	—
5-yr survival (%)	0	0	—
Resectable but not resected	—	n = 62	n = 60
Median survival (mos)	—	14	—
5-yr survival (%)	—	0	0
Noncurative resection	n = 18	n = 43	—
Median survival (mos)	21	13	—
5-year survival (%)	0	0	—
Curative resection	n = 69	n = 184	n = 116
Median survival (mos)	36	—	—
5-yr survival (%)	37	40	25
5-yr disease-free survival (%)	23	—	—

[a]GITSG = Gastrointestinal Tumor Study Group.
[b]Data from Scheele J, Stangle R, Attendorf-Hofmann A. Hepatic metastases from colorectal carcinoma: Impact of surgical resection on the natural history. *Br J Surg* 1990; 77(11):1241–1246.
[c]Data from Wagner JS et al. The natural history of hepatic metastases from colorectal cancer: A comparison with resective treatment. *Ann Surg* 1983; 199(5): 502–507.

reaching a better understanding of the effect of resection of hepatic metastases from colorectal carcinoma. This retrospective review involved 859 patients from 24 institutions across the United States and West Germany who underwent resection of hepatic metastases between 1948 and 1985 (Hughes et al.). The Registry data revealed a 5-year actuarial survival rate of 33% and a 5-year actuarial disease-free survival rate of 21% (Fig. 14-3).

The Gastrointestinal Tumor Study Group (GITSG) carried out a prospective evaluation of hepatic resection for colorectal carcinoma metastases to the liver. This study involved 156 patients from 15 institutions treated prospectively between July 1984 and May 1988. With a median follow-up of 3.2 years, this group found a 5-year disease-free survival rate of 23% among 69 patients who underwent "curative resection" of hepatic metastases (see Table 14-3).

PROGNOSTIC FACTORS

Wagner et al. in 1983 reported that the presence of extrahepatic metastases implied an unfavorable prognosis. An advanced stage of the primary colorectal carcinoma was also associated with a poor prognosis. Duke's B primary lesions with resected

hepatic metastases had a 5-year survival rate of 32%, compared with 18% in patients with Duke's C lesions. There was no difference in survival between patients with resected solitary or multiple hepatic metastases. The location, grade, and size of the primary lesion did not affect prognosis after hepatic resection.

Factors found to have a negative prognostic significance from the Registry of Hepatic Metastases affirmed and expanded upon the findings of Adson. Negative prognostic factors included tumor involvement of lymph nodes in the hepatoduodenal ligament and celiac axis, discontinuous extrahepatic metastases, more than four metastatic lesions within the liver, a margin of resection less than or equal to 1 cm, an advanced stage of primary colon or rectal carcinoma, and a disease-free interval of less than 1 year from diagnosis of primary colorectal carcinoma (Figs. 14-4, 14-5).

PATTERNS OF RECURRENCE

The Registry of Hepatic Metastases also analyzed the patterns of recurrence following resection of hepatic metastases. Forty-three percent of the patients had recurrence in the liver, and 31% had recurrence in the lung. Patients with bilobar me-

Figure 14-3. Postresectional 5-year overall survival and disease-free survival rates. (Data from the Registry of Hepatic Metastases.)

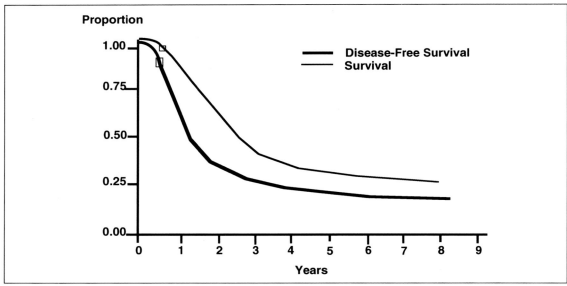

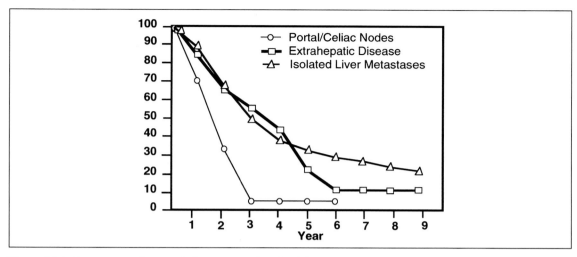

Figure 14-4. Postresectional survival of patients with isolated liver metastases, extrahepatic disease, and disease in portal/celiac lymph nodes. (Data from the Registry of Hepatic Metastases.)

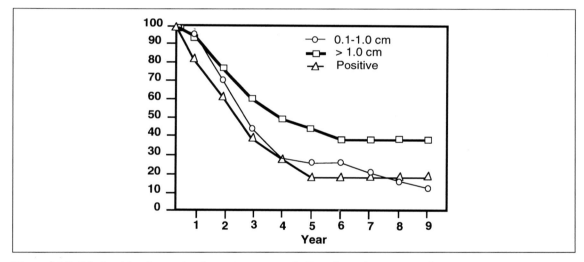

Figure 14-5. Relationship of resectional margin to survival. (Data from the Registry of Hepatic Metastases.)

tastases and positive pathologic margins at the initial hepatic resection were at increased risk of recurrence in the liver (64% and 68%, respectively). Thirty-six percent of the patients had recurrences in the first year after hepatic resection; 17% recurred in the liver, 8% recurred in the lung, 7% had local regional recurrence at the primary tumor site, and 2% had recurrence in the bone.

NATURAL HISTORY

In selecting patients for hepatic resection, are we only treating those patients who are likely to live longer anyway? Is the prolonged survival a result of surgical resection or a reflection of a less aggressive biologic nature of the patient's neoplasm?

Wagner and Adson in 1984 reported no 5-year survivors among 70 patients seen at the Mayo Clinic between 1943 and 1976 with resectable but unresected hepatic metastases from colorectal primaries. On the contrary, as already mentioned, in 116 patients who underwent hepatic resection during the same period and were rendered grossly disease-free, a 25% 5-year survival rate was observed ($p = 0.0001$) (see Table 14-3). Likewise, Scheele et al. in 1990 reported no 5-year survivors among 62 patients seen between 1960 and 1987 with resectable but unresected hepatic metastases. In 183 patients who were resected and rendered grossly disease-free, they found a 5-year survival rate of 40% ($p < 0.0001$). They further noted that survival patterns of patients who underwent resection but had gross disease left behind were the same as the patients who had resectable disease but were not resected. Median survival was 13 to 14 months, and 5-year survival was zero (see Table 14-3).

No prospective randomized studies comparing results of hepatic resection versus no resection in matched patients with proven resectable hepatic metastases from colorectal carcinoma have been reported. Rosen et al., in 1992, performed a statistical estimation showing that in order to achieve statistical significance, a randomized trial of nonresection versus resection for resectable hepatic metastases would require the accrual of an unrealistic number of patients. Furthermore, denying a patient who has potentially resectable disease and is eager to seek treatment the only chance of prolonged survival, and perhaps a 20% to 30% chance of cure, is not ethically sound.

MORBIDITY AND MORTALITY

Currently, in the hands of experienced hepatic surgeons, the mortality of elective hepatic resection is less than 2%, and the morbidity is around 16%. The average length of postoperative hospital stay is about 7 days. In patients with resectable hepatic metastases with no severe comorbid medical diseases, the risks of hepatic resection per se should not be a deterrent to hepatic resection.

SYNCHRONOUS METASTASES

In patients with synchronous hepatic metastases, Cady and Stone, in 1991, advocated a waiting period of 4 to 6 months to allow for declaration of the biologic character of the hepatic metastases. The authors agree, in principle, with Cady and Stone

that a waiting period to allow for better characterization of the liver lesion(s) and for recovery from the primary operation is appropriate. There are, however, no data giving clear guidelines as to the most appropriate waiting interval. The authors generally study these patients at 8 weeks postoperatively from surgery of primary colorectal carcinoma.

ADJUVANT CHEMOTHERAPY

Currently, no data demonstrate any survival benefits in patients who have received adjuvant chemotherapy following complete resection of hepatic metastases. Studies are presently under way, however, to answer this question.

Resection of Hepatic Metastases from Noncolorectal Carcinoma

Wolf et al. in 1991 reviewed 151 cases of resection of noncolorectal hepatic metastases performed at multiple institutions. They found that resection of hepatic metastases led to a 5-year survival rate of 40% in patients with Wilms' tumor and carcinoid tumor. An overall 15% 5-year survival rate was found in patients with hepatic metastases from carcinoma of the breast, kidney, adrenal, and stomach, and from melanoma and visceral leiomyosarcomas. However, resection of hepatic metastases from primary neoplasms of the pancreas (exocrine), ovary, endometrium, and cervix did not result in any long-term survivors.

Significant palliation of symptoms has been reported with debulking of carcinoid tumors and pancreatic islet cell tumors even when total tumor extirpation is not possible. Symptomatic carcinoid disease of the liver can also be successfully managed by operative hepatic artery ligation or percutaneous hepatic artery embolization. Symptomatic improvement has been achieved in 87% of patients who were embolized or dearterialized.

Cryosurgery

Cryosurgery is a technique by which tumors are destroyed using liquid nitrogen at $-196°C$. Two or three freeze and thaw cycles are used. The mechanism of action is by nonspecific tissue destruction because there is no tumor-specific effect. Real-time intraoperative ultrasound is used to monitor the effects of hepatic cryosurgery. Potential indications for hepatic cryosurgery are small solitary lesions located deep within the hepatic parenchyma; bilateral disease otherwise unresectable, for which a combined approach is indicated with resection of the portion of liver predominantly involved and freezing of lesions in the remaining liver; and limited recurrent disease when repeat hepatic resection is not feasible. Potential side effects of cryosurgery are perioperative hypothermia, thrombocytopenia, myoglobinuria, hepatic parenchymal hemorrhage, and bile leak.

Ravikumar et al. reported in 1991 the results of 24 patients with surgically unresectable hepatic metastases who underwent cryosurgery. At a median follow-up of 2 years, they found that 29% of the patients were disease-free, another 34% were alive with disease, and 38% died. Onik reported in 1991 that among 18 patients who underwent cryosurgery, 33% were alive at a mean follow-up of 29 months. These preliminary results of cryosurgery are promising. The application of cryosurgery in patients with surgically unresectable metastases is worth further investigation.

Percutaneous Ethanol Injection Therapy

Percutaneous ethanol injection therapy (PEIT) involves the percutaneous placement of 20- to 22-gauge needles into hepatic lesions under ultrasound guidance, much as in fine-needle aspiration biopsy. Absolute ethanol is injected through the needle directly into the tumor, causing small vessel thrombosis and cellular dehydration and resulting in tumor necrosis. Different sites within the hepatic lesion are injected during approximately two to six biweekly sessions until ethanol has been injected throughout the entire lesion or lesions.

PEIT has been shown to improve survival of patients with small primary hepatocellular neoplasms, with relatively little morbidity. There has been limited experience with PEIT for colorectal metastases to the liver. Livraghi et al. reported the results of 14 patients with liver metastases, including 7 patients with colorectal metastases. Carcinoembryonic antigen (CEA) levels transiently decreased after PEIT in 6 of 7 patients. Imaging studies showed complete response in most small (1–2 cm) lesions. Larger lesions did not respond as completely as was usually seen in hepatocellular carci-

noma. The authors attributed the lower rate of tumor necrosis to the varied consistency of the metastatic lesions, resulting in less homogeneous distribution of the injected alcohol. In another series in which 8 patients underwent PEIT for colorectal liver metastases, a partial (60%–80%) response on follow-up imaging studies and a decrease in CEA level were observed in all patients. However, local recurrences or new hepatic lesions were detected in all patients during follow-up.

No reports on the long-term survival of patients undergoing PEIT for colorectal metastases have been published. The usual multicentricity of hepatic metastases from colorectal carcinoma will probably limit the effectiveness of PEIT. However, many centers are performing PEIT on selected cases, especially single, small but inoperable lesions.

Interstitial Laser Hyperthermia Therapy

Interstitial laser hyperthermia, also called interstitial laser photocoagulation, is a new, minimally invasive technique for treatment of hepatic neoplasms. Ultrasound guidance is used for the percutaneous placement of 18- or 19-gauge needles into the hepatic lesion or lesions. Small-caliber laser fibers are then placed through the needles with the tips of the fibers within the tumor. Multiple laser fibers are used for larger lesions. Low-power laser energy is then delivered to the fibers; this causes hyperthermia around the fiber tip and results in coagulative necrosis of the surrounding tumor tissue. Real-time ultrasonography is used to monitor the development of thermal changes.

Two recent studies have examined interstitial laser hyperthermia in hepatic metastases. Nolsoe et al. treated 11 patients with 16 colorectal hepatic metastases. Twelve of 16 lesions were considered completely destroyed on the basis of follow-up imaging, fine-needle biopsy, or operative findings. The 4 incompletely treated lesions had a larger mean diameter (3.4 cm) than the 12 which were completely treated (2.4 cm). Amin et al. treated 55 liver metastases in 21 patients, 15 of whom had colorectal metastases. Complications included severe abdominal pain in 4 patients, asymptomatic subcapsular hematoma in 4 patients, and pleural effusion in 6 patients. Tumor necrosis of more than 50% of the lesion was seen on follow-up CT scan in 45 of 55 lesions (82%), and 100% necrosis was seen in 21 of 55 lesions (38%). As in the previous study, smaller metastases (< 4 cm) had more complete necrosis and required fewer treatment sessions than larger lesions. The small numbers of patients and concurrent chemotherapy precluded reliable evaluation of a survival benefit. On the basis of these encouraging preliminary trials, a randomized multicenter study is being planned.

Interstitial Radiotherapy

Interstitial radiotherapy using ultrasound-guided percutaneous placement of iridium 192 sources into colorectal liver metastases has been reported safe in a small series, but there was no long-term follow-up. Radioactive implants may have a role in the treatment of deep-seated lesions or those located around major vessels.

Hepatic Arterial Embolization and Hepatic Chemoembolization

Hepatic arterial embolization (HAE) and hepatic chemoembolization (HCE) are transcatheter therapies for the treatment of liver neoplasms. These therapies take advantage of the fact that the blood supply to hepatic neoplasms is primarily from the hepatic artery rather than from the portal vein, as in normal liver. In HAE the intra-arterial injection of small particulate embolic material interrupts the primary blood supply to the tumor in an attempt to induce ischemia and necrosis. HCE combines the infusion of both embolic and chemotherapeutic agents. The goal of HCE is to induce tumor ischemia and to prolong the dwell time of the chemotherapeutic drug within the hepatic neoplasm. The morbidity of the procedure is low. However, a post–hepatic-embolization syndrome consisting of nausea, vomiting, pain, fever, elevated leukocyte count, and elevation in liver function tests occurs to a varying degree in all patients.

Evidence suggests that patients with hypervascular hepatic neoplasms such as hepatocellular carcinoma, carcinoid metastases, ocular melanoma metastases, and hormone-secreting tumor metastases benefit from HAE and HCE. Varied, but generally less promising, results have been reported with HAE and HCE for colorectal metastases. In a series

of liver lesions treated with HAE, Allison et al. reported that patients with metastatic nonendocrine tumors (primarily of colorectal origin) had a lower response rate and survival (median 7 months) than patients with hepatocellular carcinoma (median 10 months) or functioning endocrine metastases (15 months). In a randomized controlled trial of patients with colorectal metastases, no survival benefit from HAE over a control group receiving no therapy (median survival of 8.7 months for HAE and 9.6 months for controls) was observed. In the same trial there was a trend toward prolonged survival in a third group of patients treated with HCE (median survival 13 months). Early studies from M.D. Anderson Cancer Center also showed encouraging results of HAE and HCE for colorectal metastases. However, a recent review of their experience has showed no evidence of significant tumor response or of prolonged survival with HCE over that seen with less aggressive hepatic artery infusion therapy.

The rationale for treating colorectal metastases with HCE seems sound. However, the results have been disappointing. Because of the lack of good therapeutic alternatives in these patients, further study of HCE is warranted. There may be a different chemotherapeutic or embolic agent which would prove more efficacious. Also, a subset of patients may be found (e.g., patients with relatively hypervascular metastases) who might benefit from this therapy.

Chemotherapy for Unresectable Hepatic Metastases

The most effective single agent in the management of advanced colorectal carcinoma is 5-fluorouracil (5-FU). Most trials report a 10% to 15% objective response rate with standard intermittent intravenous administration of fluorouracil for metastatic colorectal carcinoma. Various dosage schedules and methods of fluorouracil administration, including bolus, short-term continuous infusion, and protracted intravenous infusion via ambulatory infusion pumps, have been reported. With increasing doses of fluorouracil and prolongation of infusion, response rates have increased, but fluorouracil alone has failed to improve survival rates in patients with metastatic colorectal cancer. Toxicities of fluorouracil, including mucositis, diarrhea, and leucopenia, often become dose-limiting factors in therapy.

Other agents showing activity against colorectal carcinoma include chloroethylnitrosoureas, mitomycin, and several newly identified agents such as CPT-11 (a semisynthetic derivative of camptothecin, a topoisomerase inhibitor). Multiple-combination chemotherapy regimens have been tried, but none have produced a survival advantage over single-agent therapy with fluorouracil.

Recently, modulation of fluorouracil has produced higher response rates than fluorouracil alone in previously untreated patients with advanced colorectal cancer. Agents with known modulating effects upon fluorouracil include methotrexate, leucovorin, and interferon. Clinical studies have shown a 40% response rate and a 4- to 5-month extension of the median survival in patients receiving 5-FU combined with leucovorin. On the basis of such data, the Food and Drug Administration has approved leucovorin for use in combination with 5-FU for the palliative treatment of patients with advanced colorectal carcinoma.

Hepatic Artery Infusion

Several centers have used hepatic artery infusion (HAI) of fluorodeoxyuride (FUDR) in patients with metastases which are confined to the liver but anatomically not resectable. Hepatic artery infusion is achieved with a surgically implanted catheter in the hepatic artery; the catheter is connected to a pump or port-a-cath placed subcutaneously. As an alternative to a surgically placed catheter, percutaneous catheterization of the hepatic artery through the transaxillary or transbrachial routes has been employed.

Even though HAI offers the theoretical advantages of higher drug concentration in the tumor area and potentially decreased systemic toxicity, results of therapy have been palliative only, and the systemic toxicity rates are similar. A high response rate, over 50% complete or partial response, has been reported with HAI. However, survival benefits of HAI are limited and last no more than 6 to 9 months. One specific complication of HAI is chemically induced sclerosing cholangitis.

Combined Cytoreduction Protocol

For the group of patients who have isolated hepatic metastases not amenable to resection because of their location or distribution within the liver, Sugarbaker and Steves, in 1993, described a hepatic cytoreduction protocol using combined multimodality therapy. Percutaneous radiologic or operative catheterization of the hepatic artery is done. 5-FU is given intra-arterially at 20 mg/kg for 5 consecutive days. Two cycles of mitomycin C at 20 mg/m² are given systemically via a peripheral vein on the third day of the treatment. After the toxic side effects of chemotherapy have resolved, in patients who did not have disease progression, a variety of surgical techniques were used for extirpation of all diagnosable lesions of the liver. These techniques included surgical resection, cryosurgery, alcohol injection, and implantation of radioactive iridium. If the patient did not respond to chemotherapy or if there was an interval detection of systemic cancer, the patient was spared an aggressive surgical tumor extirpation procedure.

This protocol offers the theoretical advantages of combined systemic and regional chemotherapy and mechanical tumor ablation within the liver. Preliminary results showed that 4 of 7 patients had a complete response; these 4 patients had a median survival of over 30 months. Longer follow-up and larger patient samples are needed to evaluate the efficacy and applicability of such a protocol; furthermore, the cost-benefit ratio of the combined treatments must be considered.

Conclusions

Resectable Hepatic Metastases from Colorectal Carcinoma

More sophisticated preoperative and intraoperative imaging has ushered in a new era of preresection diagnostic capability; this advance has aided in the selection of patients for surgery whose disease is limited to a resectable portion of the liver. In the hands of experienced hepatic surgeons, hepatic resection for metastatic colorectal carcinoma is associated with a low morbidity and mortality and a significant prolongation of survival in 25% to 35% of the patients. In carefully selected patients with hepatic metastases from colorectal primaries, hepatic resection remains the mainstay of therapy.

The goal of surgical resection of hepatic metastases from colorectal primaries is to prolong survival and perhaps to effect a cure by achieving a tumor-free state in the liver. To achieve this goal requires accurate preoperative and intraoperative imaging techniques, meticulous visual and tactile inspection by the surgeon at the time of laparotomy, and sound clinical judgment and decision making prior to and during the operation regarding the indications for and extent of hepatic resection. Appropriate use of diagnostic laparoscopy and IOUS may minimize the chances of noncurative resection. The surgeon must acquire the technical expertise required to perform an anatomic as well as a nonanatomic hepatic resection, and must have a thorough knowledge of the anatomy of the hepatic hilum and the retrohepatic vasculature. A radiologist with special expertise in ultrasonography is very helpful in the operating room. During the performance of IOUS, the coordinated efforts of the surgeon and the radiologist often yield useful additional information which may have bearing on the surgical approach. Finally, the decision whether or not to proceed with resection must be made in the patient's best interest and not based on "surgical momentum."

Unresectable Hepatic Metastases from Colorectal Carcinoma

Patients with evidence of unresectable extrahepatic disease such as concomitant liver and lung metastases or discontiguous intra-abdominal metastases are treated with systemic 5-fluorouracil and leucovorin.

A group of patients with isolated hepatic metastases exists for whom there is no established treatment pattern. These patients have metastases which are unresectable because of their location or distribution within the liver. Palliation is possible with hepatic artery infusion of FUDR. Cryosurgery has shown some favorable results on short-term follow-up in small patient samples. Investigative protocols combining systemic and regional chemotherapy, as well as mechanical tumor ablation, are ongoing and may offer a promise for the future.

Resectable Hepatic Metastases from Noncolorectal Malignant Neoplasms

Resection of hepatic metastases appears to prolong survival in very selected patients with noncolorectal primary malignant neoplasms. Current data suggest that patients with primary pancreatic (exocrine) and gynecologic malignant diseases would not be candidates for resection of hepatic metastases because the long-term survival probability is dismal. In patients with melanoma, visceral leiomyosarcoma, and malignant neoplasms of the breast, kidney, adrenal, and stomach who present with a possible resectable metastatic hepatic lesion, thorough imaging studies must be done to verify the liver as the sole site of metastasis. This regimen includes imaging of the lungs, brain, and bone. Furthermore, imaging studies to characterize the hepatic lesion and to determine resectability must be done preoperatively, just as for resection of colorectal metastases. Since very few patients with noncolorectal malignant neoplasms present with metastases limited to a resectable portion of the liver, careful patient selection is essential.

Patients with carcinoid tumor and pancreatic islet cell tumor metastatic to the liver should be considered for palliative resection to reduce local pain and systemic symptoms. Symptomatic carcinoid disease of the liver can also be successfully managed by surgical hepatic artery ligation and/or percutaneous hepatic artery embolization.

Selected Readings

Bernardino ME, Galambos JT. Computed tomography and magnetic resonance imaging of the liver. *Semin Liver Dis* 1989; 9(1):32–49.

Castaing D, Emond J, Bismuth H. Utility of operative ultrasound in the surgical management of liver tumors. *Ann Surg* 1986; 204(5):600–605.

Hughes KS and participants of the Registry of Hepatic Metastases. Resection of the liver for colorectal carcinoma metastases: A multi-institutional study of indications for resection. *Surgery* 1988; 103(3): 278–288.

Hughes KS and participants of the Registry of Hepatic Metastases. Resection of the liver for colorectal carcinoma metastases: A multi-institutional study of patterns of recurrence. *Surgery* 1986; 100(2):278–284.

Ravikumar TS, et al. Experimental and clinical observations on hepatic cryosurgery for colorectal metastases. *Cancer Res* 1991; 51:6323–6327.

Scheele J, Stangle R, Altendorf-Hofmann A. Hepatic metastases from colorectal carcinoma: Impact of surgical resection on the natural history. *Br J Surg* 1990; 77(11):1241–1246.

Sugarbaker PH, Steves MA. A cytoreductive approach to treatment of multiple liver metastases. *J Surg Oncol Suppl* 1993; 3:161–165.

Tsao JI, et al. Trends in morbidity and mortality of hepatic resection for malignant disease: A matched comparative analysis. *Ann Surg* (in press).

Wagner JS, et al. The natural history of hepatic metastases from colorectal cancer: A comparison with resective treatment. *Ann Surg* 1983; 199(5):502–507.

Willett CG, et al. Failure patterns following curative resection of colonic carcinoma. *Ann Surg* 1984; 200 (6):685–690.

15

Biliary Atresia

FRANCISCO G. CIGARROA
KATHLEEN B. SCHWARZ
PAUL M. COLOMBANI

Biliary atresia is defined as a progressive obliteration of patent bile ducts in the perinatal period. The etiology of this disease is unknown. The incidence in the United States has been estimated to be approximately 1 in 15,000 live births, and treatment requires early diagnosis and biliary reconstruction by hepatic portoenterostomy. Patients with biliary atresia will progress to biliary cirrhosis, portal hypertension, and eventual death if untreated. Liver transplantation can now salvage many children who fail to improve following hepaticoportoenterostomy.

Etiology and Pathogenesis

Embryology

The liver primordium appears as a ventral outgrowth of the foregut during the third week of embryogenesis. The hepatic diverticulum consists of two parts: the pars cranialis (hepatica), from which the liver arises, and the pars caudalis (cystica). The extrahepatic biliary ductal system, including the gallbladder, arises from the pars cystica during the fourth week. The bile ducts go through a solid phase during elongation and rapid epithelial proliferation. The bile duct lumens are re-established during the sixth week beginning with the common hepatic duct and proceeding distally. The most commonly held theory of development of the hepatobiliary system is that hepatocyte precursor cells give rise to the intrahepatic biliary system, which then joins the extrahepatic biliary bud at the hilum. Biliary atresia may result if the bile ducts

fail to recanalize. This cause of biliary atresia is a rare event supported only by a few stillborn and newborn infants identified with atretic bile ducts.

The etiology of biliary atresia remains unknown. The fact that it is a progressive disease and that there is acute and chronic inflammation within the portal triads suggests a postnatal insult. In fact, Landing believes that neonatal hepatitis and biliary atresia may be alternative outcomes of one underlying disorder "infantile obliterative cholangiopathy." Excitement occurred when observations were made that mice infected with reovirus-3 developed obliterative inflammation of the extrahepatic ducts. Unfortunately, infection with this virus could not be established as a cause of biliary atresia in humans.

Miyano proposed an anatomic variant as a cause of biliary atresia. Postmortem studies of infants with biliary atresia demonstrated a high incidence of a long common channel at the junction of the bile and pancreatic ducts. He suggested that reflux of pancreatic juices into the biliary tree resulted in damage to the ducts, with resultant atresia. This argument has been weakened by the fact that many patients with biliary atresia have normal anatomy.

Fetal and neonatal animal models have demonstrated that hepatobiliary defects similar to biliary atresia can result from mechanical obstruction of the bile ducts, ligation of fetal arteries supplying the biliary tree, and chemical exposure in utero. Clinical support for a vascular accident as the cause of some cases of biliary atresia exists from the occasional association with intestinal atresia. Other

causative theories include bile duct injury secondary to a cell-mediated immune event and bile duct
regression secondary to an imbalance of paracrine
growth factors.

The cause of biliary atresia is probably the end
result of various mechanisms operating at different
periods in gestation and infancy. In support of a
prenatal event is the fact that there exists a 20%
incidence of associated anomalies with biliary atresia. These include cardiac and genitourinary malformations, preduodenal portal vein, intestinal malro-
tation, and polysplenia. Several isolated reports of
affected siblings have been published, but the evidence is lacking for biliary atresia being an inherited disorder.

Pathology

The histologic pattern of biliary atresia demonstrates bile duct proliferation with an associated
inflammatory cell infiltrate (Fig. 15-1). Cholestasis
is prominent. These changes progress to fibrosis
with end-stage cirrhotic changes if obstruction is
not relieved (Fig. 15-2). The findings may be similar
to those in neonatal hepatitis, although in idiopathic

neonatal hepatitis, giant cells and hepatocellular
necrosis are more common than they are in biliary
atresia. Likewise, alpha$_1$-antitrypsin deficiency may
sometimes mimic biliary atresia histologically except that this metabolic disease can be distinguished
by the presence of periodic acid-Schiff (PAS) positive diastase resistant granules.

There are various forms of biliary atresia (Fig
15-3).

A.   The proximal extrahepatic ducts are patent and
     the distal ducts are fibrosed.
B.   The proximal ducts are obliterated and the gall-
     bladder, cystic duct, and common bile duct
     are patent.
C.   The proximal and distal bile ducts are oblit-
     erated.

Diagnosis

Clinical Presentation

Infants with biliary atresia are usually active and of
normal weight. They do not appear ill. Suspicion
for an underlying problem occurs when jaundice

Figure 15-1. Liver biopsy demonstrating bile duct proliferation in a patient with biliary atresia.

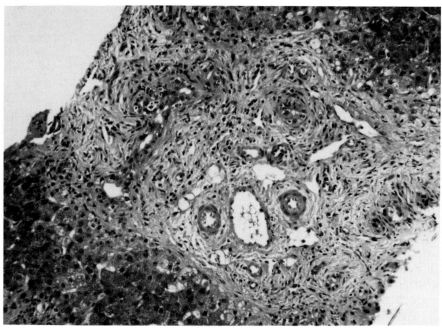

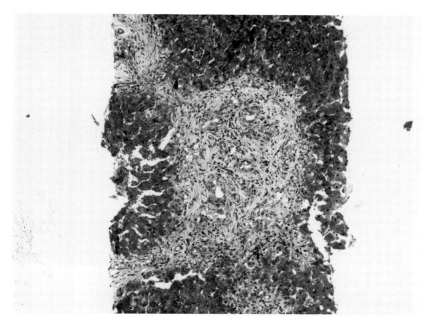

Figure 15-2. Liver biopsy demonstrating periportal fibrosis in a patient with biliary atresia.

persists after the second week of life, especially if the hyperbilirubinemia is predominantly conjugated. The differential diagnosis for conjugated hyperbilirubinemia is broad, including infections, metabolic disorders, idiopathic neonatal hepatitis, biliary hypoplasia secondary to Alagille's syndrome or non-syndromatic bile duct paucity, choledochal cyst, and extrinsic compression of the biliary tree. Infections leading to conjugated hyperbilirubinemia in the neonatal period include the following:

Cytomegalovirus
Rubella virus
Hepatitis B virus
Herpes simplex
Coxsackie B virus
Varicella-zoster virus
Gram-negative sepsis and urinary tract infections
Treponema pallidum
Toxoplasma gondii

Metabolic diseases leading to conjugated hyperbilirubinemia include the following:

Alpha$_1$-antitrypsin deficiency
Galactosemia
Fructose intolerance
Tyrosinemia
Cystic fibrosis
Niemann-Pick disease
Hypothyroidism

Physical examination of an infant with biliary atresia often reveals a jaundiced but otherwise well-appearing patient. Abdominal examination is significant for hepatosplenomegaly and ascites. Stools are usually acholic.

Appropriate Workup

Serology should be done for toxoplasmosis, rubella, syphilis, cytomegalovirus (CMV), herpes, and hepatitis B. IgM titers are preferable since IgG can be transferred across the placenta. Urine should be cultured for bacteria and CMV. A serum alpha$_1$-antitrypsin and thyroxine assay should be done, as should an assay for plasma amino acids. Urine-reducing substances should be tested to rule out galactosemia (if the formula contains lactose or if the infant is breast-fed) or fructose intolerance (if the formula contains sucrose). An ultrasound of the liver and gallbladder should be performed to rule

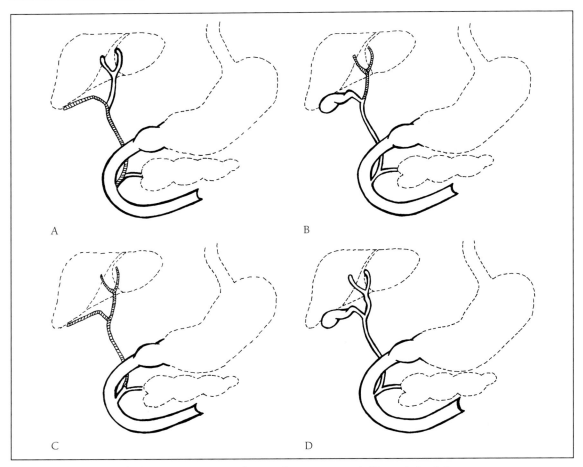

Figure 15-3. Variants of biliary atresia. A. Extrahepatic ducts patent with fibrosed distal ducts.
B. Proximal ducts obliterated with patent gallbladder, cystic duct, and common bile duct.
C. Obliteration of proximal and distal bile ducts. D. Normal liver anatomy.

out any cause of obstructive jaundice such as a choledochal cyst or a mass impinging upon the portal triad, resulting in bile duct dilatation. Patients with biliary atresia generally have a shrunken or absent gallbladder without visible extrahepatic bile ducts.

If there exists no anatomic cause for hyperbilirubinemia, a sweat chloride test should be done to rule out cystic fibrosis. A technetium Tc 99m–iminodiacetic acid (Tc-IDA) nuclear scan is then performed to investigate the ability of the hepatobiliary system to take up and excrete this marker. Phenobarbital is used to enhance the accuracy of differentiating other causes of neonatal cholestasis

from biliary atresia. Phenobarbital upregulates hepatic enzymes, facilitating bilirubin conjugation and excretion as well as improving the uptake and excretion of Tc-IDA tracer.

The infant is administered 5 mg/kg of phenobarbital in two divided doses for 5 consecutive days before intravenous administration of Tc-IDA. Images are obtained every 10 minutes for 1 hour, and delayed images are obtained at 6 and 24 hours (Fig. 15-4). The diagnosis of biliary atresia is excluded if the hepatobiliary scan demonstrates passage of radiotracer into the bowel. If tracer cannot be identified in the lumen of the bowel, the distinction between other causes of cholestasis and biliary atre-

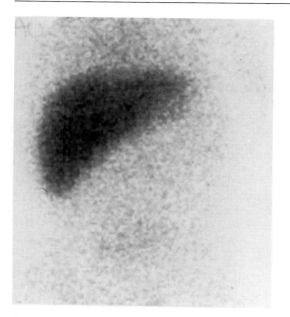

Figure 15-4. Tc-IDA nuclear scan demonstrating no tracer in the small bowel consistent with either biliary atresia or other cause of severe cholestasis.

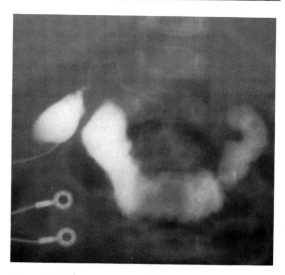

Figure 15-5. Intraoperative cholangiogram demonstrating obliteration of the proximal duct and patency of the gallbladder, cystic duct, and common bile duct.

sia cannot be made with certainty. In these cases, a percutaneous liver biopsy is recommended if the coagulation parameters are within safe limits (platelet count > 50,000/mm³, prothrombin time < 1.4 × control). If findings are consistent with biliary atresia, exploratory laparotomy with intraoperative cholangiogram should be performed as expeditiously as possible, usually the day following the liver biopsy. The cholangiogram is done via the gallbladder (Fig. 15-5). The visualization of the intrahepatic ducts and the passage of contrast into the duodenum exclude the diagnosis of biliary atresia. However, it should be noted that persistence of jaundice for weeks following the diagnosis of neonatal hepatitis might signal the progression of "hepatitis" to biliary atresia, and re-exploration might be indicated.

Management

The success of surgical correction of patients with biliary atresia is directly dependent upon the infant's age. Ohi et al. reported a 10-year survival rate of 73% for infants operated on before 61 days of age, 35% at 61 to 71 days, 23% at 71 to 90 days,

and only 13% when surgery was performed on patients older than 90 days of age. Timing is critical. The entire evaluation of a child with conjugated hyperbilirubinemia should take no longer than a week, and prompt surgical correction of obstructive jaundice should be undertaken.

Surgical Correction

In 1916 Holmes published the observation that 16% of patients with biliary atresia had bile duct anatomy that could be corrected. These patients had patent proximal bile ducts with an obliterated common bile duct. Ladd performed the first successful reconstruction of the correctable type of biliary atresia in 1928. However, since the majority of patients had noncorrectable forms of biliary atresia, the surgical results in these patients were dismal, leading to a pessimistic outlook.

A number of surgical procedures were attempted during the mid-1950s in patients with obliterated proximal ducts. These operations included placing metal tubes into the liver parenchyma as well as partial hepatectomies in an attempt to form biliary fistulas which would allow for bile drainage. The mortality was so great in these patients that arguments were made to defer surgery.

Unfortunately, infants with correctable forms of biliary atresia were seriously hurt by these techniques, as well as by surgical delay. Swenson and Fisher advocated early exploratory laparotomy and operative cholangiography in order to salvage patients with correctable biliary atresia. Reconstruction of the bile ducts was recommended in infants with patent proximal ducts. Thaler and Gellis strongly disagreed with Swenson and Fisher because they felt that laparotomy harmed infants with neonatal hepatitis. They proposed that surgery should be deferred until the child was at least 4 months of age. This argument regrettably was accepted in the United States; this practice probably resulted in irreversible cirrhosis for many patients with biliary atresia.

In 1959 Kasai and Suzuki introduced hepaticoportoenterostomy for the treatment of biliary atresia. They understood that biliary atresia was not a static process and that there was progressive fibrosis of the extrahepatic biliary tree. Kasai recommended an early surgical approach with high transection of the extrahepatic bile ducts at the level of the portal vein bifurcation, thereby maximizing the potential for exposing patent intrahepatic bile ducts. More than 50% of the infants who underwent surgery before 2 months of age achieved bile drainage. Less than 7% of the infants achieved bile drainage if hepaticoportoenterostomy was delayed beyond 4 months of age.

Preoperatively, the patient's prothrombin time should be measured. If elevated, vitamin K (2 mg IM) should be administered and the prothrombin time repeated 12 to 24 hours later to establish normalization. Fresh-frozen plasma should be available to correct the child's coagulopathy if unresponsive to vitamin K.

A right subcostal incision is recommended with visual assessment of the gallbladder and the extrahepatic biliary tree. An intraoperative cholangiogram via the gallbladder is then performed to define options for surgical reconstruction. The gallbladder can be used as a conduit for reconstruction as a portocholecystostomy if the gallbladder, cystic duct, and common bile duct are patent. If these ducts are obliterated, then a Roux-en-Y hepaticoportoenterostomy is the only option available for reconstruction. A significant number of patients will have complete obliteration of the gallbladder lumen, obviating the ability to perform a cholangiogram.

In Kasai's operation, the gallbladder, cystic duct, and extrahepatic duct remnants are gently mobilized (Fig. 15-6). The common duct is divided distally and mobilized toward the liver hilum up to the bifurcation of the portal vein. In this area the common hepatic duct broadens into a cone of fibrous tissue which is transected flush with the liver parenchyma. This tissue is sent for frozen section to define patency of intrahepatic ducts. A more proximal dissection and re-excision of the porta hepatis is required if patent ducts are absent. After identification of patent intrahepatic bile ducts, the operation is completed by directly anastomosing to this area a Roux-en-Y limb of jejunum 30 to 40 cm in length; hence the term *hepaticoportoenterostomy*. The chance of long-term effective bile drainage is negligible if the intrahepatic ducts measure less than 100 μm in diameter. If the ducts are greater than 150 μm in diameter, the chance of bile drainage is 80% if the infant is less than 8 weeks of age.

Figure 15-6. Hepaticoportoenterostomy (Kasai procedure).

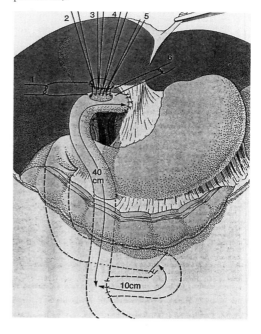

The major postoperative complication of the Kasai procedure is cholangitis as a result of bile stasis and bacterial contamination from the intestinal conduit. Cholangitis is a significant clinical problem since recurrent inflammation of the bile ducts can lead to sclerosis, with resultant failure in continued bile drainage. Several reconstruction options have therefore been devised to decrease bacterial contamination via the intestinal conduit.

Infants with a patent gallbladder, cystic duct, and common bile duct can undergo reconstruction via a portocholecystostomy (Fig. 15-7). The advantage is that cholangitis is infrequent via this approach, probably because the intact Oddi's sphincter prevents reflux of intestinal contents. Because the gallbladder and cystic duct are small and at risk for a "blowout," tube decompression of the gallbladder is recommended for approximately 4 to 6 weeks. This approach has not been popular among pediatric surgeons because of the inadequacy of the gallbladder as a conduit and technical problems with kinking of the cystic duct.

Other options exist that attempt to decrease the incidence of cholangitis when the gallbladder cannot be utilized for reconstruction. These methods all utilize the principle of exteriorizing the conduit in order to decrease intraluminal pressure and thereby diminish any resistance to bile flow. The double-barreled hepaticoportoenterostomy is known as the Surgura I procedure. The Surgura

Figure 15-7. Hepaticoportocholecystostomy.

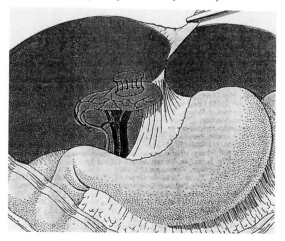

II procedure uses a subcutaneous enterostomy for the distal jejunal limb with the insertion of a jejunal tube, in the hope that the intestinal flora is completely diverted from the biliary anastomosis. Kasai later recommended a double Roux-en-Y hepaticoportoenterostomy. The most recent technical modification has been the construction of an intussusception valve in the distal intestinal conduit in order to further decrease the chance of bacterial contamination from enteric flora. Intestinal stomas, if created at the time of surgery, should be closed when bile flow reaches a steady state, because infants who develop portal hypertension can have significant variceal bleeding from these sites.

The evidence is not clear that exteriorization of the Roux-en-Y portoenterostomy reliably diminishes the frequency of cholangitis. Exteriorization, however, permits precise measurement of bilirubin output and treatment of declining bile output. Recently, a nonrefluxing biliary appendicoduodenostomy has been used in an attempt to diminish cholangitis.

Results

Kasai Procedure

Successful bile drainage can be achieved in more than 70% of infants with biliary atresia if portoenterostomy is performed prior to 10 weeks of age. Portoenterostomy is curative for one third of patients with biliary atresia. One third of patients will have minimal bile flow following reconstruction and will experience a rapid deterioration secondary to biliary cirrhosis unless hepatic transplantation is available. The other one third of patients who undergo portoenterostomy achieve moderate bile drainage, but will have progressive biliary cirrhosis and portal hypertension ultimately requiring liver transplantation, probably during school age or adolescent years.

Postoperative Management

A high index of suspicion must exist for the development of cholangitis, since this is a common problem following portoenterostomy. In infants with biliary atresia, cholangitis damages the existing bile ducts, causing deterioration in bile flow. Unfortunately, the incidence of cholangitis has not been reliably decreased by the administration of prophylactic antibiotics or choleretics.

Children who develop a fever following a Kasai procedure should be promptly evaluated and aggressively treated if cholangitis is suspected because of fever, rising serum bilirubin and amino transferase levels, and tender hepatomegaly. Therapy includes hydration, intravenous antibiotics, pulse steroids, and occasional exploration of the portoenterostomy. The use of pulse steroids in this clinical setting is controversial. Steroids act by decreasing the inflammatory reaction in the bile ducts and thereby promoting bile flow. However, they should not be used if the child has evidence of bacteremia. The portoenterostomy should be explored only in patients who have abrupt cessation of normal bile flow. In these patients, inspissated sludge or granulation tissue may block the portoenterostomy; removal of the obstructing material may result in resumption of bile flow and salvage of the portoenterostomy. The disadvantage of re-exploration is that it will eventually make liver transplantation more difficult from a technical standpoint. For this reason, indications for re-exploration are few, and repeated re-exploration should be avoided.

Two thirds of children treated with a Kasai procedure will have progressive hepatic fibrosis with resultant portal hypertension. Infants who never have establishment of bile flow have a rapid onset of cirrhosis and sequelae of portal hypertension. The remainder develop complications of portal hypertension over several years, including malnutrition, ascites, and esophageal varices. Ascites can often be managed with salt restriction and spironolactone or furosemide. Esophageal varices may be controlled with sclerotherapy or banding. Portosystemic shunting procedures should only be used in very selective circumstances where liver transplantation is contraindicated. Aggressive medical management should be continued if hepatic function is stable and the child is able to maintain a growth curve.

Nutrition

Infants with biliary atresia are often malnourished because of a deficient enterohepatic circulation of bile salts. These patients do not efficiently absorb fat or fat-soluble vitamins. In children who do not drain significant bile into their portoenterostomy, these deficits may become severe if not supplemented. All children with biliary atresia should be provided with vitamins A, D, E, and K. Nutritional supplementation should also include formulas with the majority of fat calories provided as medium-chain triglycerides, since they can be directly absorbed without bile-salt–dependent micellar stabilization. Inadequate monitoring of the nutritional profile of these infants will result in rickets secondary to vitamin D deficiency. Ataxic neuromyopathy results from vitamin E deficiency. Vitamin K deficiency results in abnormal levels of factors II, VII, IX, and X with a resultant coagulopathy. Inadequate levels of vitamin A can result in dermatitis, night blindness, keratomalacia, and xerophthalmia. It is recommended that infants with biliary atresia be given 5000 to 15,000 IU/d of water-miscible vitamin A, 5 to 7 mcg/kg/d of 25-hydroxy vitamin D, and 5 to 15 mg/d of vitamin K. A new vitamin E preparation (tocopherol polyethylene glycol succinate, 15 to 25 IU/kg/d) is thought to be more effective in preventing vitamin E deficiency syndrome in infants with biliary atresia than older formulations.

Transplantation

Infants who fail to drain bile should be referred for early transplantation. Patients who do well initially but whose growth curves become inadequate or whose hepatic function deteriorates should also be considered for liver transplantation. Fortunately, this situation may not happen until the child is 3 years of age or older, thereby optimizing the success rate of liver transplantation. Since portoenterostomy has little to no success after the child is 4 months of age, an infant at this age should be referred for liver transplantation, rather than put through a portoenterostomy, upon confirmation of biliary atresia.

The advent of cyclosporin A and now Prograf have made liver transplantation a success in children; 5-year survival rates approach 85% in most centers. The importance of timely referral cannot be overemphasized. Transplantation should be done before the child has progressed toward end-stage liver failure, since the mortality of transplantation is substantially increased by delay. A significant problem to date, however, remains an organ shortage for children. Inability to obtain adequate donor organs is directly responsible for the death of many children awaiting transplantation. This serious problem has led to the development of reduced-size liver transplants and from cadavers living-related liver transplants utilizing the left lateral segment of the living donor.

The advent of more selective immunosuppressants has allowed improvement in the management of rejection. Early tapering of steroids reduces susceptibility to infection and helps normalize growth curves. It is now possible for many children to live active and productive lives following liver transplantation, but there must be a commitment by both patient and physician for long-term follow-up. A team approach with input from surgery, general pediatrics, hepatology, psychiatry, social services, and nutrition is essential in the construction of a successful pediatric transplantation program.

Conclusions

Biliary atresia occurs in only 1 in 15,000 live births in the United States. The etiology remains unknown, although several theories have been proposed. Patients can be grouped into three broad anatomic categories. The differential diagnosis of neonatal conjugated hyperbilirubinemia is large. As a result, the workup may be extensive, but it should take no longer than a week because timing of surgical correction is critical. The results of a Roux-en-Y portoenterostomy (Kasai procedure) are best when the operation is performed before 2 months of age. Modifications of the Kasai procedure designed to prevent cholangitis are now most frequently employed. However, objective data documenting fewer problems with cholangitis are not available. Management of nutritional deficits is important before and after surgery. Revision of a portoenterostomy is now rarely indicated because the results of liver transplantation have improved. In most centers the 5-year survival rate after transplantation for biliary atresia is around 85%.

Selected Readings

Landing BH: Considerations of the pathogenesis of neonatal hepatitis, biliary atresia, and choledochal cysts—the concept of infantile obstructive cholangiopathy. Progr Pediatr Surg 1974; 6:113–139.

Miyano T, Suruga K, Suda K: Abnormal choledocho-pancreatico-ductal junction related to etiology of infantile obstructive jaundice diseases. J Pediatr Surg 1979; 14:16–26.

Ohi R, Nio M, Chiba T, et al: Long term follow up after surgery for patients with biliary atresia. J Pediatr Surg 1990; 25:442–445.

Holmes JB: Congenital obliteration of the bile ducts: Diagnosis and suggestions for treatment. Am J Dis Child 1916; 11:405–431.

Ladd WE: Congenital atresia and stenosis of the bile ducts. JAMA 1928; 91:1082–1085.

Swenson O, Fisher JH: Utilization of cholangiogram during exploration for biliary atresia. N Eng J Med 1952; 249:247.

Thaler MM, Gellis SS: Studies in neonatal hepatitis and biliary atresia: II. The effect of diagnostic laparotomy on long term prognosis of neonatal hepatitis. Am J Dis Child 1968; 116:262–270.

Kasai M, Suzuki S: A new operation for non-correctable biliary atresia-hepatic portoenterostomy. Shujutsu 1959; 13:733–739.

Matory YL, Miyano T, Suruga K: Hepaticoportoenterostomy for biliary atresia. Surgery, Gynecology, and Obstetrics 1985; 161:541–545.

Kasai M: Details of operative techniques of hepatic portoenterostomy. Abstract, Pacific Association of Pediatric Surgeons, Fukuoka, Japan, May 15, 1983.

16

Biliary Cysts

Pamela A. Lipsett
Anthony N. Kalloo
Scott J. Savader
Henry A. Pitt

Biliary cystic disease includes choledochal cyst disease, gallbladder cysts, and cystic duct cysts. Choledochal cysts are themselves a wide spectrum of diseases that involve isolated or combined intrahepatic or extrahepatic cysts. Some choledochal cysts are confined to the distal common bile duct and are better known as choledochoceles, whereas isolated intrahepatic duct cysts are commonly called Caroli's disease. Since both gallbladder and cystic duct cysts are rare and are treated by cholecystectomy alone, these diseases will not be discussed further. This chapter will review the etiology, classification, diagnosis, management options, and results of therapy for choledochal cysts, paying particular attention to the type of cyst and the therapy best suited to that cyst type.

Etiology and Classification

Etiology

Three theories have been proposed to explain the pathogenesis of choledochal cysts: (1) an anomalous pancreatobiliary duct junction, (2) abnormal canalization of the bile duct, and (3) abnormalities of autonomic innervation of the extrahepatic bile duct. Clinical and experimental data support some aspects of each of these theories. Babbitt proposed that an abnormal pancreatobiliary duct junction (APBDJ) could expose the bile duct to both pancreatic juice and to pressures higher than normally seen when the choledochopancreatic duct junction

is within the sphincter of Oddi. To support this theory, he found 19 patients with choledochal cysts in whom the pancreatic duct joined the bile duct 2.0 to 3.5 cm away from the ampulla. Other authors have noted a correlation between the type of cyst (fusiform or cystic) and the presence and type of anomalous choledochopancreatic duct junction. Although this abnormality of the junction is seen in most patients with choledochal cyst disease, an abnormal junction can occasionally be seen in normal individuals. However, an APBDJ has also been noted in patients with gallbladder cancer without choledochal cyst disease. Thus, this congenital abnormality may eventually lead to some form of biliary pathology in most patients.

Experiments in young lambs and rats demonstrate that ligation of the common bile duct leads to the development of biliary cystic dilatation much like the fusiform structure of a type I choledochal cyst. If these experiments are performed on adult animals, diffuse extrahepatic and intrahepatic cystic dilatation occurs, and a choledochal cyst does not form. These experiments support the concept that during embryogenesis abnormal canalization of the bile duct can occur when distal obstruction is present. Increased pressure can then lead to further weakening of the cyst wall.

The last theory of choledochal cyst development centers around abnormalities of autonomic innervation of the extrahepatic biliary tree. A reduced number of postganglionic cholinergic cells have been noted in the narrow distal portion of

173

the choledochal cyst as compared with the dilated proximal portion. In addition, cholecystokinin has produced smaller contractions in the muscle of the narrow portion of the cyst. The prokinetic agents gamma-aminobutyric acid and nicotine did not produce contractions of the bile duct, indicating intrinsic dysfunction of the postganglionic neurons. These three theories are all plausible and suggest that the pathogenesis of choledochal cysts may be multifactorial.

Classification

In 1959 Alonso-Lej et al. reviewed the world's experience with choledochal cyst disease and proposed a classification system for cystic biliary dilatation. Todani et al. modified that classification system in 1977 to account for the combination of intra- and extrahepatic cystic dilatation. This classification system is used by most authors today (Fig. 16-1). Type I cysts are extrahepatic cysts that can be subdivided into (a) cystic, (b) focal, and (c) fusiform. Type I cysts are the most common, accounting for 40% to 60% of all cases. The cystic subtype is five times more common than the fusiform variety. A type II choledochal cyst is a saccular diverticulum of the extrahepatic tree and is rare. Type III choledochal cysts are also known as choledochoceles and are also quite rare.

Type IV cysts are divided into two types: (A) dilatation of both the extrahepatic and intrahepatic biliary tree and (B) multiple extrahepatic cysts. Type IVA cysts are common, accounting for 20% to 40% of all cysts. Type V cysts are intrahepatic cysts only and are also known as Caroli's disease. Caroli described two types of congenital intrahepatic dilatation, a "simple" type and a "periportal fibrosis" type. Patients with the simple type have cholangitis, recurrent liver abscesses, pain, and fever but do not have hepatic fibrosis, cirrhosis, or portal hypertension. End-stage liver disease develops in the periportal fibrosis type. Caroli's disease, or isolated intrahepatic cysts, is uncommon in most series.

Both intrahepatic and extrahepatic biliary dilatation can be acquired. For example, patients with Oriental cholangiohepatitis or recurrent pyogenic cholangitis frequently form intrahepatic saccular dilatations that are associated with parasites such as *Clonorchis sinensis* or *Ascaris lumbricoides*. These pa-

tients also have intrahepatic strictures and stones. Similarly, patients who have sphincter of Oddi dysfunction or a distal bile duct obstruction may also have a cholangiographic appearance similar to a type I cyst, but acquired distal bile duct disease should probably be considered separately from choledochal cyst disease.

Diagnosis

Clinical Presentation

The classic presentation of choledochal cyst disease is the triad of abdominal pain, jaundice, and a right upper quadrant mass in a young Asian female. However, this triad of symptoms and signs is uncommon and in most series accounts for only 10% to 33% of all patients. The disease is three to eight times more common in females than in males, and more than half of the reported patients with choledochal cysts have been identified before 10 years of age. However, the authors and others have reported an increased number of adult patients who have choledochal cyst disease. During the last 16 years, 42 patients with choledochal cysts were identified and treated at Johns Hopkins Hospital. Thirty-one of these 42 patients (74%) presented for initial treatment as adults. Of the 11 children, 8 were treated prior to age 4, and the adult patients were identified and treated at a median age of 30 years (range 17 to 62). Children and adults presented with different symptoms (Fig. 16-2). A palpable abdominal mass was significantly more common in children, whereas abdominal pain, a history of pancreatitis, or a history of cholecystectomy for biliary symptoms was more common in adults. The classic triad of abdominal pain, jaundice, and a right upper quadrant mass was seen in only one child and no adult. However, two of these findings were present in 8 of 11 children (73%), but in only 7 of 31 adults (23%) ($P < 0.05$).

Radiology

Both ultrasonography and computerized tomography can easily identify cystic dilatation of the biliary tree (Fig. 16-3). Ultrasonography should be sufficient to identify most abnormalities, but biliary cystic abnormalities may be overlooked when they are

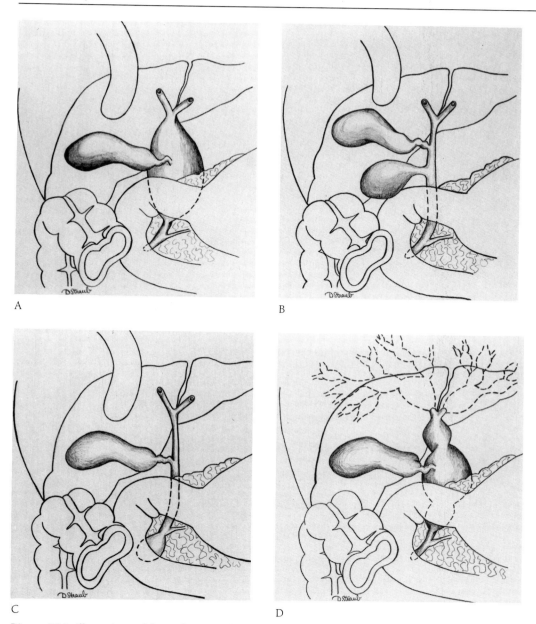

A

B

C

D

Figure 16-1. Illustrations of the Todani modification of the Alonso-Lej classification of choledochal cyst disease. A. Type I. B. Type II. C. Type III (choledochocele). D. Type IVA. (*Figure continues.*)

unsuspected. Computerized tomography has the advantage of excellent intrahepatic evaluation, particularly if a type IV or type V cyst is suspected (see Fig. 16-3). Though a radionuclide scan is often included in the evaluation of a choledochal cyst, this examination is not sufficient to adequately define the biliary anatomy, and direct cholangiography is usually necessary.

The biliary tree can be adequately visualized preoperatively by either endoscopic retrograde cho-

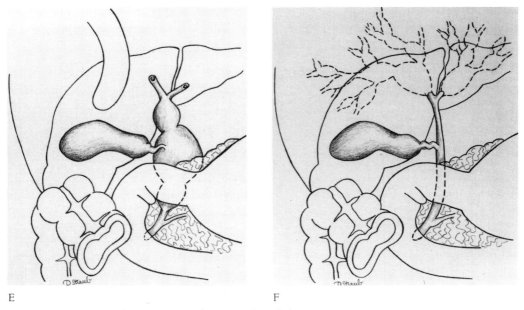

E   F

Figure 16-1. (*continued*) E. Type IVB. F. Type V (Caroli's).

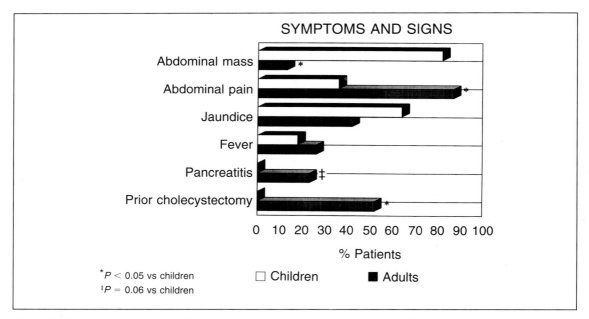

Figure 16-2. Symptoms and signs of choledochal cyst disease at presentation in children and adults at Johns Hopkins Hospital.

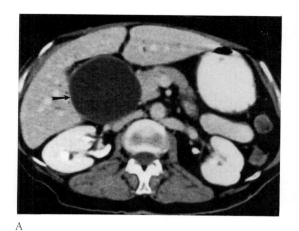
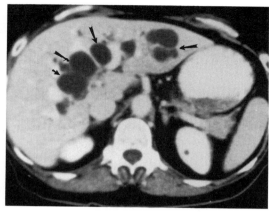

A   B

Figure 16-3. A. CT image below the level of the hepatic hilum demonstrates a large, low-density, well-circumscribed lesion (arrow) in the region of the portahepatitis. B. CT section through the liver demonstrates multiple low-density structures (arrows) within both the right and left lobe of the liver compatible with a grossly dilated intrahepatic biliary system. The findings are consistent with a type IVA choledochal cyst (extrahepatic choledochal cyst with intrahepatic extension).

langiopancreatography (ERCP) or by percutaneous transhepatic cholangiography (PTC). The exact biliary anatomy will establish the location and type of choledochal cyst and will exclude dilatation secondary to a benign stricture or a malignant process. ERCP is best suited for analysis and possible treatment of a choledochocele (type III) as well as for identification and definition of the union of the pancreatic and common bile ducts (Fig. 16-4).

The duodenoscopic appearance of a choledochocele is variable but characteristically includes a smooth, soft, compressible periampullary protrusion into the lumen with an eccentric papillary orifice. Injection of contrast reveals a "clublike" distal common bile duct and further protrusion of the intraluminal component into the duodenum. It is important to differentiate the duodenoscopic appearance of type III cysts from inflammatory and neoplastic disorders of the papilla and duodenal duplication cysts. Biopsy and brushing of the papilla help identify the former, whereas the latter characteristically fail to opacify when contrast is injected into the biliary tree. PTC may be best suited for visualizing the intrahepatic biliary tree, since that portion of the cyst may be quite extensive and may require a large volume of contrast to fill. PTC may also be used to establish preoperative drainage

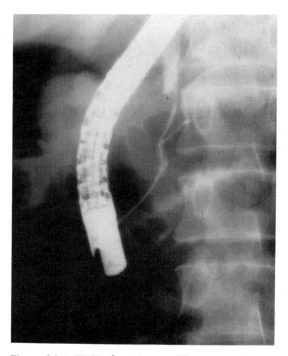

Figure 16-4. ERCP of an 18-year-old woman with a type I choledochal cyst (not shown). The long common channel with the anomalous takeoff of the pancreatic duct high above the sphincter is demonstrated.

(PTD), which can aid in the intraoperative and post-operative management of these patients. Furthermore, in patients who present with cholangitis, PTD may facilitate rapid and effective biliary drainage. If a PTD catheter is placed, it should be left above the anomalous pancreatobiliary duct junction because pancreatitis may be more likely if the stent is passed into the duodenum.

Complications

Complications of biliary cystic disease are common and may be the symptoms for which patients seek medical therapy. Gallstones, acute cholecystitis, pancreatitis, jaundice, recurrent cholangitis, and carcinoma of both the gallbladder and biliary tree have been reported. Rare complications of choledochal cyst disease include portal hypertension, portal vein thrombosis, and spontaneous cyst rupture, with or without pregnancy. Hepatic fibrosis and cirrhosis can also occur as the result of long-standing extrahepatic obstruction.

Cancers of the biliary tree, gallbladder, and pancreas have all been associated with choledochal cyst disease. The most common associated cancer is cholangiocarcinoma; thus complete excision of the cyst is warranted. Patients with cholangiocarcinoma associated with choledochal cyst disease are often in the fourth decade of life, 30 years younger than the typical patient with cholangiocarcinoma. Teenagers have been reported with disseminated cholangiocarcinoma arising in a choledochal cyst. The young age of these patients with cholangiocarcinoma and choledochal cysts is believed to be related to the anomalous pancreatobiliary duct junction and the reflux of pancreatic juice into the cyst.

Reveille has demonstrated changes in the bile acid profile of a patient with a choledochal cyst. In that patient the secondary bile acids deoxycholate and lithocholate were increased. These bile acids have demonstrated mutagenicity in a standard model of carcinogenesis. Furthermore, genetic mutation of the K ras oncogene, which has been associated with many human cancers, has been found in one patient with biliary papillomatosis and a choledochal cyst. Thus the combination of a genetically susceptible patient and a carcinogen may explain the 18% to 35% incidence of carcinoma in this patient population.

Management

Initial Treatment

The initial management of patients with a choledochal cyst will depend upon the age, the presentation, and the type of cyst. Children who present with a palpable mass may be scheduled for surgery electively, whereas those with obstructive jaundice should be treated more urgently. Similarly, adults with biliary colic can be treated electively, whereas those who present with acute cholecystitis, gallstone pancreatitis, or cholangitis will usually require urgent treatment. Most patients with acute cholecystitis should undergo cholecystectomy within the first few days of the illness. However, if an underlying choledochal cyst is diagnosed, an argument can be made for initial medical management and subsequent definitive treatment of the choledochal cyst along with removal of the gallbladder. Similarly, if the patient presents with gallstone pancreatitis, initial nonoperative management followed by resection of the choledochal cyst and the gallbladder is the ideal management option.

In patients with acute cholangitis and a choledochal cyst, broad-spectrum antibiotics and intravenous hydration should be initiated. In septic patients biliary decompression is warranted to help prevent worsening gram-negative sepsis. This goal may be accomplished using either endoscopic or percutaneous biliary drainage techniques. Endoscopy can be used for transduodenal retrograde placement of a stent into the biliary tree. However, in these patients, the altered anatomy at the pancreatobiliary junction can make access to the ampulla difficult and increase the risk of pancreatitis. Repeated unsuccessful instrumentations at the ampulla can also exacerbate biliary sepsis, and the small-caliber stents typically placed can quickly occlude if the bile is laden with debris as the result of long-standing stasis. However, altered pancreatobiliary anatomy is not a hindrance to achieving successful percutaneous transhepatic drainage (PTD). PTD can be accomplished with nearly a 100% technical success rate, and the risk of worsening gram-negative sepsis during the procedure is low.

After access is gained to the intrahepatic biliary tree, bile should be allowed to drain by gravity or under gentle suction to decrease the intrahepatic biliary pressure. A bile specimen should be collected for culture, sensitivity, and Gram's stain. Gentle contrast opacification of the biliary tract should be performed only to the degree which allows final placement of a drainage catheter. Septic patients do not require a complete cholangiogram during this initial procedure. In this setting adequate external drainage is the primary goal.

All biliary tubes should be left to external drainage with fluid and electrolytes being replaced with a volume of lactated Ringer's solution equal to the amount of bile drained every 8 hours. Broad-spectrum antibiotic therapy should be employed prophylactically in all patients. In septic patients, adjustments in the antibiotics should be made depending on the results of bile cultures and changes in the patient's clinical status. After the patient has defervesced for at least 24 hours, and while the patient is still on antibiotic therapy, a detailed low-pressure cholangiogram should be performed to fully evaluate the intra- and extrahepatic biliary tree (Figs. 16-5, 16-6). In addition, care must be taken to evaluate and document the presence of concurrent biliary tract pathology such as strictures, calculi, and abscesses in communication with the biliary tree.

The decision to perform PTD preoperatively will depend upon the anatomy of the cyst and the patient's presentation. Although randomized trials have not proven that preoperative biliary drainage improves outcome, these percutaneous transhepatic catheters can be a significant technical aid during and after the operation. An anastomosis to large duct(s) at the bifurcation can be decompressed postoperatively by the transhepatic catheter, which provides easy access for cholangiography. Moreover, in patients with intrahepatic strictures or stones, the percutaneous catheter can facilitate intraoperative placement of larger polymeric silicone (Silastic) transhepatic stents. These stents can then be used for postoperative choledochoscopy, balloon dilatation, or stone removal.

Options

In the past, enteric drainage of a choledochal cyst was considered appropriate therapy. However, this option is no longer favored, for two reasons. First, anastomotic difficulties following cyst-enteric anas-

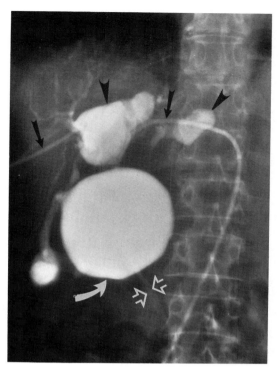

Figure 16-5. Type IVA choledochal cyst in a 60-year-old Caucasian female presenting with right upper quadrant pain, jaundice, nausea, and vomiting. Bilateral percutaneous biliary drainage catheters (arrows) were placed in this patient, who had extensive intrahepatic biliary duct dilatation (arrowheads) and a huge extrahepatic choledochal cyst (curved arrows). Note that the PTD catheters (open arrows) exit the cyst and enter the duodenum.

tomosis are common. Rattner et al. reported that strictures developed in 68% of these patients. This high rate of stricture formation and subsequent development of acute cholangitis are probably related to the lack of a mucosa-to-mucosa anastomosis, since the cyst wall is often denuded of epithelium. Second, if the cyst or the gallbladder is retained, the risk of developing a carcinoma is not eliminated. Thus patients who have had a prior cyst bypass procedure should have the cyst and the gallbladder excised to prevent the development of cholangiocarcinoma or gallbladder cancer.

The treatment of choice for type I and type IV cysts is surgical excision of the extrahepatic cyst with Roux-en-Y hepaticojejunostomy. Details of these surgical procedures will be discussed below. Type

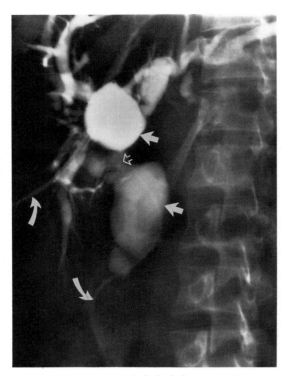

Figure 16-6. Type IVA choledochal cyst in a 24-year-old Caucasian female who presented with right upper quadrant pain and jaundice. The extrahepatic biliary tree (solid arrows) is grossly dilated, as is the intrahepatic biliary tree. The dilated intrahepatic biliary tree facilitated placement of a PTD catheter (curved arrows). A stricture (open arrow) is present between this focal dilatation and the remainder of the extrahepatic biliary ductal system.

II cysts, which are diverticula extending from the otherwise normal biliary tree, should also be excised, but Roux-en-Y reconstruction is not required. A T tube should be placed to decompress the bile duct in the early postoperative period after the excision of a type II cyst. In all patients undergoing surgery for choledochal cyst disease, the gallbladder should be removed to prevent subsequent acute cholecystitis or carcinoma of the gallbladder.

After cholecystectomy in patients with cyst types I and IV, the distal common bile duct is identified and transected above the pancreas. A balance must be achieved between complete excision of the cyst and preservation of the pancreatic duct, which enters the bile duct well above the sphincter of Oddi in these patients. The lower end of the choledochal cyst is oversewn to prevent a pancreatic

fistula. The plane between the cyst wall and the portal vein is identified, and the dissection proceeds from caudad to cephalad. In type I cysts the dissection proceeds to the normal common hepatic duct usually just below the hepatic duct bifurcation.

In patients with a type IVA cyst, the bifurcation and/or hepatic ducts are also involved. If hepatic duct strictures are present, resection of these areas may be necessary, and separate anastomosis may be required. If resection of strictured areas cannot be performed, biopsies are necessary to rule out associated malignancy, and long-term stenting will be required. A standard Roux-en-Y biliary anastomosis is performed, as stated previously. Preoperatively placed percutaneous stents are used to facilitate placement of larger polymeric silicone stents, if necessary, or are used for postoperative decompression and cholangiography. Closed suction drains are placed at the distal pancreatic duct site, the anastomosis, and the exit site(s) from the liver if larger polymeric silicone stents have been used.

For type III choledochal cysts, management options depend on the symptoms. Malignant degeneration of the cyst has been reported in only one case of a choledochocele. Thus complete excision may not be as important as in cyst types I, II, and IV. The presenting symptoms may be isolated to the biliary tree or pancreas. If jaundice, cholangitis, or pancreatitis is the only symptom, endoscopic sphincterotomy, sphincteroplasty, or biliary bypass may all be appropriate treatment. These various options will be discussed in more detail in the section on controversies. However, patients with choledochoceles may also have signs of duodenal obstruction rather than pancreatic or biliary obstruction. If vomiting and weight loss are the presenting symptoms, then surgical excision is the preferred treatment.

The management of patients with type V choledochal cysts (Caroli's disease) must be individualized, and consideration must be given to the patient's underlying hepatic function, general medical condition, and indication for surgery. In general, the indications for treatment are recurrent cholangitis, intrahepatic stones, or persistent pain. Some patients can be treated initially with percutaneous transhepatic tubes, percutaneous cholangioscopy, stone extraction, and biliary dilatation. Caroli's disease may be confined to an isolated hepatic segment or to a hepatic lobe. If a hepatic abscess or cirrhosis with atrophy has developed, hepatic resection may be the preferred treatment. In the absence of multiple abscesses or cirrhosis, the treatment should be designed to (1) remove all stones and debris from the intrahepatic cysts, (2) dilate intrahepatic strictures, and (3) rule out associated cholangiocarcinoma. These principles apply to patients with both unilateral and bilateral disease in the absence of cirrhosis.

In patients with type IVA and type V cysts with intrahepatic ductal dilatation, percutaneous transhepatic drainage can facilitate intraoperative management (Fig. 16-7). At operation, PTD catheters can provide excellent physical landmarks which can be easily palpated in patients with distorted or confusing anatomy. After the gallbladder is removed, the extrahepatic biliary tree is divided distally and excised up to the hepatic duct bifurcation. In the presence of intrahepatic stones, intraoperative cholangioscopy can facilitate stone removal as

well as examination and biopsy of the biliary tree. Additional helpful tools for stone removal are pressurized irrigation, graspers, baskets, and balloon catheters. However, pressurized irrigation should be used with caution in patients who have any degree of ongoing biliary sepsis because bacteremia can rapidly ensue. After the stones have been cleared, preoperatively placed stents are replaced first by catheters coudé, which are used to progressively dilate the tube tract, and finally by 16 to 20 French polymeric silicone catheters. More proximal biliary resection will occasionally be necessary for patients with cyst type IVA or V who have strictured component(s) of the biliary tree above the bifurcation.

Standard Roux-en-Y hepaticojejunostomies are performed after stone removal, stricture dilatation, or resection and stent placement. Near the completion of the anastomosis, the large-bore polymeric silicone stents are positioned so that the fenestrated portions pass through the intrahepatic biliary tree and into the jejunum (Fig. 16-8). The nonfenestrated portions of the stents are brought out over the anterior surface of the liver and are subsequently brought through the abdominal wall via new stab wounds. The Roux-en-Y is completed by performing an end-to-side jejunojejunostomy approximately 50 cm distal to the hepaticojejunostomies. Drains are placed at the exit site of the liver and

Figure 16-7. Percutaneous transhepatic cholangiogram of a 30-year-old Asian female who presented with right upper quadrant pain, nausea, and jaundice. A large choledochal cyst (solid arrow) involves the extrahepatic biliary tree. Note the intrahepatic extension of the biliary dilatation and the strictured segment (open arrow) inferior to the dilated hepatic duct confluence.

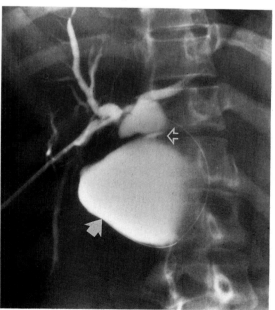

Figure 16-8. Illustration of a Roux-en-Y hepaticojejunostomy. The posterior row of the anastomosis has been completed, and the preoperatively placed transhepatic stents have been placed into the lumen of the jejunum.

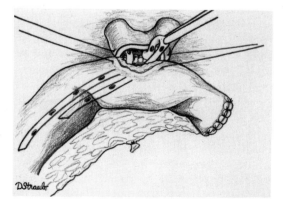

also at the anastomosis. The majority of patients with Caroli's disease can be effectively managed by these techniques. However, a minority of patients may develop unremitting sepsis or cirrhosis, and hepatic transplantation may be required for a small subset of patients. The decision to perform a transplantation should be made on the basis of hepatic synthetic function, portal hypertensive complications, and degree of unremitting sepsis.

Postoperative Management

During the immediate postprocedure period, the stents prevent cholangitis that may result from edema and provide decompression if a bile leak occurs. Prior to discharge from the hospital, all patients should have a cholangiogram to ensure that the stents are properly positioned within the biliary tract. These stents also provide long-term protection against anastomotic scarring and continue to dilate intrahepatic strictures. In addition, the stents provide access to the biliary tree for postoperative removal of residual stones, balloon dilatation of strictures, and biopsy of areas suspicious for malignancy. The length of stenting will depend upon the presence of residual intrahepatic pathology. If no stones or strictures are present, large-bore catheters may not be required, and a preoperatively placed stent may be removed in 3 to 6 weeks. Patients with multiple intrahepatic strictures will usually require long-term stenting. In these patients, stents are usually changed every 3 or 4 months.

These stents are maintained on internal drainage and are flushed two times a day with 10 to 20 cc of normal saline to help prevent occlusion with biliary sludge. Chronic antibiotic therapy is generally not used because of concerns over emergence of resistant organisms. Tubes are changed electively every 3 or 4 months or sooner if the patient experiences (1) fever, (2) chills, (3) nausea and vomiting, (4) right upper quadrant or abdominal pain, (5) an inability to flush the stents, or (6) pericatheter bile leakage.

Patients with intrahepatic strictures or residual stones usually have transhepatic stents kept in place for at least 12 months. After this period, a "clinical trial" may be instituted by placing modified drainage catheters which are positioned above the surgical anastomosis. These tubes are capped and provide no form of drainage but function simply to maintain access to the biliary tree. Patients are discharged, observed at home for 2 to 3 weeks, and asked to return if any symptoms of obstruction occur. If problems arise, these patients generally require restenting with larger biliary catheters. Patients who complete their clinical trial without symptoms can usually have their biliary tubes removed.

Alternately, patients can undergo a biliary manometric perfusion test in order to objectively assess intrahepatic biliodynamics. For this test, an angiographic injector is used to infuse 30% contrast into the intrahepatic biliary tree through the modified catheter(s) at rates ranging from 2 to 20 cc/min. During these infusions, the intrabiliary pressure is monitored via the second biliary catheter, or if only one catheter is present, a three-way stopcock is used to allow for both pressure monitoring and contrast infusion. If the intrahepatic biliary pressure is less than 20 cm water throughout the exam, the test is considered to be normal. Patients who pass a biliary manometric perfusion test or a clinical trial have a probability of being symptom-free at 1 year of 90% and 86%, respectively.

Since both the clinical trial and the manometric test are equal predictors of success, either test can be performed to determine an endpoint of treatment. However, the manometric perfusion test takes less time to complete and costs less. Patients who have inconclusive results following the completion of either test should have the other test performed. These results should be correlated with the clinical course, liver function tests, and the cholangiographic appearance of the biliary-enteric anastomosis before the biliary intubation is discontinued.

Controversies

Surgical resection of cyst types I, II, and IV is generally accepted as the treatment of choice. More controversy exists regarding the proper management of cyst types III (choledochocele) and V (Caroli's). Type III cysts presenting with biliary or pancreatic symptoms can be managed with endoscopic sphincterotomy. If these patients also have gallstones, the gallbladder should be removed, because most of these patients are relatively young and remain at risk for acute cholecystitis and gallbladder cancer. In these patients laparoscopic cholecystectomy may be performed in addition to endoscopic sphincterotomy. Whether these patients would be better served with an open cholecystectomy and surgical sphincteroplasty remains a matter of debate. In addition, choledochoduodenectomy and choledochojejunostomy are options if the bile duct is dilated above the choledochocele. As mentioned above, the cyst will have to be resected if duodenal obstruction is the problem. The specifics of biliary and pancreatic duct reconstruction will depend upon the individual circumstances.

The main controversy regarding cyst types IVA and V that involve the intrahepatic ducts is whether to treat intrahepatic stones and strictures or to resect the involved liver. This decision will depend upon the degree of hepatic fibrosis or cirrhosis and whether the disease involves one or both lobes. In general, the authors' philosophy has been to preserve noncirrhotic parenchyma. Others argue that resection of the diseased area reduces the risk of subsequent cholangiocarcinoma. However, if both lobes are involved, as is often the case, resection will require hepatic transplantation. In general, the authors have been reluctant to transplant patients without severe parenchymal liver disease.

Preferred Approach

Types I and IVB choledochal cysts which are completely extrahepatic should be excised with Roux-en-Y biliary reconstruction. Long-term transhepatic stenting will usually not be required in these patients. Type II cysts are simply excised, and the bile duct is reconstructed with temporary use of a T-tube while the choledochotomy is healing. The preferred approach for type III cysts will depend upon the presentation. In general, endoscopic sphincterotomy will usually suffice for biliary or pancreatic symptoms, whereas resection will be required for duodenal obstruction. In all of these patients the gallbladder should be removed to prevent sepsis and cancer. Cyst types IVA and V will usually be managed with extrahepatic bile duct resection, large-bore transhepatic stents, and Roux-en-Y hepaticojejunostomies. In these patients preoperative percutaneous transhepatic stents are very helpful, and postoperative percutaneous choledochoscopy,

balloon dilatation, stone removal, and stricture biopsy may all be required. Some of these types IVA and V patients will require liver resection for unilateral disease or hepatic transplantation for bilateral disease if severe recurrent sepsis or end-stage liver disease develops.

Results

A recent report from Johns Hopkins University suggests that relatively more adults with biliary cysts are being diagnosed after they present with acute cholecystitis or gallstone pancreatitis. Some of these patients have undergone cholecystectomy before the presence of a choledochal cyst is appreciated. This situation should be avoidable with careful ultrasonography or preoperative cholangiography when patients present with jaundice or cholangitis. Numerous reports suggest that bypass operations that do not remove the cyst have a poor long-term outcome. These patients are prone to recurrent cholangitis and remain at risk for cholangiocarcinoma.

Most recent reports of patients with choledochal cysts suggest that the short- and long-term outcome from surgical resection is excellent. Moreover, surgery should be performed early to prevent biliary cirrhosis and cancer. Postoperatively, the most common problems are recurrent cholangitis and progression of hepatic disease to cirrhosis. However, these problems can be minimized with early diagnosis and appropriate resection of types I, II, and IVB choledochal cysts. Results of endoscopic sphincterotomy for type III cysts have also been excellent. In patients with complex type IVA and type V biliary cystic disease, the combined efforts of surgery and interventional radiology can preserve hepatic function and prevent sepsis. Furthermore, in patients with poor hepatic function or ongoing biliary sepsis, hepatic resection or transplantation can offer long-term survival. Patients with biliary cystic disease who have cholangiocarcinoma or gallbladder cancer at the time of presentation rarely survive more than 3 years.

Conclusions

Biliary cysts are common in Japan but occur rarely in Western countries. Debate continues regarding their etiology, which may be multifactorial. However, the majority of patients have an abnormal pancreatobiliary duct junction (APBDJ). The classification system proposed by Todani in 1977 is used most often and includes types I, II, III (choledochocele), IVA, IVB, and V (Caroli's) cysts. Presentation differs between children and adults and can be confused with routine cholecystitis or gallstone pancreatitis in adults. Ultrasound and CT will usually establish the diagnosis. ERCP will define the APBDJ, but PTC may be more useful in defining intrahepatic anatomy. These patients are at significantly increased risk of developing bile duct and gallbladder cancer.

Initial management depends upon the patient's age, the presentation, and the type of cyst. Preoperative percutaneous transhepatic drainage may be very useful in adult patients who present with cholangitis or have type IVA or V cysts which involve the intrahepatic ducts. Resection of the cyst and removal of the gallbladder is the treatment of choice for cyst types I, II, and IVB. Management of type III cysts may be accomplished by the endoscopist or the surgeon, depending upon the presenting symptoms. Cyst types IVA and V are best managed by a team effort involving interventional radiologists and biliary surgeons with the occasional aid of hepatologists and transplant surgeons.

Selected Readings

Alonso-Lej F, Rever WB Jr, Pessagno DJ. Congenital choledochal cysts, with a report of 2, and an analysis of 94 cases. *Surg Gynecol Obstet* 1959; 108: 1–30.

Chijiiwa K, Koga A. Surgical management and long term followup of patients with choledochal cysts. *Am J Surg* 1993; 165:238–242.

Iwai N, et al. Congenital choledochal dilatation with emphasis on pathophysiology of the biliary tract. *Ann Surg* 1992; 215:27–30.

Lipsett PA, et al. Choledochal cyst disease: A changing pattern of presentation. *Ann Surg* 1994; 220:644–652.

Lopez RR, et al. Variation in management based on type of choledochal cyst. *Am J Surg* 1991; 161:612–615.

Okada A, et al. Congenital dilatation of the bile duct in 100 instances and its relationship with anomalous junction. *Surg Gynecol Obstet* 1990; 171:291–298.

Pitt HA. Biliary cysts: Choledochal cysts and Caroli's disease. In Cameron JL (ed), *Current Surgical Therapy* (4th ed). St. Louis: Mosby, 1992. Pp. 367–372.

Todani T, et al. Carcinoma related to choledochal cysts with internal drainage operations. *Surg Gynecol Obstet* 1987; 164:61–64.

Venu RP, et al. Role of endoscopic retrograde cholangiopancreatography in the diagnosis and treatment of choledochocele. *Gastroenterology* 1984; 87:1144–1149.

Yamaguchi M. Congenital choledochal cyst. Analysis of 1,433 patients in the Japanese literature. *Am J Surg* 1980; 140:653–657.

17

Gallbladder Stones

Nathaniel J. Soper
Giuseppe Aliperti
Steven A. Edmundowicz
Daniel Picus
Steven M. Strasberg

Until relatively recently, traditional "open" cholecystectomy was the preferred therapy for gallstone disease. The morbidity of this operation, however, led to a search for other means to manage gallstones. Many techniques have been described to remove, dissolve, or destroy gallstones while leaving the gallbladder in situ. The recent introduction of "minimally invasive" techniques to remove the gallbladder has revolutionized the surgical approach to cholelithiasis as well as to other abdominal diseases. This chapter will discuss the current approach to gallstone disease, detail the different methods for treating cholecystolithiasis, and outline a multidisciplinary approach to the management of the patient with gallstone disease.

Etiology and Pathogenesis

Gallstones may be classified as cholesterol, black pigment stones, or brown pigment stones. All three types of stones have distinct mechanisms of formation. Cholesterol gallstones are the commonest type, accounting for 85% of stones in the United States. About 20% of women and 10% of men develop stones by the age of 60. A Western diet, age, obesity, female gender, parity, and some forms of hyperlipidemia are risk factors. Three conditions must be met for cholesterol stones to form (Fig. 17-1). The bile must become supersaturated with cholesterol, crystals must nucleate from the super-

saturated bile, and the crystals must become agglomerated into macroscopic stones.

Cholesterol is a very insoluble lipid. The main route of excretion of cholesterol is in the bile, where it is solubilized in phospholipid vesicles or bile-salt–phospholipid micelles. Excess cholesterol secretion into bile can overwhelm the carrying capacity of the system and result in supersaturation. Excess secretion is caused by an imbalance in cholesterol metabolism so that either excess cholesterol is synthesized in the liver or there is a reduction in other cholesterol-metabolizing steps so that more is available for biliary secretion. Enzymes control these metabolic steps, and, interestingly, risk factors for cholesterol stones such as age, gender, pregnancy, and obesity have been found to influence these enzymes.

Supersaturation is very common, especially in industrialized countries. Many persons have supersaturated bile but do not form stones because they lack a nucleating defect. Supersaturated bile will nucleate cholesterol crystals slowly over many days, but in order for nucleation to occur in the time during which bile remains in the biliary tree, nucleating agents are required. Actually, bile normally contains nucleating and antinucleating agents, with the balance favoring slow nucleation. In the pathological state the balance shifts to rapid nucleation. Many different nucleating and antinucleating molecules have been identified, and their exact role is

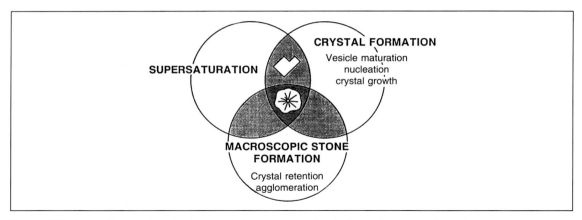

Figure 17-1. Venn diagram showing the conditions necessary for cholesterol gallstone formation (From Strasberg SM, Clavien P-A, Harvey PRC. Pathogenesis of cholesterol gallstones. *HPB Surg* 1991; 3:79–102. Reproduced by permission of publisher.)

not yet understood. A motility defect in the bowel may lead to an excess of the relatively toxic secondary bile acid deoxycholate in the bile, which in turn irritates and inflames the gallbladder, leading to the secretion of pronucleating substances such as mucous glycoprotein and immunoglobulins. Nucleating agents accelerate the production of cholesterol-enriched unilamellar phospholipid vesicles, which appear to aggregate and fuse into multilamellar structures (onion skin form). Cholesterol crystals appear from this phase. Patients who form multiple stones appear to have a greater nucleating defect than patients who form single stones.

For crystals to form into stones, they must be retained in the gallbladder. Good evidence exists for a motility defect in the gallbladder of patients with stones. Their gallbladder muscle appears to contract abnormally, and this defect may be induced by supersaturation. Cholesterol stones are complex structures containing many different molecules, and the exact mechanism of packing is not understood. It appears that mucous glycoprotein is the scaffolding for the packing arrangement.

Black pigment stones are brittle, spiculated, shiny black objects that form as a result of an excess of calcium salts in bile, including calcium bilirubinate, calcium phosphate, or calcium carbonate. Supersaturation of bile with these salts is not uncommon, especially in hepatic bile. Gallbladder bile is usually not supersaturated. Nucleating agents are certainly also involved in calcium stone forma-

tion, and one such agent, calcium-binding protein (CBP), has recently been identified in bile. Hemolysis is the main clinical mechanism of inducing calcium bilirubinate supersaturation in bile, and black pigment stones are commonly found in chronic hemolytic states such as sickle cell anemia, spherocytosis, and thalassemia. Such stones are also found in cirrhotics and patients with Crohn's disease.

Brown pigment stones are composed of calcium bilirubinate, calcium palmitate, and bacterial cell walls. The palmitate is also of bacterial origin. These stones form in the gallbladder or bile duct, as opposed to the other types of stones, which form almost exclusively in the gallbladder. Stasis is the initiating factor and may be due to strictures or foreign bodies such as parasites and other types of stones that have moved into the ducts. Stasis leads to bacterial overgrowth and secretion of enzymes that deconjugate bilirubin, rendering it insoluble in bile. The unconjugated bilirubin and dead bacteria coalesce into a soft, brownish yellow stone. Such stones are associated with recurrent cholangitis, new stricture formation, and eventual destruction of the biliary tree and liver.

Diagnosis

The diagnosis of gallbladder stones requiring therapy is influenced by the high prevalence of gallstones in the population, the fact that most patients with gallstones are asymptomatic, and the presence of many disorders that have symptoms similar to those caused by gallstones. The three clinical stages of cholelithiasis are asymptomatic, symptomatic, and complicated. The diagnosis of symptomatic gallbladder stones, or more appropriately gallstone disease, depends on two equally important features: the detection of gallstones and the presence of symptoms felt to be due to gallstones. The presence or absence of gallbladder stones is usually easily documented in patients using abdominal ultrasonography. Unfortunately, no highly specific and sensitive test exists for symptom correlation in patients with documented gallstones. The diagnosis of symptomatic cholelithiasis must therefore be based on both detection of gallstones and clinical suspicion that the patient's symptoms are indeed related to gallstones.

Symptoms of Gallstone Disease

Although many symptoms have been attributed to gallstone disease, it is often difficult to distinguish gallstone symptoms from those of other gastrointestinal disorders. In fact, when symptoms were compared in several epidemiologic studies of varying design, only abdominal pain is reliably relieved by cholecystectomy. Biliary pain is usually characterized as episodic, severe, and localized in the epigastrium or right upper quadrant, and may radiate to the back. Pain often wakes the patient from sleep or comes after meals. Other symptoms, such as fatty food intolerance, flatulence, indigestion, and belching, were found to be equally prevalent in patients with and without gallstones and are unlikely to be relieved by gallstone treatment.

Liver Function Tests

A patient presenting with biliary colic should undergo a diagnostic evaluation to document the presence of gallstones in the gallbladder and to exclude other conditions that could lead to a similar presentation. Liver function tests are usually normal in patients with uncomplicated gallstone disease. They may be elevated in acute cholecystitis or when choledocholithiasis is present. Serum bilirubin levels rarely rise above 3 mg/dl with acute cholecystitis, but are frequently higher with choledocholithiasis.

Roentgenologic Tests

Ultrasonography remains the most useful test for detecting cholelithiasis but is highly operator-dependent (Fig. 17-2). The sensitivity and specificity for gallstone detection are both greater than 95% in expert hands. The resolution of modern ultrasound equipment allows for the detection of stones as small as 1 mm. Stones in the gallbladder neck or cystic duct are more difficult to image, as are stones in the bile duct. Choledocholithiasis is usually diagnosed indirectly by the presence of ductal dilatation on ultrasound.

Oral cholecystography was revitalized during the 1980s in the era of gallstone lithotripsy as a diagnostic test to assess cystic duct patency, magnitude of stone burden, and cholesterol stone content, but it is rarely used now. Gallbladder visualization should occur after the ingestion, intestinal absorption, hepatic excretion, and gallbladder concentration of the agent. A patent cystic duct is required for entry of the contrast into the gallbladder. Sensitivity and specificity for detecting gallstones are less than with ultrasonography. Stones of high cholesterol content have a low density and sometimes float in the contrast layer during imaging. Of all patients with symptomatic gallstones, 15% to 20% are sufficiently calcified to be visible on plain abdominal films.

Figure 17-2. Ultrasonogram of the gallbladder showing a gallstone with acoustic shadowing (arrows).

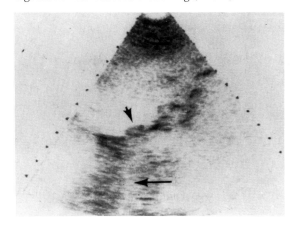

Diagnostic Evaluation

Patients with symptoms of recurrent right upper quadrant or epigastric pain are evaluated with a careful history and thorough physical examination. If the presentation suggests biliary pain, a gallbladder ultrasound examination should be performed to assess the presence of cholelithiasis or other diseases in the upper abdomen. The differential diagnosis includes peptic ulcer disease, esophagitis, gastritis, and pancreatitis, and these conditions should be considered and excluded. In the straightforward patient with typical biliary colic and sonographic evidence of cholecystolithiasis, additional diagnostic tests are unnecessary. Patients with symptomatic cholelithiasis should be offered therapy because there is a high incidence of recurrent symptoms and the possibility of developing a significant complication from gallstones.

Management and Results

Oral Bile Acids

The principal advantage of nonoperative therapy is that it avoids surgery. Candidates for the dissolution of gallstones with oral bile acids are those in whom advanced age or comorbid conditions increase the risk of surgery, or those who refuse cholecystectomy. Two bile acids are clinically available and are approved for oral gallstone dissolution. Both chenodeoxycholic acid, a primary human bile acid, and its epimer, ursodeoxycholic acid, reduce concentrations of cholesterol in bile. Chenodeoxycholic acid was the first to be used in clinical trials, and was associated with a significant incidence of diarrhea and abnormal liver enzymes. Greater efficacy and virtual absence of side effects have made ursodeoxycholic acid the agent of choice for oral gallstone dissolution. This bile acid causes biliary cholesterol desaturation by reducing both hepatic synthesis and secretion of cholesterol into bile, without inhibiting the synthesis of endogenous bile acids. Ursodeoxycholic acid also prolongs nucleation time in the gallbladder bile by shifting cholesterol from vesicles to micelles, and competitively reduces reabsorption of endogenous bile acids by the terminal ileum. The combination of these effects does not influence serum cholesterol levels.

The dissolution of cholesterol gallstones with oral bile acids is a lengthy process. A decrease in diameter of 1 mm/mo is typical. The low efficiency prevents its use in the phase of acute cholecystitis or in patients with bile duct stones, where more immediate results are needed. The success of dissolution is maximized by strict patient selection, which should be directed to high-cholesterol-content stones, small stone burden by both individual size and total number, a functioning gallbladder (patent cystic duct on cholecystography), and stable symptoms that allow for prolonged therapy. Oral cholecystography should be used to assess both gallstone composition and cystic duct patency. Small (< 5 mm) noncalcified gallstones that float are ideal for bile acid dissolution. Even in the most favorable circumstances, complete dissolution occurs in only half of patients. A meta-analysis performed on the recent randomized trials of bile acid therapy revealed that both bile acids were more effective at higher doses. When used for longer than 6 months, high doses of ursodeoxycholic acid achieved complete dissolution in 37% of patients, and low doses in 20%. Chenodeoxycholic acid achieved complete dissolution in 18% of patients at high doses, and in 8% at low doses. Combination therapy was more effective, completely dissolving stones in more than 60% of patients in one series of selected patients. The size of stones significantly influenced therapeutic success, since stones smaller than 10 mm were dissolved more frequently than larger ones.

Extracorporeal Shock Wave Lithotripsy

Biliary extracorporeal shock wave lithotripsy has been evaluated alone and with bile salt therapy as an adjunct. Sound waves are focused from an external generator and aimed at the stones using ultrasonography or fluoroscopy. The shocks are of sufficient amplitude when summated at the focal point to fragment hard stones, while passing relatively harmlessly through softer surrounding tissues. Fragmentation per se is fairly successful, with success rates of over 40%, especially if patients have been selected to have no more than three noncalcified gallstones, each with a maximal diameter of 30 mm. Only 15% to 20% of patients with gallstones meet this criteria. The reported complication rate is low, in the order of 2% to 3%. Elimination of residual stone fragments via the common duct into the small intestine has been problematic, since it relies upon gallbladder contractions. Poor gallbladder muscular function, common in gallstone patients, prevents complete clearance of fragments in many patients after successful lithotripsy. Some of the retained fragments have been reported to have even increased in size over time. Combining lithotripsy with oral bile acids has improved gallbladder clearance rates in patients with cholesterol gallstones. Narrowing the selection criteria to include only single stones less than 20 mm in diameter increases the efficacy but decreases the number of patients likely to benefit from lithotripsy to about 5% of all patients with gallstones. This low applicability, added to the high cost and high recurrence rates for gallstones, has made the use of extracorporeal biliary lithotripsy virtually obsolete in the United States.

After successful dissolution, gallstones form again in 50% of cases initially presenting with multiple stones but in only 15% to 20% of patients with single stones. However, only a small proportion of the reformed stones are reported to be symptomatic, and the new stones appear to be as easily treated as the primary stones. Despite this low efficacy and the potential for recurrence, there remains a role for oral dissolution therapy in selected candidates who refuse surgery, as well as in elderly and debilitated patients with stable symptoms.

Endoscopic Sphincterotomy

Patients with simultaneous cholelithiasis and choledocholithiasis may be adequately treated by endoscopic sphincterotomy and stone removal from the bile duct. The gallbladder may be intentionally left in place after endoscopic sphincterotomy if laparotomy and general anesthesia are deemed too risky in elderly or otherwise debilitated patients. Cholecystectomy, usually not urgent, has been required in 10% of these patients, most often in the first 1 or 2 years after sphincterotomy. Lack of gallbladder filling at the time of endoscopic retrograde cholangiopancreatography (ERCP) does not appear to be a reliable predictor for symptoms or complications requiring cholecystectomy. Acute pancreatitis as the initial manifestation of gallstone disease, on the other hand, has been associated with an increased need for subsequent cholecystectomy following endoscopic sphincterotomy.

Endoscopic Cholecystostomy

The gallbladder itself can also be accessed by peroral endoscopy, via the common bile duct and cystic duct, for interventional purposes. This approach is technically challenging and somewhat indirect, since any type of therapy needs to overcome the small size and tortuosity of the cystic duct. Endoscopic retrograde cannulation of the gallbladder has recently been reported with success rates as high as 75% of specialty centers. Transpapillary drainage of the gallbladder has been used to drain gallbladder empyemas and mucoceles, and to treat acalculous cholecystitis. Endoscopically placed nasocystic drains have also been used as a means of delivering methyl-tert-butyl ether for contact dissolution of stones. This technique has been reported alone and combined with extracorporeal shock wave lithotripsy. With these approaches, the gallbladder has been cleared of gallstones in 50% to 75% of patients, with complication rates no higher than expected for endoscopic retrograde cholangiography alone.

Early experience at Washington University Medical Center with dislodging cystic duct stones and draining gallbladder empyemas has allowed the authors to change their operative management from urgent to elective by allowing resolution of the acute inflammatory process. Patients at high risk for surgery may be managed by endoscopic gallbladder clearance alone. The use of this technique is limited to patients with combined disease of the gallbladder and common bile duct who have clear indications for endoscopic retrograde cholangiography, since patients with gallbladder disease alone can be managed more directly by operative or percutaneous approaches. Further experience is desirable before endoscopic management of gallbladder diseases gains widespread acceptance. The intrinsic difficulties of the technique and the small number of patients likely to benefit from this approach will probably limit its application to tertiary centers with advanced endoscopic expertise.

Percutaneous Gallstone Removal
(Cholecystolithotomy)

In otherwise healthy patients, surgical cholecystectomy is an excellent procedure with a low rate of morbidity and mortality. However, in elderly and debilitated patients, both the morbidity and mortality of cholecystectomy are significantly greater and may be as great as 10% to 30%. In these high-risk patients, percutaneous gallstone removal (cholecystolithotomy) has potential benefit as a less invasive therapeutic alternative.

The most common indication for percutaneous cholecystolithotomy is a patient at high risk for general anesthesia, usually because of severe cardiac or pulmonary disease. Percutaneous gallstone removal in the authors' practice is always performed using local anesthesia and intravenous analgesia (e.g., morphine sulfate and midazolam). Therefore, the procedure is very well tolerated by even the most severely medically compromised patients. In extremely ill patients, the procedure can be staged into smaller components and tailored to the patient's ability to withstand the intervention. Percutaneous gallstone removal consists of four steps: (1) percutaneous cholecystostomy, (2) tract dilatation, (3) gallstone removal, and finally (4) tract evaluation with tube removal (Fig. 17-3).

The technical details of the initial percutaneous access into the gallbladder (percutaneous cholecystostomy) are covered in Chapter 20. Frequently, the percutaneous cholecystostomy catheter has already been placed to decompress an acutely inflamed gallbladder in a patient too ill for surgical intervention. In these patients, the gallbladder is allowed to drain externally until the symptoms of acute cholecystitis resolve. In patients with cholelithiasis for whom elective gallstone removal is undertaken, percutaneous cholecystostomy is usually performed on day 1, with subsequent stone removal the next day.

When the patient is ready for gallstone removal, tract dilatation is performed. Using standard interventional radiology techniques, a safety wire is placed within the gallbladder lumen and stitched to the skin. Over the primary wire, coaxial polytef (Teflon) dilators (Cook Inc., Bloomington, Ind.) are used to establish an 18 French tract to the gallbladder. Through this tract, an 18 French

polytef sheath is placed into the gallbladder lumen. All subsequent manipulations are then performed through this sheath. The use of a sheath protects against bile leaking into the peritoneal space and also tamponades any small bleeding that may occur in the tract.

Actual gallstone removal is performed using a combination of fluoroscopy and flexible choledochoscopy. The authors use a 15 French flexible choledochonephroscope (Olympus, Inc.). This scope has a 5 French working channel which allows the use of standard baskets, graspers, and irrigation. Stones too large to remove intact are fragmented with electrohydraulic lithotripsy through the working channel of the choledochoscope. Electrohydraulic lithotripsy is an intracorporeal shock wave technique that has been used extensively by urologists for fragmenting stones in the bladder and ureter. The authors have found that most gallstones can be removed with simple irrigation and basket retrieval. In patients with an extremely large stone burden, several sessions may be needed to render the gallbladder stone-free. This practice is particularly necessary in severely ill patients with significant cardiac or pulmonary compromise.

Stone removal is successful when direct-vision choledochoscopy shows no further stones within the gallbladder. Cholangiography is performed to exclude stones in the cystic duct or common bile duct. Usually stones in the cystic duct and common bile duct can be removed through the transhepatic gallbladder tract. However, occasionally common duct stones may require endoscopic retrograde techniques for removal. Following the stone removal session, a 14 French retention pigtail catheter is replaced within the gallbladder lumen. Patients are sent home with the cholecystostomy tube in place. This cholecystostomy tube is left to external drainage for 1 to 2 weeks and then capped to internal drainage for an additional 1 to 2 weeks.

Prior to removing the cholecystostomy tube, a tract evaluation is performed. It is critical that a fibrous tract has formed between the gallbladder lumen and the skin. Unless such a fibrous tract is present, bile will leak into the peritoneal cavity, causing intense pain and possibly bile peritonitis. To ensure tract maturity, the cholecystostomy tube is removed over a guidewire, and contrast is injected into the tract. The cholecystostomy tube is removed

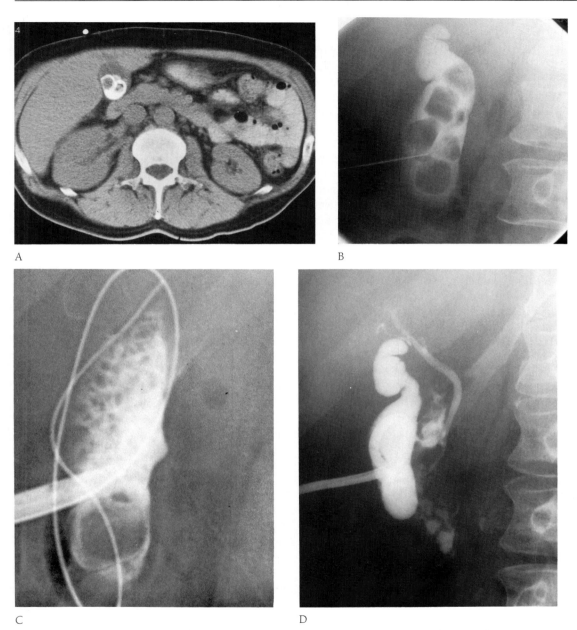

A

B

C

D

Figure 17-3. Images of a 57-year-old patient with severe three-vessel coronary artery disease and chronic recurrent attacks of severe biliary colic. A. CT scan shows calcified gallstones with a marker defining a transhepatic tract to the gallbladder. B. Contrast injection performed at the time of percutaneous cholecystostomy shows at least seven large gallstones. C. Several of the gallstones have been fragmented with electrohydraulic lithotripsy. Note the safety wire coiled in the gallbladder as well as the 18 French polytef (Teflon) sheath. D. Final cholangiogram demonstrates the biliary system to be stone-free. At this point the cholecystostomy tube was capped to internal drainage for 1 week prior to tract evaluation and tube removal. (From Picus D, et al. Percutaneous cholecystolithotomy: Analysis of results and complications in 58 consecutive patients. *Radiology* 1992; 183:779–784. Reproduced by permission of the publisher.)

only if this tract evaluation shows an intact tract to the skin. If intraperitoneal spill of contrast is noted, the tube is replaced over the guidewire, and the tract is allowed to mature for another week or two, at which time a repeat tract evaluation is performed.

Several large series of percutaneous gallstone removals using a variety of techniques have been reported. To date, the authors have performed percutaneous gallstone removal on 91 patients ranging in age from 29 to 97 years. All patients had symptomatic gallstones and a strong contraindication to cholecystectomy. The stones in these patients ranged from 1 to over 500 in number, and ranged from 3 mm to more than 4 cm in size. Twenty-two patients had cystic duct stones, and 18 patients had additional common bile duct stones. All stones were successfully removed in 89 of 91 patients (98%). Often two or more stone-removal sessions were required to clear the gallbladder, cystic duct, and common bile duct of stones. Major complications were encountered in 5 of the 91 patients (5%). Three of the 5 problems were related to the percutaneous tract and occurred prior to institution of a standard policy of tract evaluation prior to tube removal. Since then, major complications resulting from immature tracts have not occurred.

The primary advantage of percutaneous gallstone removal is that it does not require general anesthesia and therefore can be used to treat even the sickest patients with symptomatic gallstones. The technique is applicable to patients with acute or chronic cholecystitis, as well as to patients with any type, number, or size of stones. The major disadvantage of the procedure is that the gallbladder is left in place, allowing a risk of stone recurrence as well as possible gallbladder malignancy. However, these disadvantages are true of all nonsurgical approaches to gallbladder disease. Because of these considerations, the authors have chosen to limit this procedure to nonsurgical candidates. The shorter life expectancy in these patients makes recurrent gallbladder disease less of a concern. Percutaneous gallstone removal is the nonsurgical treatment of choice in the authors' institution for patients with symptomatic gallstones who are at high risk for surgery and who are not candidates for oral dissolution therapy.

Surgical Approach

Open cholecystectomy had been the primary mode of therapy of symptomatic cholelithiasis since shortly after its introduction in 1882 by Karl Langenbuch of Berlin, Germany. Langenbuch made the now famous statement that "the gallbladder should be removed, not because it contains stones but because it forms them." The mortality rates for open cholecystectomy have declined progressively over the succeeding years, and it is not uncommon to find large series without mortality. However, in the era of open cholecystectomy, the incidence of minor morbidity ranged from 10% to 20%, and duration of postoperative hospitalization was generally between 3 to 7 days. Removal of the gallbladder using laparoscopic guidance was first performed in France in 1987 but was not widely publicized until it was performed in the United States in 1988. Many published reports have appeared since 1989. Laparoscopic cholecystectomy diminishes postoperative pain and duration of hospitalization and disability more than its "open" counterpart, and it has rapidly become the preferred technique for surgical removal of the gallbladder. An estimated 85% of all cholecystectomies were done laparoscopically in 1993 (Figure 17-5). This change has also been seen at the authors' institution, where more than 95% of patients undergoing cholecystectomy have been treated by the laparoscopic approach since its clinical introduction in November 1989.

The ability to perform laparoscopic cholecystectomy depends upon all members of the operating team viewing the same operative field on a video monitor projected from a miniature television camera attached to the eyepiece of a laparoscope. Usually the procedure is performed after insufflating the peritoneal cavity with carbon dioxide to a pressure of 10 to 15 mm Hg and inserting the video laparoscope through an umbilical trocar. Operating instruments are then inserted through three other laparoscopic ports positioned in the right subcostal region and epigastrium. The supine patient is positioned in a steep reverse Trendelenburg position and rolled to the left to allow the intra-abdominal viscera to fall away from the right upper quadrant (Fig. 17-4A,B). The gallbladder is grasped and elevated in a lateral and cephalad direction, and the

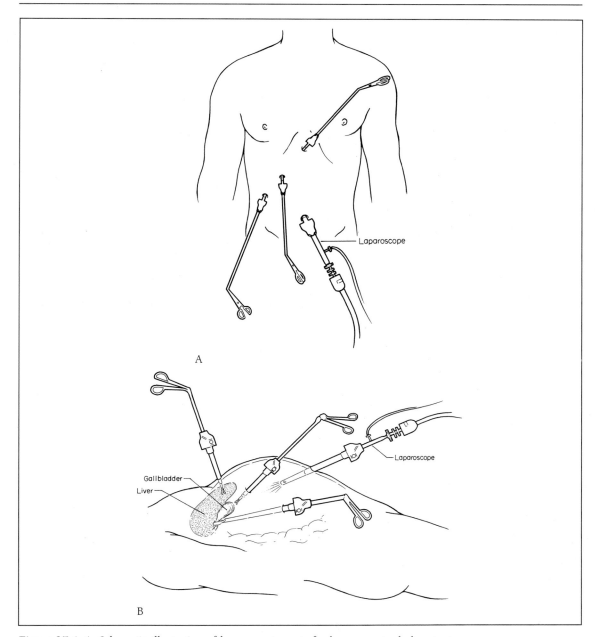

Figure 17-4. A. Schematic illustration of laparoscopic ports for laparoscopic cholecystectomy.
B. Cross-sectional view of abdomen after creation of the pneumoperitoneum and insertion of
instruments for laparoscopic cholecystectomy. (From Soper NJ, Brunt LM, Kerbl K. Laparoscopic
general surgery. *N Eng J Med* 1994; 330:409–419. Reprinted by permission of the *New England
Journal of Medicine.*)

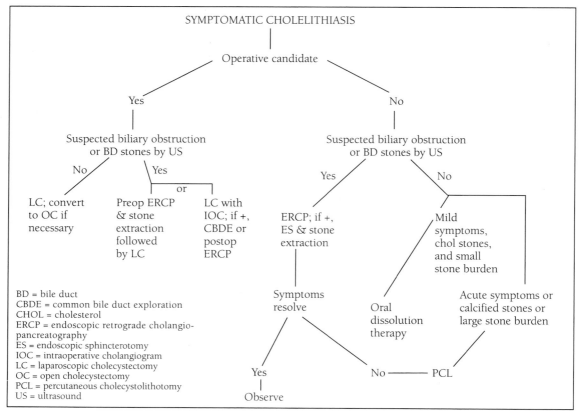

Figure 17-5. Management of symptomatic cholelithiasis.

entire right lobe of the liver is rolled cranially to expose the gallbladder neck and porta hepatis. The neck of the gallbladder is dissected from the surrounding tissue to expose the origin of the cystic duct from the infundibulum of the gallbladder.

Because of the limitations inherent in the current phase of laparoscopic technology, that is, limited tactile discrimination and two-dimensional imaging, great care must be taken while dissecting the infundibulum of the gallbladder to avoid injuring the structures contained within the porta hepatis. It is critical to assess the neck of the gallbladder and cystic duct both from the classical ventral aspect of Calot's triangle (while placing traction on the gallbladder in a lateral direction) as well as from the dorsal aspect of Calot's triangle (while placing tension on the infundibulum in a superior and medial direction). When meticulous dissection is un-

dertaken in this region, the risk of bile duct injury is low, and a selective approach to operative cholangiography is reasonable. However, both for training purposes and for becoming facile at transcystic access to the common bile duct (utilized during laparoscopic management of choledocholithiasis), the authors perform routine fluoroscopic intraoperative cholangiography. The cystic duct and cystic artery are ligated with clips and divided, and the gallbladder is removed from its hepatic bed using electrocautery. Generally, the gallbladder is extracted through the umbilical incision, which may require stretching or lengthening in cases of large stone burdens or a markedly thickened gallbladder wall. Fascial sutures are required only in the umbilical incision. Patients are generally discharged the morning following the operation and are allowed to return to full activity as tolerated.

Indications for laparoscopic cholecystectomy should be the same as those for open cholecystectomy. Concerns have been raised that laparoscopic cholecystectomy may have decreased the threshold for the performance of cholecystectomy, resulting in an increased number of cholecystectomies in the United States. Whether this represents an ongoing phenomenon or merely the treatment of a "reservoir" of patients who had been symptomatic but reluctant to seek operative therapy previously is undetermined. The authors perform laparoscopic cholecystectomy in patients who have symptomatic gallstones and occasionally in those patients with stones but no symptoms (*Salmonella* carriers, patients immunosuppressed because of organ transplantation, those whose occupations remove them from readily available medical care, and those with a porcelain gallbladder). Patients with typical biliary colic but no visible stones may also be offered laparoscopic cholecystectomy, particularly those with a low ejection fraction on a cholecystokinin-stimulated radionuclide hepatobiliary scan.

Contraindications to cholecystectomy relate to the patient's medical status and not to the characteristics of the gallstones; that is, all types and numbers of gallstones may be thus treated. Open cholecystectomy is contraindicated only in those patients with severe underlying medical conditions that would preclude a general anesthetic or laparotomy. Contraindications to laparoscopic cholecystectomy have diminished considerably as experience has been gained with this technique (Table 17-1). Absolute contraindications to laparoscopic cholecystectomy are similar to those for open cholecystectomy. Relative contraindications reflect the surgeon's experience with the laparoscopic approach as well as

the potentially deleterious effects of absorbed carbon dioxide from the pneumoperitoneum. Thus the vast majority of patients are candidates for either laparoscopic or open cholecystectomy.

The results of laparoscopic cholecystectomy have generally been excellent. Table 17-2 details a number of laparoscopic cholecystectomy series that have been reported over the last few years. In these series, major complications have occurred in less than 5% of patients, and mortality is rare. Some patients, ranging from 2% to 9%, will require conversion of the operation from a laparoscopic to an open approach, generally because of adhesions or inflammation interfering with a clear view of the operative field when laparoscopic techniques for dissection and visualization are used. Because conversion from a laparoscopic to an open operation is always possible, patients who are not candidates for open cholecystectomy should not be considered for laparoscopic cholecystectomy.

The reported incidence of bile duct injuries with laparoscopic cholecystectomy has been as high as 0.7%, a rate greater than that accepted for open cholecystectomy, which has ranged from 0.1% to 0.2%. It has been proposed that these common bile duct injuries are attributable to the "learning curve" and that the incidence of laparoscopic bile duct injury should ultimately approach that of open cholecystectomy. However, because of concerns regarding an increase in complications of cholecystectomy after initiation of the laparoscopic operation, an NIH Consensus Development Conference was held in September 1992 entitled "Gallstones and Laparoscopic Cholecystectomy." The consensus statement concluded that "laparoscopic cholecystectomy provides a safe and effective treatment for

Table 17-1. Contraindications to Laparoscopic Cholecystectomy

Absolute	Relative
Unable to tolerate general anesthesia or laparotomy	Severe acute cholecystitis
Uncorrected coagulopathy	Biliary fistula
Generalized peritonitis or cholangitis	Suspected gallbladder carcinoma
Concomitant disease requiring laparotomy	Previous upper abdominal surgery
	Cirrhosis/portal hypertension
	Severe chronic obstructive lung disease
	Pregnancy

Table 17-2. Outcome of Laparoscopic Cholecystectomy: Compiled Results

Series	Number of Patients	Converted[a] (%)	Mortality (%)	Major Complications (%)	CBD[b] Injury (%)
Southern Surgeons (1991)[c]	1518	4.7	0.07	1.5	0.5
European Surgeons (1991)[d]	1236	3.6	0	1.6	0.3
Soper et al (1992)[e]	618	2.9	0	1.6	0.2
Spaw, Reddick, Olsen (1991)[f]	500	1.8	0	1	0
Wolfe et al (1991)[g]	381	3	0.9	3.4	0
Bailey et al (1991)[h]	375	5	0.3	0.6	0.3
Schirmer et al (1991)[i]	152	8.5	0	4	0.7

[a]Converted to open laparotomy.
[b]CBD = common bile duct
[c]Data from The Southern Surgeons Club. A prospective analysis of 1518 laparoscopic cholecystectomies. *N Engl J Med* 1991; 324:1073–1078.
[d]Data from May GR, et al. Efficacy of bile acid therapy for gallstone dissolution: A meta-analysis of randomized trials. *Ailment Pharmacol Ther* 1993; 7:139–148.
[e]Data from Soper NJ, et al. Laparoscopic cholecystectomy: The new "gold standard"? *Arch Surg* 1992; 127:917–921.
[f]Data from Spaw AT, Reddick EJ, Olsen DO. Laparoscopic laser cholecystectomy: Analysis of 500 procedures. *Surg Laparosc and Endosc* 1991; 1:2–7.
[g]Data from Wolfe BM, et al. Endoscopic cholecystectomy: An analysis of complications. *Arch Surg* 1991; 126:1192–1196.
[h]Data from Bailey RW, et al. Laparoscopic cholecystectomy: Experience with 375 consecutive patients. *Ann Surg* 1991; 214:531–540.
[i]Data from Schirmer BD, et al. Laparoscopic cholecystectomy: Treatment of choice for symptomatic cholelithiasis. *Ann Surg* 1991; 213:665–676.

Table 17-3. Outcomes of Treatment Modalities for Gallbladder (GB) Stones

	Gallbladder Extirpation		Gallstone Ablation		
	Open Cholecystectomy	Laparoscopic Cholecystectomy	Lithotripsy	Oral Bile Acid Therapy	Cholecystolithotomy
Applicability (%)	98	90–95	7–16	15–30	1–5
Efficacy: rate of initial GB stone clearance (%)	100	100	60–95	40–90	100
Adverse outcomes					
Mortality (%)	<1	<1	~0	~0	~0
Overall morbidity (%)	4–8	2–5	~5	~0	~2.5
Bile duct injury	0.1–0.2	0.2–0.6	0	0	0
Recurrence of GB stones	0	0	<50	~50	~50
Costs					
Medical care costs	X[b]	0.9X–X	~X	~X	~.7X
Disability (d)[a]	20–40	7–14	1–2	<1	<1
Patient preference issues					
Length of hospital stay (d)	2–7	1–2	<1	0	1–2
Discomfort	Severe	Mild	Mild	None	Mild
Scar	Moderate	Minimal	None	None	None

[a](d) = day(s)
[b]X = $10,000
Source: Adapted from Kalser SC, et al. National Institutes of Health Consensus Development Conference statement on gallstones and laparoscopic cholecystectomy. *Am J Surg* 1993; 165:390–396.

most patients with symptomatic gallstones" and has "distinct advantages over open cholecystectomy." However, "because of its wide applicability and low mortality and morbidity, open cholecystectomy remains the standard against which new treatment should be judged."

Conclusions

From the preceding narrative, it is obvious that many choices exist for treating the patient with gallstones. An overview of the outcomes of different treatment modalities is shown in Table 17-3. In the patient with symptomatic gallstones, the first consideration is whether the patient is a candidate for operation (Fig. 17-5). If the patient can undergo operative resection and agrees to this therapy, laparoscopic cholecystectomy is attempted, but if the anatomy precludes this approach, an open cholecystectomy is performed. Gallbladder resection is generally advised because the technique is applicable to the vast majority of patients, is not influenced by the size, number, or composition of gallstones, and is immediately (and permanently) successful with a relatively low morbidity and mortality.

In patients who are unable or unwilling to undergo cholecystectomy, the gallstones may be ablated or removed using oral bile acid therapy or percutaneous cholecystolithotomy. The authors restrict oral bile acid therapy to those patients who have small (< 10 mm) cholesterol gallstones contained within a functioning gallbladder and who are experiencing relatively mild symptoms. High-risk patients with stones in both the gallbladder and common bile duct may be treated by endoscopic sphincterotomy alone or, rarely, in combination with transcystic drainage of the gallbladder. The remainder of patients, particularly those at high risk for operation, will be offered cholecystolithotomy. Although the optimal choice of treatment for most patients is relatively clear-cut, the authors' group of gastroenterologists, interventional radiologists, and surgeons often discuss the care of the complex patient and work together to maximize the clinical outcome. If this multidisciplinary approach is used, patients with cholelithiasis may be treated with safety and efficacy in the 1990s.

Selected Readings

Barkun JS, et al. Laparoscopic vs. open cholecystectomy: The Canadian experience. *Am J Surg* 1993; 165: 455–458.

Feretis CB, et al. Endoscopic transpapillary catheterization of the gallbladder followed by external shock wave lithotripsy and solvent infusion for the treatment of gallstone disease. *Gastrointest Endosc* 1992; 38(1):19–22.

Johlin FC, Neil GA. Drainage of the gallbladder in patients with acute acalculous cholecystitis by transpapillary endoscopic cholecystectomy. *Gastrointest Endosc* 1993; 39:645–651.

Johnston DE, Kaplan MM. Pathogenesis and treatment of gallstones. *N Engl J Med* 1993; 328:412–421.

Kalser SC, et al. National Institutes of Health Consensus Development Conference statement on gallstones and laparoscopic cholecystectomy. *Am J Surg* 1993; 165:390–396.

May GR, Sutherland LR, Shaffer EA. Efficacy of bile acid therapy for gallstone dissolution: A meta-analysis of randomized trials. *Aliment Pharmacol Ther* 1993; 7:139–148.

Picus D, et al. Percutaneous cholecystolithotomy: Analysis of results and complications in 58 consecutive patients. *Radiology* 1992; 183:779–784.

Soper NJ, Dunnegan DL. Routine versus selective intraoperative cholangiography during laparoscopic cholecystectomy. *World J Surg* 1992; 16:1133–1140.

Soper NJ, et al. Laparoscopic cholecystectomy: The new "gold standard"? *Arch Surg* 1992; 127:917–921.

Strasberg SM, Clavien PA. Cholecystolithiasis: Lithotherapy for the 1990's. *Hepatology* 1992; 16:820–839.

18

Choledocholithiasis

Alfred D. Roston
David R. Lichtenstein
David C. Brooks
David L. Carr-Locke

Choledocholithiasis and its attendant complications have traditionally fallen under the purview of surgical management. With the advent of endoscopic retrograde cholangiopancreatography (ERCP) in 1968 and the first use of endoscopic sphincterotomy (ES) in 1974, newer treatment options and plans for the optimal management of choledocholithiasis have emerged. The widespread use of ultrasonography (US) and computerized tomography (CT) has enhanced the clinician's ability to more accurately diagnose common bile duct stones. The popularity of laparoscopic cholecystectomy has furthered a minimally invasive approach to the management of choledocholithiasis. Given the variety of therapeutic approaches, it is clear that a multidisciplinary team approach is best. This team, in addition to the primary care physician, should consist of a gastroenterologist, radiologist, and surgeon. Management strategies should be viewed in the context of available local expertise.

With the improvement in therapeutic endoscopic techniques, the role of ERCP in the management of common bile duct stones has greatly expanded. General agreement exists among surgeons and gastroenterologists that common bile duct stone removal should be endoscopic rather than surgical in the following clinical scenarios: (1) previously cholecystectomy or bile duct exploration, (2) severe acute cholangitis, (3) severe acute biliary pancreatitis, (4) high-risk surgical patients with gallbladder in situ, and (5) low-risk surgical patients with suspected common bile duct stones prior to or immediately following laparoscopic cholecystectomy.

Etiology and Pathogenesis

Common bile duct stones are classified into primary (arising de novo in the bile duct) and secondary (forming in the gallbladder and migrating into the common bile duct). Primary duct stones are composed primarily of calcium bilirubinate and have a cholesterol content less than that of gallbladder stones. Although their precise pathogenesis is not known, bacterial or parasitic infection, bile stasis due to strictures or obstructing lesions, and dietary factors contribute to their formation. Secondary bile duct stones are the more prevalent form in the Western world, and cholesterol stones are the most common type. Of patients with "Western" choledocholithiasis, 80% to 90% have concomitant gallbladder stones.

As many as 15% of patients undergoing cholecystectomy harbor bile duct stones. In those patients undergoing bile duct exploration, up to 5% have retained bile duct stones. Although most patients with cholelithiasis will not become symptomatic, patients with bile duct stones will characteristically develop complications such as cholangitis, pancreatitis, biliary pain, or jaundice. Thus the discovery of choledocholithiasis, whether incidental or intentional, argues for active intervention, not expectant management.

Diagnosis

The clinical presentation of choledocholithiasis is broad, and may range from asymptomatic with incidental discovery to abrupt, critical illness. Perhaps the most common presentation is that of biliary pain syndrome. The pain is usually in the epigastrium or right upper quadrant, and is not colicky but continuous. The pain may radiate to the interscapular area and may be associated with nausea and vomiting. The pain syndrome is indistinguishable from that of a stone migrating through the cystic duct. If a stone obstructs the common bile duct and infection supervenes, acute cholangitis ensues. Eponymous associations such as Charcot's triad (fever/chills, pain, and jaundice) or Reynold's pentad (the addition of hypotension and mental status change) are not uniformly present, and a high index of suspicion must be maintained, especially in subtler situations where the serum bilirubin level may be only slightly elevated and fever is minimal. Pain may be mild and jaundice absent in up to 20% of patients.

In the absence of cholangitis, painless jaundice may be the predominant clinical scenario. The serum bilirubin level is usually elevated to less than 15 mg/dl, and the alkaline phosphatase level may be normal or elevated to many times normal. In addition, if a stone traverses or impacts at the papilla, biliary pancreatitis may be the dominant clinical picture. Pancreatitis and cholangitis may coexist. Clinical and laboratory data, although suggestive, are not sufficient to diagnose common bile duct stones. Levels of bilirubin, alkaline phosphatase, and serum transaminases may be elevated to various degrees. Normal liver tests do not preclude the presence of choledocholithiasis. Their pattern of rise or fall may prove to be the best predictor in symptomatic choledocholithiasis.

The use of both noninvasive and invasive imaging modalities is crucial in the diagnosis and management of choledocholithiasis. US is useful in documenting the presence of cholelithiasis and bile duct dilatation, but cannot reliably exclude bile duct stones (Fig. 18-1). Sensitivities in the range of 10% to 81% have been reported. Body habitus and surrounding bowel gas may preclude optimal visualization of the distal common bile duct. CT scanning also demonstrates biliary ductal dilatation

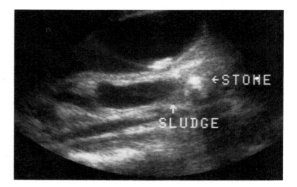

Figure 18-1. Ultrasonogram (sagittal view) showing a 1.0-cm common bile duct stone with acoustic shadowing, intraductal sludge, and proximal ductal dilatation (1.2 cm). The gallbladder contains echogenic material. (Provided by Faye Laing, MD, Department of Radiology, Brigham & Women's Hospital.)

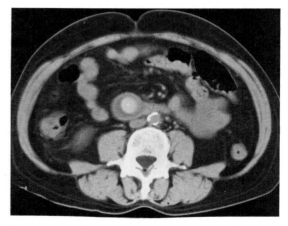

Figure 18-2. CT scan showing markedly dilated bile duct containing a large stone of higher attenuation than the surrounding bile (white cross).

and may afford better visualization of the distal common bile duct, but cholesterol stones may not be adequately distinguished from the surrounding bile (Fig. 18-2). Its accuracy in detecting common duct stones has been reported in the range of 50% to 90%.

Intravenous cholangiography (IVC) and nuclear scintigraphic techniques have been suboptimal for diagnosing common bile duct stones, but are being revisited with newer agents. Percutaneous transhepatic cholangiography (PTC) and ERCP are usually applied to those patients with suspected stones but with unrevealing noninvasive imaging. The choice of modality is guided by the presence or absence of a dilated biliary tree and local expertise. The main advantage of these modalities is the ability to employ therapeutic options in removing stones. Bile duct stones may first be diagnosed intraoperatively by palpation, intraoperative cholangiography, or ductal exploration.

Management and Results

Choices in the multidisciplinary management of choledocholithiasis are dependent on a number of factors, including the overall success and complication rates for the different techniques. Direct comparisons between endoscopic and surgical management are difficult because of patient selection and lack of randomized comparative trials. In expert hands open surgical bile duct exploration is expected to be at least 95% successful in duct clearance at the expense of mortality rates, which range from 0% in low-risk patients to 28% in elderly high-risk patients. Stone recurrence rates after open surgery vary from 5% to 21%, depending on the length of follow-up. Encouraging results for laparoscopic management are emerging from a small number of pioneering centers, but whether these results will be confirmed remains unanswered.

Equivalent results for endoscopic management in expert centers are duct clearance rates of at least 95% of patients and 30-day mortality rates 0% to 3%. Stones seem to recur in less than 5% of patients. The management of specific subsets of patients will be discussed below.

Postcholecystectomy with T Tube in Situ

T tube cholangiograms obtained in the early postoperative period may demonstrate bile duct stones. Those with a diameter of less than 10 mm may pass spontaneously or with active perfusion. However, many will require mechanical manipulation to facilitate passage. Since consequent surgical bile duct exploration may impart considerable morbidity and mortality, a variety of other techniques may be employed. These methods include vigorous irrigation and simultaneous use of sphincteric relaxants (e.g., glucagon, nitrates), T tube track choledochoscopy,

or percutaneous stone extraction through a mature track. Reported success rates of 77% to 96% are encouraging, but multiple sessions are usually required, and complications such as sepsis, trauma, and bile leak may occur in the range of 4% to 8%. When a mature T tube track is necessary, delays of up to 4 to 6 weeks are required. Early sphincterotomy is safe and can be applied without track maturation, thus facilitating timely hospital discharge (Fig. 18-3). Although no controlled trials of the various therapeutic options have been performed, endoscopic success rates of 90% with morbidity and mortality rates of 7% and 0.6%, respectively, have been documented. When available, it would

Figure 18-3. T tube cholangiogram revealing a distal CBD stone subsequently removed after endoscopic sphincterotomy.

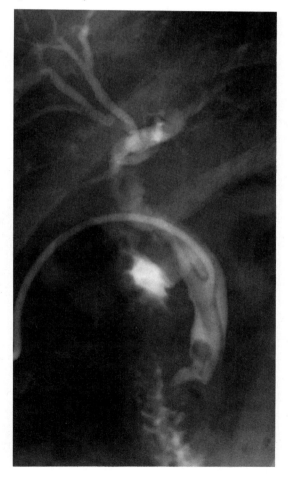

appear that early ERCP, with ES as necessary, is an attractive option.

Postcholecystectomy Without T Tube

Common bile duct stones have been found in up to 15% of all patients undergoing open cholecystectomy for symptomatic cholelithiasis, and the incidence of retained common bile duct stones has approached 15% even after open duct exploration. Available data suggest that ES for retained common duct stones in the postcholecystectomy elderly patient remains the treatment of choice (Fig. 18-4). Reoperation with ductal exploration may carry significant morbidity and mortality in elderly patients or those with comorbidity. Similarly, ES is also recommended in the young, otherwise fit postcholecystectomy patient. These data are extrapolated

from the follow-up data obtained for the elderly, and long-term follow-up of sphincterotomy in the young will be required. However, no theoretical or practical reasons exist to suspect that these results would differ.

Gallbladder in Situ

After ES and common bile duct stone removal in the elderly, the clinical situation may dictate that subsequent cholecystectomy may impose an unnecessary surgical risk. Because of the shorter life expectancy in this population, the decision can be made to leave the gallbladder intact (Fig. 18-5). Outcome measures (short-term, long-term, and complications) observed in those patients with gallbladder in situ do not differ from those in the postcholecystectomy elderly patient. These patients are often

Figure 18-4. ERCP in postcholecystectomy patient showing three bile duct stones being removed by basket extraction after endoscopic sphincterotomy.

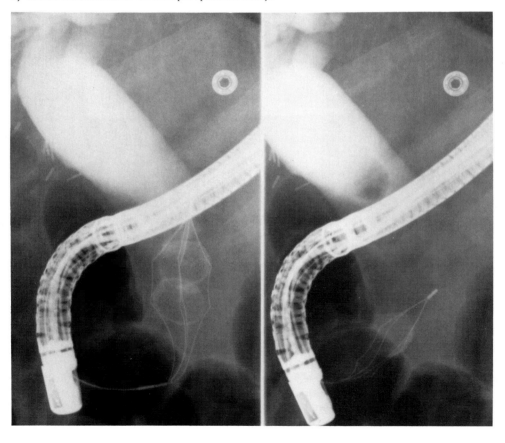

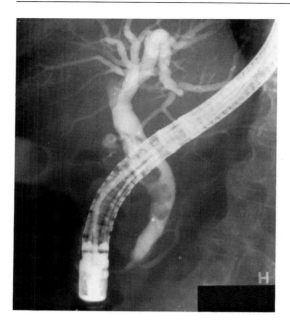

Figure 18-5. ERCP showing cholelithiasis and choledocholithiasis, the latter being removed after sphincterotomy.

managed expectantly unless the clinical situation dictates otherwise. Follow-up data reveal that about 10% develop symptoms severe enough to warrant cholecystectomy, usually within the first year, and most often nonemergently.

The continued presence of stones within the gallbladder is probably necessary for the development of gallbladder complications following ES and common bile duct clearance. Since this overall risk is low, and if close follow-up is possible, it would appear prudent to forego routine cholecystectomy in this population, given the higher risk.

In the otherwise fit patient under age 60, with greater potential for long-term survival, the likelihood of developing future symptoms related to cholelithiasis requiring an operation is greater than the risk of elective cholecystectomy. This patient population benefits from cholecystectomy.

The role of routine preoperative ES in the young, fit patient with choledocholithiasis and cholelithiasis is more controversial. Earlier trials that evaluated the role of preoperative ES and any advantage related to morbidity, mortality, and hospital stay compared to open cholecystectomy and ductal exploration found no option superior. However,

these studies did not employ a laparoscopic approach, nor did they include poor-surgical-risk patients. In the era of laparoscopic cholecystectomy, these conclusions require re-evaluation.

Laparoscopic Cholecystectomy

Although laparoscopic cholecystectomy (LC) has rapidly become the method of choice for gallbladder removal in the majority of patients with symptomatic cholelithiasis, its role in the optimal management of bile duct stones remains to be determined. The options available for managing bile duct stones intraoperatively continue to evolve and include laparoscopic transcystic extraction, transcystic choledochoscopy with stone extraction, and laparoscopic choledochotomy. The last-mentioned technique is still under development and is available only at specialized surgical centers. Novel transpapillary methods are being explored. The small caliber of the cystic duct makes instrumentation, lithotripsy, and stone retrieval relatively difficult. Thus peroral endoscopic therapy is still needed in the preoperative and postoperative periods. Its application is determined by institutional expertise with, in general, predominantly postoperative ERCP in those centers where reliable endoscopic management is available with or without intraoperative expertise, and with preoperative ERCP when endoscopic success is less consistent or laparoscopic techniques are limited.

If preoperative identification is desired, it is useful to incorporate clinical and biochemical indicators in an attempt to identify those patients who are at low, intermediate, and high risk of harboring bile duct stones (Table 18-1). These indicators include abnormal liver tests (both absolute elevation and the pattern of their rise or fall), sonographic evidence of common bile duct (CBD) dilatation of more than 8 mm, and past history of jaundice or presentation with cholangitis. Although some centers have advocated routine preoperative or intraoperative cholangiography (IOC) in order to document aberrant anatomy or silent stones, the authors do not support this position, since good surgical technique should obviate the demonstration of variant ductal anatomy, which rarely influences operative strategy. Additionally, in those low-risk patients without appropriate clinical, biochemical, or sono-

Table 18-1. Risk Factors for Choledocholithiasis

High
  Bile duct stone or bile duct dilatation on US or CT
  Presentation with cholangitis or jaundice
  Rising liver tests after presentation
  Bilirubin > 2 dl
  Alkaline phosphatase > 150 U/I
Intermediate
  Recent jaundice
  Bilirubin 1.5–2.0 dl
  Alkaline phosphatase 110–150 U/I
  Improving liver tests after presentation
Low
  Normal liver tests
  Absence of ductal dilatation on US or CT
  Absence or remote history of jaundice or pancreatitis
  Normalized liver tests after presentation

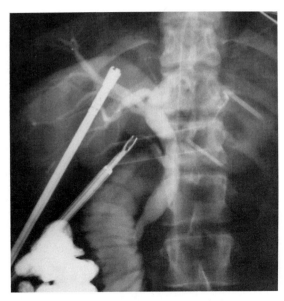

Figure 18-6. Transcystic intraoperative cholangiogram during laparoscopic cholecystectomy.

graphic predictors, CBD stones are present in only 2% to 3% of patients. The authors therefore recommend IOC only in those patients who are intermediate or high risk for choledocholithiasis (Fig. 18-6). Figure 18-7 outlines the optimal use of the available treatment modalities in those patients with suspected choledocholithiasis.

Total surgical management with only one procedure, obviating preoperative or postoperative attempts at stone extraction, may carry a higher conversion rate to open bile duct exploration, thus countering the objective of minimal invasion, unless reliable methods are available for transcystic extraction or laparoscopic common bile duct exploration (CBDE).

Prelaparoscopic ductal clearance by ERCP is particularly well suited to the patient at high risk for harboring bile duct stones, since a minimally invasive approach can be maintained by avoiding the need for conversion to open duct exploration. In addition, small duct stones of up to 8 mm in diameter can be removed during ERCP through an intact papilla. This method would serve to protect the patient from the putative short-term and long-term risks related to ES. The authors recommend performing a prelaparoscopic cholecystectomy ERCP 24 to 48 hours prior to the planned surgery whenever possible in order to avoid the infrequent occurrence of stone migration into a previously clear common bile duct during the ERCP–LC interval.

Duct stones identified intraoperatively may also be treated at postoperative ERCP. This approach relies heavily on the available endoscopic expertise, since failed endoscopic stone extraction will require either referral to a more experienced endoscopist or an open operative procedure. The choice of management strategy in the patient of intermediate risk is influenced by the ability of available endoscopic or surgical team members.

Until laparoscopic modalities are developed that permit easy and reliable duct exploration by most surgeons, the options for CBD stone extraction remain pre-LC or post-LC endoscopic sphincterotomy and duct clearance or conversion to open cholecystectomy with CBDE.

Cholangitis

The most common cause of suppurative cholangitis is calculous ductal obstruction with consequent cholangiovenous reflux due to elevated intrabiliary pressure. Most patients present with mild disease and respond rapidly to treatment with intravenous fluids and antibiotics. Subsequent management options are dictated by their surgical risk. The poor-risk patient should undergo ERCP with ES and stone extraction and retain the gallbladder, whereas the low-risk patient should undergo either ES with

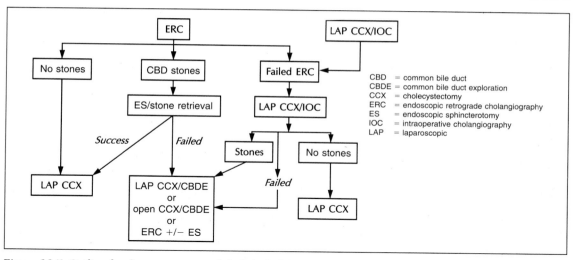

Figure 18-7. Outline for the management of choledocholithiasis in the era of laparoscopic cholecystectomy.

subsequent laparoscopic cholecystectomy or open cholecystectomy with CBDE.

Emergency ERCP is the treatment of choice for those patients with severe acute cholangitis at presentation or those failing to respond to conventional therapy within 24 hours. Since conventional surgical management is associated with morbidity and mortality rates between 10% and 50% in these patients, it should be reserved for those patients failing endoscopic therapy. Endoscopic biliary decompression is successful in 85% to 95% of cases and is associated with lower morbidity and mortality than percutaneous or surgical drainage. Most biliary endoscopists agree that some of the most gratifying procedures they perform are in this setting, since rapid clinical improvement is the rule after successful decompression.

In the critically ill patient, only brief or no attempts at stone retrieval should be attempted, and the establishment of adequate drainage via the use of a nasobiliary tube (NBT) (Fig. 18-8) or endoprosthesis (Fig. 18-9) is of paramount importance. This technique will also serve to temporize matters in those patients with failed or incomplete duct clearance and allow for safe removal on a semielective basis. NBTs may be placed without sphincterotomy and thus may prevent potential bleeding because of coagulopathy associated with sepsis. If the patient also suffers from mental confusion, one may

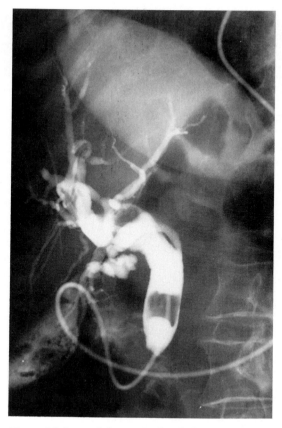

Figure 18-8. Nasobiliary tube for cholangitis caused by square bile duct stone.

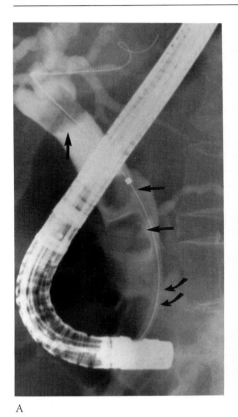
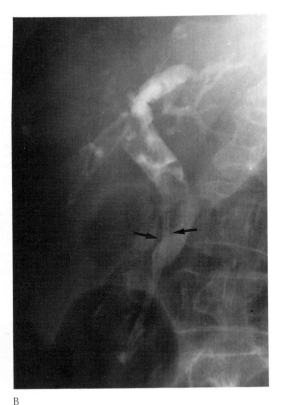

A   B

Figure 18-9. A. Endoprosthesis (curved arrows) placed over guidewire for acute cholangitis caused by multiple large stones (arrows). B. Endoprosthesis in place showing immediate drainage.

elect to place both an NBT and an endoprosthesis. This procedure would afford continued decompression if the NBT is accidentally dislodged.

Retrospective comparisons from Lease et al. and Leung et al. of surgical and endoscopic management of severe acute cholangitis have revealed 30-day mortalities of 21.4% and 4.7%, respectively. A prospective study of endoscopic biliary drainage and surgical decompression in 82 patients with severe acute cholangitis from Lai et al. reported mortality rates (10% vs. 32%), complications (34% vs. 66%), need for mechanical ventilation (29% vs. 63%), and presence of retained ductal stones (7% vs. 29%) all lower in the endoscopic group. Thus the data support the conclusion that endoscopic decompression is safer and more effective than surgery for acute severe cholangitis related to common bile duct stones.

Biliary Pancreatitis

Acute pancreatitis due to gallstone disease is thought to occur during stone migration from the gallbladder to or across the papilla, with pancreatic duct obstruction, bile reflux into the pancreatic duct, and duodenopancreatic reflux as possible sequelae. Recovery of stones in the feces in a majority of these patients, coupled with the relatively high incidence of bile duct stones in those undergoing urgent therapeutic intervention for severe pancreatitis, lends credence to these concepts. It is particularly useful to rank patients by the severity of their illness using a prognostic scoring system (e.g., Ranson, Imrie, Glasgow, or APACHE) and thereby predict those at greatest risk for local or systemic complications. Most patients follow a mild course and spontaneous resolution with supportive care. The available data indicate that these patients are least likely to benefit from acute intervention. In stark contrast, those patients with a predicted severe course are most likely to benefit from urgent stone extraction, which will possibly halt further progression or reverse the consequences of the acute attack. Urgent surgical intervention in the subgroup with severe biliary pancreatitis carries high operative mortality (48% for emergency surgery vs. 11% in delayed surgery) as compared with those with a mild attack (3.3% for emergency surgery vs. 0). The trend has been to avoid early biliary surgical intervention unless local complications dictate otherwise.

An early endoscopic approach, however, offers the advantage of immediate ductal clearance without the risks associated with early surgical intervention. Once uncontrolled data became available documenting the apparent safety of ERCP in acute pancreatitis, the initial reluctance toward performing ERCP in severe biliary pancreatitis was overcome. The Neoptolemos et al. group carried out the first randomized, controlled trial of urgent ERCP within 72 hours of admission in patients with acute biliary pancreatitis. Common bile duct stones were found in 63% of those with predicted severe attacks and in 26% of those with predicted mild attacks. Those with predicted mild attacks had favorable outcomes irrespective of treatment strategies. Urgent ES in those patients with severe attacks, as predicted by the Glasgow criteria, significantly reduced morbidity (61% to 24%) and length of stay (17 to 9.5 days) versus conservatively managed patients. Mortality was lower in the ERCP group, but did not attain statistical significance (4% vs. 18%).

In the more recent Hong Kong study, emergency ERCP with ES and stone extraction within 24 hours of admission reduced biliary sepsis from 12% to 0% as compared to the conservatively treated group. Although no significant reduction in the overall rate of local or systemic complications was observed, in the subgroup of patients with a predicted severe course, emergent ES decreased the combined incidence of local and systemic complications from 21% to 5.3%. Mortality rates were decreased from 68.8% to 25% as compared to the conservatively managed group.

These data provide the rationale for early endoscopic intervention in patients with predicted se-

vere acute biliary pancreatitis. Subsequent elective cholecystectomy should be performed in the low-risk surgical patient, whereas leaving the gallbladder in situ should be considered in the high-risk surgical patient. In the subgroup with mild pancreatitis, immediate intervention is not indicated. Should cholelithiasis or microlithiasis be documented, elective laparoscopic cholecystectomy with intraoperative cholangiography should be performed during the initial hospitalization. Preoperative ERCP has a low yield in such patients. In those patients with previous cholecystectomy, ES is definitive therapy. The role of sphincterotomy as the only therapy for the high-risk surgical patient with intact gallbladder and no documented choledocholithiasis remains to be evaluated.

Pregnancy

Symptomatic choledocholithiasis during pregnancy poses a particularly challenging diagnostic and therapeutic scenario. ERCP and sphincterotomy may be safely performed provided that specific precautions are strictly followed to minimize fetal radiation exposure. Consultation with radiologic colleagues, including a radiation physicist, is imperative. During ERCP, the fetus is shielded with a lead apron, dosimetry is performed to estimate fetal exposure, fluoroscopic imaging is minimized, and no radiographs are taken. These patients should undergo elective cholecystectomy in the postpartum period in order to prevent recurrence.

Difficult Bile Duct Stones

The most challenging circumstances encountered in endoscopic, surgical, and radiologic stone extraction are related to technical considerations and aberrations of anatomy and pathology. Difficult endoscopic access may be the result of altered duodenal anatomy, periampullary diverticula, or prior surgery (e.g., Billroth II anastomosis or Roux-en-Y reconstruction) (Fig. 18-10). Employment of modified accessories and techniques such as needle-knife papillotomy and reverse sphincterotomy have enhanced the success rates.

Following successful ES, factors such as narrow distal CBD, square stones, stones larger than 1.5 cm, stones located above strictures, or multi-

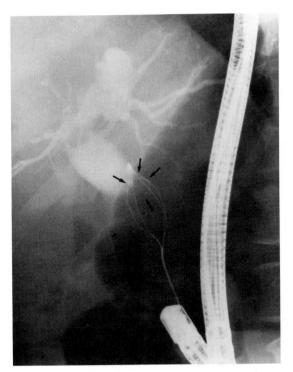

Figure 18-10. ERC in patient with Billroth II anastomosis. Endoscope is within afferent loop, showing basket extraction of stones (arrows) after sphincterotomy.

ple stones may still pose considerable difficulty in successful extraction. Application of adjuvant techniques such as mechanical lithotripsy, extracorporeal shock wave lithotripsy (ESWL), and intracorporeal lithotripsy may facilitate successful stone extraction. Selection of the most appropriate options will depend entirely on the experience and availability of experienced endoscopists, surgeons, and interventional radiologists.

Mechanical lithotripsy is usually the most appropriate option (Fig. 18-11). Mechanical lithotripters are modifications of the standard basket device that have increased tensile strength and a covering metal sheath. Once in place, a cranking system is employed that traps the stone against the distal tip of the metal sheath and fractures it. The fragments can then be removed using either balloon catheters or baskets. Successful stone extraction using mechanical lithotripsy ranges from 80% to 94% in the difficult bile duct stones refractory to stan-

dard techniques, and increases overall bile duct clearance in expert centers to about 98%.

The choice of ESWL or intracorporeal techniques (laser or electrohydraulic) or surgery is dependent upon local expertise, since high success rates are reported in expert hands. Adequate stone targeting is the major obstacle to the successful application of these methods. Shock wave focusing may be accomplished using a "mother-daughter" endoscope system for peroral cholangioscopy or using intraductal or extraductal sonographic or fluoroscopic targeting. Multiple treatment sessions may be required to achieve duct clearance. Percutaneous cholangioscopy may also play a limited role for difficult stones where transpapillary access has failed or is impossible.

Laser systems have been more recently employed to facilitate stone fragmentation. Initial use of Nd:YAG systems were ineffective and posed considerable risk of thermal bile duct injury. Newer systems use flash-lamp pulsed dye technology. Early studies used "mother-daughter" endoscope systems to facilitate contact with the stone under direct visualization. Most recently, fluoroscopic guidance has achieved laser-stone contact, and the "smart" laser can distinguish stone from tissue. The overall success rate for ductal clearance of the difficult common bile duct stone by laser lithotripsy ranges from 80% to 90%.

Electrohydraulic lithotripsy experience is limited in the United States, but published data, mostly from Europe, show overall success rates of up to 86%. Multiple sessions are often required, but the cost is much less than for laser lithotripsy.

ESWL does not require direct contact with the common bile duct stone. Instead, a previously placed nasobiliary catheter is used to perfuse the CBD with contrast, and fluoroscopic focusing is then possible. The overall success rate for fragmentation is 53% to 91%, and duct clearance is 58% to 86%. Multiple sessions are often required, and follow-up ERCP is required for fragment extraction. Minor complications are frequently encountered, including hematuria, pain, hemobilia, cutaneous petechiae, and transient liver test abnormalities.

Chemical dissolution for bile duct stones has little application. Catheter delivery systems, which have included a nasobiliary tube (NBT), percuta-

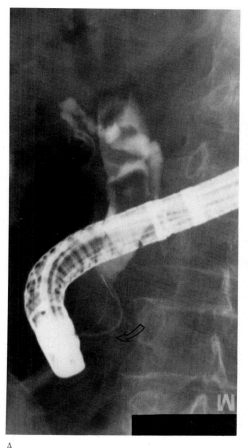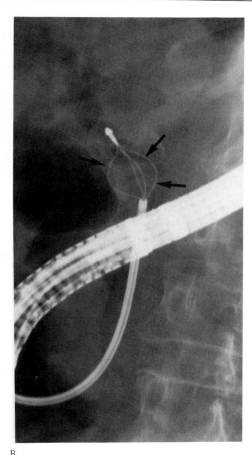

A   B

Figure 18-11. A. Endoscopic sphincterotomy (open arrow) in same patient as Fig. 18-9. B. Followed by mechanical lithotripsy with stone in basket (arrows).

neous transhepatic catheter, or an existing T tube, have been used to perfuse the bile duct agents such as mono-octanoin and MTBE (methyl-tert-butyl-ethyl ether). With the former, complete clearance has been achieved in 25.6% with additional partial success rates of 28%. Five percent of patients experienced serious side effects (hemorrhage, pancreatitis, pulmonary edema, sepsis, and anaphylaxis). Results with MTBE have also been disappointing, with complete dissolution seen in 30% to 45% of patients. Since large common bile duct stones contain smaller concentrations of cholesterol and greater concentrations of bile pigments, high ductal clearance rates are unlikely with only organic solvents. The addition of metal chelators may enhance thera-

peutic efficacy. The combination of poor efficacy and high morbidity has limited the role of dissolution therapy to patients with refractory stone disease who have failed other techniques and are poor surgical risks.

When stone extraction is incomplete or not possible because of anatomical factors, bleeding diathesis, or incomplete sphincterotomy, a nasobiliary catheter should be placed to afford decompression of the biliary tree and prevent stone impaction in the distal CBD (see Fig. 18-8). This maneuver is temporizing and in the case of cholangitis may allow for clinical improvement, which then may allow for additional endoscopic therapy or surgery in a more elective setting. A follow-up cholangiogram can be obtained via the NBT without additional ERCP. These catheters are well tolerated, but their major limitation is that patients accidentally or intentionally remove them.

Alternatively, a biliary endoprosthesis may be placed in addition to an NBT. When aggressive endoscopic measures have failed to achieve duct clearance and surgery is considered of high risk, long-term biliary endoprosthesis therapy may be an acceptable alternative. Stent patency is not of paramount importance in this situation, because sphincterotomy allows for bile drainage, and the stent prevents distal stone impaction. In many series of elderly, poor-risk surgical patients, long-term stent therapy with 5 years of follow-up has proven efficacious, with only 6% of patients requiring surgery for biliary complications, and an additional 2% requiring elective surgery for stent occlusion or migration. Some experts recommend ursodeoxycholic acid to enhance stone dissolution and choleresis in this setting, but prospective trials are needed to document the true efficacy of this approach.

Conclusions

In the last 20 years diagnostic and therapeutic strategies for choledocholithiasis have changed dramatically from a purely surgical approach to one in which endoscopists, interventional radiologists, and surgeons play an integrated and active role in management. New treatment modalities are being developed, but the optimum selection of established therapies must be clarified, since this will have the greatest impact on patient management. Many questions remain unanswered: What is the natural history of small, asymptomatic bile duct stones? What are the long-term complications of ES and balloon dilatation of the papilla in the young? What is the exact role of ERCP in an era of minimally invasive surgery? Will laparoscopic techniques become disseminated sufficiently to become the primary mode of management of nonemergent bile duct stone disease?

Selected Readings

Baillie J, Cairns S, Cotton P. Endoscopic management of choledocholithiasis during pregnancy. *Surgery* 1990; 171:1–4.

Cotton PB. Removing duct stones without sphincterotomy. *Gastrointest Endosc* 1993; 39:312.

Davidson BR, Neoptolemos JP, Carr-Locke DL. Endoscopic sphincterotomy for common bile duct calculi in patients with gallbladder in situ considered unfit for surgery. *Gut* 1988 29:114–120.

Fan ST, et al. Early treatment of acute biliary pancreatitis by endoscopic papillotomy. *N Engl J Med* 1993; 328:228–232.

Hunter JG. Laparoscopic transcystic common bile duct exploration. *Am J Surg* 1992; 163:53–56.

Lai ECS, et al. Endoscopic biliary drainage for severe acute cholangitis. *N Engl J Med* 1992; 326:1582–1586.

Leese T, et al. Management of acute cholangitis and the impact of endoscopic sphincterotomy. *Br J Surg* 1986; 73:988–992.

Neoptolemos JP, et al. Controlled trial of urgent endoscopic retrograde cholangiopancreatography and endoscopic sphincterotomy versus conservative treatment for acute pancreatitis due to gallstones. *Lancet* 1988; 2:979–983.

NIH Consensus Conference on Gallstones and Laparoscopic Cholecystectomy. *Am J Surg* 1993; 390–547.

Siegel JH, Ben-Zvi JS, Pullano WE. Mechanical lithotripsy of common duct stones. *Gastrointest Endosc* 1990; 36:351–356.

19

Hepatolithiasis

GERHARD R. WITTICH
ERIC VANSONNENBERG
WILLIAM H. NEALON
DAVID T. WALDEN

Although common in the Far East, intrahepatic stone disease is relatively rare in the Western world. Hepatolithiasis may result in cholangitis and severe septic complications. Therefore, intervention is frequently required. In many hepatobiliary centers traditional surgical treatment has been replaced by a multidisciplinary approach that combines the expertise of surgeons, radiologists, and gastroenterologists. This chapter outlines this modern team approach to diagnosing and treating patients with hepatolithiasis.

Etiology and Pathogenesis

Bacterial infection is one of the main pathogenetic factors contributing to hepatolithiasis. This fact is evident by the presence of bacterial casts which may be found within brown pigment stones. The other important factor is bile stasis, which may result from the formation of biliary strictures. Benign strictures can be caused by prior surgery such as cholecystectomy, hepaticojejunostomy, partial hepatectomy, or liver transplantation. Furthermore, strictures can be associated with sclerosing cholangitis, ischemic damage to bile ducts secondary to radiation therapy, chemoembolization of hepatic tumors, or chronic pancreatitis. Malignant strictures such as those caused by a slow-growing cholangiocarcinoma are less common causes of biliary calculi. Bile stasis is also a sequela of congenital ectasia of the biliary system as seen in patients with choledochoceles or Caroli's disease. Oriental cholangiohepatitis is a common cause of hepatolithiasis in the Far East and may be encountered in Asian immigrants.

Diagnosis

The spectrum of symptoms in patients with hepatolithiasis ranges from pain in the right upper quadrant to jaundice with pruritus, cholangitis, and sepsis. After an initial clinical evaluation, noninvasive imaging with ultrasonography is helpful in jaundiced patients to confirm biliary obstruction, to determine the level of obstruction, and to rule out an underlying tumor. Computerized tomography is indicated if ultrasound is inconclusive and if staging is needed for a suspected tumor. Patients with clinical symptoms of bile duct stones without jaundice are best assessed by direct cholangiography. Percutaneous transhepatic cholangiography (PTC) is the preferred method in patients with prior hepatobiliary surgery.

Endoscopic retrograde cholangiopancreatography (ERCP) is often performed first in patients with an intact common bile duct and nondilated intrahepatic ducts. Diagnostic ERCP may be followed by attempts to remove intrahepatic stones. However, percutaneous transhepatic intervention is frequently required in these patients. Diagnostic tests which may be indicated after establishing percutaneous access to the biliary system include transluminal biopsy to rule out a malignant stricture, perfusion manometry to confirm the presence of a significant benign stricture and to determine the result of balloon dilatation, and percutaneous cholangioscopy, which is of value in monitoring stone fragmentation. Intraluminal ultrasonography also may be useful in detecting residual stone fragments and in guiding transluminal biopsy of abnormal bile ducts.

Management

Surgical techniques used for treatment of patients with hepatolithiasis include hepaticojejunostomy or hepaticocutaneous jejunostomy, which results in a stoma that allows repeat retrograde access for percutaneous interventions in the biliary system. Other procedures include partial hepatectomy or selective central hepatic resection. Although surgical management is effective and safe in most patients, surgery alone is somewhat flawed by a relatively high incidence of residual or recurrent stones. This fact underscores the need for less aggressive complementary or alternative interventional procedures.

Endoscopic retrograde cholangiography followed by sphincterotomy and stone extraction is standard treatment for many patients with common bile duct stones. This method is less successful for removing intrahepatic calculi. Therefore, the majority of these patients are candidates for transhepatic biliary intervention, which will be described in detail. After a history and physical examination are obtained, liver and kidney function as well as clotting factors are checked and corrected if abnormal. Broad-spectrum antibiotics are administered therapeutically in patients with symptoms of cholangitis and are given prophylactically before the procedure if signs of infection are absent. Prior imaging studies obtained by ultrasonography, computerized tomography, or ERCP are reviewed, if available. Most percutaneous biliary procedures are performed using a combination of local anesthesia, systemic pain control, and conscious sedation combined with periprocedural monitoring of the patient's blood pressure, heart rate, and oxygen saturation. Anesthesia support is very valuable in patients with high anxiety, in unstable patients, or in cases where extensive procedures such as one-step tract dilatation, stone removal, or balloon dilatation of strictures are planned.

The authors commonly start a de novo percutaneous biliary intervention using portable ultrasonography to optimize planning of access. Real-time ultrasound guidance may allow rapid access to dilated bile ducts, often with a single fine needle stick. Fluoroscopic guidance is essential for safe manipulation of needles, guidewires, introducer sheaths, drainage tubes, and other devices such as balloon catheters. The availability of modern C-arm fluoroscopy equipment with the capability of magnification and digital image processing is valuable and allows interventional radiologists who are well versed in segmental biliary anatomy to gain access to selected bile ducts with a technical success rate of well over 90%.

For right-sided PTC the authors select a puncture site in the midclavicular line inferior to the tenth rib to minimize the risk of transgression of the pleura. After performing PTC, one then determines whether the punctured and opacified duct is suitable for biliary drainage and subsequent stone removal. Preferred strategies include either direct puncture of the affected bile duct peripheral to the obstructing stones or access to the contralateral biliary system (Fig. 19-1). In patients with prior hepaticojejunostomy a third option for percutaneous removal of intrahepatic stones is access via percutaneous jejunostomy (Fig. 19-2). Refinements of instrumentation available for percutaneous biliary drainage (PBD) include so-called one stick access sets, which consist of a combination of fine needles, small-diameter guidewires, and coaxial dilator introducer systems. These sets allow for relatively atraumatic insertion of biliary drainage tubes and other instruments.

Most commonly transhepatic biliary stone removal is planned as a two- or multistage procedure. The initial session aims at gaining safe access with a small (8 or 9 French) drainage catheter to minimize the risk of bacteremia. Tract dilatation and stone removal are performed in the absence of clinical symptoms of cholangitis. Findings at the initial cholangiogram determine technical details of further manipulations. For instance, stones up to 6 mm in diameter can be extracted through 18 French sheaths, which can be placed after serial coaxial dilatations during the second session. This step usually takes place within a few days after initial biliary drainage.

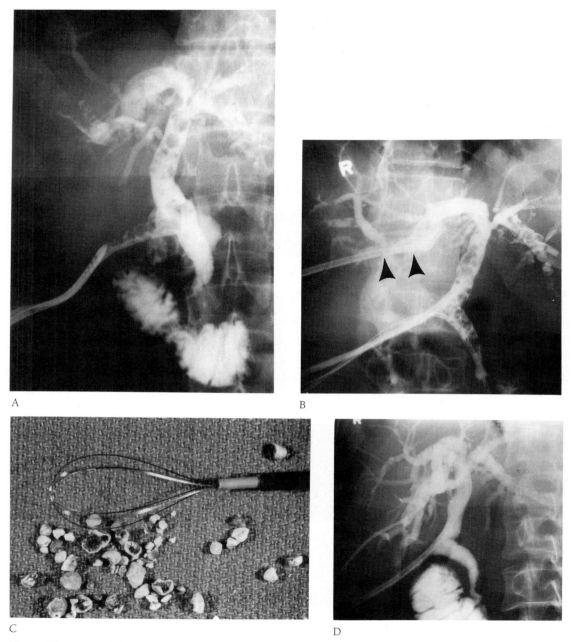

A

B

C

D

Figure 19-1. Hepatolithiasis secondary to benign common bile duct stricture. Sixty-eight-year-old patient with history of chronic pancreatitis, status postcholecystectomy and common bile duct exploration. Multiple stones were removed surgically and a T tube was placed for subsequent percutaneous removal of stones. Four weeks later the patient presented with acute cholangitis and a dislodged T tube. A. A cholangiogram was obtained by cannulating the T tube tract. Multiple calculi are seen within the tract, the common bile duct, and intrahepatic ducts. Several segmental ducts are not opacified because of impaction with stones. B. Biliary drainage was optimized by transhepatic insertion of a catheter into the right posterior segmental duct (arrowheads) and by catheters inserted through the T tube tract. C. After sepsis was controlled by external drainage, stone removal was performed with a nitinol retrieval basket. D. Complete stone clearance of the biliary system was achieved. The distal common bile duct stricture was treated with balloon dilatation.

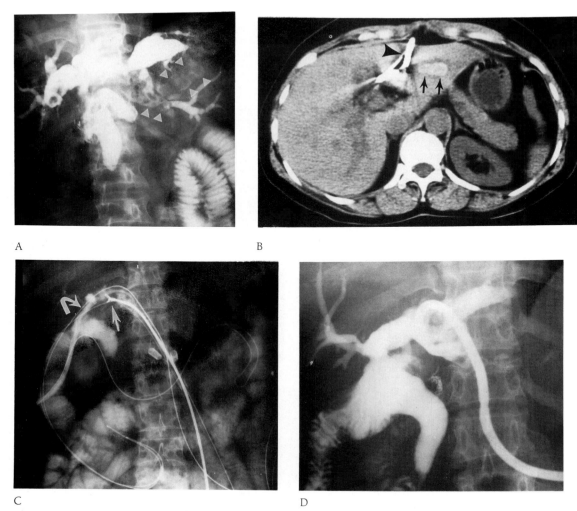

A   B

C   D

Figure 19-2. Hepatolithiasis secondary to cholangiohepatitis. Forty-three-year-old patient with a history of choledochojejunostomy. A. PTC demonstrates strictures, dilated bile ducts and extensive hepatolithiasis (arrowheads). Cholangitis was effectively treated by left-sided percutaneous biliary drainage. B. CT scan after left biliary drainage (arrowhead) demonstrates large calcified calculi in bile duct III (arrows). C. Percutaneous jejunostomy was performed to gain retrograde access to multiple intrahepatic ducts. A grasping forceps (arrow) has been inserted through a sheath in the left lobe for fragmentation of soft bilirubinate stones. A 16 French choledochoscope (curved arrow) has been inserted via the jejunostomy access to monitor stone fragmentation and removal. D. Tube cholangiogram after stone removal and stricture dilatation demonstrates complete stone clearance and rapid drainage of contrast material into the jejunum. (The patient returned 3 years later with recurrent hepatolithiasis and was again managed successfully using percutaneous techniques.)

The authors have used a variety of baskets for stone extraction and have found a nitinol retrieval basket to be particularly useful. Percutaneous removal of larger stones can be performed by prior fragmentation with "heavy-duty" baskets for mechanical lithotripsy or by contact lithotripsy using electrohydraulic or laser-induced shock waves. Alternative methods include extracorporeal shock wave lithotripsy (ESWL) or contact dissolution. ESWL and the use of potent cholesterol solvents such as methyl-tert-butyl-ethyl ether (MTBE) or other investigational substances have to date not been approved by the Food and Drug Administration.

Frequently, the authors combine stone removal with percutaneous cholangioscopy using flexible 9 to 16 French endoscopes. Direct endoscopic visualization is important for monitoring contact lithotripsy when using laser or electrohydraulic lithotripsy probes. Conversely, basket fragmentation can easily be performed under fluoroscopic guidance. After successful stone fragmentation and retrieval of fragments, cholangioscopy is often used to rule out residual stones. Tube cholangiography may be combined with manometry to evaluate associated biliary strictures. These strictures are treated with a trial of percutaneous balloon dilatation and temporary stenting using internal and/or external biliary drainage catheters. Catheters are removed if the patient is free of stones and without residual biliary obstruction.

Results

Patients with hepatolithiasis often present with partial biliary obstruction and thus with only mildly dilated bile ducts. In these cases, gaining percutaneous access to the biliary system may be challenging. The authors have reviewed their experience with percutaneous biliary drainage in patients with non- or minimally dilated ducts. In 48 of 50 patients (96%) they were able to successfully insert biliary drainage catheters. Indications for PBD in these patients included malignant obstruction, stone disease, and various other benign disorders.

In a series of 41 patients referred for treatment of intrahepatic or combined intra- and extrahepatic bile duct calculi, the authors were able to gain access to the biliary system in 40 patients (97%). Sixty-eight percent of these patients had prior biliary surgery. Eighty-eight percent presented with cholangitis (including 8 patients with oriental cholangiohepatitis). Transhepatic stone removal was attempted and was successful in all 40 patients, in whom access was gained. In 22 of these 40 patients (55%), stone size exceeded 6 mm, and fragmentation was therefore required. Methods of stone fragmentation are listed in Table 19-1. The only

Table 19-1. Methods Used for Fragmentation of Bile Duct Calculi

Mechanical lithotripsy	18
Laser lithotripsy	3
Rotational lithotripsy	1
(Fragmentation not required	18)
NUMBER OF PATIENTS	40

significant complication occurred in a patient who presented with acute cholangitis due to a stricture and stones impacted in a left segmental duct. This duct was punctured successfully, but attempts to advance a guidewire past the stones failed. The patient developed bacteremia requiring intensive care. He improved clinically and was subsequently treated with left hemihepatectomy. Signs of mild bacteremia were noticed in 3 other patients, who responded well to antibiotic therapy. In addition to the patient described above, surgical intervention was required in 2 other patients. A liver transplant recipient with ischemic damage to the biliary system required retransplantation because of rejection. One patient with extensive hepatolithiasis secondary to chronic pancreatitis and stricture of the common bile duct did not respond to balloon dilatation and was treated with elective hepaticojejunostomy.

A few other series of transhepatic removal of bile duct stones have been reported by American, European, and Asian authors. Pitt et al. presented their experience with 54 patients treated over an 18-year period. Fourteen of these patients (26%) were managed exclusively with percutaneous techniques. More than half of the remaining patients who were treated surgically had preoperative percutaneous transhepatic drainage. The most common surgical technique used was a Roux-en-Y hepaticojejunostomy. Efforts were made to remove stones during surgery with the aid of choledochoscopy. Partial hepatic resection was required in only 1 patient with cirrhosis and chronic sepsis. Forty-five percent of patients treated surgically required additional percutaneous procedures for removal of residual intrahepatic stones or for dilatation of intrahepatic strictures. The stone clearance rate in this series was 94% with a 30-day mortality of zero. Complications were rare and included bacteremia due to cholangitis, wound infections, bile fistulae, pancreatitis, and liver abscesses.

Bonnel et al. described their experience with transhepatic electrohydraulic lithotripsy in 50 patients. Of 27 patients with common bile duct stones, 20 had undergone previous endoscopic sphincterotomy, but attempts at endoscopic stone removal had failed. Of the remaining 23 patients with intrahepatic stones, 9 had associated biliary strictures. Percutaneous stone removal was successful in 92% of patients. However, these authors encountered severe complications, including massive hemobilia, bile duct perforation, and hemothorax, in 22% of their patients. This initially high complication rate was subsequently reduced by replacing their one-step technique with a staged approach. During the initial procedure, a drainage tube up to 14 French in size was inserted. Several days later the tract was dilated to a 20 French size, followed by contact lithotripsy and stone removal.

Han et al. reported an overall success rate of 73% in 96 patients referred for percutaneous removal of retained intrahepatic stones. This number includes patients with complete (50%) and partial (23%) stone removal. Techniques used for stone removal and disintegration included angled catheters, irrigation and suction, mechanical fragmentation of stones, and ESWL. These authors encountered no significant complications.

Several other investigators have focused on ESWL for fragmentation of bile duct calculi. Choi et al. performed ESWL using a piezoelectric lithotripter combined with stone extraction through a T tube tract in 11 patients. Complete stone clearance was achieved in 54% and partial clearance in 27% of their patients. Reasons for failure were severe bile duct strictures in some patients and difficulties in targeting stones for lithotripsy in others. These authors observed no major complications. Others have published their results with contact lithotripsy using laser energy transmitted via optical fibers. Regardless of the access—via ERCP, via a T tube tract, or via a percutaneous transhepatic tract—laser lithotripsy can be used effectively and safely when applied under direct endoscopic vision. Complete clearance of stones was achieved in 75% to 88% of patients. Clinically relevant complications in these series were rare.

Conclusions

Close cooperation among surgeons, radiologists, and endoscopists is an efficient way to establish the diagnosis of hepatolithiasis and to initiate safe and successful therapy. This chapter has discussed the authors' experience and that of other authors who emphasize the value of minimally invasive percutaneous and conventional surgical techniques. The percentage of surgical interventions in the series reported by Pitt et al. was higher than in the authors' series. This difference may in part be explained by the fact that their series extends back to 1976 and therefore includes a period during which percutaneous radiological techniques were either not yet available or not yet sufficiently refined. Today, percutaneous transhepatic access can be gained in most patients. Subsequent tract dilatation performed in two or more stages allows for retrieval of smaller stones with baskets or insertion of devices which allow fragmentation of larger stones.

In the authors' experience mechanical lithotripsy with baskets is highly successful. The availability of additional techniques such as laser lithotripsy or electrohydraulic lithotripsy—both performed under percutaneous cholangioscopic control—ensures a very high success rate in fragmentation and subsequent removal of stones. Biliary strictures, if present, can be dilated percutaneously with a success rate of approximately 70%. Thus the authors feel that surgical interventions can be reserved for patients in whom less invasive percutaneous techniques fail. The majority of these patients can be treated with hepaticojejunostomy or hepaticocutaneous jejunostomy followed by percutaneous interventions if necessary. Partial hepatectomy may be indicated in a minority of patients with extensive focal cirrhosis and recurrent sepsis.

Selected Readings

Bonnel DH, et al. Common bile duct and intrahepatic stones: Results of transhepatic electrohydraulic lithotripsy in 50 patients. *Radiology* 1991; 180:345–348.

Choi BI, et al. Retained intrahepatic stones: Treatment with piezoelectric lithotripsy combined with stone extraction. *Radiology* 1991; 178:105–108.

Dawson SL, et al. Treatment of bile duct stones by laser

lithotripsy: Results in 12 patients. *AJR* 1992; 158: 1007–1009.

Fan ST, et al. Appraisal of hepaticocutaneous jejunostomy in the management of hepatolithiasis. *Am J Surg* 1993; 165:332–335.

Han JK, et al. Percutaneous removal of retained intrahepatic stones with a pre-shaped angulated catheter: Review of 96 patients. *Br J Radiol* 1992; 65:9–13.

Nakayama F, et al. Hepatolithiasis in East Asia: Comparison between Japan and China. *J Gastroenterol Hepatol* 1991; 6:155–158.

Pitt HA, et al. Intrahepatic stones: The transhepatic team approach. *Ann Surg* 1994; 219:527–535.

Ponchon T, et al. Pulsed dye laser lithotripsy of bile duct stones. *Gastroenterology* 1991; 100:1730–1736.

Rubin GD, et al. Percutaneous removal of small gallstones—in vitro comparison of baskets. *J Intervent Radiol* 1992; 7:29–31.

Su HC, et al. Treatment of bilateral intrahepatic stones with high duct strictures through selective central hepatic resection. *Surgery* 1991; 110:8–12.

20

Acute Cholecystitis

Joseph T. Ferrucci
Ewa Kuligowska
Desmond H. Birkett

Cholecystectomy, either open or laparascopic, remains the treatment of choice for uncomplicated acute cholecystitis. In the well patient, cholecystectomy remains a safe and totally curative procedure with an operative mortality of 0.5% to 1.0%. Acute cholecystitis in the medically compromised patient, however, carries a formidable 13% operative mortality when treated by open cholecystectomy. Whether cholecystitis results from gallstone disease or bile stasis (acalculous cholecystitis), such high-risk patients often succumb to cardiovascular disease or respiratory failure.

Less invasive therapeutic alternatives, therefore, are critically important. The operative placement of a cholecystostomy tube in the gallbladder has been the traditional alternative to cholecystectomy. After 1 to 2 weeks of tube drainage, elective interval cholecystectomy or transtube stone removal (endoscopic and/or radiologic) may be performed. However, the initial surgical placement of the catheter usually requires general anesthesia with its attendant risks.

Over the last several years percutaneous cholecystostomy (PC), a radiologic ultrasound-guided gallbladder drainage procedure, has been widely accepted as a safe method for accessing the gallbladder without general anesthesia. The feasibility, technique, and clinical efficacy of PC for acute cholecystitis were established by several radiology groups in the early 1980s. Subsequently, gastroenterologists and radiologists at the Mayo Clinic performed PC electively in order to administer methyl-tert-butyl ether (MTBE) for solvent dissolution of cholesterol

gallstones. Despite its effectiveness, percutaneous MTBE dissolution has since been largely eclipsed by the advent of laparascopic cholecystectomy. The demonstrated safety and wide availability of ultrasound-guided PC for gallbladder access make this the preferred approach for achieving therapeutic gallbladder drainage in medically compromised patients with acute cholecystitis at the present time. For high-risk patients who subsequently prove to have underlying gallstones, interval cholecystectomy or percutaneous stone extraction remain options. For those critically ill patients with primary acalculous cholecystitis, PC followed by catheter drainage is often curative. This chapter focuses on the percutaneous management of the acute gallbladder in critically ill patients and provides a special focus on the problem of acute acalculous cholecystitis.

Etiology and Pathogenesis

Acute cholecystitis usually results from gallstone obstruction of the cystic duct. Bile stasis, gallbladder distention, and secondary bacterial overgrowth in the gallbladder bile eventually lead to acute inflammation of the gallbladder wall. Hyperemia, edema, and tissue friability ensue. Perforation and pericholecystic abscess are occasional late sequelae.

In patients without gallstones, primary acalculous cholecystitis may occur by a somewhat similar mechanism. The underlying process begins again with bile stasis. The clinical preconditions include serious illness or trauma requiring prolonged bedrest. Gallbladder hypomotility results from a lack of oral intake (parenteral nutrition), narcotic analgesic drugs, and other factors. Gallbladder sludge is commonly present, but it is not a requisite for the development of acalculous cholecystitis. Presumably, the thick bile, accumulating sludge crystals, and poor emptying lead to progressive distention of the gallbladder lumen, followed by hypoperfusion of the mucosa and subsequently of the full thickness of the gallbladder wall.

Diagnosis

Classic acute cholecystitis is manifested clinically by the onset of epigastric pain which moves to the right upper quadrant of the abdomen. The pain is made worse by movement. The patient feels systemically unwell and on examination has a fever with localized tenderness and guarding of the right upper quadrant of the abdomen. The patient may or may not have a history of previous gallbladder disease or gallbladder calculi. Plain abdominal radiographs may show calcified stones or air in the gallbladder wall (emphysematous cholecystitis). Ultrasonography demonstrates gallstones with or without thickening of the wall and with or without pericholecystic fluid (Fig. 20-1). Radionuclide scintigraphy discloses no filling of the gallbladder lumen 1 to 2 hours after injection. Each of these studies is sufficient to confirm the diagnosis of acute cholecystitis in most cases. Whether the patient was previously

well or was medically compromised, the imaging features of acute calculous cholecystitis are essentially identical.

Ultrasonography (US) has emerged as the single most useful technique for assessing patients with suspected acute cholecystitis. Gallbladder distention, the presence of gallstones or sludge, the thickness of the gallbladder wall, and the presence of pericholecystic fluid are easily assessed by US even at the patient's bedside (Fig. 20-2). There are many causes for thickening of the gallbladder wall (Fig. 20-3) which need to be excluded. They include hepatitis, hypoalbuminemia with gallbladder wall edema, and ascites. Pericholecystic fluid is a useful sign of acute cholecystitis provided that ascites elsewhere in the abdomen has been excluded by ultrasound. The sonographic Murphy's sign has been recognized as being more specific and more useful than the clinical Murphy's sign when the transducer is placed directly over the sonographically localized gallbladder fundus and pressure is applied which elicits a recoil response of acute pain. Color flow Doppler sonography has recently been used to demonstrate the hyperemic pericholecystic flow of blood associated with acute inflammation in the gallbladder fossa.

The diagnosis of acute acalculous cholecystitis is often very difficult. The typical patient resides in an intensive care unit, presents with spiking fevers despite antibiotic therapy, and often complains of vague right upper quadrant distress. Ultrasound

Figure 20-1. Ultrasonograms of a patient with acalculous acute cholecystitis showing a distended gallbladder with a layer of sludge in the dependent portion with multiple stones. The gallbladder wall is thickened, measuring approximately 1 cm.

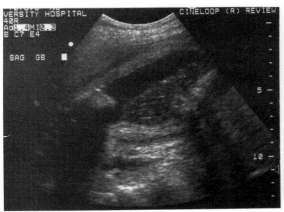
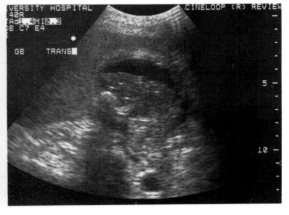

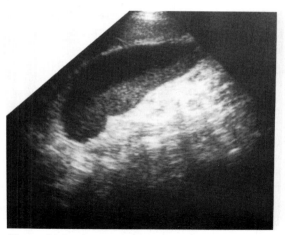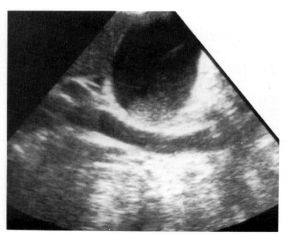

Figure 20-2. Ultrasonograms of the gallbladder, longitudinal views, showing the gallbladder to be distended with a layer of sludge along the dependent portion. No discrete stones, wall thickening, or pericholecystic fluid is visible. The findings are compatible but not diagnostic of acalculous cholecystitis.

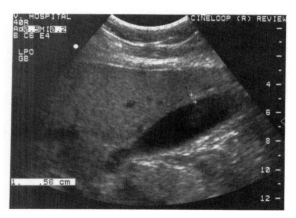

Figure 20-3. Thickened gallbladder wall (5 mm) noted on ultrasonogram longitudinal view.

tive rate in these patients. Clinical history and physical examination are also often unreliable because of the impaired mental status of these critically ill individuals. Nevertheless, the decision to drain the gallbladder percutaneously must be made by the clinicians managing the patient. If the situation deteriorates, a more accurate assessment of surgical complications can be made.

Laboratory tests are similarly of little value in establishing the diagnosis of acalculous cholecystitis. Many patients with sepsis and multiorgan failure have leucocytosis and elevated liver fuction tests. Needle aspiration of bile for culture is also unreliable, since 50% of patients with proven cholecystitis have negative bile cultures, presumably due to concurrent antibiotic therapy.

examination usually visualizes a distended gallbladder with or without sludge (see Figs. 20-1, 20-2).

Distended sludge-filled gallbladders are common in patients on total parenteral nitrition (TPN) in intensive care unit settings. Despite these US findings, acute acalculous cholecystitis is present in only 60% to 70% of these patients. The majority of these patients, with no clinical evidence of cholecystitis, will also have an abnormal radionuclide scintigraphic study with no flow of bile into the gallbladder. Even cholecystokinin morphine-augmented cholescintigraphy carries a 60% false-posi-

Management

Cholecystectomy

The best treatment for symptomatic gallbladder disease is removal of the gallbladder, the first successful operation being described by Langenbuch in 1886. This operation, performed most commonly through a right subcostal incision, became the "gold standard" for just over 100 years. However, in 1987, Mouret of Lyon performed the first laparoscopic cholecystectomy, opening up a new era in abdominal surgery. Over the last few years, laparoscopic cholecystectomy has matured into the preferred method for treating symptomatic gallbladder disease. In only a small proportion of patients is it combined with common duct exploration when common duct stones are found. The laparoscopic approach results in a faster postoperative recovery from cholecystectomy than the open approach, with quicker return to normal intestinal function, less postoperative use of pain medications, a shorter hospital stay of 1 to 2 days as opposed to 4 to 6 days with the open procedure, and a faster return to work. However, in a poor-risk patient minimal access approaches to the biliary tree may be the more appropriate and preferable method of management.

Percutaneous Cholecystostomy

The seriously ill patient, particularly one with comorbidities and unexplained sepsis with an abnormal gallbladder on ultrasonography, presents a difficult management dilemma. The traditional surgical options of open cholecystectomy or operative placement of a cholecystostomy tube usually require a general anesthetic and have a significant morbidity and mortality. For this reason, they are increasingly being supplanted by the less invasive technique of percutaneous ultrasound-guided cholecystostomy. The threshold for performing radiologic catheter drainage is lower than for these conventional surgical interventions because of the wider margin of safety. When the diagnosis is uncertain, a therapeutic trial of catheter drainage can be performed which is, in effect, a prophylactic decompression. If the patient responds, the diagnosis is essentially substantiated. If the patient fails to respond, at least the gallbladder is eliminated as a source of concern, and other foci of sepsis can then be sought.

Percutaneous cholecystostomy is a well established and standard procedure. The materials, techniques, and results are well described (Tables 20-1, 20-2). Depending upon the radiologist's experience and the patient's clinical status, the procedure may

Table 20-1. Percutaneous Gallbladder Introduction Systems

Name	Manufacturer	Catheter Size (Fr) O.D.[a]	Largest Guidewire Accepted (in.)
Cope Introduction Catheter System	Cook Inc.	6.3	.035
Accustick Introducer System	Boston Scientific	6.0	.038
Hawkins Needle Guide Access Set	Cook Inc.	Preloaded 4 or 5	.035

[a]O.D. = outer diameter

Table 20-2. Percutaneous Gallbladder Drainage Catheter*

Catheter	Material	Size (FR)	Guidewire (in.)	Number of Side Holes
Elecath-One Step (TM)	Polyethylene	5.5	0.25	6
Sacks Single Step Self Retaining Catheter Medi-Tech (Boston Scientific)	Polyethylene	6.7	0.25	8
Cope-Loop Self Retaining (Cook)	Polyethylene	8.5, 10.2, 12, 14	.038	4
Special Pigtail (Cook)	Polyethylene	5	.035	32
		6.3	.038	32
		7	.038	32
VanSonnenberg (Trocar) Self Retaining Catheter (Boston Scientific)	Polyethylene	7	.038	4
McGahan Multipurpose Drainage Catheter (Cook)	Polyethylene	6.7	.028	8
		8.3	.038	8

*Will not dissolve in MTBE.

be performed using either a one-step percutaneous cholecystostomy method under portable ultrasound guidance at the patient's bedside or a two-step guidewire exchange (Seldinger) method in the fluoroscopy suite.

SINGLE-STEP TROCAR TECHNIQUE

Catheter drainage under ultrasound guidance is the preferred method of performing emergency percutaneous cholecystostomy. Use of ultrasound guidance as opposed to CT or fluoroscopy allows the majority of these procedures to be performed at the patient's bedside in the intensive care unit or on the ward. In many of these cases the patients are desperately ill and cannot be moved easily because of clinical instability.

After appropriate premedication with intravenous analgesics and antibiotics, a sterile field is prepared and infiltrated with local 1% lidocaine (Xylocaine). The patient usually is placed in the left posterior oblique position. The ultrasound transducer with a biopsy-guided attachment is inserted inside a sterile covering, and the gallbladder is visualized in relationship to the liver, kidney, hepatic flexure, and duodenum. The optimal path and depth for planning to introduce the trocar to the gallbladder are then determined by real-time monitoring (Fig. 20-4A).

The puncture site should be chosen so that the catheter route traverses liver parenchyma and enters the body of the gallbladder across the superior-lateral nonperitonealized surface of the liver, which

Figure 20-4. Visualization of the one-step procedure for percutaneous cholecystostomy under ultrasound guidance. A. Planning the optimal path and depth for placing the trocar to the gallbladder. B. Transhepatic insertion of the trocar (arrow) to the gallbladder. C. Diagnostic aspiration of bile. D. Placement of the pigtail catheter into the gallbladder. E. Decompression and evacuation of all bile from the gallbladder. F. Lavage of the gallbladder with saline; note the increased echogenicity of air bubble in the saline.

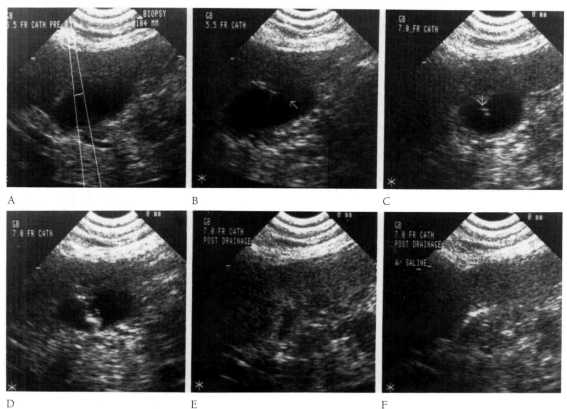

is in contact with the gallbladder in most patients. The nonperitoneal upper surface of the gallbladder is attached to connective tissue in a shallow fossa in the liver located between the right and quadrate lobe. The theoretical advantage of this transhepatic approach in these patients over a more caudal transperitoneal approach is that any bile leaking around the catheter puncture site will be contained within the confines of the gallbladder fossa and will not leak out into the free peritoneal cavity to produce bile peritonitis. The gallbladder is almost completely invested by peritoneum in some patients, however, and may be suspended from the liver, producing a "floating" gallbladder. A transhepatic approach cannot be performed in this situation. A caudal transperitoneal approach must be used for percutaneous drainage in these patients. Recent data suggest that either approach can be used safely.

Although many commercial catheter drainage sets are available, the authors routinely use a small single-step Sacks catheter (5.5, 6, or 7 French, 20- to 28-cm pigtail), which is composed of three coaxial parts: a stiffening cannula, a trocar stylet, and the catheter itself. Some commercially available one-step trocar-catheter systems have retention devices such as a locking suture or loop to prevent catheter dislodgement. The assembly is advanced transhepatically (if possible) into the middle portion of the gallbladder under continuous ultrasound guidance. The trocar is removed, and bile is aspirated from the cannula to confirm that the gallbladder has been entered (see Fig. 20-4B, C). The cannula should then be held firmly, and the catheter should be advanced over it into the gallbladder to allow the pigtail to reform and to ensure the placement of the catheter tip with its drainage holes in the gallbladder lumen (see Fig. 20-4D). When the trocar and cannula are removed, bile is aspirated. Specimens of bile are submitted for culture and cytology. All of the bile is aspirated by hand suction under real-time ultrasound monitoring (see Fig. 20-4E). The gallbladder is then lavaged several times with a volume of sterile saline that never exceeds half of the volume of the bile that was aspirated (see Fig. 20-4F). The catheter is secured on the skin by a retention disc and additional sutures if necessary. A closed drainage system is applied. After 24 hours or more, a contrast cholecystogram can be performed under fluoroscopic control

to assess the status of the cystic and common bile ducts (Fig. 20-5).

TWO-STEP SELDINGER GUIDEWIRE EXCHANGE TECHNIQUE

A Seldinger guidewire exchange technique can also be utilized. Through the initial 20-gauge spinal needle inserted into the gallbladder under ultrasound, a 0.028-in. floppy-tipped guidewire is advanced and coiled in the gallbladder lumen. The cannula-catheter assembly is then advanced over the wire and the cannula is removed, allowing the catheter to coil comfortably within the gallbladder fundus. A variety of different commercially available gallbladder puncture and catheter systems are available for the Seldinger approach (see Tables 20-1, 20-2). A self-retaining anchor locking design minimizes inadvertent dislodgement of the drainage catheter.

The catheter is then fixed to the lateral abdominal wall, and all the bile and contrast is aspirated from the gallbladder lumen. Specimens are sent for culture and bile cytology. A gravity drainage bag is attached, and delayed radiographic study is carried out as above. A postprocedure CT scan is presented (Fig. 20-6).

Figure 20-5. Contrast cholecystography performed via a catheter injection. A percutaneous cholecystostomy was performed 10 days earlier for acute acalculous cholecystitis. Note the free flow through the cystic duct into a normal-appearing common bile duct. The catheter was removed in 2 weeks.

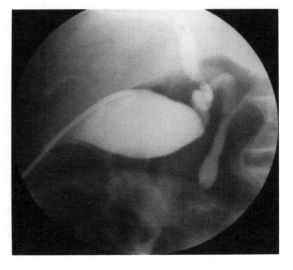

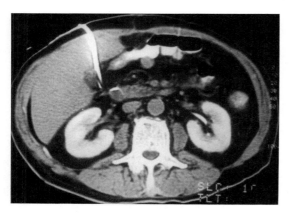

Figure 20-6. Postprocedure CT scan showing the cholecystostomy drainage catheter traversing the left liver lobe with its tip in a contracted decompressed gallbladder lumen.

Table 20-3. Complications of Percutaneous Cholecystostomy

Catheter dislodgement
Hematoma
Vasovagal reaction
Bile peritonitis
Intestinal perforation
Septicemia
Death

Table 20-4. Contraindications to Percutaneous Cholecystectomy

Unfavorable right upper quadrant anatomy
Contracted, thick-walled gallbladder
Colon interposition
Severe fibrotic liver disease
Irreversible coagulopathy

Some workers use an even simpler technique, confining the entire procedure to a single stick aspiration and avoiding catheter placement entirely. If pus or cloudy bile is retrieved, saline lavage is carried out and the procedure terminated. Verbanck et al. and Kiss et al. treated 18 and 21 high-risk patients, respectively, with this approach with excellent results.

COMPLICATIONS

The complications of percutaneous cholecystostomy are well described in the literature and are summarized in Table 20-3. Minimal complications occur after the one-step ultrasound technique. In the authors' experience, they include catheter dislodgement and minor hematoma formation. Septicemia and bile peritonitis are rare but always possible complications.

The major complications of the Seldinger technique are also listed in Table 20-3. Vasovagal reactions can be avoided by limiting manipulation of catheters and guidewires in the presence of an acutely inflamed gallbladder. Management includes atropine, IV fluids, pressors, and cardiac monitoring. Bile leaks cause acute right upper quadrant or right shoulder pain for 10 to 15 minutes after initial catheter insertion. Severe bile peritonitis often indicates faulty technique. Ultrasound demonstration of free fluid in the gallbladder fossa in the presence of persistent right flank pain supports the diagnosis.

Puncture of the right colon or duodenum, septic shock, and death have also been reported with this technique.

CONTRAINDICATIONS

Anatomic factors interfering with free catheter passage into the gallbladder constitute the principle contraindications to percutaneous cholecystostomy. A contracted gallbladder or an obviously thickened wall on ultrasound diminishes the likelihood of successful catheter insertion (Table 20-4). Similarly, an interposed loop of colon or a chronically scarred segment of liver parenchyma may also obstruct easy catheter passage (Fig. 20-7).

CATHETER MANAGEMENT

Postprocedure ultrasonography immediately confirms adequate gallbladder decompression. Contrast cholecystography is required to demonstrate gallstones in the cystic duct and cystic duct patency. This study should generally be performed at 2 to 10 days. If no stones are present, the catheter may be removed. The small catheter used in the one-step ultrasound technique can be removed as soon as the patient's overall condition is improved, if gallstones are not present and patency of the cystic duct is documented. Catheters usually are removed between 3 and 14 days after insertion.

The larger catheters used in the Seldinger technique are removed after 3 to 4 weeks. This delay

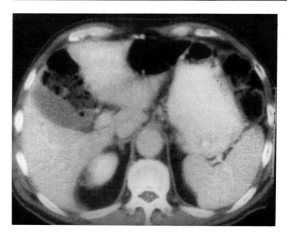

Figure 20-7. CT scan showing gas-filled right colon interposed adjacent to the gallbladder. This unfavorable anatomy constitutes a relative contraindication to percutaneous cholecystostomy. The indication for the CT scan was poor visualization of the gallbladder at ultrasonography because of adjacent gas.

allows sufficient time for a mature tract to form. Without a well-formed tract, bile leakage is a potential risk once these catheters are withdrawn. Demonstration of a mature tract can be achieved by contrast injection under fluoroscopic control as the catheter is gradually withdrawn. If a well-formed tract is not demonstrated, the catheter should be left in place for a longer interval. If stones are detected, treatment can be carried out by either direct trans-tract extraction using radiologic or endoscopic control or by installation of solvents such as MTBE for cholesterol stone dissolution. Because the direct method of nonoperative gallstone therapy is a separate free-standing procedure, the reader is referred to Chapter 17 for further detail.

PREFERRED TECHNIQUE

The combination of ultrasound and fluoroscopy has been utilized for gallbladder decompression at some centers. The initial catheter insertion can be followed by formal fluoroscopic contrast injection for cholecystography. This procedure requires the use of a fluoroscopy suite, exposure of the patient to radiation, and multistage manipulation of catheters and guidewires, and it is much more time-consuming and has more complications than ultrasound guidance alone. One-step percutaneous cholecys-

tostomy performed under ultrasound guidance usually requires 5 to 10 minutes to perform and is extremely safe. Thus the one-step technique is the preferred approach for decompressing the gallbladder in acute cholecystitis.

Results

Percutaneous catheter cholecystostomy is a much safer means than surgical cholecystectomy for controlling gallbladder sepsis in the acutely ill, high-risk patient. No deaths were reported in a cumulative series of 322 patients undergoing PC in whom the predominant indication for gallbladder drainage was sepsis. This result is in contrast to the 13% operative mortality noted previously from large surgical series. As with successful drainage of any purulent fluid collection, response is usually dramatic and prompt, often within 24 hours. Pain subsides, and leucocytosis and fever diminish. Successful weaning from pressor support is also achieved.

When percutaneous cholecystostomy was used as a therapeutic trial for critically ill patients with sepsis of unknown source, Lee et al. found a 58% response rate in a prospective series of 24 patients. In the 10 patients (42%) who failed to respond to PC, a respiratory source of infection was ultimately found in 3, and 5 eventually died of unrelated causes. However, underscoring the difficulty in making the diagnosis, no correlation existed between the ultrasound findings (pericholecystic fluid, thick gallbladder wall, or sludge) in responders versus nonresponders. Given the safety and high efficacy of percutaneous gallbladder drainage, these authors suggest that there should be a very low threshold for performing PC in this difficult clinical setting.

Conclusions

Cholecystectomy remains the treatment of choice for acute cholecystitis. Approximately 75% of these patients can have the gallbladder removed by the laparoscopic technique. Acute cholecystitis in the medically compromised intensive care unit patient, on the other hand, is often of the acalculous variety and may present a perplexing dilemma in terms of diagnosis and appropriate therapy. The development of ultrasound-guided percutaneous catheter drainage affords a safe, minimally invasive alternative to surgery which can be used as a therapeutic trial for patients in whom the diagnosis is not totally clear. Clinical improvement after percutaneous catheter drainage in patients with acute acalculous cholecystitis is prompt and decisive. In nonresponders, the gallbladder is removed as a cause for continuing concern. An aggressive approach to gallbladder diversion is warranted in critically ill patients with multiorgan failure, uncontrolled sepsis, and distended gallbladders.

Selected Readings

Jeffrey RB, Sommer FG. Follow-up sonography in suspected acalculous cholecystitis: Preliminary clinical experience. *J Ultrasound Med* 1993; 4:183–187.

Kiss J, et al. The role of ultrasound guided percutaneous aspiration of the gallbladder in the management of hydrops/empyema caused by acute cholecystitis. *Int Surg* 1988; 73:35.

Lee MJ, et al. Treatment of critically ill patients with sepsis of unknown cause: Value of percutaneous cholecystostomy. *AJR* 1991; 156:1163.

Long TN, Heimbach DM, Carrko CJ. Acalculous cholecystitis in critically ill patients. *Am J Surg* 1987; 136:31.

Malone DE. Interventional radiologic alternatives to cholecystostomy. *Rad Clinics,* No. America 1990; 28: 1145.

McGahan JP, Lindfors KK. Acute cholecystitis: Diagnostic accuracy of percutaneous aspiration of the gallbladder. *Radiology* 1988; 167:669.

McGahan JP, Lindfors KK. Percutaneous cholecystostomy: An alternative to surgical cholecystostomy for acute cholecystitis. *Radiology* 1989; 173:48.

Mirvis SE, et al. The diagnosis of acute acalculous cholecystitis: A comparison of sonography, scintigraphy and CT. *AJR* 1986; 147:1171.

VanSonnenberg E, et al. Diagnostic and therapeutic gallbladder procedures. *Radiology* 1986; 160:23.

Verbanck JJ, et al. Ultrasound guided puncture of the gallbladder for acute cholecystitis. *Lancet* 1993; 341:1132.

21

Acute Cholangitis

EDWARD C. S. LAI
KENT-MAN CHU
HENRY NGAN

Etiology and Pathogenesis

A cholangitic attack often develops among patients with proven biliary obstruction secondary to either benign or malignant pathology. In the presence of bile stasis and bacterial overgrowth, biliary sepsis follows. With the increase in intraductal pressure, reflux of bacteria into the portal venous circulation and the lymphatic system causes bacteremia, with or without septicemia.

Irrespective of the nature of the obstruction, whether benign or malignant, biliary sepsis fails to resolve with conservative measures in about 15% to 19% of patients who present initially with acute cholangitis. Different terminologies, such as *acute suppurative cholangitis* and *acute obstructive suppurative cholangitis,* which reflect the degree of biliary suppuration, have been used to describe the life-threatening condition. However, past experiences have shown that even among patients with fulminating cholangitis, no pus and occasionally a negative bacteriologic culture could be obtained from the bile aspirated during surgery. Terms such as *toxic cholangitis* or *severe acute cholangitis* are probably better because they accurately depict the clinical condition of these patients, rather than a physical finding.

Diagnosis

The clinical diagnosis of acute cholangitis can usually be made on clinical grounds, whereas the presence of all three classical features of the Charcot's triad (jaundice, abdominal pain, and fever) may not always be present. Although up to one third of these patients can be afebrile, both jaundice and abdominal pain are found in over 90% of patients who have fulminant calculous cholangitis. Among patients with hepatolithiasis, obstruction may be limited to a few segmental ducts, and an apparently unexplained septicemic shock may be the only significant presentation. The use of liver biochemistry is helpful because it is unusual to find entirely normal results in the presence of frank clinical cholangitis.

Ultrasonography (US) should be the first method of investigation for all patients with suspected biliary sepsis. In the presence of a dilated ductal system together with the clinical symptoms and signs, a diagnosis can be made with certainty (Fig. 21-1). Occasionally, intrahepatic ductal calculi (Fig. 21-2), liver atrophy, and liver abscess can be found. Although percutaneous US often fails to localize an intraductal pathology located in the distal common duct because of the overlying duodenal gas, the approximate level of obstruction can be determined with fair certainty. Moreover, US can usually differentiate whether the obstruction is due to a stone or a tumor, since the former invariably produces an acoustic shadow (Figs. 21-3, 21-4).

The value of computerized tomography (CT) for patients with cholangitis is often limited, but it may occasionally provide useful information, especially on patients with cholangitis secondary to hepatolithiasis. The presence of pneumobilia from a previous bili-enteric anastomosis or endoscopic

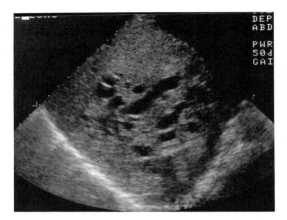

Figure 21-1. Ultrasonogram showing dilated bile ducts in the right lobe of liver.

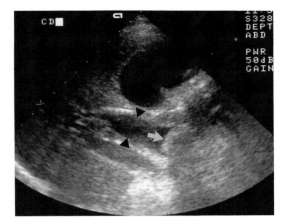

Figure 21-3. Ultrasonogram showing a stone (white arrow) impacted in the dilated common bile duct (black arrowheads) casting an acoustic shadow.

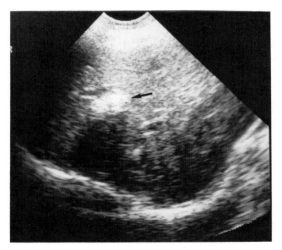

Figure 21-2. Ultrasonogram showing an intrahepatic ductal calculus (arrow) casting an acoustic shadow.

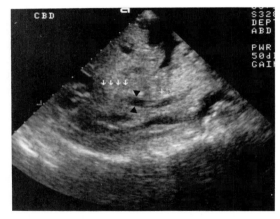

Figure 21-4. Ultrasonogram showing a tumor (four white arrows) obstructing the common bile duct (black arrowheads). Note that no acoustic shadow is present.

sphincterotomy may make the interpretation of a direct cholangiogram difficult. Segmental obstruction from stone impaction or strictured ductal orifices may result in the incomplete opacification of all the major intrahepatic branches, which may not be obvious on cholangiography. These problems can usually be overcome with CT. Intrahepatic stones are denser than the hepatic parenchyma on precontrast CT but may become less obvious against the parenchyma after intravenous contrast (Fig. 21-5A, B). If nonfilling of a segmental intrahepatic duct is present on cholangiography, CT may

demonstrate dilated hepatic ducts in that segment with a stone responsible for the obstruction (Figs. 21-6A, B; 21-7A, B). When unexplained sepsis continues in cholangitis in spite of treatment, CT may reveal a liver abscess missed by US or situated in an occult site such as the caudate lobe. Moreover, CT may show segmental liver atrophy secondary to repeated infection with compensatory hypertrophy in the opposite lobe.

A direct cholangiographic examination to delineate the exact ductal pathology is mandatory before deciding on the appropriate treatment. The

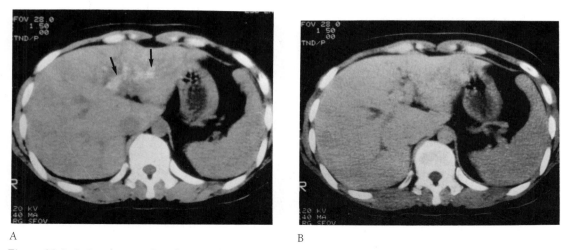

A   B

Figure 21-5. A. Intrahepatic ductal stones (arrows) are present in the left lobe in a precontrast CT scan. B. The stones are less obvious on CT scan after intravenous contrast. Note that the intrahepatic bile ducts are slightly dilated.

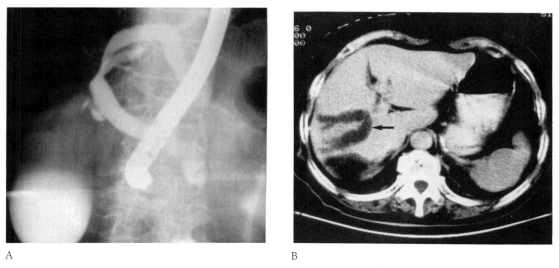

A   B

Figure 21-6. A. ERCP showing nonfilling of the intrahepatic bile ducts in the right lobe. B. CT scan showing dilated bile ducts (arrow) in the right lobe, which is slightly atrophic.

choice between percutaneous transhepatic cholangiography (PTC) and endoscopic retrograde cholangiopancreatography (ERCP) depends on the level and nature of the ductal obstruction and the availability of expertise in these examinations.

Since ERCP opacifies the common bile duct, the intrahepatic branches, and the gallbladder, dilatation of the biliary system, stones, strictures, and nonfilling of segmental ducts can usually be detected unless severe pneumobilia is present (Fig. 21-8). In obstruction of the biliary tract, the exact level of obstruction can invariably be determined (Fig. 21-9). For patients whose biliary obstruction is secondary to choledocholithiasis, ERCP has the advantage that therapeutic measures can be offered immediately at the same setting.

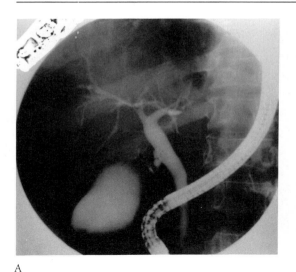
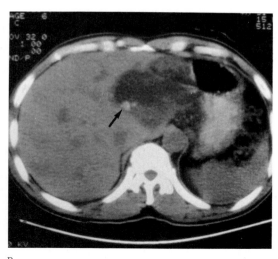

A   B

Figure 21-7. A. ERCP showing less obvious nonfilling of segmental intrahepatic ducts in the left lobe. B. CT scan showing grossly dilated bile ducts in left lobe with a stone (arrow) causing obstruction.

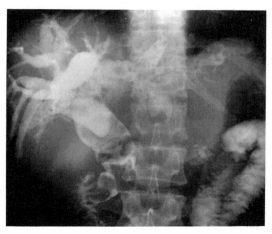

Figure 21-8. ERCP showing dilatation of the common bile duct and intrahepatic ducts with many stones present in the common bile duct and left intrahepatic ducts.

PTC is another useful technique in demonstrating the status of the biliary tree (Fig. 21-10). PTC is an alternative procedure when the patient has had a previous Polya's partial gastrectomy or a choledochoenterostomy. When nonopacification of a segmental duct is demonstrated by ERCP, a puncture into this segment will confirm the presence of dilated ducts with complete obstruction. However,

PTC is more invasive than ERCP and can produce intraperitoneal hemorrhage, intrahepatic hematoma which occasionally results in hemobilia, intrahepatic arteriovenous shunting, bile peritonitis, and exacerbation of the cholangitis. Percutaneous transhepatic biliary drainage and the insertion of a plastic or metallic stent can also be undertaken at the same setting to decompress the obstructed biliary tree.

Caution should be exercised in deciding on the appropriate timing of direct cholangiography following a recent attack of cholangitis if early biliary drainage is not possible. The introduction of bacteria, especially in patients with malignant strictures, as a consequence of increased intraductal pressure following the injection of hyperosmotic contrast medium into the obstructed ductal system, poses a definite risk of precipitating a cholangitic attack. Although the overall incidence of acute cholangitis complicating a diagnostic ERCP is about 7% among patients with confirmed ductal obstruction, patients with an underlying malignant obstruction and evidence of low-grade biliary sepsis are at a higher risk. However, the necessity of a prophylactic biliary drainage immediately following the radiologic examination is debatable. If the patient is afebrile, the estimated risk of cholangitis after a diagnostic ERCP is about 3%, irrespective of the

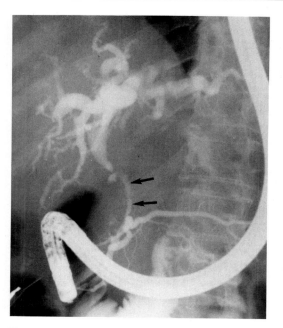

Figure 21-9. ERCP showing a malignant stricture in the middle of the common bile duct (arrows) with dilatation of intrahepatic ducts.

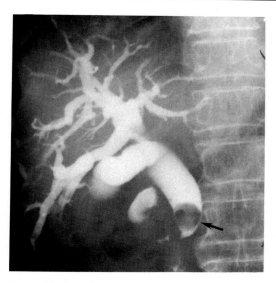

Figure 21-10. PTC showing a stone (arrow) impacted in the lower end of the common bile duct causing obstruction.

nature of the underlying ductal obstruction. In contrast, complication rates associated with either endoscopic papillotomy or percutaneous transhepatic drainage are about 7% to 20%. Precautions such as limiting the amount of contrast medium injected to a minimum and commencing antibiotics immediately after the examination should be adequate to prevent a cholangitic attack. Whenever possible, the diagnostic examination should be scheduled as close as possible to the time of the definitive procedure. Otherwise, cholangiography should be deferred for about 72 hours or more after the febrile attack has completely resolved.

Management and Results

When a patient presents with acute cholangitis, conservative treatment with antibiotics is the accepted initial measure. The pattern of microbiology varies with the period of the respective studies and the individual medical center. Mixed bacterial growths are frequent, and the antimicrobial agents chosen should cover common organisms such as *Escherichia coli, Klebsiella* spp., *Pseudomonas,* and

the enterococci. Although the patient's condition might initially be stable, close monitoring is important to detect any rapid deterioration. In one series from Hong Kong by Lai ECS et al. in 1990, emergency surgical exploration was necessary in 49% of the 86 patients with severe cholangitis within the first 24 hours of admission. The corresponding figures from the United States varied from 15% to 17% within the initial 72 hours.

The diagnosis of severe acute cholangitis and thus the timing of urgent ductal drainage depend entirely on the clinical features. The presence of mental confusion, a history of hypotension, and persistent swinging fever despite antibiotic treatment for 48 hours are clear indications for urgent biliary decompression. Warning signs of impending septicemic shock such as progressive tachycardia, a fall in blood pressure, and oliguria should also prompt early therapeutic intervention. Irrespective of the mode of urgent biliary decompression, the prime objective is to reduce the intraductal pressure by a safe, expeditious, and effective measure instead of eliminating the offending obstructive lesion. Experimental canine studies have shown that the reflux of microorganisms into the lymphatic or venous stream will be interrupted once the pressure is reduced to 25 cm H_2O or below.

In the following discussion, which examines the various therapeutic options and their individual merits in the management of acute cholangitis, patients with malignant obstruction are omitted, since they carry a significantly worse prognosis than those with calculous disease, although sepsis occurs infrequently in these patients if direct cholangiography is avoided.

Therapeutic Options

Until recently, surgery has been the only therapeutic option for urgent biliary decompression. The extent and the duration of the operation that are feasible should be judged judiciously according to the condition of the patient during emergency surgery. Drainage of the common bile duct by a choledochotomy and placement of a T tube of the largest possible caliber are the minimum procedures required. In areas where hepatolithiasis is endemic, the presence of a proximal stricture close to the confluence of the hepatic ducts must be excluded if direct cholangiography is not available before surgery. A biliary sound can be gently passed into both intrahepatic ductal systems, and in case of doubt one limb of the T tube should be left to splint the duct after dilatation.

During the common duct exploration, all ductal calculi should be extracted as far as possible. However, intraoperative T tube cholangiography or choledochoscopy to ensure complete ductal clearance is not necessary for these critically ill patients. Residual stones can be safely removed in the postoperative period using flexible choledochoscopy. In a retrospective review of 103 patients with residual stones, ductal clearance was achieved with no morbidity in 95% and 82% of patients with common duct stones and intrahepatic calculi, respectively. With the aid of adjunctive measures such as electrohydraulic lithotripsy, which helps to fragment the stones, the likelihood of ductal clearance can be increased. In selected patients who are hemodynamically stable and have no serious concomitant medical problems, an intraoperative choledochoscopy is justified because it helps to reduce the incidence of retained stones. A flexible choledochoscope is the preferred instrument because it can visualize the proximal ducts better than a rigid one. Caution should be exercised, however, to restrict the pressure applied for fluid irrigation to 80 mm Hg or below during the examination. Otherwise, the intraductal pressure can easily exceed the safety limit, at which point cholangiovenous reflux of bacteria will begin.

Percutaneous transhepatic biliary drainage (PTBD) and endoscopic intervention are proven alternatives for urgent biliary decompression during an attack of severe acute cholangitis. An effective PTBD can be established safely with low procedure-related morbidity (about 7%) using small catheters. Sepsis usually resolves following a successful procedure. Nonetheless, most clinicians consider PTBD to be a temporizing measure in the management of ductal calculi because the removal of these calculi via the percutaneous catheter or its tract is restricted when compared with the endoscopic route.

The use of therapeutic endoscopy in the management of patients with choledocholithiasis is well established, and different approaches are available. The most effective way to secure a proper ductal decompression is to completely remove all ductal calculi at the time of emergency endoscopy. To allow for subsequent active instrumentation, a complete endoscopic papillotomy whereby the ampulla of Vater is severed from the ductal orifice to the duodenal wall is necessary. The duration of the endoscopic procedure depends on the size and number of the common duct stones encountered. An alternate approach for patients with fulminant biliary cholangitis is the insertion of either an endoscopic stent or a nasobiliary catheter (Fig. 21-11) into the ductal system for decompression. Since immediate removal of the offending calculi is not contemplated, a limited endoscopic papillotomy or even occasionally no papillotomy is required if the ampulla is patulous. The endoscopist must be certain, however, that the tip of the catheter has been placed proximal to the site of the obstruction irrespective of the choice of drainage catheters. In experienced hands, a simple endoscopic papillotomy followed by a drainage procedure can be accomplished within half an hour. Despite the small caliber of these endoscopic catheters, usually 7 French, resolution of the biliary sepsis is certain after the endoscopic decompression. If the patient remains septic after a successful endoscopic drainage, other occult septic foci such as concomitant intrahepatic abscesses must be considered. Further definitive

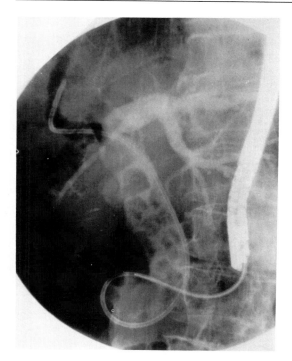

Figure 21-11. A patient with severe acute cholangitis managed by endoscopic nasobiliary drainage. Multiple calculi were found. The tip of the catheter was placed into the right ductal system and proximal to the stones. Care should be taken to maintain the distal alpha loop of the nasobiliary catheter to prevent accidental dislodgement during removal of the endoscope.

treatment, surgery, or repeated endoscopic intervention can be decided on according to the general condition and past medical history of the patient after the cholangitic attack has completely subsided.

As in emergency surgical exploration, the extent of emergency endoscopy is governed by the condition of the patient. If the patient is stable and mentally orientated, a complete endoscopic papillotomy followed by stone extraction using a Dormia basket is warranted because it could save the patient a second endoscopic procedure. However, if the patient is hemodynamically unstable and has a complicated ductal pathology, a quick drainage procedure which serves as an initial temporizing measure would be a better option. Regarding the choice of catheter, an indwelling nasobiliary catheter is better if a complete endoscopic papillotomy has been done because it permits irrigation of the biliary

tree with saline or other stone dissolution agents and a repeated cholangiogram without another endoscopic examination. On the other hand, an endoscopic stent is free from the risk of accidental dislodgment, especially when the patient is mentally confused. Furthermore, subsequent definitive measures can be deferred to a suitable time when the vital signs or any concomitant medical problems have been dealt with. A pigtail stent, whether single or double in configuration (Fig. 21-12), should be used to avoid stent migration as the common duct is usually dilated, especially when the sphincter of Oddi has been disrupted by an endoscopic papillotomy.

Figure 21-12. Emergency endoscopic drainage was established using a 7 French double-pigtail endoprosthesis. Much as with a nasobiliary catheter, the proximal tip was positioned well within the intrahepatic ducts. At such an ideal location, stent migration is unlikely and satisfactory ductal decompression can be ascertained.

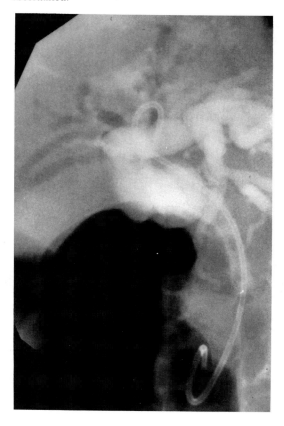

Controversy

Since the advent of various nonoperative measures, the data published on their application for patients with severe acute cholangitis have been impressive. After an emergency endoscopic drainage for patients with calculous cholangitis, mortality rates ranging from 0 to 7.7% were reported (Table 21-1). On the other hand, the overall figure reported for patients who had undergone emergency surgery was in the order of 20% to 40% (Table 21-2). In view of these favorable results, the question of whether emergency endoscopic decompression should be offered routinely to all patients with severe calculous cholangitis was raised.

The definite superiority of therapeutic endoscopy was not certain when the data on emergency surgery were reviewed. On the basis of the clinical data of 86 consecutive patients in one unit who had surgery for their fulminant calculous cholangitis, five independent risk factors for postoperative

mortality were identified on multivariate analysis. These five factors were the presence of concomitant medical problems, arterial blood pH less than 7.4, total serum bilirubin level over 5.5 mg/dl, platelet count less than 150×10^9/liter, and serum albumin level less than 3.0 mg/dl. Among patients with two or fewer of these risk factors, the mortality rate of emergency surgery was 6%, which compared favorably with that of therapeutic endoscopy reported in the literature. Moreover, in another retrospective study from the same unit, the morbidity rates of surgery and therapeutic endoscopy were comparable, although a much lower mortality rate was achieved by the use of therapeutic endoscopy. When the issue of whether an emergency endoscopy is a superior option for patients with severe acute cholangitis was examined by a randomized controlled trial, the significant reduction in mortality rate and duration of ventilator support verified the definite advantage of initial therapeutic endoscopy over emergency surgery for these patients.

Table 21-1. Summary of Morbidity and Mortality Rates of Patients with Severe Acute Cholangitis Managed by Emergency Nonoperative Biliary Drainage

Author	Mode of Nonoperative Drainage	Number of Patients		Morbidity Rate (%)	Mortality Rate (%)
		Total	Calculous Obstruction		
Kinoshita et al (1984)[a]	Percutaneous	11	NA[k]	NA	36
Gould et al (1985)[b]	Percutaneous	7	3	NA	28.6
Pessa et al (1987)[c]	Percutaneous	42	12	58	41.7
Ikeda et al (1981)[d]	Endoscopic	3	3	0	0
Delmotte et al (1982)[e]	Endoscopic	18	18	NA	0
Leese et al (1986)[f]	Endoscopic	43	43	27.9	4.6
Gogel et al (1987)[g]	Endoscopic	13	13	0	7.7
Leung et al (1989)[h]	Endoscopic	105	105	4.7	4.7
Lai et al (1990)[i]	Endoscopic	15	15	40	6.7
Lai et al (1992)[j]	Endoscopic	41	41	34	10

[a]Data from Kinoshita H et al. Cholangitis. *World J Surg* 1984;8:963–969.
[b]Data from Gould RJ et al. Percutaneous biliary drainage as an initial therapy in sepsis of the biliary tract. *Surg Gynecol Obstet* 1985;160:523–527.
[c]Data from Pessa ME, Hawkins IF, Vogel SB. The treatment of acute cholangitis. Percutaneous transhepatic biliary drainage before definitive therapy. *Ann Surg* 1987;205:389–392.
[d]Data from Ikeda S et al. Emergency decompression of bile duct in acute obstructive suppurative cholangitis by duodenoscopic cannulation: a lifesaving procedure. *World J Surg* 1981;5:587–593.
[e]Data from Delmotte JS et al. Initial duodenoscopic sphincterotomy in patients with acute cholangitis or pancreatitis complicating biliary stones. *Gastroenterology* 1982;82:1042.
[f]Data from Leese T et al. Management of acute cholangitis and the impact of endoscopic sphincterotomy *Br J Surg* 1986;73:988–992.
[g]Data from Gogel HK et al. Acute suppurative obstructive cholangitis due to stones: treatment by urgent endoscopic sphincterotomy. *Gastrointest Endoscopy* 1987;33:210–213.
[h]Data from Leung JWC et al. Urgent endoscopic drainage for acute suppurative cholangitis. *Lancet* 1989;1:1307–1309.
[i]Data from Lai ECS et al. Severe acute cholangitis: the role of emergency nasobiliary drainage. *Surgery* 1990;107:268–272.
[j]Data from Lai ECS et al. Endoscopic biliary drainage for severe acute cholangitis. *N Engl J Med* 1992;326:1582–1586.
[k]NA = not available.

Table 21-2. Summary of Morbidity and Mortality Rates of Patients with Severe Acute Cholangitis Managed by Emergency Surgery

| Author | Number of Patients | | Morbidity Rate (%) | Mortality Rate (%) |
	Total	Calculous Obstruction		
Welch and Donaldson (1976)[a]	15	15	44	25
O'Connor et al (1976)[b]	19	NA[f]	NA	50
Boey and Way (1980)[c]	30	19	NA	40
Thompson et al (1982)[d]	2	NA	NA	9
Lai et al (1990)[e]	86	86	50	20

[a]Data from Welch JP, Donaldson GA. The urgency of diagnosis and surgical treatment of acute suppurative cholangitis. *Am J Surg* 1976; 131:527–532.
[b]Data from O'Connor MJ et al. Acute bacterial cholangitis. *Arch Surg* 1982; 117:437–441.
[c]Data from Boey JH, Way LW. Acute cholangitis. *Ann Surg* 1980; 191:264–270.
[d]Data from Thompson JE et al. Factors in management of acute cholangitis. *Ann Surg* 1982; 195:137–145.
[e]Data from Lai ECS, et al. Emergency surgery for severe acute cholangitis. *Ann Surg* 1990; 211:55–59.
[f]NA = not available.

Preferred Approach

When patients present with acute cholangitis, intravenous antibiotics should be commenced, once the necessary septic workup has been completed, using a third-generation cephalosporin, either alone or in combination with an aminoglycoside. A US examination of the hepatobiliary system should be performed within 24 hours after admission to confirm the clinical diagnosis. If the cholangitic attack subsides, an early elective ERCP should be scheduled about 72 hours later.

If the biliary sepsis progresses despite an adequate trial of antibiotics, an emergency ERCP by a competent endoscopist should be arranged. While the endoscopic examination is done in the usual manner under local anesthesia applied to the pharynx, the use of intravenous sedation should be reduced to the minimum, especially when the condition of the patient is unstable. Oxygen supplement via a nasal prong and close monitoring of both the blood pressure and oxygen saturation should be routinely carried out throughout the entire examination. Once the ductal pathology has been clearly delineated, an immediate decision is made with regard to the appropriate mode of biliary drainage to be initiated. In the presence of common duct stones, endoscopic drainage, at least as an initial measure, should be carried out, since in Hong Kong and elsewhere in Asia, patients with complicated intrahepatic calculi or strictures are not infrequently encountered. Although attempts at initial endoscopic drainage for such patients is occasionally worthwhile, suitable candidates have been few.

In one series of 26 patients who had fulminant cholangitis secondary to hepatolithiasis, only 1 patient with an isolated common hepatic duct stricture was considered a suitable candidate for urgent endoscopic decompression. Under such circumstances effective drainage to the proximal segmental ducts would be difficult and unsatisfactory, and surgery would be a better option for securing biliary drainage. Nevertheless, an initial attempt at endoscopic drainage is still worthwhile, because when successful, definitive reconstruction can be conducted as an elective one-stage operation. Even when adequate endoscopic decompression is unsuccessful, a preoperative cholangiogram is most valuable in deciding on the appropriate surgical procedure.

At the time of emergency endoscopy, a conservative approach is advisable. Although immediate instrumental extraction of all ductal calculi was widely practiced, such an aggressive approach carried an increased morbidity of 28% even in experienced hands. Complications such as bleeding and retroduodenal perforations, which require emergency exploration, are highly undesirable, especially at the time of a fulminant cholangitic attack. Approximately 10% of patients who were subjected to endoscopic drainage for their biliary sepsis did not require a papillotomy for the insertion of a drainage catheter.

Conclusions

The successful management of patients with acute calculous cholangitis depends primarily on the timing of biliary decompression. Despite the documented advantage of initial nonoperative biliary drainage, early surgical intervention can have an equally good result if the appropriate expertise in nonoperative biliary drainage is not available. Conversely, if the cholangitic attack is allowed to progress to a morbid stage, the morbidity and mortality rates remain formidable in spite of successful endoscopic treatment.

The use of therapeutic endoscopy has the distinct advantage of being able to offer definitive treatment. Besides having technical competency, the endoscopist responsible for the urgent ductal drainage should understand the limitation of therapeutic endoscopy when confronted with patients who have complicated intrahepatic ductal pathology. The availability of an interventional radiologist as part of the team is ideal, since even if endoscopic decompression fails, immediate drainage can be established percutaneously. The latter is of particular importance when patients with malignant biliary obstruction are considered. When confronted with patients who have multiple intrahepatic stones confined to a segmental duct or concomitant liver abscess, emergency surgery remains the best therapeutic option. After reviewing the data from a randomized controlled trial, the authors are disappointed at the high mortality rate of 10% among patients who had initial endoscopic drainage. Conceivably, an earlier endoscopic intervention soon after presentation, irrespective of the outcome of the trial of initial conservative management, might help to reduce the mortality. Further prospective studies are necessary to validate such a hypothesis.

Selected Readings

Boey JH, Way LW. Acute cholangitis. *Ann Surg* 1980; 191:264–270.

Gigot JF, et al. Acute cholangitis: Multivariate analysis of risk factors. *Ann Surg* 1989; 209:435–438.

Himal HS, Lindsay T. Ascending cholangitis: Surgery versus endoscopic or percutaneous drainage. *Surgery* 1990; 108:629–634.

Lai ECS. Management of severe acute cholangitis. *Br J Surg* 1990; 77:604–605.

Lai ECS, et al. Emergency surgery for severe acute cholangitis. *Ann Surg* 1990; 211:55–59.

Lai ECS, et al. Endoscopic biliary drainage for severe acute cholangitis. *N Engl J Med* 1992; 326:1582–1586.

22

Biliary Parasites

Chen-Guo Ker
Pai-Ching Sheen
Chang-Yi Chen
Eng-Rin Chen

Biliary parasites are common in many areas in East Asia but are rare in more developed parts of the world. In Taiwan biliary ascariasis was commonly encountered in the 1960s, but this problem is rarely seen in the 1990s. However, endemic infection with *Clonorchis sinensis* is still a problem in Taiwan. The association between ascariasis and clonorchiasis and biliary stone formation was appreciated by Maki in the early 1960s. The incidence of ascaris elements was reported at 10% among gallstones examined in Japan at that time. Around the same time Tech also discovered liver flukes in the center of gallstones and suggested that these parasites played an important role in gallstone formation. Subsequent studies of the ultrastructure of calcium bilirubinate, brown pigment stones in Taiwan, have confirmed that parasitic elements play a direct role in the formation of these stones.

In general, the treatment of biliary parasites is medical. However, when stones form in the gallbladder or the extra- or intrahepatic bile ducts, surgery is often indicated. If the patient presents with severe cholangitis, this disease process may be life-threatening. Therefore, early diagnosis is key to a good outcome. However, in developed countries, where biliary parasites are an infrequent disease, early diagnosis may be difficult.

Etiology and Pathogenesis

Prevalence of Gallstones in Clonorchiasis

To determine whether gallstones are associated with clonorchiasis, an ultrasound survey was performed in an endemic area in southern Taiwan. Of 947 Kakkanese people with proven clonorchiasis, 89 people were found to have biliary stones, including 85 gallbladder stones (9.0%), 3 common duct stones (0.4%), and 1 intrahepatic stone (0.1%) (Table 22-1). Control populations in Kaohsiung, a nonendemic area of southern Taiwan, and in the aborigines have also been studied with ultrasound. The prevalence of gallbladder stones in these two populations was 4.5% and 1.5%, respectively. Comparison of these rates with those found in the clonorchis-infected population demonstrated a statistically significant difference (see Table 22-1). Thus the high prevalence of gallstones may be the result of clonorchis infection, although ethnic differences may also be important.

Pathogenesis and Clonorchis Stones

The authors have studied four cases of gallbladder stones from patients infected with *Clonorchis sinensis*. During the operations, pigment stones and liver

Table 22-1. Incidence of Gallstones by Sonography

Stone	Clonorchiasis Patients ($n=947$)	Kaohsiung Controls ($n=1166$)	Aborigine Controls ($n=870$)
Gallbladder stones	85 (9.0%)*	52 (4.5%)	13 (1.5%)
Intrahepatic duct stones	1 (0.4%)	22 (1.9%)	1 (0.2%)

*$P < 0.05$ versus controls.

flukes were found in the gallbladder and/or the common duct. In each patient, bile-stained mucus was found around clonorchis ova (Fig. 22-1A). Numerous clonorchis eggs were also seen on light microscopic study of the bile (see Fig. 22-1B). In three of the patients thin slices of the stones also revealed clonorchis ova in the matrix (Fig. 22-2). Based on these observations, a possible schema for the pathogenesis of clonorchis stones is presented in Fig. 22-3. Adult flukes producing ova may cause increased mucus secretion and cholecystitis. A combination of dead liver flukes, ova, inflammatory cells, and exfoliated epithelium may cause gallbladder stasis. In this setting calcium bilirubinate may precipitate with the dead liver flukes and clonorchis ova as a nidus for stone formation in either the gallbladder or the common duct.

Pathogenesis of Ascaris Stones

The authors have also studied five patients with *Ascaris lumbricoides* in gallstones, including ascaris ova in three and dead adult liver flukes in two. In each case the stones were obtained from the common bile duct. The stones were prepared for light and scanning electron microscopy. In addition, element analysis was performed by calcium ion line scanning. Calcium bilirubinate particles were observed on the surface of either the liver fluke carcass or the ascaris ova.

A schema for the pathogenesis of ascaris stones is depicted in Fig. 22-4. This schema is similar to that described above for clonorchis stones but takes place in the bile ducts rather than the gallbladder. Either the dead ascaris worm or a combination of ascaris ova and mucus may be the nidus for stone formation. Mucus secretion may be increased as

the result of chronic irritation of the ductal wall and of infection, ascardic cholangitis. Again, stasis of bile flow occurs, and the precipitation of calcium bilirubinate with mucus and ascaris ova forms a stone (Fig. 22-5, see also Fig. 22-4). Several studies have documented a high incidence of ascaris elements in biliary stones in East Asia. A 1961 study from Japan found ascaris worms or ova in 10% of the patients studied. the authors' 1985 report found ascaris elements in 12% of Taiwanese patients' stones. The highest reported incidence of ascaris stones was 38% in a 1984 analysis from mainland China.

Diagnosis

Biliary Clonorchiasis

When a good history is available in a young adult with a heavy infection, the diagnosis can be obtained easily. The diagnosis may be proven by demonstration of eggs in the patient's stool or by an enzyme-linked immunosorbent assay (ELISA) test. However, these flukes may survive in a patient for many years, possibly as long as 20 years or more, without causing clinical problems. In endemic areas many cases have been diagnosed at autopsy in patients who had no history of any complaint.

In patients who develop biliary tract symptoms, ultrasound may demonstrate diffuse dilatation of the small intrahepatic bile ducts with no or minimal dilatation of the large intra- or extrahepatic ducts. Lim et al. have suggested that clonorchiasis should be considered when sonography discloses this characteristic pattern of bile duct dilatation with increased wall echogenicity and nonshadowing discrete, echogenic foci in the gallbladder lumen.

The stones that form with clonorchiasis are most likely to be found in the gallbladder. However, as the disease progresses, the bile ducts and the whole liver may become involved with the disease. Thus small liver flukes may occasionally be visualized in the bile ducts with endoscopic or operative cholangiography. Stones may also be seen in the extrahepatic or, more rarely, in the intrahepatic ducts. When stones obstruct the bile ducts, secondary bacterial infection, especially with *Escherichia coli*, exacerbates the problem and leads to cholan-

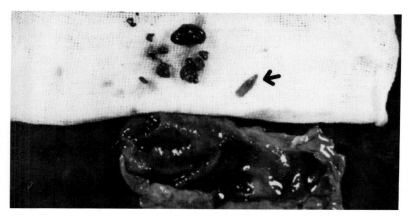

A

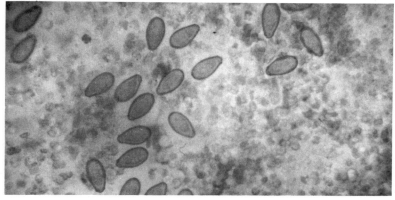

B

Figure 22-1. A. Liver fluke (arrow) and gallbladder stones found from resected gallbladder. B. Numerous clonorchis eggs found in the bile.

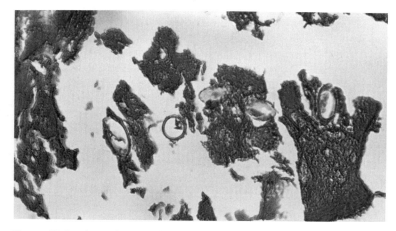

Figure 22-2. Clonorchis eggs found in the section of a gallstone.

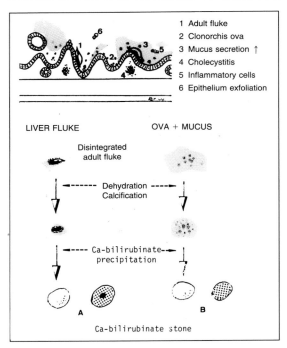

1 Adult fluke
2 Clonorchis ova
3 Mucus secretion ↑
4 Cholecystitis
5 Inflammatory cells
6 Epithelium exfoliation

Figure 22-3. Schema of stone formation from clonorchis as nidus (A) and the ova mixed with mucus and calcium bilirubinate (B).

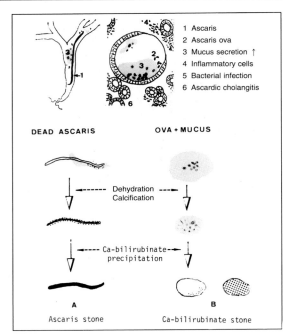

1 Ascaris
2 Ascaris ova
3 Mucus secretion ↑
4 Inflammatory cells
5 Bacterial infection
6 Ascardic cholangitis

Figure 22-4. Schema of stone formation from ascaris (A) and eggs mixed with mucus and calcium bilirubinate (B).

gitis. Clonorchiasis has also been reported to have an etiologic role in cholangiocarcinoma. However, the authors have not found any relation between clonorchiasis and cholangiocarcinoma in the endemic area in Taiwan.

Biliary Ascariasis

Biliary ascariasis is a helminthic infection caused by the migration of the nematode *Ascaris lumbricoides* into the biliary tract. The clinical manifestations vary in severity depending on the number of parasites migrating into the ducts, remaining in the ducts, or returning to the duodenum. Clinically, the patients are seized suddenly by acute, agonizing, throbbing epigastric or right upper quadrant pain that usually radiates to the shoulder, back, or hypogastrium. Nausea and vomiting are common, and the patient will try bending over to relieve the acute distress. The pain may last for 20 minutes or longer and then slowly abates. The patient will become exhausted and rest quietly until the beginning of the

next attack. The pain may recur at short intervals or after rather prolonged periods of remission.

In approximately 90% of the patients the ascaris is found in the common duct. Less often, this liver fluke is found in the intrahepatic ducts, with the left more often involved than the right. Ascaris is rarely located in the gallbladder. In one report by Hsu, 63% of the ascarides found during operations were alive. When the adult parasite is trapped in the intrahepatic bile ducts, thousands of eggs are released upon disintegration of the worm, causing an acute and chronic suppurative cholangitis. With time the symptoms become more severe and persistent. In the patient suffering from extensive ascaridic cholangitis, the prognosis is poor without adequate treatment. Although ascariasis is an infrequent disease in developed countries, Eymeri and colleagues reported a case of biliary ascariasis from France.

In the past the diagnosis of biliary ascariasis was made chiefly by intravenous cholangiography. More recently, direct cholangiography has become more useful in the diagnosis of this disease. In the

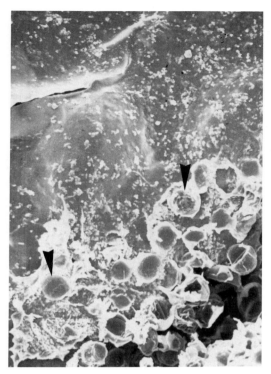

Figure 22-5. A cluster of ascaris eggs (arrowheads) in the center of a gallstone obtained from an intrahepatic duct studied by scanning electron microscopy.

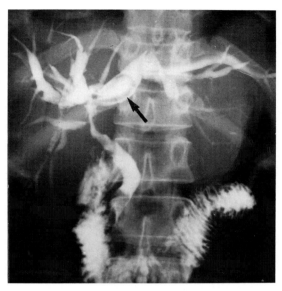

Figure 22-6. Cholangiogram demonstrating a live ascaris worm in the left hepatic duct, a stricture at the hilum, and a stone in the common bile duct.

authors' department, 13 recent patients with biliary ascariasis were diagnosed by direct cholangiography, including percutaneous transhepatic cholangiography (PTC) in 3 cases and endoscopic retrograde cholangiopancreatography (ERCP) in 10 cases. According to the location of the worms, 4 cases (31%) were classified as intrahepatic and 9 cases (69%) as extrahepatic. The clinical manifestations were much more severe in the intrahepatic than in the extrahepatic group. Obstructive jaundice was encountered in 80% of the intrahepatic group but in none of the extrahepatic group. Stenosis of a hepatic duct was observed in all 4 patients in the intrahepatic group but in none of the extrahepatic group. One patient died from sepsis and severe jaundice after almost complete obstruction of the hepatic duct, as shown in Fig. 22-6. Pancreatitis is another complication that may occur with biliary ascariasis. In addition, the migration of a worm into the pan-

creatic duct may result in acute necrotizing pancreatitis.

Management and Results

Clonorchiasis

The initial treatment of clonorchiasis is medical. Since 1975, praziquantel has been the primary medical treatment for clonorchiasis in Taiwan and Korea. Praziquantel is a pyrzinoquinoline compound which is also an effective agent for schistosomiasis and tapeworms. Since praziquantel is relatively nontoxic, the patient can be treated at home. In some cases, however, drug treatment will be unsatisfactory because clonorchis flukes remain viable in the bile ducts.

Ascariasis

The treatment of biliary ascariasis remains controversial. Usually, medical treatment is attempted when biliary ascariasis is first diagnosed and the patient is not severely ill. After 2 weeks, an ERCP can be repeated to determine whether the worm has escaped from the biliary tract. However, if the

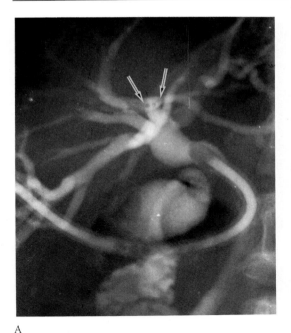

A

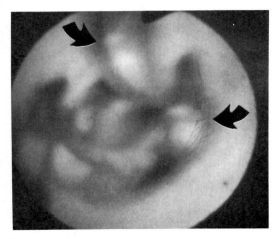

B

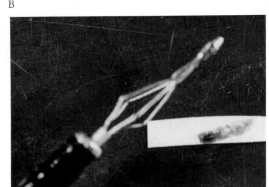

Figure 22-7. Postoperative cholangiography (A) showing several small defects (arrows) which were liver flukes proven by choledochoscopy (B). The liver flukes were removed with the aid of a choledochoscopic basket (C).

C

patient presents with severe cholangitis or if the ascaris is located in a dilated intrahepatic duct with a stenotic orifice so that it cannot return to the duodenum, early surgery may be indicated.

In general, the indications for surgery in biliary ascariasis are (1) failure of medical treatment, (2) persistence of a worm in the biliary system on a second cholangiogram, and (3) obstructive jaundice, cholangitis, or gross hepatomegaly. At surgery, the ascaris worm should be removed from the bile duct, and a T tube should be left for postoperative cholangiography and, if necessary, percutaneous choledochoscopy. In a recent report from Kashmir, India, Chrungoo et al. found that surgery was required in 214 of 876 cases (24%) of biliary ascariasis. The overall mortality rate in this series was 4.3%.

Postoperative Choledochoscopy

As stated above, biliary clonorchiasis is mainly treated by nonoperative methods. However, the authors have operated on 30 patients with proven clonorchiasis and bile duct stones. Postoperative choledochoscopy was performed routinely in these patients. Residual liver flukes were washed out and removed through the T tube sinus tract with a stone basket (Fig. 22-7). Follow-up examinations were performed until eggs were no longer found in the stool and no more liver flukes were found in the bile ducts by choledochoscopy.

Postoperative choledochoscopy has been performed by the authors in 982 patients (Table 22-2). In 30 patients the indication was residual liver flukes, whereas 723 patients had residual in-

Table 22-2. Residual Stones and Liver Flukes
Removed by Postoperative Choledochoscopy

	Number of Patients	Successful Rate (%)
Residual common bile duct stones	228	100
Residual intrahepatic duct stones	723	95
Residual liver flukes	30	100
Fish bone	1	100
TOTAL	982	96

trahepatic stones, and 228 patients had residual common bile duct stones. Postoperative choledochoscopy was successful in all 30 patients with liver flukes and overall in 96% of the patients. The complications of percutaneous choledochoscopy were minimal, and this procedure was very useful for both diagnosis and treatment. Thus the authors believe that postoperative choledochoscopy is very effective for removing residual material and for direct observation of the bile duct mucosa in various biliary tract diseases.

Conclusions

The two most common biliary parasites are *Clonorchis sinensis* and *Ascaris lumbricoides*. *C. sinensis* is an endemic parasite in East Asia, and man is the most suitable definitive host. *A. lumbricoides* is a helminthic parasite which is the most prevalent and largest of human parasites. Both of these parasites can cause stones to form in the biliary system. The diagnosis can be made by finding eggs in the stool, and initial treatment is usually nonoperative. Surgery is indicated in patients who have failed medical treatment and in patients who present with obstructive jaundice or cholangitis. Prognosis is generally good except in unusual patients who develop suppurative cholangitis. Postoperative choledochoscopy via a T tube tract may be very helpful in patients with residual parasites or bile duct stones.

Selected Readings

Chen HH, et al. Twenty-two year experience with the diagnosis and treatment of the intrahepatic calculi. *Surg Gynecol Obstet* 1984; 159:519–524.

Chrungoo RK, et al. Surgical manifestations and management of ascariasis in Kashmir. *J Indian Med Assoc* 1992; 90:171–174.

Eymeri JC, et al. Biliary ascariasis: A case of massive infestation: The importance of the preoperative choledochoscopy. *Chir Pediatr* 1989; 30:178–180.

Ker CG, Huang TJ, Sheen PC. Obstructive jaundice in clonorchiasis. *J Formosan Med Assoc* 1980; 79:1144–1148.

Ker CG, Sheen PC. Ultrastructure and electron microanalysis at the core of human gallstones II: Calcium bilirubinate stones. *Kaohsiung J Med Sci* 1985; 1:744–753.

Ker CG, et al. Direct cholangiographic features and therapeutic methods of biliary ascariasis. *Kaohsiung J Med Sci* 1985; 1:334–342.

Ker CG, et al. Ultrasound survey of hepatobiliary lesions in Kaohsiung, Taiwan. *Trans R Soc Trop Med Hyg* 1984; 78:758–760.

Lee KT, et al. The ultrasonic survey of gallstone disease in Taiwan Aborigines. *J Surg Assoc ROC* 1987; 20:396–400.

Lim JH, et al. Clonorchiasis: Sonographic findings in 59 proved cases. *AJR* 1989; 152:761–764.

Tech TB. A study of gallstones and included worms in recurrent pyogenic cholangitis. *J Pathol Bact* 1963; 86:123–129.

23

Sclerosing Cholangitis

Stanley G. Alexander
Thomas J. Howard
Kenyon K. Kopecky
Glen A. Lehman
Lawrence Lumeng
Rene Male
Stuart Sherman

The number of new cases of primary sclerosing cholangitis (PSC) diagnosed annually has markedly increased in recent years, largely as a result of the more widespread use of screening liver chemistries and the availability of endoscopic retrograde cholangiopancreatography (ERCP). The disease severity varies from asymptomatic individuals with normal or minimal elevations of serum alkaline phosphatase levels to secondary biliary cirrhosis which may be complicated by liver failure and portal hypertension. The disease course of PSC is also quite variable. Although a subset of patients who are asymptomatic at the time of diagnosis may remain stable for many years, the course is most often progressive, leading to advanced cholestatic liver disease. Despite progress in earlier recognition, optimal management of patients with primary sclerosing cholangitis remains a major challenge for hepatologists, endoscopists, gastroenterologists, interventional radiologists, and surgeons.

Etiology and Pathogenesis

The syndrome of sclerosing cholangitis may be broadly divided into primary and secondary forms based upon etiology. In primary sclerosing cholangitis, the most common form, the underlying cause of the inflammatory and fibrotic ductal lesions remain largely unknown. Although the cholangiographic and histologic features may be similar in both forms, they are generally distinguishable following a detailed history. The multiple etiologies of secondary sclerosing cholangitis are listed in Table 23-1. Several mechanisms have been proposed as potentially important in the pathogenesis of PSC, including (1) portal bacteremia, (2) absorption of bacterial toxins or toxic bile acids, (3) copper accumulation, (4) genetic factors, (5) immunologic factors, (6) infectious agents, and (7) ischemia. Autoimmune mechanisms appear to be the most important. Indeed, PSC is strongly associated with human leukocyte antigen (HLA)-B8, DR3 phenotype, a well-established marker of other chronic autoimmune disorders. PSC occurs with a 2:1 male-to-female predominance. Approximately 70% of cases occur in patients with inflammatory bowel disease (IBD), especially chronic ulcerative colitis, but may also be associated with Crohn's colitis. Interestingly, the occurrence and severity of PSC do not parallel disease activity in the colon. Persistent or recurrent liver enzyme abnormalities in patients with inflammatory bowel disease, even if unassociated with symptoms, should raise suspicion to the possibility of concomitant biliary disease. Conclusive evidence as to the etiology of PSC remains elusive, but recent studies show that PSC

247

23-1. Conditions Producing Cholangiograms ich May Mimic Primary Sclerosing Cholangitis

Neoplasms
  Metastatic carcinoma
  Cholangiocarcinoma
  Lymphoma
Cirrhosis
Polycystic liver disease
Caroli's disease
Multiple hepatic abscesses
Systemic fungal infection
Bacterial cholangitis
Secondary sclerosing cholangitis
  Associated with bacterial infection and impacted intrahepatic
    ductal stones
  Associated with immunodeficiency congenital syndromes,
    opportunistic infections (e.g., cytomegalovirus)
Acquired immunodeficiency syndrome
  Associated with CMV, *Cryptosporidium*, papillary stenosis
Graft-versus-host disease
Hepatic arterial ischemia
  Posttraumatic
  Postsurgical (including intentional or inadvertent ligation of
    hepatic artery and complications from liver transplantation)
  Associated with intra-arterial 5-fluorodeoxyuridine (5-FUDR)
  Preservation injury of biliary tract in the donor liver
  Chronic allograft rejection in liver transplantations

patients have antibodies directed toward a shared peptide found in the biliary tract and the colon.

Diagnosis

The diagnosis of PSC is generally based upon a combination of clinical, biochemical, radiologic, and histologic abnormalities.

Symptoms

The onset of symptoms of PSC is typically insidious, with variable manifestations including pruritus, fatigue, jaundice, weight loss, fever, and mild right upper quadrant discomfort. Modest weight loss may result from anorexia or malabsorption due to cholestasis; however, profound or rapid weight loss suggests the possibility of a superimposed cholangiocarcinoma. Overt bacterial cholangitis is unusual as an initial manifestation in the absence of prior biliary tract manipulations such as ERCP or surgical procedures. Approximately 25% of patients have no hepatobiliary symptoms at the time of diagnosis. Detection at earlier stages has resulted from in-

creased awareness of the association between PSC and IBD and appropriate use of endoscopic retrograde cholangiography. Despite limited symptoms, fairly advanced disease may be detected by ERCP or liver biopsy. A small portion of patients may present with complications of portal hypertension, especially hemorrhage from esophageal or gastric varices.

Liver Chemistries

A cholestatic biochemical profile will be found in most cases. Initially, mild elevations in the levels of serum alkaline phosphatase and gamma-glutamyl transpeptidase (two to four times the upper limits of normal) are common. With more advanced disease, higher elevations of these enzymes are common, along with mild to moderate hyperbilirubinemia. Sustained hyperbilirubinemia connotes advanced disease and poor prognosis. Serum transaminase levels are often abnormal, but usually to a lesser extent. As in other liver diseases, low serum albumin levels may reflect more advanced disease or poorer nutritional status. Autoimmune factors are thought to be important in the pathogenesis of PSC; however, specific autoantibodies with diagnostic usefulness have not been found. Less specific autoantibodies, such as anti–neutrophil peripheral cytoplasmic antibodies (p ANCA) are found in 60% of patients with PSC. Antimitochondrial antibodies are nearly always absent in PSC, which is a helpful distinguishing feature in cases where primary biliary cirrhosis is also a concern.

Noninvasive Imaging ?

All patients with cholestasis should have liver parenchymal and/or biliary imaging with transcutaneous ultrasound or computerized tomography (CT) imaging. Ultrasound evaluates the gallbladder and ducts better for calculi, but CT gives better liver parenchymal and adjacent organ information.

Liver Biopsy

Histologic changes found on liver biopsy may be helpful but are more often nonspecific. Segmental involvement of the intrahepatic bile ducts is sometimes seen and may limit the diagnostic value of liver biopsy because of sampling error. Needle biopsies of the liver are primarily useful for staging the severity of liver disease, which is helpful in determining prognosis. Biopsies may also be helpful in excluding malignancy and in the minority of patients who may have "small duct PSC," in which characteristic histologic findings are present without associated cholangiographic abnormalities. The proportion of PSC patients in the latter category is unclear.

Cholangiography

Cholangiographic imaging of the biliary tree is essential for the definitive diagnosis of PSC. Initial cholangiography serves to establish a diagnosis and to evaluate for other mechanical diseases causing cholestasis, and also serves as a guide for future therapy. Both percutaneous transhepatic cholangiography (PTC) and ERCP may be used to show the characteristic changes. Intravenous cholangiography is usually not adequate. The choice between PTC and ERCP will depend on local or regional expertise and availability. When available, ERCP is generally considered the procedure of choice because (1) the often small fibrotic ducts of PSC may be difficult to puncture via the percutaneous route and (2) problems with traversing the peritoneal cavity (and potentially the pleural space) and the liver capsule are avoided. The disadvantage of ERCP is that it is generally more technically demanding and may provoke pancreatitis or cholangitis. Both techniques allow for tissue sampling of any lesions suspicious of malignancy and for the application of therapy if treatable obstructions are found. In difficult cases, both techniques may be required.

Preparation for Diagnostic Cholangiography

Percutaneous cholangiography can be performed safely, without decompression, even if treatable obstructions are found. By contrast, ERCP involves injection of bacterially contaminated contrast media, which may provoke cholangitis and an urgent need for simultaneous therapy if treatable lesions are found. Administration of prophylactic antibiotics, such as third-generation cephalosporins, is recommended. If at all possible, patients with overt cholangitis should generally be treated for 1 to 2 days with full therapeutic antibiotic doses before proceeding with cholangiography. Alternatively, a septic patient may require urgent decompression. A careful bleeding history is needed, and coagulation parameters should be checked on all patients. Prothrombin time greater than 3 seconds over control, partial thromboplastin time greater than 5 seconds over control, and platelet count less than 50,000 generally warrant correction of coagulopathy before proceeding. Relatively dilute contrast media (e.g., 20% to 30% meglumine diatrizoate) are preferable for demonstrating stones and biliary debris which may be present and significantly contributing to jaundice or cholangitis. More concentrated contrast media (e.g., 60% meglumine diatrizoate) are preferred for defining strictures and details of peripheral biliary radicles. The patient should be questioned regarding his or her previous history of contrast reactions. Blood pressure and pulse oximetry monitoring are recommended during sedative or analgesic administration.

The informed consent process should review risks, benefits, and alternatives. The authors recommend obtaining simultaneous consent for ERCP and PTC if needed. It should be emphasized to the patient and care givers that stents and percutaneous drainage catheters may be needed for an extended period of time and that the latter will require appropriate home care.

Technique of Diagnostic ERCP

Successful standard major papilla cannulation is required at ERCP. Aggressive cannulation techniques are generally warranted in this group because detailed cholangiography is essential. Use of precutting is warranted in experienced hands. Once cannulation is achieved, full cholangiography of the intrahepatic and extrahepatic biliary tree is generally required. If therapeutic techniques are not immediately available, care should be taken to not put more than 2 to 3 ml of contrast media above high-grade strictures. Not uncommonly, contrast media will take the path of least resistance and enter the cystic duct and normal gallbladder. Intrahepatic filling is therefore limited. Preferably, a balloon catheter is then manipulated above the cystic duct take-off, and higher pressure injection of the intrahepatic radicles is undertaken. Extra care should be taken to keep catheters and equipment in their least contaminated state.

Cholangiographic Findings

Typical changes of sclerosing cholangitis are a combination of stricturing and upstream saccular dilatations. Although focal segmental narrowings are typical, diffuse narrowing is not uncommon. Involved ducts commonly have a beaded appearance. Pseudodiverticula of the common bile duct or common hepatic duct are seen in approximately one fourth of cases and are essentially diagnostic. Intrahepatic radicles may have a pruned appearance, since small ductules do not fill. Diffuse involvement of the intrahepatic and extrahepatic duct is typical and is seen in approximately 75% to 80% of affected patients. Isolated involvement of the intrahepatic ducts is seen in 10% to 20%, and predominant extrahepatic involvement occurs in 10% to 20%. The gallbladder and cystic duct are usually spared. Chronic pancreatitis changes at pancreatography are seen in 10% to 20% of patients and are generally asymptomatic. Extrahepatic strictures which severely compromise the duct lumen (greater than 90% decrease in diameter) are referred to as dominant strictures, and such strictures generally contribute to cholestasis. Brush cytology or fine-needle or forceps biopsy should generally be obtained from all dominant strictures or polypoid lesions, since cholangiocarcinoma occurs in up to 40% of sclerosing cholangitis patients in their terminal (pretransplant) state. The sensitivity of these tissue sampling methods in this setting needs clarification.

Differential Diagnosis

Several other disease conditions may cause cholangiographic findings which mimic PSC or cause secondary sclerosing cholangitis (see Table 23-1). Multiple liver metastases or abscesses may cause compression of the intrahepatic ducts, simulating PSC. Infectious cholangitis, either in the immunosuppressed patient (e.g., AIDS patients with cytomegalovirus [CMV] or *Cryptosporidium*) or patients with gallstones (bacterial cholangitis), may mimic PSC. Untreated chronic biliary obstruction, as from gallstones or extrahepatic strictures, may cause chronic stasis, bacterial infection, and strictures. Oriental subjects are particularly prone to this prob-

lem. Graft-versus-host disease following bone marrow transplantation and ischemic injury, as occurs from hepatic arterial chemotherapy with 5-fluorodeoxyuridine, or compromise of nutrient vessels to the common bile duct wall, as from liver transplant, may cause a PSC-like picture. Chronic allograft rejection can also cause a PSC-like complication after liver transplantation.

No single test should be used alone in establishing a diagnosis of PSC or secondary cholangitis. The total history, noninvasive images, and serum liver tests must be taken into account.

Management and Results

Therapy of PSC clearly requires multidisciplinary input. Initial (usually medical) management is provided by the gastroenterologist/hepatologist. As the disease progresses, other specialists are commonly needed.

No firm guidelines are available to tell the clinician when to intervene in the search for and treatment of dominant strictures. The authors' general practice has been to perform diagnostic cholangiography (with potential to proceed to therapy) in persons who have unexplained alkaline phosphatase levels of more than twice normal or gammaglutamyl transpeptidase levels of more than three times normal (assuming the patient otherwise has anticipated longevity). In patients with documented PSC and alkaline phosphatase levels more than three to four times the upper limit of normal, a bilirubin level greater than 1.5, or cholangitis, search for dominant strictures seems clearly warranted. Good evidence exists that stricture therapy in patients with cholangitis decreases cholestasis symptoms and cholangitis frequency. It is presumed, but not proven, that such therapy slows the rate of parenchymal destruction and progression of cirrhosis.

Medical Therapy

Most medical treatments, including corticosteroids, cholestyramine, colchicine, penicillamine, azathioprine, and antibiotics, have no proven benefit. Recent follow-up reports of the use of methotrexate have also failed to show benefit. Ursodeoxycholic acid (ursodiol) may improve biochemical parameters but has no definite effect on histology or the natural course of the disease. In addition to ursodiol, pruritus can be ameliorated by cholestyramine, antihistamines, phenobarbital, and rifampin (10 mg/kg/d). Nutritional therapy may include supplemental calories (using medium-chain triglycerides), vitamins (parenteral vitamins A, D, and K and oral water-soluble vitamin E), and minerals (particularly calcium and zinc).

Interventional Radiology   ? when is this ? an option?

Interventional radiologic techniques in the management of PSC serve to complement endoscopy and surgery. Percutaneous access and procedures are usually employed when endoscopic access is impossible because of prior surgery (e.g., Roux-en-Y gastrojejunostomy) or has been unsuccessful in demonstrating or treating the disease. Likewise, when surgery needs to be delayed, is contraindicated, or has been tried and the patient manifests recurrent symptoms, percutaneous techniques may provide palliation or salvage the surgical correction.

The history of interventional radiology in the management of PSC is a subset of the broader history of biliary interventions in the management of other benign and malignant diseases. Although many studies of biliary interventions included a small number of cases of PSC in their study populations, results are difficult to extrapolate given the relatively small case material. Contraindications for intervention are few and mostly relative: incorrectable coagulation defects, massive ascites, anatomy that precludes percutaneous access such as interposed bowel, or end-stage cirrhosis.

Imaging of the liver preoperatively with ultrasound or CT is useful to define the biliary anatomy and pathology (Figs. 23-1, 23-2). Because sclerosing cholangitis does not uniformly affect all bile ducts, there may be biliary dilatation in some areas and not in others. Knowledge of this anatomy prior to percutaneous transhepatic cholangiography (PTC) can improve the efficacy of the intervention by guiding the PTC (and drainage procedure) to the areas of most severe biliary dilatation. In patients with signs and symptoms of bacterial cholangitis, CT can detect the presence of associated abscesses (Fig. 23-3). Occasionally, the larger ab-

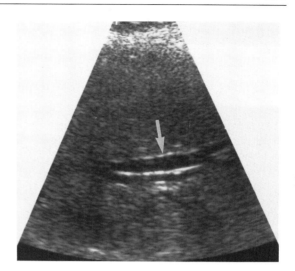

Figure 23-1. Ultrasound shows a dilated left hepatic duct (arrow) lying just anterior to the left portal vein. Doppler sonography (not shown) is useful to distinguish between the duct and vein.

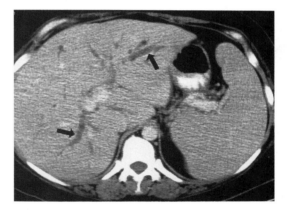

Figure 23-2. Enhanced CT scan shows dilated bile ducts (arrows) in both lobes of the liver.

scesses require percutaneous drainage in addition to drainage of the obstructed bile ducts.

Unless a T tube or other biliary catheter is in place, the percutaneous transhepatic cholangiogram is the usual de novo approach to gain access to the biliary tree. A fine (22-gauge) needle is advanced into the liver from a percutaneous entry site identified by ultrasound guidance and/or fluoroscopic observation. Once the needle tip is confirmed as being intraductal, sufficient contrast is then intro-

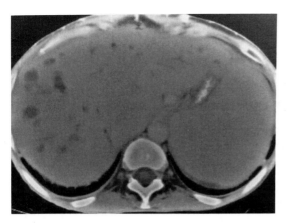

Figure 23-3. CT scan without intravenous contrast material shows focal abscesses in the right lobe of the liver, slight biliary dilatation in the left lobe, and splenomegaly. More inferior scans showed dilated right lobe ducts as well. This patient with sclerosing cholangitis had superimposed acute bacterial infection with liver abscesses.

duced into the biliary tree to opacify the radicles and central ducts. Radiographs are obtained in multiple projections.

The PTC (Fig. 23-4A) is utilized in diagnosis and planning for intervention and serves as the platform from which to launch other procedures. The PTC needle usually enters the biliary tree in a large duct near the center of the liver, and the needle may have passed through a large branch of the portal vein or hepatic artery before entering the bile duct; therefore, it may be dangerous to introduce a guidewire and catheter from the initial central biliary access site because of the risk of creating a portal vein to biliary fistula. Thus, after the PTC, a second fine-needle access is performed utilizing the now opacified biliary tree to specifically select a small peripherally located duct. This process requires multidirectional fluoroscopy. The second access approach is from below the tenth rib, if possible, for right lobe access and below the xyphoid for left lobe access. Intercostal access above the tenth rib is acceptable if a more caudal pathway is not possible, with the recognition that pleural fluid collections may result. A wire is introduced into the desired duct, and then exchanges can be performed for larger working catheters, guidewires, and devices.

After catheterization of the biliary tree, it is desirable to pass a wire and catheter through the stricture(s) and into the intestine. Most strictures can be traversed easily with a torque-stable, hydrophilic-coated guidewire with an angled tip. In the unusual event that a stricture cannot be traversed in the initial session, an external drain can be placed above the level of the stricture. Once the obstructed system is decompressed and inflammation has subsided, the stricture can usually be crossed in a second session.

Combined internal and external drainage is preferred to external drainage alone because the tube position is more stable and accidental catheter dislodgement is less likely. The catheter is directed through the strictured biliary segment into the common bile duct and then into the duodenum (or jejunum if the patient has a choledochojejunostomy). The process of passing sequentially larger-sized catheters through a stenosis serves to dilate it. Secure positioning of the catheter is facilitated by depositing a sufficient length within the small bowel. Specialized catheters with a pigtail-shaped loop at the tip which is placed inside the bowel lumen add more security to the catheter position. Because these tubes have side holes both at the level of the bile ducts and at the level of the intestine, bile can flow into the intestine or externally into a bag, or in both directions simultaneously. The external hub of the catheter can be capped once the patient has clinically stabilized, and subsequently the bile will flow exclusively enterically. Internal drainage is preferable to external drainage for several reasons: (1) fluids are conserved, preventing dehydration; (2) bile salts are preserved, maintaining enterohepatic circulation; and (3) the patients do not have to wear a bag.

The patients are told that if pain or fever develop, they are to connect the external catheter to bag drainage and call, because the tube may have become clogged. After administration of fluids and antibiotics, a diagnostic cholangiogram is obtained by injecting contrast material through the tube. If the tube is partially or totally occluded, it is replaced over a guidewire for a new one. To prevent episodes of cholangitis due to sludge accumulation within the tubes, the tubes are routinely replaced every 3 or 4 months. Chronic antibiotic prophylaxis is not used for patients with indwelling biliary catheters.

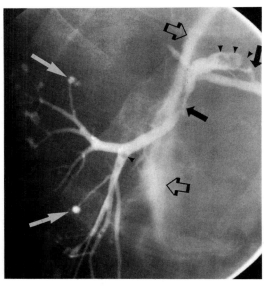
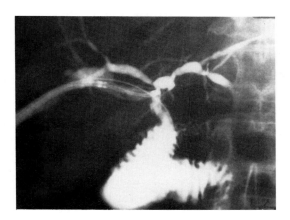

A   B

Figure 23-4. A. PTC shows two focal biliary strictures (black arrows). Bile duct stones (arrowheads) are seen as filling defects within the contrast material upstream from the strictures. Small abscesses (white arrows) are also seen in this patient with acute bacterial infection. Extravasation of contrast material (open arrows) occurred from the needle entry site into the bile duct; however, this leakage caused no clinical sequelae. A percutaneous catheter was placed through the two strictures and into the jejunum. B. Six weeks later, after the percutaneous tract had matured, percutaneous endoscopy was performed, and the stones were fragmented with a pulsed dye laser and removed.

Antibiotics are reserved for episodes of clinically evident cholangitis.

Transhepatic balloon dilatation or cholangioplasty may be used to treat biliary strictures, including those due to PSC. High-pressure balloons are introduced into the stricture and dilatations are performed, expanding the stenosis to diameters typically between 4 and 10 mm, determined by measuring adjacent nondiseased ducts. Attention should be focused on one or more dominant strictures, if present. These strategic strictures are typically located at or near the junction of the right and left hepatic ducts. Subsequently, these stenoses are stented following cholangioplasty and over the course of several sessions, the stents are gradually increased in diameter, usually to 8 to 16 French. The optimal time for stents to remain in place after cholangioplasty is unknown. Because of the progressive nature of the disease, sometimes the stents are left in place for the life of the patient or until the patient receives a liver transplant. Stents are

removed prior to this time with the understanding that they may have to be replaced if the strictures recur.

Overall, improvement in cholestasis or cholangitis is seen in approximately 80% of PSC patients with dominant strictures. Gradual subsequent deterioration is common, and repeat dilatations are needed during the next 3 years in more than half of the patients. Complications reported from radiologic interventional biliary procedures include cholangitis (the most commonly experienced complication) sepsis, hemobilia, hemorrhage, pneumothorax, liver abscess, retroperitoneal abscess, hepatic artery pseudoaneurysm, and subphrenic fluid collections. Pleural effusions, some containing bile, have been reported where transhepatic access has been attained via a transpleural approach. Overall, major complications occur in 5% to 10% of patients, and deaths have been reported.

In cases of recurrent benign biliary strictures where other therapies have failed or are contraindicated, self-expanding metallic stents may provide an effective method of achieving patency across strictures. In two benign stricture series totalling 24 patients, metal stents were successful in relieving symptoms and normalizing liver-related tests in approximately 80% of patients. PSC patients generally responded less well than patients with strictures of other etiologies. These stents become incorporated in bile duct mucosa and cannot be removed. Because restenosis eventually develops in bile ducts containing metal stents, and because the stents may interfere with or prevent subsequent surgery, most physicians are extremely reluctant to use them for benign disease. Such stents are easily removed with the diseased liver during transplantation, as long as they do not extend into the common bile duct.

New devices and techniques continue to be developed for the potential management of PSC patients. Percutaneous transhepatic access has been utilized to introduce small ultrasound transducers within bile ducts. Such devices may quantitate periductular fibrosis and characterize the composition of intraluminal filling defects (clot versus stone versus tumor). In the future, they may prove helpful in differentiating benign from malignant strictures. Transhepatic tracts can be utilized to introduce fiberoptic endoscopes into the biliary tree. Percutaneous choledochoscopy can be used in conjunction with pulsed dye laser lithotripsy to treat intrahepatic stones (see Fig. 23-4B). Endoscopy can guide stone basketing and biopsy procedures. Biopsies have been performed using needles, brushes, forceps, and atherectomy devices. Stents and drainage catheters which resist biofilm accumulation and occlusion are being tested. Catheters with one-way valves may inhibit enterobiliary reflux.

In some patients with a choledochojejunostomy or a hepatojejunostomy, it is possible to access the biliary tree without a transhepatic approach. Percutaneous needle access to a loop of jejunum near the porta hepatis has been reported. Through this entry, catheters have been guided in a retrograde direction across the biliary-jejunal anastomosis. To facilitate retrograde percutaneous access, some surgeons, at the time of creation of the hepatojejunostomy, have sutured the surface of the small bowel to the anterior abdominal wall. By placing radiopaque markers around this site, subsequent

percutaneous entry under fluoroscopic guidance is facilitated.

Collaboration involving the radiologist and the endoscopist in a combined effort offers opportunities to address complex biliary interventions using the strengths and advantages of each approach. Combined procedures permit passage of a guidewire percutaneously into the biliary tree, through a stricture, and into the intestine, where the other end of the wire is grasped endoscopically. This control of both ends of the wire permits passage of catheters and balloons through severe stenoses that may be otherwise untreatable.

Sounds like the best course of action?

Endoscopic Therapy

Endoscopic stricture dilation has been reported in PSC over the last 10 years, but published series total less than 200 patients. Favorable anatomic cholangiographic features include one or more extrahepatic short strictures associated with obstructing stone material and sparing of intrahepatic radicles. Such ideal anatomy is uncommon. Patients less likely to respond are those with severe diffuse narrowing of the intrahepatic ducts without focal extrahepatic strictures. Sphincterotomy is routinely performed to permit easier access to the biliary tree. It is unknown whether the enteric-biliary reflux created by the sphincterotomy is hazardous in the long run. Like the interventional radiologist, the endoscopist uses dilating catheters, stone extraction baskets, and stents. Nasobiliary tubes may be used for saline or steroid lavage. Series vary, but generally they show that one fourth to one half of PSC patients will have an endoscopically treatable lesion.

Overall, the technique is relatively simple, in that a guidewire must be passed through a narrowed segment (hydrophilic wires are very helpful) and subsequently balloons (preferably low-profile or no-profile) or Soehendra-type push catheters are advanced. Newer high-pressure balloons permitting inflation to 10 to 12 atm have decreased the frequency of failure to obliterate the waistline for endoscopically passed balloons, but may have a higher risk of duct perforation (Fig. 23-5). Strictures are generally dilated to match the size of adjacent normal ducts (i.e., generally 4 to 6 mm for

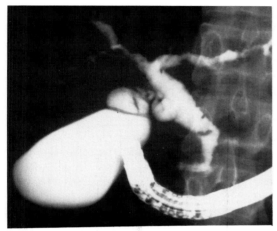

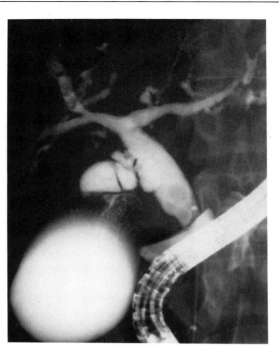

A   B

Figure 23-5. A. ERCP of patient with sclerosing cholangitis. Irregularities of the intrahepatic and extrahepatic ducts are seen, along with stricturing of the right and left hepatic ducts. B. An 8-mm hydrostatic balloon is present in the distal common bile duct. Strictures of the right hepatic duct and left hepatic duct have already been dilated and show considerable improvement in diameter compared to the baseline study. Intrahepatic stones are still evident in a branch of the right hepatic duct. The bilirubin level dropped from 1.5 down to normal, and the alkaline phosphatase level dropped after therapy from 800 IU/dl to 325 IU/dl.

intrahepatic ducts and 6 to 10 mm for extrahepatic ducts). Strictures which are too tight to pass anything other than a guidewire can generally be managed by leaving the guidewire in overnight and returning the next day for passage of at least a 5 French catheter.

Overall, approximately 80% of desired strictures can be endoscopically treated. Endoscopic failures are generally referred for percutaneous approach or assistance. Leaving a nasobiliary catheter in the extrahepatic duct below the stricture of interest can be useful to the percutaneous interventionalist to aid in cholangiography immediately prior to percutaneous puncture. Placement of a balloon catheter in this position is optimal. Approximately three fourths of patients undergoing stricture dilation will have obvious clinical benefit, with a lowering of serum bilirubin or alkaline phosphatase levels by at least 50% or a decrease or elimination of cholangitis episodes.

If stricture dilation shows good postdilatation cholangiographic effect, no stents are generally placed. If significant stricture remains, placement of 7 to 10 French stents is recommended. Removal of stents and further dilation are recommended in 2 or 3 months. Once the desired dilatation is achieved, some authorities ask patients to return at 6- to 12-month intervals for empiric redilatation (the authors' approach) rather than return only for deteriorating liver serum chemistries or recurrent pruritus, jaundice, or cholangitis. Minimal data are available on irrigating the biliary tree with steroids or saline. To date, the value of such irrigations is inconclusive.

Overall endoscopic therapy, like percutaneous therapy, appears to temporize the downhill course of PSC patients with dominant strictures. Such therapy has not been applied long enough to know if patients can be salvaged from death or liver transplant.

is this an option now or in

Surgical Therapy *Secondary stage only?*

Early surgical experience with PSC was disappointing, but surgical management has evolved steadily over the last decade. Current surgical aims are to improve the quality of life and long-term survival rates in patients by applying one of the two surgical options to properly selected patients: (1) extrahepatic biliary resection and biliary-enteric bypass, with or without long-term transhepatic stenting (nontransplant surgery for PSC); or (2) orthotopic liver transplantation. No role exists for prophylactic protocolectomy in the treatment of PSC when it coexists with ulcerative colitis.

Although nontransplant surgery has a longer history than radiologic and endoscopic interventions, the increasing availability of experienced interventional radiologists and therapeutic endoscopists and the lesser morbidity associated with catheter methods currently give nontransplant surgery for PSC a very limited role. No prospective randomized studies have been published comparing any of the therapeutic modalities. In selected settings where skilled interventional radiologists or endoscopists are not available or in patients who are intolerant to or unable to travel to locations for repeated catheter interventions, nontransplant surgical approaches should be considered. Occasionally, concern over malignancy in a dominant stricture may warrant resection.

In 1982, Pitt and colleagues reported an aggressive approach to the extrahepatic biliary system in patients with PSC. In their series, 17 of 22 patients (77%) from 1974 to 1980 underwent extrahepatic biliary resection and choledochoenteric anastomosis. Thirteen of these patients (77%) had a good or excellent result following surgery. In addition, 18 of these patients (82%) were alive with a mean of 52 months after operation and 64 months following establishment of the diagnosis. This series represented a definite change in surgical management

and, although uncontrolled, suggested a probable improvement in long-term survival rates.

Cameron and colleagues noted that hepatic hilar stricturing was nearly universal in PSC and that this area was most severely involved in 67% of patients. They therefore resected the hepatic duct bifurcation, dilated the intrahepatic biliary tree, and permanently stented the ductal system with polymeric silicone (Silastic) transhepatic biliary stents in 31 patients with a bilirubin level equal to or greater than 5 mg/dl or severe recurrent bouts of cholangitis and a dominant extrahepatic bile duct stricture. The overall operative mortality rate for this series was 9.7% (40% for 5 cirrhotic patients and 4% for 26 noncirrhotic patients). Overall actuarial survival rates at 1, 3, and 5 years were 80%, 76%, and 63%, respectively. Among the 26 patients without cirrhosis, actuarial 1-, 3-, and 5-year survival rates were 92%, 87%, and 71%, respectively. Four patients in this series whose hepatic function deteriorated during follow-up have subsequently gone on to have a successful liver transplant.

These data support the use of extrahepatic bile duct resection and hepaticojejunostomy or intrahepatic choledochojejunostomy as an effective method of palliation for a very selected group of patients with PSC. Close follow-up must be maintained, since approximately 15% of these patients will go on to require liver transplantation for progressive hepatic dysfunction, despite adequate extrahepatic biliary drainage. This option should, however, be limited to those patients who have failed endoscopic and radiologic stricture therapies and who exhibit no evidence of biliary cirrhosis on liver biopsy. Hepatic transplantation in the setting of a prior hepaticojejunostomy is technically demanding. Experiences vary, but there is evidence that both morbidity and mortality of liver transplantation are adversely affected by prior hepatobiliary surgery.

Liver Transplantation

Selecting the optimal timing for liver transplantation is difficult because the natural history of PSC is poorly understood. In the Mayo Clinic experience, 174 patients with established PSC were followed for 6 years, during which time 34% died. The median survival from the time of diagnosis of PSC was 11.9 years. Subsequently, five major medical centers combined data on 426 PSC patients. Cox proportional hazard regression modeling was used to identify clinical variables most important in predicting survival. Multivariate analysis revealed that the following variables were independent survival predictors: total serum bilirubin level,

age, histological stage, and the presence or absence of splenomegaly. Studies are currently under way to further evaluate these models in regard to optimal timing for liver transplantation.

In general, a patient should be evaluated for liver transplantation when any of the following manifestations exist: (1) gastrointestinal bleeding from portal hypertension; (2) persistent jaundice (> 5 mg/dl); (3) spontaneous bacterial peritonitis

Figure 23-6. Scheme for the management of sclerosing cholangitis patients. ＊ *Where is Jim on this tree?*

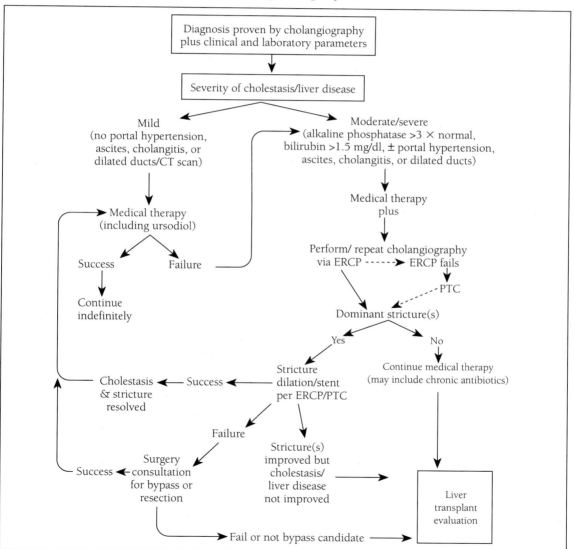

or intractable ascites; (4) repeated bouts of cholangitis not readily controlled by catheter techniques; (5) evidence of liver failure (encephalopathy or loss of synthetic function); or (6) poor quality of life (intractable pruritus, intense fatigue, bone pain associated with hepatic osteodystrophy). These patients should be referred in early stages of the disease to transplantation centers to get them involved in the process and for a close follow-up to determine the best timing. Appropriate financial and social support is essential for this costly and complex intervention.

Liver transplantation is a standard form of treatment for end-stage liver diseases. Recent success and refinement of technique have made this the best option in patients with PSC in terminal stages or with poor quality of life. In the largest series, from the University of Pittsburgh, PSC was the third most common indication for orthotopic liver transplantation in adults, preceded only by postnecrotic cirrhosis and primary biliary cirrhosis. This series included 55 patients with PSC who had liver transplantation. Seventeen patients had a previous unsuccessful surgical attempt to drain the biliary tract, and 8 others had T tube or percutaneous transhepatic catheter drainage before transplantation. The survival rates after transplantation at 1 and 3 years were 71% and 57%, respectively. Previously unrecognized cholangiocarcinoma was found in 10% of the patients. This complication, together with very advanced disease and the high incidence of pretransplantation surgical procedures, was probably responsible for the 29% mortality rate in the first year.

Several series have reviewed the recurrence rate of PSC in the transplanted liver. Biliary complications, especially strictures, do appear to be slightly more frequent in patients with PSC after transplantation when compared to other transplant indications.

In conclusion, the best and only major treatment available for terminal PSC is liver transplantation. Appropriate follow-up in a pretransplant clinic is recommended to optimize management and the potential timing of transplantation.

Therapy of Secondary Sclerosing Cholangitis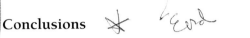

Therapy of this group of diseases is largely directed toward management (if possible) of the underlying disease. Alternatively, stricture management methods outlined for PSC often apply here as well. Selectively, these patients may be candidates for liver transplantation or retransplantation.

Conclusions

Sclerosing cholangitis remains a challenging disease for all physicians involved. A multidisciplinary approach clearly appears optimal. A schema for patient management is outlined in Fig. 23-6. Further research into the etiology, prevention, and other improved treatments for this disease is awaited.

Selected Readings

Ament A, et al. Primary sclerosing cholangitis: CT findings. *J Comput Assist Tomogr* 1983; 7:795–800.

Cameron JL, et al. Resection of the hepatic duct bifurcation and transhepatic stenting for sclerosing cholangitis. *Ann Surg* 1988; 207:614–622.

Carroll BA, Oppenheimer DA. Sclerosing cholangitis: Sonographic demonstration of bile duct wall thickening. *AJR* 1982; 139:1016–1018.

Chaspak LW, et al. Multidisciplinary approach to complex endoscopic biliary intervention. *Radiology* 1989; 170:995–997.

Cotton PB, Nickl N. Endoscopic and radiologic approaches to therapy in primary sclerosing cholangitis. *Semin Liver Dis* 1991; 11:40–48.

Knox TA, Kaplan MM. A double-blind, controlled trial of oral-pulse methotrexate therapy in the treatment of primary sclerosing cholangitis. *Gastroenterology* 1994; 106:494–499.

O'Brien CB, et al. Ursodeoxycholic acid for the treatment of primary sclerosing cholangitis: A 30-month pilot study. *Hepatology* 1991; 14:838–847.

Rahn NH, et al. CT appearance of sclerosing cholangitis. *AJR* 1983; 141:549–552.

Pitt HA, et al. Primary sclerosing cholangitis: Results of an aggressive surgical approach. *Ann Surg* 1982; 196:259–268.

Wiesner RH, et al. Selection and timing of liver transplantation in primary biliary cirrhosis and primary sclerosing cholangitis. *Hepatology* 1992; 16(5):1290–1299.

24

Benign Strictures

KEITH D. LILLEMOE
ADAM B. WINICK
ANTHONY N. KALLOO

A benign bile duct stricture is a serious and potentially devastating complication which usually occurs as the result of a technical mishap associated with cholecystectomy. If it is unrecognized or managed improperly, life-threatening complications such as biliary cirrhosis, portal hypertension, and cholangitis may develop. Prompt recognition and treatment are essential to ensure optimal results. In recent years numerous technological developments have facilitated the diagnosis and management of bile duct strictures. Bile duct strictures can be managed successfully by surgeons, radiologists, or gastroenterologists; however, in most cases a combined modality approach will lead to optimal management.

Etiology and Pathogenesis

Benign bile duct strictures have numerous causes (Table 24-1). Most benign strictures occur following primary operations on the gallbladder or biliary tree. With the introduction of laparoscopic cholecystectomy in recent years, bile duct injuries and associated strictures have been seen more frequently. Injury to the bile ducts can also occur during nonbiliary operations or as a result of penetrating or blunt abdominal trauma. Inflammatory conditions such as chronic pancreatitis, gallstones within the gallbladder or bile duct, stenosis of the sphincter of Oddi, duodenal ulcers, or biliary tract infections can cause benign bile duct strictures. Finally, primary sclerosing cholangitis, a rare disease of unknown etiology, can result in multiple strictures to the intrahepatic and extrahepatic bile ducts. This chapter will focus on the management of postoperative bile duct strictures.

The majority of benign bile duct strictures occur as a result of an iatrogenic injury to the biliary tree during cholecystectomy. The exact incidence of bile duct injury is unknown, since many go unreported in the literature. Data gathered from the pre–laparoscopic cholecystectomy years suggest that the incidence of bile duct injury during open cholecystectomy is approximately 0.1% to 0.2%. The incidence of bile duct injury following laparoscopic cholecystectomy is clearly higher. A wide range in the incidence of such injuries has been reported; however, many reports reflect either the early learning curve with the procedure or the results of large personal series. The most accurate data for the true incidence of such injuries following laparoscopic cholecystectomy probably come from surveys encompassing thousands of patients. The incidence reported in such series is in the range of 0.4% to 0.6%.

A number of factors appear to be associated with bile duct injuries during cholecystectomy, including significant acute or chronic inflammation of the gallbladder, congenital ductal anomalies, and patient obesity. Technical factors associated with laparoscopic cholecystectomy may also increase the risk of bile duct injury when compared to the open procedure. These factors include the use of an end-viewing laparoscope, which alters the surgeon's perspective of the operative field. Excessive cephalad retraction of the gallbladder fundus may cause the

259

Table 24-1. Causes of Benign Bile Duct Strictures

Postoperative Strictures
   Injuries occurring at primary biliary operations
      Laparoscopic cholecystectomy
      Open cholecystectomy
      Common bile duct exploration
   Injuries at other operative procedures
      Gastrectomy
      Hepatic resection
      Portacaval shunt
      Pancreatic procedures
   Strictures of a biliary-enteric anastomosis
   Blunt or penetrating trauma
Strictures Due to Inflammatory Conditions
   Chronic pancreatitis
   Cholelithiasis and choledocholithiasis
   Primary sclerosing cholangitis
   Sphincter of Oddi stenosis
   Duodenal ulcer
   Crohn's disease
   Viral infections
   Toxic drugs

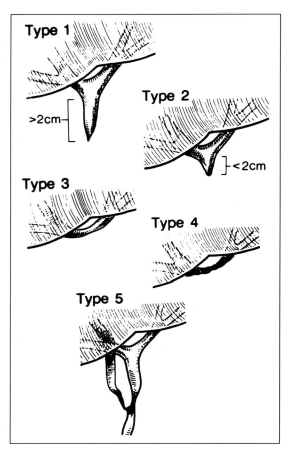

Figure 24-2. Classification of bile duct strictures based on the level of the stricture related to the confluence of the hepatic ducts. (From Bismuth H. Postoperative strictures of the bile duct. In Blumgart LH (ed), *The Biliary Tract*. Clinical Surgery International, vol. 5. Edinburgh: Churchill-Livingstone, 1982. Pp. 209–218. Reproduced by permission.)

Figure 24-1. Classic laparoscopic bile duct injury. A portion of the extrahepatic biliary tree is removed with those ducts transected. The right hepatic artery, in the background, is also usually injured. (From Branum G, et al. Management of major biliary complications after laparoscopic cholecystectomy. *Ann Surg* 1993; 217:532–541. Reproduced by permission.)

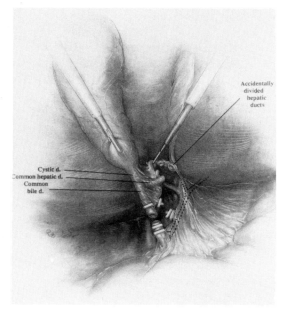

cystic duct and common bile duct to become aligned in the same plane. This distortion often results in the "classic laparoscopic injury," in which the common bile duct is mistaken for the cystic duct and clipped and divided (Fig. 24-1). Finally, the experience of a surgeon in performing laparoscopic cholecystectomy can be correlated with the risk of bile duct injury.

In addition to iatrogenic bile duct injury occurring during cholecystectomy or other operations, postoperative bile duct strictures can occur at a previous biliary anastomosis. Such strictures can occur at a biliary-enteric anastomosis performed for reconstruction after resection for benign or malignant disease of the pancreaticobiliary system or following an end-to-end bile duct anastomosis for repair of a traumatic injury or following liver transplantation. Ischemia of the anastomosis due to excessive skeletonization of the duct in preparation for the anastomosis is probably an important factor in such strictures. Finally, the recurrence of a bile duct stricture following an initial attempt at repair is common. Factors associated with recurrent bile duct stricture include the length of follow-up, multiple previous attempts at repair, the type of repair performed, and the use of perioperative stenting of the biliary anastomosis. The location of a bile duct stricture is also of primary importance in dictating management and predicting outcome. In recognition of the importance of the stricture location, Bismuth has developed a classification of bile duct strictures based on the anatomical pattern of involvement (Fig. 24-2). In general, the higher the location of the stricture, the greater the recurrence rate.

Diagnosis

Most patients with benign postoperative bile duct strictures present soon after their initial operation (Fig. 24-3). Following open cholecystectomy, only about 10% of patients with postoperative strictures are actually suspected within the first week, however; nearly 70% are diagnosed within the first 6 months and over 80% within 1 year of surgery. In the few series reporting bile duct injuries following laparoscopic cholecystectomy, recognition usually occurs either during the procedure or more commonly in the early postoperative period.

Those patients suspected of having postoperative bile duct strictures within days to weeks of the initial operation usually present in one of two ways. The first mode of presentation is the progressive elevation of liver function tests, particularly total bilirubin and alkaline phosphatase levels. These changes can be seen as early as the second or third postoperative day. The development of jaundice may or may not be associated with biliary sepsis. The second mode of early presentation relates to leakage of bile from the injured bile ducts. Bilious drainage from operatively placed drains or through the wound following cholecystectomy is abnormal and undoubtedly represents some form of bile duct injury. When the injury is associated with distal bile duct obstruction, the amount of bilious drainage can represent the entire bile production and can be associated with the development of fluid and electrolyte abnormalities. In those patients without

Figure 24-3. Cumulative percentage of patients developing symptoms with respect to the time interval from the procedure where the injury occurred until the presentation of symptoms. (From Pitt HA, et al. Factors influencing outcome in patients with postoperative biliary strictures. *Am J Surg* 1982; 144:14–21. Reproduced by permission.)

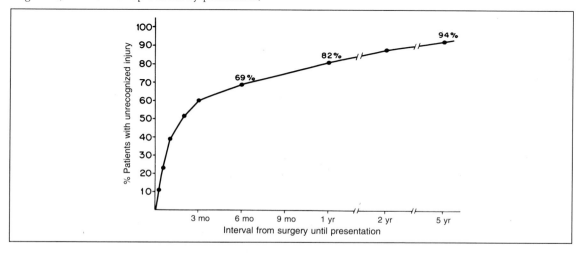

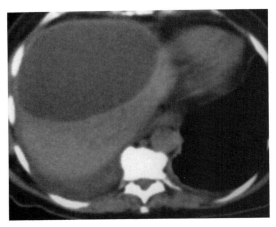

Figure 24-4. Large bile collection (biloma) occurring following bile duct injury. (From Lillemoe KD, Pitt HA, Cameron JL: Current management of benign bile duct strictures. *Adv Surg* 1992; 25:119–174. Reproduced by permission.)

drains or in whom the drains have been removed, the bile may leak freely into the peritoneal cavity as bile ascites or may loculate as a subhepatic or subphrenic collection (Fig. 24-4). This mode of presentation appears to be quite common in patients presenting with bile duct injuries after laparoscopic cholecystectomy.

Patients with postoperative bile duct strictures diagnosed months or years after the initial operation frequently present with cholangitis. Symptoms of fever, chills, abdominal pain, and jaundice can be found in most of these patients. Episodes of cholangitis are frequently mild and respond to antibiotic therapy. Repetitive episodes usually occur prior to definitive diagnosis. Less commonly, patients may present with painless jaundice and no evidence of sepsis. In such cases, malignancy must be considered in the differential diagnosis as the etiology of the biliary obstruction.

The laboratory investigations useful in the diagnosis of a bile duct stricture include liver function tests, which will show evidence of cholestasis. The serum bilirubin level may fluctuate and may occasionally even be normal. Elevations of serum bilirubin are often associated with cholangitis and may represent obstruction of the narrow bile duct lumen by biliary sludge, which forms proximal to the stricture. Serum alkaline phosphatase is usually elevated. Serum transaminase levels may be normal or minimally elevated, but during the episodes of cholangitis, transaminase levels may transiently become very elevated. If advanced liver disease exists with impaired hepatic function, the serum albumin and prothrombin time may become abnormal.

Computerized tomography (CT) is valuable in the initial evaluation of patients with benign postoperative bile duct strictures. In those patients presenting in the early postoperative period with evidence of a bile leak or biliary sepsis, CT is useful for ruling out the presence of intra-abdominal collections which may require drainage (see Fig. 24-4). Moreover, in patients presenting with jaundice months or years after the operation, a CT scan can confirm biliary obstruction by demonstrating a dilated biliary tree and can often predict the site of obstruction based on the extent of dilatation of the extrahepatic bile duct. Finally, in those patients in whom the presentation is remote from their cholecystectomy, a CT scan can also be useful to rule out pancreatic or biliary neoplasms as the cause of jaundice. In patients suspected of having an early postoperative bile duct injury, a radionucleotide biliary scan with iminodiacetic acid may confirm a bile leak. Such studies can quickly and noninvasively confirm the presence of a biliary fistula but may lack the sensitivity to delineate anatomy or the actual site of a leak.

The gold standard for diagnosing a bile duct stricture is cholangiography. Either percutaneous transhepatic cholangiography (PTC) or endoscopic retrograde cholangiography (ERC) can confirm the site of the injury or stricture. ERC is most often the initial route of cholangiography for early bile duct injuries in that the biliary tree may often not be dilated, making PTC technically more difficult. ERC, however, is often limited in that discontinuity of the extrahepatic bile duct usually prevents adequate filling of the proximal biliary tree (Fig. 24-5). In many cases, especially following laparoscopic bile duct injury, ERC may demonstrate a normal-sized distal bile duct up to the site of obstruction. PTC may be more useful in such patients in that it defines the anatomy of the proximal biliary tree, which is used in the surgical reconstruction (Fig. 24-6).

A biliary stent can be placed through the stricture by either the endoscopic or percutaneous transhepatic route. However, for successful endoscopic

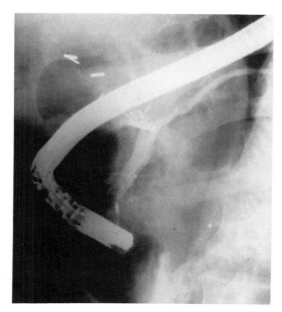

Figure 24-5. Endoscopic retrograde cholangio-pancreatogram showing filling of a normal pancreatic duct; however, the common bile duct does not fill beyond the large ligaclip which appears to be placed across the duct. (From Lillemoe KD, Pitt HA, Cameron JL. Postoperative bile duct strictures. *Surg Clin North Am* 1990; 70:1355–1380. Reproduced by permission.)

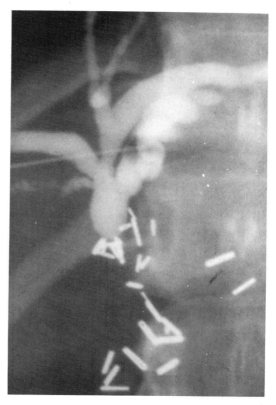

Figure 24-6. Percutaneous transhepatic cholangiogram (PTC) demonstrating a bile duct stricture at the hepatic duct bifurcation with proximal duct dilatation.

stent placement, the bile duct must be in continuity, which is often not the case in patients with the most common forms of laparoscopic injury. Therefore, in most patients, the percutaneous route for cholangiography and placement of transhepatic biliary catheters is most useful in decompressing the biliary system to treat or prevent cholangitis and to control biliary leaks. Finally, these catheters are also of great assistance in surgical reconstruction or to provide access to the biliary tree for nonoperative dilatation.

Management

Injury Recognized at Cholecystectomy

In many cases, the recognition and repair of a bile duct injury at the time of cholecystectomy can prevent the development of a bile duct stricture. Unfortunately, recognition of a bile duct injury is uncommon during either open or laparoscopic cholecystectomy. It must be emphasized that if abnormal bile leakage is noted or if "atypical" anatomy is

encountered, early conversion to an open technique and prompt cholangiography is imperative. If the recognized injury involves the common hepatic duct or common bile duct, repair should be carried out immediately. The aims of any repair should be to maintain ductal length and not sacrifice tissue, as well as to affect a repair which will not result in postoperative bile leakage. To accomplish these goals, all repairs at the time of the initial operation should involve some form of external drainage.

Lateral bile duct injuries, without significant loss of length, are unusual but must be recognized and repaired to avoid a bile leak. If such a defect is small, as with the avulsion injury of the cystic duct, direct repair over a T tube can often be accomplished without the development of a late stricture. Unfortunately, in most cases the bile duct is transected with or without excising a segment of the injured duct. If the injured segment of bile duct is short, generally less than 1 cm, and the two ends can be opposed without tension, then an end-to-end anastomosis can be performed with placement of a T tube through a separate choledochotomy either above or below the anastomosis. An end-to-end repair, however, should be avoided if the ductal injury is high, near the hepatic duct bifurcation. For proximal injuries or if the injured segment of the bile duct is greater than 1 cm in length, an end-to-end anastomosis should be avoided because of the excessive tension which usually exists in these situations. In these circumstances the distal bile duct should be oversewn and the proximal bile duct should be debrided of injured tissue and re-anastomosed in end-to-side fashion to a Roux-en-Y loop of jejunum. Regardless of the type of anastomosis, the area should be drained externally with a closed suction drain.

Initial Management of a Bile Duct Injury or Stricture

The initial management of a patient with postoperative bile duct stricture depends primarily on the timing and presentation. Patients presenting in the early postoperative period may be septic with either cholangitis or intra-abdominal bile collections. Sepsis must be controlled first with broad-spectrum parenteral antibiotics, percutaneous or endoscopic biliary drainage to control the biliary leak, and percutaneous or operative drainage of biliary collections. A combination of proximal biliary decompression and external drainage will allow most biliary fistulas to be controlled or even closed. Once biliary drainage has been achieved and sepsis is controlled, there is **no hurry** in proceeding with definitive management of the bile duct stricture. Attention should be paid to correcting fluid and electrolyte abnormalities, anemia, and nutritional deficits.

In patients presenting with a biliary stricture remote from the initial operation, symptoms of cholangitis or jaundice may lead to cholangiography. If the patient is septic or deeply jaundiced, the placement of either a percutaneous or endoscopic stent to accomplish biliary drainage is essential before proceeding with definitive management. The routine use of preoperative biliary decompression prior to surgical management is controversial, but in most patients prolonged biliary decompression appears to be unnecessary.

Definitive Management

The goal of definitive management of a bile duct stricture is the establishment of bile flow into the proximal gastrointestinal tract in a manner that prevents cholangitis, sludge or stone formation, restricturing, and progressive liver injury. Currently, three options are available for the definitive management of benign postoperative bile duct strictures. These include surgical reconstruction or balloon dilatation and stenting by either the percutaneous or endoscopic route.

SURGICAL RECONSTRUCTION

Several principles are associated with successful surgical repair of a biliary stricture. First, the healthy proximal bile ducts which provide drainage of the entire liver should be exposed. Second, a suitable segment of intestine which can be brought to the area of stricture without tension should be prepared. Most frequently, a Roux-en-Y jejunal limb, at least 40 cm long to avoid reflux of intestinal contents, should be used to provide such a conduit. Finally, a direct biliary-enteric mucosal-to-mucosal anastomosis needs to be created.

The role of a transanastomotic stent of such an anastomosis, however, is controversial. It is the opinion of the authors that a transanastomotic stent is helpful in almost all cases. The placement of transhepatic stents is greatly facilitated with the placement of preoperative percutaneously placed transhepatic catheters. If the stent is near or involves the hepatic bifurcation, at least two preoperative stents should be placed. The valuable aspects of transanastomotic stents are numerous. In the early postoperative period, the stent is useful in decompressing the biliary tree and in providing access for cholangiography or removal of retained intrahepatic stones. Over the long term, the use of a nonreactive silastic stent ensures a stable biliary anastomosis during the period of healing and scar contracture. Finally, the stent allows for follow-up assessment of the anastomosis to ensure an adequate lumen and may provide access for subsequent dilatation if indicated.

After early postoperative cholangiography is performed to document anastomotic integrity and the absence of a biliary leak, the stent can be internalized prior to hospital discharge (Fig. 24-7). After hospital discharge, routine periodic stent changes are recommended, since the side holes of the transhepatic stents can be occluded by biliary sludge and secretions. The stents should be exchanged fluoroscopically over guidewires every 3 to 4 months. This procedure can usually be performed on an outpatient basis, although prophylactic antibiotics are recommended to prevent cholangitis.

In patients with a large bile duct in which circumferential mucosa is available, the period of stenting can be relatively short, usually 6 to 12 weeks. However, when the anastomosis is performed in the hilum of the liver, where the bile ducts are small and only a one-layer anastomosis is possible, the authors have employed transhepatic silastic stents for at least 1 year postoperatively. Prior to stent removal, a Whittaker test, which assesses biliary pressure in response to saline infusion at varying pressures, should be performed to ensure that the anastomosis is patent and will accept a reasonable bile flow. Finally, the stent can be pulled back above the anastomosis and left in place for a 2- to 3-week clinical trial prior to its ultimate removal.

Repairs of bile duct strictures are performed primarily in major medical centers by experienced surgeons. Nevertheless, these operations are still associated with significant morbidity. In the last decade most centers have reported mortality rates of less than 5%, with postoperative morbidity approaching 20% to 30%. Factors such as advanced age, coexistent disease, and a history of major biliary tract infection are associated with increased postoperative complications. However, the state of underlying liver disease is the most important determinant of operative morbidity and mortality. Complications following biliary reconstruction include the usual postoperative problems, such as hemorrhage, cardiopulmonary complications, and infection. Specific complications related to the repair of the bile duct stricture include bile leak at the site of the biliary-enteric anastomosis or at the hepatic exit site of the transhepatic stents, cholangitis, hepatic insufficiency from pre-existing biliary cirrhosis, and hemobilia. Most anastomotic leaks are documented by postoperative cholangiography or by

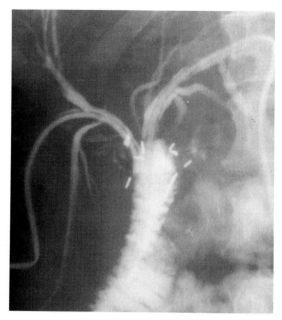

Figure 24-7. Postoperative cholangiogram performed through polymeric silicone biliary stents showing no evidence of anastomotic leak. (From Lillemoe KD, Pitt HA, Cameron JL. Postoperative bile leak strictures. *Surg Clin North Amer* 1990; 70:1355–1380. Reproduced by permission.)

bilious drainage from intraoperatively placed drains and can be successfully managed nonoperatively. Transhepatic stenting externally diverts biliary secretions in the face of the leak and is one of the major advantages to this technique. In the vast majority of these cases, the bile leak heals in short order with no long-term consequences.

Operative management of bile duct strictures is technically difficult and, as already stated, is associated with significant postoperative morbidity. Furthermore, the psychological problems to the patient produced by the need for reoperation has led many groups to support a nonoperative approach to bile duct strictures. Technical advances in the fields of interventional radiology and endoscopy have led to the development of such nonoperative techniques.

NONOPERATIVE MANAGEMENT: PERCUTANEOUS DILATATION

The largest experience in the nonoperative management of benign bile duct strictures is via the percu-

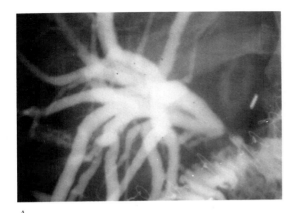

A

Figure 24-8. A. Transhepatic cholangiogram demonstrating stricture at a previous choledochojejunostomy. B. Progressive dilatation of the strictured anastomosis with an angioplasty balloon catheter. C. Postdilatation stenting of the anastomotic stricture for prolonged periods. D. Subsequent cholangiogram demonstrating resolution of the anastomotic stricture. (From Pitt HA, et al. Benign postoperative biliary strictures: Operate or dilate? *Ann Surg* 1989; 210:417–427. Reproduced by permission.)

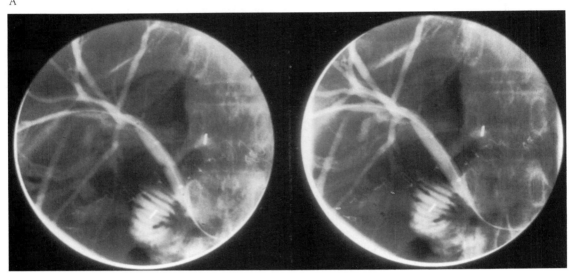

B

taneous transhepatic route. In this technique, access to the proximal biliary tree is gained and the stricture is traversed with a guidewire under fluoroscopic guidance. At this point, the stricture is dilated using angioplasty-type balloon catheters, chosen on the basis of the location of the stricture and the diameter of the normal duct (Fig. 24-8). The balloon is inflated to 10 to 12 atm, or higher if necessary, for at least 30 sec, and the process is repeated until "no waist deformity" is noted during the inflation. After the procedure, a transhepatic silastic stent is left in place across the stricture to allow access to the biliary tree for follow-up cholangiography, repeat dilatation, and maintenance of

the lumen during the healing process. In most series, numerous sittings for dilatation are required.

Alternatively, there has been recent investigation into the use of metallic stents for treatment of benign biliary strictures. Three stents are commercially available: the balloon-expandable Palmaz stent and the self-expandable Wallstent and Gianturco Z-stent. Although significant experience with these stents has been reported for the palliation of malignant strictures, their placement in benign disease is controversial. Metallic stent placement for benign biliary strictures appears to be primarily indicated in patients who have failed previous attempts at surgical reconstruction or percutaneous

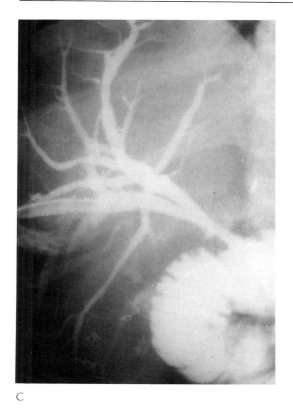

C

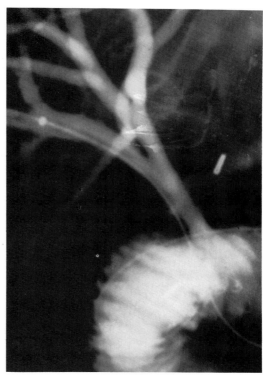

D

Figure 24-8. (continued)

balloon dilatation with prolonged stenting. Finally, metallic stent placement may be appropriate in patients with biliary cirrhosis and portal hypertension from long-standing bile duct obstruction.

Relative contraindications to the use of metallic stents include secondary sclerosing cholangitis due to an increased incidence of stent occlusion. The presence of intrahepatic stone disease also is a relative contraindication because the stones may occlude the stents. Therefore, attempts should be made to remove all calculi before placing stents. Finally, before placing a metallic stent, it must be made clear that attempts at surgical reconstruction or even liver transplantation are not future options because the presence of a metallic stent may make surgery technically difficult.

Short-term complications associated with either balloon dilatation or the placement of metal stents are similar. Cholangitis, hemobilia, and bile leaks can occur in up to 20% of patients. Antibiotic

coverage is necessary before and after the procedure for 24 hours to help prevent cholangitis. Hemobilia occurs frequently but is usually self-limited. However, if bleeding becomes significant, arteriography and arterial embolization may be necessary. Significant bile leakage is rare and is usually due to acute occlusion or migration of the stent. The major long-term complication of metallic stents is occlusion. Occlusion is rarely due to bile encrustation, which is seen in silastic stents; rather, tissue ingrowth slowly occludes the stent. The patient will then present with jaundice and cholangitis. Tissue ingrowth has been the major concern in the use of metallic stents for benign disease. Once metallic stents occlude, they cannot be removed percutaneously and are difficult to remove surgically. Patients will need to be reaccessed percutaneously for placement of an internal/external drainage catheter through the occluded or stenotic stent lumen. Following access across the stent into the bowel, the hyperplastic ingrowth in the stent can be reangioplastied or atherectomized with an atherectomy catheter. Ultimately, however, the patient may need to have another stent placed within the previous stent to maintain patency and to allow for bile flow.

The best current patency rates with metallic stents for benign strictures have been reported with the Gianturco Z-stents. Investigation is currently under way to evaluate the use of coated metallic stents with segmented polymer or silicone membranes. Theoretically, the membranes should prevent ingrowth and occlusion of the stents. At present the use of plastic stents should be avoided because of a higher incidence of occlusion. However, investigations are under way to develop hydrogel coatings that may decrease the incidence of occlusion. Bonding of the hydrogel with antibiotics that are slowly released into the system may also prevent cholangitis.

NONOPERATIVE MANAGEMENT:
ENDOSCOPIC DILATATION

The experience with endoscopic dilatation and stenting is somewhat more limited. The endoscopic approach is favored by many groups because it avoids the more painful percutaneous access and the higher incidence of biliary infection associated with external stents. Endoscopic dilatation and stenting are possible only in patients with primary duct strictures or strictures at a choledochoduodenal anastomosis. In some cases, the combination with percutaneous transhepatic access can increase the success rate of an endoscopic approach.

The technique begins with an endoscopic retrograde cholangiogram. An endoscopic sphincterotomy may also be necessary to help gain access to the biliary tree. The stricture is traversed retrograde with an atraumatic guidewire. Sequential dilatation with 4- to 10-mm balloons is employed (Fig. 24-9). Re-evaluation with cholangiography is performed at 3 months with redilatation performed as necessary. A recent trend in endoscopic intervention is to sequentially add stents. Instead of changing stents, at 3 months a second stent is added. At 6 months a third stent may be added, and all three stents are left in place for up to 12 months. Finally, minimal experience with metallic expanding stents placed endoscopically for benign strictures has been re-

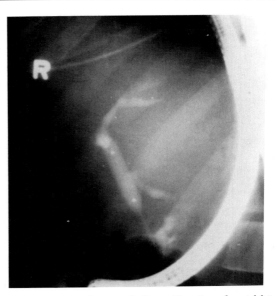

Figure 24-9. Endoscopic balloon dilatation of a mid-bile duct stricture.

ported. Complications of the endoscopic technique include acute pancreatitis and bleeding associated with the sphincterotomy, and cholangitis following biliary manipulation. Cholangitis is also a frequent late complication of stent occlusion.

Results

The long-term results for the surgical and the nonoperative approaches are shown in Table 24-2. Excellent long-term results can be achieved in 70% to 90% of patients by any of the techniques. The definition of satisfactory results in most cases requires that the patients are asymptomatic and have no jaundice or cholangitis. The length of follow-up is very important in analyzing final results because restenosis can occur up to 20 years after the initial procedure (Fig. 24-10). The chance of late restricturing requires that the patient should be followed indefinitely for the possibility of recurrence. Serum bilirubin, transaminases, and alkaline phosphatase are used to monitor for recurrent biliary obstruction. Radionucleotide scanning provides good physiologic information concerning bile flow and can be useful in follow-up examination.

Table 24-2. Results of Surgical and Nonoperative Management of Bile Duct Strictures

Technique	Year	Institution	Number of Patients	Success rate (%)	Follow-up (mos)
Surgical					
	1982	UCLA	66	86	60
	1984	UCSF	60	78	102
	1986	Cleveland Clinic	105	82	60
	1989	Johns Hopkins	25	88	57
	1993	Amsterdam	35	83	50
Nonoperative percutaneous dilatation					
	1986	Multi-institution	73	67	36
	1987	Mayo Clinic	74	78	28
	1989	Johns Hopkins	20	55	59
	1991	Emory	28	93	38
	1992	San Diego*	43	87	12
Endoscopic dilatation					
	1989	Milwaukee	25	88	48
	1993	Amsterdam	46	72	42

*Metallic stent.

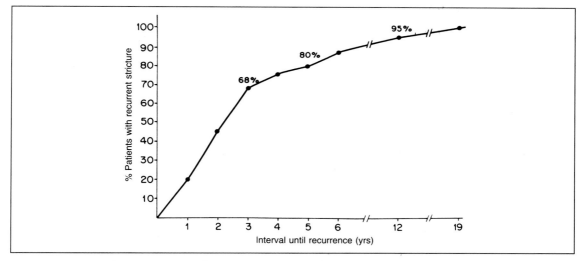

Figure 24-10. Cumulative percentage of recurrent strictures with respect to the time interval from the initial repair until the next repair. (From Pitt HA, et al. Factors influencing outcome in patients with postoperative biliary strictures. *Am J Surg* 1982; 144:14–21. Reproduced by permission.)

Comparative Results

Comparison of nonoperative techniques and surgical reconstruction has been difficult. Few centers have significant expertise with both operative and nonoperative management. Furthermore, the definition of a successful procedure, the reporting of complications, and the length of follow-up reported have not been consistent in the literature. At present, two comparative retrospective studies have been published: one comparing surgical and percutaneous management and the second comparing surgical and endoscopic treatment.

The first study is a retrospective comparison of the results of percutaneous dilatation and surgery at The Johns Hopkins Hospital between 1979 and 1987. In this report, 42 patients had 45 procedures for benign postoperative biliary strictures. Twenty-five patients underwent surgical repair with Roux-en-Y hepaticojejunostomy and postoperative transhepatic stenting for a mean of 13 ± 1.3 months. Twenty patients had balloon dilatation (a mean of 3.9 times) and were stented transhepatically for a mean of 13.3 ± 2 months. Three patients were managed with both surgery and dilatation. The two groups in the Hopkins analysis were similar with respect to multiple parameters that might have predicted outcome, including age, sex, secondary biliary cirrhosis, intrahepatic stones, and the presentation with either obstructive jaundice or biliary fistulas. Fifty-six percent of the surgical patients and 65% of the balloon dilatation patients had undergone one or more previous surgical attempts at stricture repair. The mean length of follow-up was similar for the two groups. No patient died after any of the procedures. Procedure-related morbidity occurred in 20% of the surgical patients and in 35% of the patients undergoing balloon dilatation.

For both groups, a successful outcome was defined as no evidence of cholangitis or jaundice requiring another procedure more than 12 months from the outset of treatment. A successful result was achieved in 88% of the surgical patients and in only 55% of balloon dilatation patients ($P <$ 0.02, Fig. 24-11). To further define the relative benefit of the two procedures, total hospital stay and total procedural costs were determined. As expected, initial hospitalization was longer for surgery than for balloon dilatation. However, when rehospitalizations for further dilatations, complications, or recurrences were considered, total hospital stay did not differ significantly between the two groups. Cost data paralleled hospitalization data and did not differ significantly between the two groups.

In the second comparative study, a group from The Netherlands compared endoscopic versus surgical treatment of benign bile duct strictures. Thirty-five patients were treated surgically, and 66 were treated by endoscopic stenting. Patient characteristics, initial injury, previous repairs, and the level of obstruction were comparable in both groups. Surgical therapy consisted of Roux-en-Y hepaticojejunostomy, and endoscopic therapy consisted of placement of an endoprosthesis with trimonthly elective exchange for a 1-year period. Successful stent placement was accomplished in 94% of patients managed endoscopically. Six of the 66 endo-

Figure 24-11. Actuarial success rate over 72 months for surgery (89%) and balloon dilatation (52%). The difference is statistically significant ($P < 0.01$). (From Pitt HA, et al. Benign postoperative biliary strictures: Operate or dilate? *Ann Surg* 1989; 210:417–427. Reproduced by permission.)

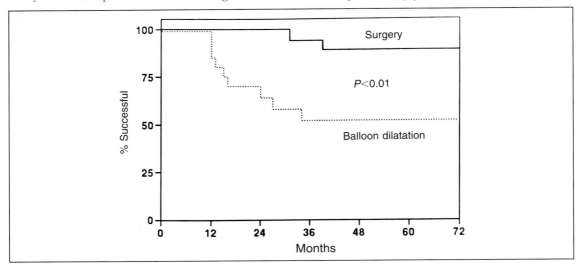

scopic patients, however, underwent surgical reconstruction for failed stent placement or other reasons. Early complications occurred more frequently in the surgically treated group (26% vs. 8%; $P < 0.03$). However, the only procedure-related death occurred in a patient who developed severe pancreatitis after endoscopic stent placement. Late complications occurred only in the endoscopic group (27%) and included primarily episodes of cholangitis. The overall complication rate, therefore, was similar: 26% for surgical patients and 35% for endoscopic patients. The mean follow-up and definitions of success applied were similar. Following surgery, excellent results were observed in 83% of patients, with 6 patients developing a recurrent stricture at a mean of 40 months after the initial operation. Following endoscopic stenting, excellent results were observed in 72% of patients, with 18% of patients developing restricture at a mean of 3 months after stent removal.

Conclusions

Management of a patient presenting with a postoperative bile duct stricture should be individualized according to the clinical situation. The ability to provide a multidisciplinary team approach is essential. The use of cholangiography by the endoscopic route, the percutaneous route, or both will be necessary in all patients for diagnosis and delineation of the stricture. Early efforts in management should focus on treating sepsis and controlling biliary leaks. The use of either percutaneous or endoscopic stents

is essential in accomplishing these goals. A nonoperative technique as the initial attempt at definitive management, in those patients suited for such an approach, is usually appropriate as an attempt to avoid another operation. However, in many patients eventual surgical management, either because of anatomic constraints or because of the failure of nonoperative techniques, will be necessary to restore bile flow to the upper gastrointestinal tract. Overall, with the combination of currently available techniques, successful long-term results can be achieved in up to 90% of patients.

Selected Readings

Branum G, et al. Management of major biliary complications after laparoscopic cholecystectomy. *Ann Surg* 1993; 217:532–541.

David PHP, et al. Benign biliary strictures: Surgery or endoscopy? *Ann Surg* 1993; 217:237–243.

Geenan DJ, et al. Endoscopic therapy for benign bile duct strictures. *Gastrointest Endosc* 1989; 35:367–371.

Lillemoe KD, Pitt HA, Cameron JL. Current management of benign bile duct strictures. *Adv Surg* 1992; 25: 119–174.

Mueller PR, et al. Biliary stricture dilatation: Multicenter review of clinical management in 73 patients. *Radiology* 1986; 160:17–22.

Pelligrini CA, Thomas MJ, Way LW. Recurrent biliary stricture: Patterns of recurrent and outcome of surgical therapy. *Am J Surg* 1984; 147:175–180.

Pitt HA, et al. Benign postoperative biliary strictures: Operate or dilate? *Ann Surg* 1989; 210:417–427.

Pitt HA, et al. Factors influencing outcome in patients with postoperative biliary strictures. *Am J Surg* 1982; 144:14–21.

25

Biliary Fistulas

ALAN M. ZUCKERMAN
STEVEN GOLDSCHMID
JOHN G. HUNTER
STEPHEN L. KAUFMAN

Etiology

The multiple causes of biliary fistulas may be divided into four broad categories: trauma, cholelithiasis, tumors, and inflammatory processes (Table 25-1). Most biliary fistulas are secondary to inadvertent operative biliary trauma. At the present time, laparoscopic cholecystectomy is one of the more common causes. Any patient that presents with signs and symptoms referable to the biliary tree after surgery should be suspected of having had a bile duct injury with a resultant fistula.

Complications of cholelithiasis can lead to the development of a biliary fistula. Stones can erode through the gallbladder into the small bowel. If the stone is large, generally greater than 2 cm, bowel obstruction can occur, producing a gallstone ileus. Stones can erode from the gallbladder to other areas of the gastrointestinal tract including the colon, stomach, and bile duct. Stones that erode into the stomach can cause gastric outlet obstruction and gastrointestinal bleeding (Bouveret's syndrome). Obstruction of the common bile duct can occur by extrinsic compression from a stone lodged in the cystic duct (Mirizzi's syndrome). These stones subsequently can erode into the biliary tree, producing a biliobiliary fistula.

Tumors and trauma can occasionally lead to the development of biliary fistulas. Patients who have recently undergone liver biopsy or have had liver trauma and subsequently develop pain, cholangitis, gastrointestinal bleeding, or biliary drainage through a skin wound should be suspected of having a biliary fistula. Other fistulous communications can occur between nonbiliary lesions that erode into a bile duct. These include gastric and duodenal ulcers, pancreatic pseudocysts, abscesses, and aneurysms.

Diagnosis

The diagnosis of a biliary fistula is generally straightforward. Patients present with signs of biliary obstruction, cholangitis, cholecystitis, hemobilia, or leakage of bile through a drain or a cutaneous wound. The successful and timely diagnosis of a biliary fistula, however, depends on the clinician's knowledge of the various disorders associated with these fistulas.

The ideal diagnostic procedure for identifying a biliary fistula depends upon the suspected etiology. Fistulas into a vascular structure that present with bleeding are best diagnosed by arteriography. Cholecystocolonic fistulas and choledochogastric fistulas can be diagnosed by endoscopy. Patients with fistulas from trauma or surgery often have collections of bile that can be identified by CT scan or sonography (Fig. 25-1). Persistent bile leakage can be demonstrated reliably and consistently by radionuclide imaging of the biliary tree with obvious extravasation of the contrast medium (Fig. 25-2).

In most instances, the successful treatment of biliary fistulas requires interventional therapy. Un-

273

Table 25-1. Causes of Biliary Fistulas

Traumas
  Operative
  Penetrating
  Blunt
  Liver biopsy
  Percutaneous manipulation
  Endoscopic manipulation
Cholelithiasis
  Cholecystoduodenal
  Cholecystocolonic
  Cholecystogastric
  Cholecystocholedochal
  Choledochoduodenal
Tumors
  Gallbladder
  Bile ducts
  Duodenum
  Pancreas
  Colon
Inflammatory processes
  Duodenal ulcer
  Gastric ulcer
  Pancreatic pseudocyst
  Subphrenic abscess

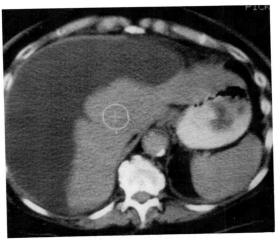

Figure 25-1. CT scan showing a large biloma after an operative bile duct injury.

der these circumstances, direct cholangiography of the biliary tree is critical to precisely identify the anatomy, and ideally the cause, of the fistula. This information is necessary for deciding on the most appropriate therapy. If the fistula is external, a catheter can be inserted into the fistulous tract and contrast can be injected to delineate the anatomy. Therapy can often be instituted at the same time the anatomy is delineated.

Endoscopic retrograde cholangiography (ERC) and percutaneous transhepatic cholangiography (PTC) are both excellent methods of visualizing abnormalities in patients with biliary fistulas. The best technique to use depends on the expertise available at an individual institution. Occasionally, if repeated cholangiograms are necessary, the percutaneous route may be preferred because a catheter can be left in place to external drainage. If there is complete disruption of the biliary tree, simultaneous endoscopic and percutaneous cholangiography are necessary to visualize all segments of the biliary tree. When both techniques are available at an institution, the endoscopic cholangiogram is preferred because patient discomfort is less and there are fewer major and minor complications. When im-

aging modalities fail to identify the etiology of the fistula, surgical exploration should be considered.

Regardless of the technique used to visualize the biliary tree, fistulas are generally readily identified when contrast media either extravasates or follows an abnormal course (Fig. 25-3). Diagnosis and therapy of these often difficult problems requires evaluation of these patients and these findings by a multidisciplinary group from surgery, radiology, and gastroenterology.

Management

Endoscopic, percutaneous transhepatic, laparoscopic, and open surgical treatment may be used in the management of biliary fistulas. Most of these fistulas are side fistulas. The flow of bile into the gut is intact; there is merely a hole in the side of the system. For this type of fistula the principles of management are (1) eliminate the source of distal obstruction, and (2) remove the foreign body, tumor, or infection from the fistula site. For a biliary fistula, elimination of distal obstruction most frequently means dividing or stenting the sphincter of Oddi. An intact, unstented sphincter of Oddi will tend to perpetuate fistula drainage by keeping the intrabiliary pressure higher than the intraabdominal pressure, thereby causing a net flux of bile out of the biliary system.

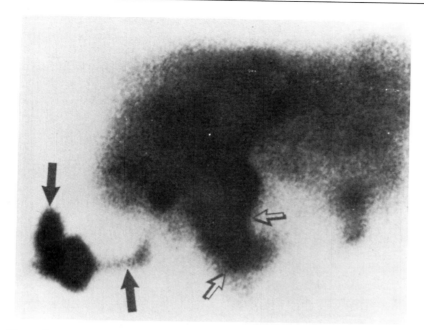

Figure 25-2. Technetium iminodiacetic acid scan demonstrating uptake by the liver and a bile leak into the subhepatic space (open arrows) and into a drain and bag (closed arrows).

Figure 25-3. Percutaneous transhepatic cholangiogram demonstrating a leak from the common duct with contrast collecting below the margin of the liver.

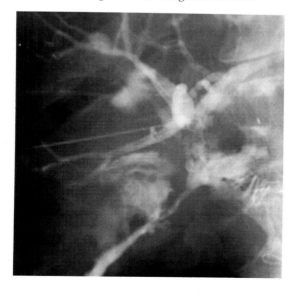

By surgically, endoscopically, or radiologically opening the sphincter, one can reduce the pressure in the biliary system to that of the intra-abdominal pressure. The path of least resistance becomes the pathway through the stent or sphincterotomy into the duodenum, resulting in diminished fistula drainage and rapid closure.

Intrabiliary obstruction may also be caused by periampullary carcinoma or chronic pancreatitis. A third cause of distal bile duct obstruction is common bile duct stones. Ideally, these stones should be removed through a sphincterectomy, a balloon-dilated sphincter muscle, or a choledochotomy. Removal of these obstructing foreign bodies will generally permit closure of the fistula. When a biliary fistula complicates a bilioenteric bypass procedure for a biliary stricture, the same principles of opening up the distal bile duct with percutaneous stenting will frequently heal the fistula.

Fistulas kept open by a foreign body, an infection, or a tumor are much rarer than those kept open by distal obstruction. Infection can generally be managed with a percutaneously placed radiologic drain. Once the infection is treated, the fistula will generally close. A foreign body, such as a misplaced stent, a suture, or a portion of a T tube, may be more difficult to remove without laparoscopy or laparotomy.

Options

SURGERY

In the past, the surgical approach to bile fistulas was the main therapeutic option. The surgical treatment employed depends on the nature of the fistula. For example, a cystic duct leak following cholecystectomy may be managed with ligation of the cystic duct stump. More difficult anastomotic bile leaks require an entirely different approach. If the fistula is large, the anastomosis should be redone. If the fistula is small, placing the drain adjacent to the fistula generally permits eventual closure of the fistula as long as downstream obstruction is not present. Lastly, a large traumatic laceration of the biliary tree is surgically managed by choledochoenterostomy. Distal injuries may be managed with choledochoduodenostomy. Most fistulas in the common hepatic or intrahepatic biliary system require Roux-en-Y hepaticojejunostomy for repair. Rarely, a suture repair of a lateral biliary fistula may be appropriate if it is coupled with a bile duct drainage procedure such as a T tube or sphincterotomy.

RADIOLOGY

Shortly after the advent of percutaneous transhepatic cholangiography, therapeutic procedures on the biliary tract that included drainage, stricture stenting, and stone removal were developed. Transhepatic radiologic placement of polyethylene stents has allowed for the spontaneous closure of most biliary side fistulas if a guidewire can be passed across the fistula into the duodenum or small bowel. Percutaneous transhepatic stenting allows for both external and internal drainage to be accomplished with the same tube. Radiologic management is also frequently needed to provide drainage of the biloma that accompanies an undetected biliary fistula. Usually percutaneous drainage diverts bile sufficiently to permit closure of a low-volume biliary fistula (Fig. 25-4).

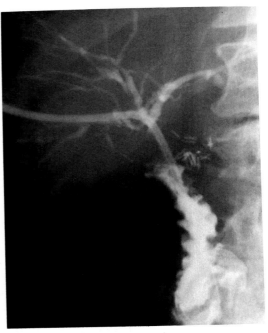

Figure 25-4. Same patient as in Fig. 25-3. This cholangiogram, performed after several months of percutaneous drainage, demonstrates closure of the previously identified leak.

ENDOSCOPY

The most recent addition to the fistula management team, the biliary endoscopist, may have the least invasive method of successfully treating the majority of biliary fistulas. Once the diagnostic endoscopic retrograde cholangiogram (ERC) documents a biliary fistula, the endoscopist may elect to (1) do nothing, (2) perform endoscopic sphincterotomy, (3) pass a nasobiliary tube, or (4) place an endoprosthesis (stent). In addition, a combination of these procedures such as sphincterotomy and stent placement may also be performed.

LAPAROSCOPY

It is more common for laparoscopy to be the procedure initiating a bile fistula rather than the mode of treatment; however, occasionally, if detected early, a leaking cystic duct stump may be managed by repeat clipping and drainage of the gallbladder fossa.

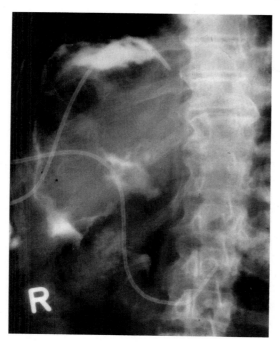

Figure 25-5. Subphrenic drainage catheter and percutaneous transhepatic catheter demonstrating persistent bile leak from operative bile duct injury.

Controversies

When a postoperative fluid collection is identified by CT scan or ultrasonography in the right upper quadrant after hepatobiliary surgery and if needle aspiration demonstrates bile, there is little argument that a percutaneous drain should be placed into the collection, unless the patient is to be immediately returned to the operating room (Fig. 25-5). After drainage is attained, the need for further immediate studies is controversial. Some individuals prefer immediate endoscopic cholangiography with ERC. Others advocate percutaneous transhepatic cholangiography, and a third camp would argue that nothing further needs to be done because most fistulas will close spontaneously. The case for cholangiography becomes stronger with persistence of the biliary fistula, which is indicated by persistent bile drainage from a percutaneously or surgically placed drain. Generally, an attempt to image the fistula through the drain is ill-advised because there is a risk of inducing cholangitis by introducing bacteria from the biloma into the biliary system. Early endoscopic or radiologic imaging and therapy are most important when the drainage is copious (> 300 ml/d) or shows no sign of lessening over the first week after drain placement. The authors' preferred approach is developed in the next section.

The second controversy surrounds the most appropriate endoscopic therapy. A diagnostic ERC is only rarely indicated but may be appropriate when a well-drained fistula is demonstrated to be nearly closed. This situation should rarely present itself because it is unnecessary to perform a cholangiogram for a low-output fistula unless chronicity of drainage is the indication. If so, a therapeutic maneuver is needed. The second option, endoscopic sphincterectomy as the sole treatment of fistulas, involves the use of a standard, side-viewing endoscope and eliminates the discomfort of a nasobiliary tube. The clear disadvantage of endoscopic sphincterotomy is the morbidity related to sphincterotomy (8%, including duodenal perforation, bleeding, stenosis, and death) and the potential long-term ramifications of a destroyed sphincter of Oddi. These problems include a greater incidence of bactobilia and cholangitis. Because of these concerns, therapeutic endoscopists are relying on nasobiliary tubes or endoscopic stents more frequently.

Nasobiliary tubes have the advantage of easy placement, the ability to perform a cholangiogram through the nasobiliary tube to document fistula healing, and the ease of removal without a second endoscopic procedure. Balanced against these advantages is the fact that the long, narrow-caliber nasobiliary tube is less effective at reducing intrabiliary pressure than a short, wide stent. In addition, the discomfort associated with a nasobiliary tube makes it less acceptable to patients. Thus the most frequent endoscopic method of dealing with side biliary fistulas today is placement of an endoprosthesis (Fig. 25-6). Ideally, this prosthesis should be of a large caliber and should cross the site of fistulous opening. It is generally not necessary to make an endoscopic sphincterotomy before placing an endoprosthesis. The only disadvantage of using an endoprosthesis is that a second procedure must be performed to remove this prosthesis. Generally, prosthesis removal can be accomplished with an end-viewing scope and is thus a much less complicated procedure than ERC.

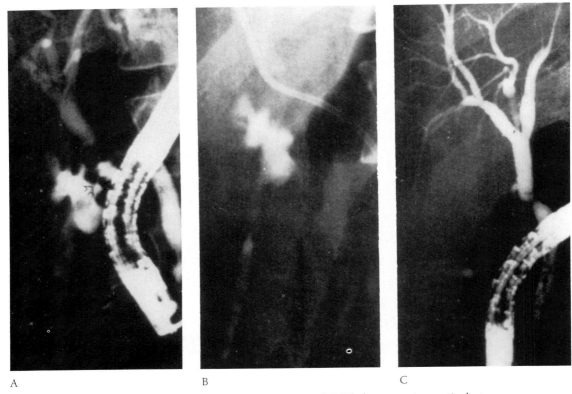

A   B   C

Figure 25-6. A. Endoscopic retrograde cholangiopancreatogram (ERCP) demonstrating cystic duct
leak. B. Endoscopic endoprosthesis placed for management. C. ERCP after stent removal.

Few controversies exist in the surgical management of biliary fistulas, largely because surgery is
so rarely necessary. A long and hotly debated issue,
that of choledochoduodenostomy versus transduodenal sphincteroplasty, is more germane to the
management of recurrent choledocholithiasis than
it is to the management of biliary fistulas. In general,
a biliary fistula sufficiently complicated as to require
surgical reintervention will rarely be managed with
either of these techniques. There is reasonably uniform agreement that for high fistulas a Roux-en-Y
hepaticojejunostomy is the treatment of choice.

Preferred Approach

A patient who presents in the period following hepatobiliary surgery with right upper quadrant pain,
fever, or jaundice should be initially evaluated with
ultrasonography. If this examination reveals fluid
in the right upper quadrant, this collection should

be aspirated. If bile or pus is present, a drain should
be placed. If a small fluid collection is not reachable
with percutaneous methods, a bile fistula can be
ruled out by performing a technetium-HIDA scan.
After placing the drain, the authors generally wait
36 to 72 hours to assess the patient's response to
therapy and to establish a curve for the diminution
or persistence of biliary drainage. With a steeply
declining curve the authors wait longer before performing intervention. Only with persistent high-
volume drainage do the authors move early to endoscopic or percutaneous imaging and therapy.

Endoscopy is usually attempted first because
of the more invasive nature and possible bleeding
complications associated with PTC. The endoscopic
therapeutic maneuver is tailored to the nature of
the fistula. Generally, the fistula is treated by placing
an endoprosthesis (minimum 10 French) across the
fistulous opening, if possible. The endoprosthesis
is removed 2 weeks after fistula drainage has ceased.

Transhepatic stenting is reserved for occasions when the retrograde (endoscopic) approach fails or is impossible because of alterations in anatomy, including the presence of a surgical bilioenteric anastomosis.

For a large-volume fistula from major duct transection, or a fistula above a fixed bile duct obstruction (e.g., surgical clip), an operation may be necessary. The surgical procedure performed is generally hepaticojejunostomy. An effort is made to anastomose all transected ducts greater than 2 to 3 mm in diameter to the jejunum. Clearly, fine 6, 7, or 8–0 monofilament suture and loop magnification are necessary to perform these more delicate anastomoses. Ducts smaller than 2 mm in diameter can generally be safely ligated without causing significant cholestasis or cholangitis. When hepaticojejunostomy is performed for biliary fistula, transhepatic stents are placed to reduce the incidence of a postoperative stricture. The authors prefer to use a soft polymeric silicone (Silastic) stent placed through the liver into the jejunum (not a U tube). If the anastomosis has been performed to a normal-caliber bile duct, this stent is left in 6 to 12 months before being removed. In addition, the Roux limb is approximated to the lateral abdominal wall and marked with clips to permit subsequent percutaneous entrance for stricture dilatation through the small bowel rather than through the liver. This approach to the anastomosis is preferable to a transhepatic approach because the likelihood of a bleeding complication, empyema, or bile fistula is diminished.

Results

Surgical trauma of the biliary tree and gallstone disease account for the vast majority of biliary fistulas, and surgery remains a well-established means for their correction. With the advent of sonographic and CT imaging in the 1970s, percutaneous drainage of bile collections became possible and presented an attractive alternative to surgery. PTC also allowed bile flow to be diverted away from the fistulous communication, increasing the likelihood that a fistulous tract would close spontaneously.

A number of published reports confirm the efficacy of the percutaneous approach. In 1983, 15 patients with postoperative biliary problems were managed by percutaneous drainage at The Johns Hopkins Hospital. Nine patients had a fistula, and 2 had complete transection of a major bile duct. All patients were initially treated with percutaneous stent placement, and fistula closure occurred in all cases. Drainage also allowed for the resolution of sepsis and clinical stabilization of the majority of patients. Of 12 patients who also had an abscess, operative drainage was necessary in 11.

Kaufman et al. treated 12 patients with fistulas and bile leaks confirmed by cholangiography. Percutaneous drainage was successful in all patients. Seven of the 12 patients had complete resolution of their bile leak within 2 months without definitive surgery on the biliary tree. Of the remaining 5 patients, 4 required biliary surgery because of complete obstruction of a major bile duct, and in 1 patient the fistula failed to resolve. Two patients had complications related to their percutaneous drainage. One patient developed arterial bleeding when the catheter was removed, and another had metabolic complications due to bile loss from the catheter.

In another study, 35 patients with biliary fistulas secondary to a variety of disorders underwent PTC with catheter drainage. Therapy was definitive in 28 patients (80%). In the remainder, failure was thought to be secondary to inadequate catheter positioning or an inability to treat the cause of the fistula.

Endoscopic therapy of biliary tract fistulas includes the placement of endoprostheses, nasobiliary drainage, biliary sphincterotomy, and combinations of these therapies. All techniques have been used successfully, and no one method has proven to be superior to the others. Ponchon et al. attempted endoscopic therapy in 24 patients with biliary fistulas. ERC was successful in all patients, and the fistulas were identified in 22 (92%). Twelve patients were treated by sphincterotomy alone. In 8 patients, external fistulas disappeared within 5 days. In 3 patients (25%), the fistulas failed to heal and required surgical intervention. Eleven patients had insertion of an endoprosthesis. Fistulas resolved quickly in 7 patients, and the prosthesis was removed after 4 months. The fistulas failed to close in 4 patients, who eventually underwent surgery. The failures were thought to be secondary to large defects and other associated medical problems.

Some of these patients also underwent percutaneous drainage of abscess collections.

More recently, Binmoeller et al. reviewed the results of endoscopic therapy in 77 cases of biliary leaks. Patients were treated with endoscopic sphincterotomy (ES) alone (23), ES and nasobiliary drainage (3), ES and endoprosthesis (34), ES and stone extraction (9), and nasobiliary drainage alone (7). The procedure was successful in 73 of the 77 cases (95%), and the fistulas healed in 63 cases (86%). The healing rate did not vary significantly with the type of procedure done (Table 25-2). Data using endoprostheses without sphincterotomy are not available. Interestingly, there was a significant difference in healing rate depending on the site of origin of the fistula. Cystic stump leaks failed to heal in 4% of patients. Leaks from the common bile duct failed to heal in 19% of patients. The greatest failure rate was in leaks from the hepatic ducts, which occurred in 31% of patients. These data suggest that fistula site may have some prognostic significance.

No randomized data exist comparing the outcome of percutaneous to endoscopic management of biliary fistulas. Between 65% and 100% of fistulas will heal as long as there is adequate drainage of the biliary tree. It is uncertain which technique lowers intraductal pressure the most and allows for the greatest diversion of bile away from the fistula. There seems to be no difference in outcome between ES, ES with endoprosthesis, and nasobiliary drainage. Complications with percutaneous and endoscopic techniques in patients with biliary fistulas are not well documented. In patients with malignant obstructive jaundice, endoscopically placed stents have a higher success rate and a lower 30-day mortality rate.

Often percutaneous or surgical drainage of abscesses is necessary, even if decompression of the biliary tree is successful. However, decompression helps to resolve jaundice and sepsis, allows for patient stabilization before surgery, and in some instances eliminates the need for a biliary operation. Because of the endoscopic and percutaneous techniques now available, fewer patients will require surgery. For patients that fail these less invasive methods, surgery remains highly successful. However, the patients that fail percutaneous and endoscopic techniques may be poorer surgical candidates and have higher morbidity and mortality.

Conclusions

Multiple causes of biliary fistulas include trauma, complications of cholelithiasis, tumors, and inflammatory processes. Of these many possibilities, operative trauma at the time of laparoscopic cholecystectomy is now the leading cause. CT is very useful in defining bilomas and bile ascites, and percutaneous drainage of perihepatic fluid collections is often indicated. Endoscopic retrograde or percutaneous transhepatic cholangiography is then performed to further define the anatomy of the fistula. Management can usually be undertaken initially by endoscopic placement of a nasobiliary catheter or endoprosthesis or by transhepatic biliary drainage. Surgery may be required to regain biliary-enteric continuity, and Roux-en-Y choledocho- or hepaticojejunostomy is usually the procedure of choice. Surgery is also usually required for definitive management of internal biliary fistulas between the gallbladder or bile duct and adjacent organs.

Table 25-2. Data Showing that Healing Rate of Fistula is not Dependent on the Type of Endoscopic Procedure Performed to Divert the Flow of Bile

Procedure	Success (%)
Nasobiliary drainage	100
ES* plus stone extraction	89
ES	87
ES plus endoprosthesis	85
ES plus nasobiliary drainage	67

*ES = endoscopic sphinctectomy.

Selected Readings

Binmoeller KF, Katon RM, Schneidman R. Endoscopic management of postoperative biliary leaks: Review of 77 cases and report of two cases with biloma formation. *Am J Gastro* 1991; 86:227–231.

Branum G, et al. Management of major biliary complications after laparoscopic cholecystectomy. *Ann Surg* 1993; 217(5):532–541.

Kaufman SL, et al. Percutaneous transhepatic biliary drainage for bile leaks and fistulas. *AJR* 1985; 144:1055–1058.

Liguory C, et al. Endoscopic treatment of postoperative biliary fistula. *Surgery* 1991; 110:779–784.

Papanicolaou N, et al. Abscess-fistula association: Radiologic recognition and management. *AJR* 1984; 143: 811–815.

Peters JH, et al. Complications of laparoscopic cholecystectomy. *Surgery* 1991; 110:769–778.

Ponchon T, et al. Endoscopic treatment of biliary tract fistulas. *Gastrointest Endosc* 1989; 35:490–498.

Speer AG, et al. Randomized trial of endoscopic versus percutaneous stent insertion in malignant obstructive jaundice. *Lancet* 1987; 2(8550):57–62.

Walker AT, et al. Bile duct disruption and biloma after laparoscopic cholecystectomy: Imaging evaluation. *AJR* 1992; 158:785–789.

Zuidema GD, et al. Percutaneous transhepatic management of complex biliary problems. *Ann Surg* 1983; 197:584–593.

26

Motility Disorders

James Toouli
Ian C. Roberts-Thomson
Allan G. Wycherley

Little controversy persists regarding the existence of motility disorders of the biliary tract and pancreas. Much of the discussion over the last decade centered around the question of incidence and recognition of these disorders. Current discussion and research are aimed at determining their pathophysiology and whether they are primary or secondary events. The clinical presentation of pancreatobiliary motility disorders occurs in one of three forms; gallbladder dyskinesia, sphincter of Oddi dysfunction of the bile duct sphincter, and sphincter of Oddi dysfunction of the pancreatic duct sphincter.

Gallbladder

Etiology and Pathogenesis

Patients with gallbladder motility disorders present with symptoms suggestive of gallstones but on investigation do not have demonstrable stones in the gallbladder. Although the pathogenesis of the motility disorder is unknown, some clues may be deduced from the etiology of acute acalculous gallbladder disease. Patients may develop acute gallbladder inflammation while on parenteral nutrition. Often these patients are being treated in an intensive care unit environment for an unrelated major illness. Ultrasonographic studies have demonstrated reduced gallbladder contractility and the development of "sludge" in the gallbladder. Rarely, this setting may lead to cystic duct obstruction and acute gangrenous cholecystitis. More frequently, acute obstruction does not occur, but these patients subsequently are at high risk for the development of gallstones.

The majority of patients with acalculous gallbladder disease, however, do not develop their symptoms following a major illness or after parenteral nutrition. However, the underlying motility disorder may be similar and may reflect changes which result in relative or absolute obstruction to the normal emptying of the gallbladder. Since the further investigation and management of patients who develop acute acalculous cholecystitis are discussed elsewhere in this book, the following discussion will be confined to patients with recurrent symptoms.

Diagnosis

Abdominal pain is the most common symptom associated with a motility disorder of the gallbladder. The pain is epigastric or in the right upper quadrant. This pain occurs in episodes and is quite severe, often lasting 2 to 3 hours or until relieved by analgesics. It may radiate to the back and under the tip of the right scapula. The pain may follow a fatty meal and may be associated with nausea and vomiting, although these are not diagnostic features. Occasionally the pain wakes the patient in the early hours of the morning and is not relieved by changing the posture or taking antacids. Examination during an episode of pain reveals tenderness under the right costal margin, and there may be localized guarding. The temperature is usually normal, and there are no changes in the white cell count or in levels of liver transaminases, bilirubin, alkaline phosphatase, or serum amylase. These symptoms occur most commonly in women in the 35- to 55-year-old age group, but they are also recognized in younger or older patients of either sex.

A diagnosis of gallbladder disease due to gallstones is usually made following the above presentation. The most appropriate first investigation is a biliary ultrasound, and in these patients the result is that of a normal gallbladder and bile duct with no evidence of stones. When other possible causes of upper abdominal pain (e.g., peptic ulcer, irritable bowel, or nonulcer dyspepsia) have been excluded, options include a second ultrasound study or an oral cholecystogram.

In patients in whom the suspicion of biliary tract disease remains strong, further investigation is warranted. Endoscopic retrograde cholangiopancreatography (ERCP) is sometimes useful and may be combined with endoscopy to exclude any gastric or duodenal pathology. ERCP is mandatory in any patient with associated changes in the levels of liver transaminase, bilirubin, alkaline phosphatase, or amylase with episodes of pain. In such patients, careful radiological screening of the biliary tract after the controlled infusion of dilute contrast material is very likely to identify small stones in either the gallbladder or bile duct. Rare causes for pain, such as sclerosing cholangitis, Caroli's disease, or choledochal cyst, will also be identified.

At the end of the endoscopic procedure, gallbladder contraction may be produced by the intravenous injection of cholecystokinin octapeptide (CCK-OP 40 ng/kg). Gallbladder bile which flows into the bile duct and duodenum can then be aspirated through the ERCP catheter and examined for the presence of cholesterol crystals. The finding of cholesterol crystals in gallbladder bile is strongly associated with the presence of small calculi in the gallbladder or cholesterolosis. Such patients may benefit from cholecystectomy. Bile from the gallbladder for examination for crystals can also be obtained from a separate procedure by aspirating through a duodenal tube after the administration of CCK-OP. However, the authors prefer to aspirate bile during endoscopy in order to limit the number of invasive upper gastrointestinal procedures.

Provocation tests have been used to reproduce pain in patients with suspected gallbladder motility disorders. The mainstay of these tests has been the administration of a fixed bolus dose of CCK-OP. A positive response is taken as the subjective reproduction of the pain. A radiological modification of this test is the "CCK oral cholecystogram." In this test, the gallbladder is opacified by oral cholecystography, and the subject is given an intravenous injection of CCK-OP (20 ng/kg). A positive response is when the patient's pain is reproduced and an exaggerated contraction is seen on x-ray. Unfortunately, the specificity and sensitivity of these tests in selecting patients for treatment have not been reproduced in prospective randomized studies. A number of studies have demonstrated that an IV bolus dose of CCK-OP is an inadequate stimulus for evaluating gallbladder emptying because of the short half-life of CCK in blood. Furthermore, the reproducibility of gallbladder emptying following bolus doses is poor. In addition, bolus injections of CCK-OP stimulate not only the gallbladder but also the colon, and pain may not necessarily arise from gallbladder contraction. For these reasons, the authors do not favor the use of the CCK provocation test in selecting patients for treatment of gallbladder motility disorders.

The introduction of the technetium-Tc-99m–labeled iminodiacetic acid derivatives has made it feasible to study the hepatobiliary system using the gamma camera computer analysis (Fig. 26-1). It is possible to estimate the gallbladder ejection fraction (GBEF) by using the formula

$$\text{GBEF (\%)} = \frac{\text{change in GB activity}}{\text{baseline GB activity}} \times 100$$

The normal gallbladder empties in excess of 50% of its volume in response to a standard meal or a 45-min intravenous infusion of CCK-OP (20 ng/kg/hr). One study demonstrated a significant difference in the GBEF of patients with gallstones when compared to controls. The gallbladder emptying in 14 of 20 patients with gallstones measured below 50% after ingestion of a corn oil meal. In another study, 24 patients with abnormal CCK-OP GBEF (< 40%) were identified from a group of patients presenting with biliary-type pain and no evidence of gallstones. Unlike in CCK-OP provocation studies, none of the patients receiving an infusion of cholecystokinin or a corn oil meal experienced pain.

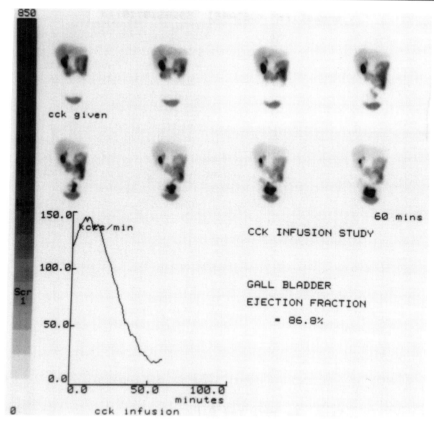

Figure 26-1. Gallbladder scintigraphy, illustrating a normal gallbladder ejection fraction (GBEF) in response to infusion of cholecystokinin octapeptide (CCK).

Management and Results

The most appropriate treatment for patients with identified gallbladder motility disorder is cholecystectomy because it permanently eliminates the organ which produces the symptoms. However, in certain situations the disorder may be transient, and it may be unnecessary to proceed to surgery.

In one small study, the prokinetic drug cisapride was used to treat symptomatic patients with gallbladder hypokinesia on ultrasonography. Long-term treatment produced relief of symptoms and a reversal of the motility changes. However, the results are preliminary, and the study has not been reproduced.

The role of cholecystectomy was evaluated in 24 patients with abnormal CCK-OP GBEF. Patients were randomized prospectively to either cholecystectomy or follow-up. All but one of the patients having cholecystectomy were cured of biliary symptoms at 3 years after the operation. Histologic examination of the gallbladders removed at operation revealed features of chronic cholecystitis such as increased gallbladder wall thickness, fibrosis, and chronic inflammatory cells. None of the patients had gallstones. Those patients who did not have cholecystectomy continued to have symptoms, and three of these patients subsequently developed gallstones.

The authors' preferred approach for patients with a suspected gallbladder motility disorder is to make the diagnosis using CCK-OP infusion scintigraphy. If the GBEF is abnormal, the authors recommend laparoscopic cholecystectomy.

Sphincter of Oddi

Over 100 years ago, Rugero Oddi proposed that the sphincter he had recently identified could malfunction, resulting in clinical symptoms. Interest in motility disorders of the sphincter has continued over the last century, and potential abnormalities have been described by the terms *biliary dyskinesia* or *dyssynergia, papillitis, Odditis,* or *papillary stenosis.* The terms *postcholecystectomy syndrome* and *idiopathic recurrent pancreatitis* also have been used to describe conditions which seem likely to be due to motility disorders of the sphincter of Oddi. In an attempt to disassociate the nomenclature from any possible pathological implications, the authors suggested that the term *sphincter of Oddi dysfunction* be adopted as an overall description of "motility disorders of the sphincter."

Etiology and Pathogenesis

The pathogenesis of sphincter of Oddi dysfunction is unknown. One possibility is the existence of primary disorders of motility perhaps related to defects in the enteric nervous system. Secondary disorders also seem likely, either from direct damage or from the indirect effects on factors which control motility of the sphincter.

The sphincter of Oddi is a smooth muscle structure approximately 1 cm in length which is situated at the junction of the bile duct, pancreatic duct, and duodenum. Its function has been characterized by manometric techniques which allow direct measurement of pressure changes using a small catheter directed into either the bile duct or pancreatic duct.

The sphincter normally produces high-pressure phasic contractions which are superimposed on a modest basal pressure. The pressure changes produce a resistance to flow while at the same time propelling small volumes of either bile or pancreatic juice into the duodenum. Most flow occurs in between the phasic contractions, but the contractions also serve to keep the sphincter segment empty. An increase in flow and a decrease in resistance across the sphincter occur when there is a fall in basal pressure and a decrease in the amplitude and frequency of phasic contractions. These changes in resistance are normally produced by neural stimuli via local refluxes from the duodenum or by circulating hormones such as cholecystokinin.

Abnormal responses to normal stimuli have been recorded. In a number of studies, cholecystokinin has been shown to produce an increase in resistance across the sphincter associated with a rise in the basal pressure and a rapid frequency of phasic contractions. This paradoxical response of the sphincter to cholecystokinin may reflect a primary motility disorder of the sphincter. Secondary damage to the sphincter may result from the passage of small stones or following inflammation in either the biliary tract or pancreas. This situation may result in repair by fibrosis which may lead to a fixed stenosis reflected manometrically by a high basal pressure. At present, however, no direct evidence exists for these pathogenetic mechanisms.

Diagnosis

Clinically, patients who present with sphincter of Oddi dysfunction divide into two broad groups. The majority of patients have symptoms which are mainly referable to the biliary tract, and a smaller group present with symptoms which are referable to the pancreas.

The majority of patients with sphincter of Oddi dysfunction are women who have had a cholecystectomy for treatment of symptomatic gallstones. The operation usually results in improvement in symptoms, but pain recurs after 2 to 10 years. The pain is situated in the epigastrium or right upper quadrant, often radiates into the back, and may be associated with nausea and vomiting. The pain generally occurs in episodes which last for up to several hours or until relieved by analgesics. These episodes may occur at intervals of weeks or months. Some patients also describe discomfort in the upper abdomen which is more frequent and may occur every day. In addition, symptoms consistent with irritable bowel syndrome may coexist with episodic biliary-type pain. Some patients are aware that their symptoms can be precipitated or aggravated by opioid analgesics, including codeine. Indeed, the first episode of pain may have been experienced following opiate medication, usually for an unrelated procedure.

Physical examination during an acute episode of pain reveals a distressed afebrile patient who is often moving on the examination couch in order to find the most comfortable position. Abdominal examination is usually noncontributory other than revealing mild to moderate tenderness in the epigastrium or right upper quadrant. Signs of local or general peritonitis are not associated with this condition.

Blood screens reveal a normal white cell count. About 10% to 20% of patients, however, show increases in serum concentrations of liver transaminases, particularly in blood specimens which are taken 3 to 4 hours after the onset of pain. This finding is occasionally accompanied by increases in the levels of serum bilirubin and alkaline phosphatase. In a subgroup of patients, the serum amylase may be elevated either solely or in conjunction with changes in liver enzymes. This group of patients often are given the clinical label of *idiopathic recurrent pancreatitis.*

Initial treatment of patients presenting with the above clinical symptoms is directed at relief of pain, which is usually achieved via administration of a systemic analgesic or butyl hyoscyamine (Buscopan). Pethidine (meperidine) hydrochloride is thought to be the most appropriate analgesic in patients with suspected sphincter of Oddi dysfunction.

All patients who present with significant postcholecystectomy biliary- or pancreatic-type symptoms should be evaluated by endoscopic retrograde cholangiopancreatography (ERCP). The majority of patients will have a cause other than sphincter of Oddi dysfunction to explain their symptoms, particularly bile duct stones. In the performance of the ERCP, it is important to correctly position the patient in order to adequately screen the bile and pancreatic ducts. It should also be noted whether pain is produced on manipulating the sphincter of Oddi with the ERCP catheter. The rate of drainage of contrast material from the bile duct after the procedure can also be evaluated. Although these signs from the bile duct have a low sensitivity and specificity for sphincter of Oddi dysfunction, they support the diagnosis in the setting of symptoms and radiological signs such as duct dilatation. A number of studies have now shown that significant

bile duct dilatation does not occur following cholecystectomy and that dilatation of the bile duct suggests a relative stenosis of the sphincter of Oddi. The authors take the corrected diameter of 12 mm as the upper limit of normal for the bile duct and diagnose duct dilatation if the maximum corrected diameter exceeds this value. Abnormal drainage is defined by the presence of contrast in the bile duct at 45 minutes after completion of the procedure.

The effect of opiates on sphincter of Oddi contractility also may be used to evaluate these patients and serves as an additional nonspecific screening test. Morphine and neostigmine are given in a dose determined by the patient's weight (in previous reports a fixed dose was used). Reproduction of pain as well as changes in liver enzymes and amylase are assessed. In a group of patients with recurrent postcholecystectomy pain thought to originate from sphincter of Oddi dysfunction, the morphine-neostigmine test was more likely to cause pain and changes in liver enzymes than results in asymptomatic controls. However, as in previous studies, its specificity and sensitivity were poor. When compared with sphincter of Oddi manometry, patients with increases in liver enzymes after a morphine-neostigmine test had a greater incidence of sphincter stenosis when compared to patients whose liver enzymes remained within the normal range.

The role of the morphine provocation test in selecting patients who will benefit from therapy to the sphincter of Oddi has not been clarified. One study concluded that it has low sensitivity for the selection of patients who will benefit from sphincterotomy. The authors use the morphine provocation test as a screening investigation which adds support to other clinical data when the diagnosis of sphincter of Oddi dysfunction is being considered. However, the test is not used to select patients for division of the sphincter of Oddi.

Two additional noninvasive investigations using ultrasonography have been developed to indirectly assess sphincter of Oddi function. Fatty meal sonography is a "real-time" ultrasound investigation designed to evaluate bile duct diameter following a standard fatty meal stimulus of 3.3 ml/kg corn oil (Lipomul). In the duodenum, corn oil releases circulating CCK that normally causes sphincter of Oddi relaxation. This response should lower sphincter of Oddi resistance and enhance bile flow into the duodenum so that the bile duct diameter either diminishes or remains unchanged. With a partial obstruction of the distal end of the bile duct, the diameter increases 1 mm or more, thus suggesting sphincter of Oddi stenosis. The test is sensitive in the presence of a significant obstruction to flow through the sphincter, such as a stone or tumor. However, this test is insensitive for diagnosing motility changes in the sphincter of Oddi. Hence, its use is confined to centers where more specific tests of sphincter of Oddi motility such as manometry are unavailable. A positive test suggests a possible motility disorder, and patients should be referred for manometric studies.

A similar investigation is used to evaluate the pancreatic portion of the sphincter of Oddi in patients with suspected pancreatic sphincter of Oddi dysfunction. The diameter of the pancreatic duct within the body of the pancreas is determined. Normally, this diameter does not exceed 1 mm. Secretin (1 u/kg) is infused intravenously over 15 minutes while the pancreatic duct diameter is monitored. As a result of the increased flow of pancreatic juice, the ductal diameter increases but rapidly returns to normal within 30 minutes. If the duct remains dilated (> 1.5 mm) at 30 minutes, it is thought to be as a result of increased resistance across the pancreatic sphincter, perhaps due to sphincter of Oddi dysfunction. Although the sensitivity and specificity of the test are undefined, it may be used as a noninvasive screen in patients with idiopathic recurrent pancreatitis.

Flow across the sphincter of Oddi may be evaluated in postcholecystectomy subjects using cholescintigraphy following the injection of a ^{99m}Tc-labeled iminodiacetic acid derivative which is excreted into bile from the liver. This test is a minimally invasive investigation which potentially may provide useful data regarding flow dynamics across the sphincter of Oddi. Unfortunately, methodological problems, including difficulty with the clear separation of liver, bile duct, and duodenum and errors induced by bile duct dilatation, make this investigation one of low sensitivity for sphincter of Oddi dysfunction. However, delay in the flow of radionuclide from the bile duct into the duodenum may represent a raised resistance to flow which could be due to sphincter of Oddi dysfunction.

The development of techniques to measure pressure across the sphincter of Oddi has enhanced our understanding of the normal physiology of the human sphincter of Oddi and has also defined with accuracy and reproducibility the presence of manometric disorders of the sphincter (Fig. 26-2). The miniaturized manometry catheters which are used for pressure measurement have three lumens and are made of either polyethylene or polytef (Teflon). They have an outer diameter of 1.5 or 1.7 mm. Three side holes are made at the recording tip of the catheter at 2-mm intervals starting at 10 mm from its distal tip. Thus the three lumens record across a length of 5 mm from within the sphincter of Oddi. The catheter is connected to a pneumohydraulic capillary perfusion system with pressure force transducers in series. The catheter is perfused with deionized bubble-free water at a pressure of 750 mm Hg, and the whole system is capable of recording accurately pressure changes of up to 300 mm Hg/sec.

A patient undergoing endoscopic sphincter of Oddi manometry is prepared for the procedure as for an ERCP. The oropharynx is anesthetized by a topical anesthetic agent. Mild sedation is achieved with intravenous diazepam. Prior to and during the manometric recording, drugs which alter sphincter motility, such as atropine and opiate analgesics, are avoided.

When the duodenoscope is in an appropriate position in relation to the papilla, the manometry catheter is inserted through the biopsy channel. The catheter is passed into either the bile duct or pancreatic duct to record the duct pressure. The catheter is then withdrawn so that all three recording ports are positioned within the sphincter segment (see Fig. 26-2). Baseline recording from the sphincter is made for approximately 3 to 5 minutes. The response to an intravenous bolus dose of cholecystokinin octapeptide 20 ng/kg is then assessed. Catheter position, in either the pancreatic or bile duct, may be assessed by injecting a small volume of contrast medium (< 1 ml) through the most distal port while briefly screening by fluoroscopy.

Endoscopic sphincter of Oddi manometry is the most objective of all available investigations in determining sphincter of Oddi motility characteristics (Table 26-1). Furthermore, in recent studies, the authors have shown that the diagnosis made as

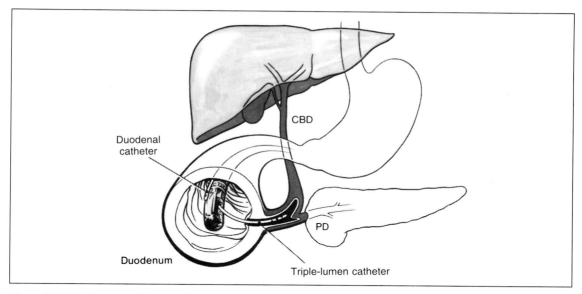

Figure 26-2. Endoscopic sphincter of Oddi manometry. The triple lumen catheter is passed through the biopsy channel of a duodenoscope and inserted into either bile duct or pancreatic duct so that the three ports record from the sphincter.

Table 26-1. Sphincter of Oddi Pressures

	Normal		Abnormal
	Median	Range	
Basal pressure (mm Hg)	15	3–35	> 40
Amplitude (mm Hg)	135	95–195	> 300
Frequency (n/min)	4	2–6	> 7
Sequences			
Antegrade (%)	80	12–100	
Simultaneous (%)	13	0–50	
Retrograde (%)	9	0–50	> 50
CCK (20 ng/kg)	Inhibits		Contracts

a result of manometry is reproducible and appears to identify normal from abnormally functioning sphincters. Manometrically, the sphincter of Oddi is characterized by regular phasic contractions which are superimposed on a modest basal pressure (Fig. 26-3). The majority of the contractions are oriented in an antegrade direction, but simultaneous and retrograde contractions can be recorded in control subjects.

Manometric abnormalities have been identified in patients with clinically suspected sphincter of Oddi dysfunction. Using the manometric findings, the authors have subdivided sphincter of Oddi dysfunction into two major groups, irrespective of whether the symptoms are primarily biliary or pancreatic (Table 26-2). This manometric division has allowed for targeting of specific therapy for patients in whom diagnosis of sphincter of Oddi dysfunction is made. The two major groups are sphincter of Oddi stenosis and sphincter of Oddi dyskinesia.

Sphincter of Oddi Stenosis

Manometrically, these patients have an abnormally elevated sphincter of Oddi basal pressure which is defined as a basal pressure above 40 mm Hg (Fig. 26-4). Patients with manometric stenosis of the sphincter of Oddi may have a dilated bile duct at ERCP and elevation of liver enzymes during episodes of pain. However, since the correlation is not strong, these signs cannot be used to predict those patients with sphincter stenosis.

The finding of sphincter of Oddi stenosis may involve the bile duct sphincter, the pancreatic duct sphincter, or both sphincters. Stenosis in the pancreatic duct sphincter is associated with pancreatic sphincter of Oddi dysfunction, and treatment of these patients requires division of not only the bile duct portion of the sphincter of Oddi but also the septum between the bile duct and pancreatic duct.

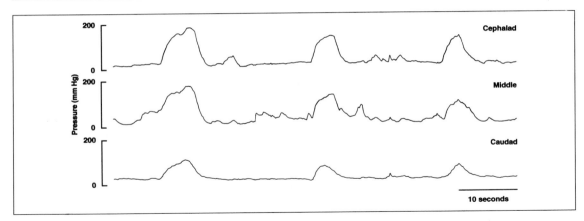

Figure 26-3. Manometric recording from the sphincter of Oddi. Prominent phasic contractions are superimposed on a modest basal pressure.

Table 26-2. Sphincter of Oddi Dysfunction

Stenosis
    Basal pressure $\geq$ 40 mm Hg
Dyskinesia
    Frequency $\geq$ 7/min
    Intermittent rise in basal pressure
    Retrograde contractions $\geq$ 50%
    Paradoxical CCK-OP response

Sphincter of Oddi Dyskinesia

In this group are placed a number of manometric abnormalities which have been described in patients with suspected sphincter of Oddi dysfunction. Their grouping may be inappropriate because they may not have a common etiology.

RAPID PHASIC CONTRACTIONS

Spontaneously occurring bursts of rapid phasic contractions may be recorded. These episodes are distinct from activity fronts which relate to the migrating motor complex (MMC) because they may extend for periods of time in excess of normal MMC activity. Furthermore, rapid contractions may be accompanied by pain. They have been likened to similar recordings which have been made in the stomach (tachygastria) and can be called "tachyoddia."

In order to make the diagnosis of tachyoddia on manometry, one should not commence the recording until the artifacts which follow the introduction of the catheter have subsided. A sustained

frequency in excess of seven contractions per minute is considered abnormal (Fig. 26-5).

INTERMITTENT EPISODES OF ELEVATED BASAL PRESSURE

An intermittent elevation of the basal pressure sometimes may be noted in association with tachyoddia. This finding is unlike the stenotic recordings in that the basal pressure returns to normal, usually spontaneously but sometimes after the inhalation of amyl nitrate. Both this problem and tachyoddia reflect what is recognized as an "irritable" sphincter which appears to readily produce "spasm," whether it be to the stimulus of a recording catheter or to other stimuli such as food in the duodenum or emotional stress.

EXCESSIVE RETROGRADE CONTRACTIONS

In normal subjects, the majority of sphincter of Oddi contractions are oriented in an antegrade direction. However, an excess of simultaneous and retrograde contractions may reflect an abnormally functioning sphincter which may impair bile flow (Fig. 26-6). This subtle manometric finding may be of low significance, and its reproducibility is poor. Taken in isolation, the direction of phasic wave propagation should not be used to make a diagnosis of sphincter of Oddi dysfunction.

PARADOXICAL RESPONSE TO CHOLECYSTOKININ

The normal response of the human sphincter of Oddi to the administration of cholecystokinin is an inhibition of phasic contractions and a fall in basal

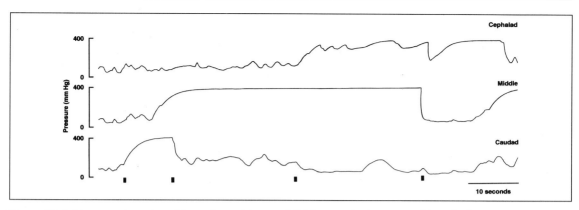

Figure 26-4. Manometric tracings illustrating sphincter of Oddi stenosis characterized by a high basal pressure. The black squares illustrate a stepwise withdrawal of the triple lumen catheter across a narrow stenosis.

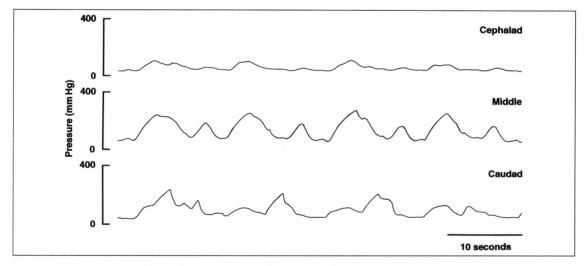

Figure 26-5. Manometric tracing illustrating rapid sphincter of Oddi contractions.

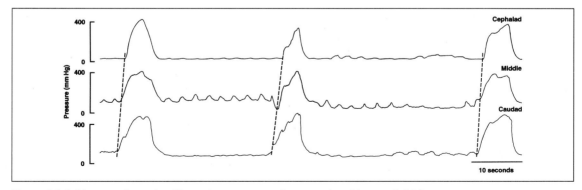

Figure 26-6. Manometric tracing illustrating an excess of retrograde sphincter of Oddi contraction.

pressure. A paradoxical response is recorded when cholecystokinin has no effect on the sphincter contractions or produces an increase in contraction frequency or a rise in basal pressure (Fig. 26-7). Cholecystokinin produces its normal action on the sphincter by stimulating nonadrenergic, noncholinergic inhibitory neurons. In patients exhibiting a paradoxical response to cholecystokinin, it is possible that inhibitory nerves are either damaged or absent and that cholecystokinin has a direct stimulatory effect on smooth muscle. This finding is similar to that seen in patients with an aganglionic segment of the esophagus (achalasia), although similar pathologic correlates have not been defined.

Management and Results

The options for management of sphincter of Oddi dysfunction are either division of the sphincter or pharmacotherapy. In the past, uncertainty in regard to the diagnosis of sphincter dysfunction has been associated with uncertainty in regard to therapy. However, the development of sphincter manometry and the recognition of abnormal motility have led to the identification of individuals who may be cured by targeted treatment.

Patients with biliary-type symptoms are subdivided into three main groups on the basis of their clinical presentation. This grouping permits a practical approach to management (Table 26-3).

Patients in group 1 have biliary pain, abnormal liver enzymes associated with episodes of pain, and a dilated bile duct on ERCP. Most of these patients (> 70%) will have abnormal manometry. Thus it might be argued that manometry is not always necessary in this group prior to sphincterotomy.

Patients in group 2 have biliary pain and either abnormal liver enzymes or a dilated bile duct. Only 50% of these patients have abnormal manometry, perhaps because the disorder is not as advanced as in group 1. Manometry should be done in this group of patients before sphincterotomy is considered.

Patients in group 3 have biliary pain and no detectable abnormalities in liver enzyme or bile duct size. Manometry is mandatory in these patients prior to treatment.

In a prospective study, patients with biliarylike pain in groups 1 and 2 were randomized into endoscopic sphincterotomy or a sham procedure. Manometry was done but was not used to determine therapy. The results of manometry were correlated with the clinical outcome. After 4 years of follow-up, patients with sphincter of Oddi stenosis treated by sphincterotomy were more likely to show improvement in symptoms than patients with sphincter stenosis who had the sham procedure (Table 26-4). If the manometric diagnosis was dyskinesia, significant differences were not observed, although there was a trend toward improvement with sphincterotomy. The results from this study led to the

Figure 26-7. Manometric tracing demonstrating a paradoxical response to cholecystokinin octapeptide (CCK-OP). An increase in contraction frequency is noted instead of inhibition of contractions.

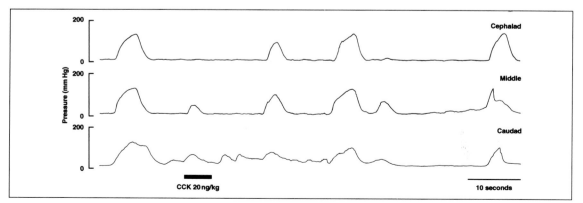

Table 26-3. Sphincter of Oddi Dysfunction Groups

	Group 1	Group 2	Group 3
Pain	+	+	+
LFT change	+	±	−
Dilated central bile duct	+	±	−
Delay in duct emptying	+	±	−

Table 26-4. Endoscopic Sphincterotomy and Sphincter of Oddi Dysfunction

	SO[a] basal pressure < 40 mm Hg		SO basal pressure > 40 mm Hg	
	Sham	ES[b]	Sham	ES
Number of patients	12	12	12	12
Improvement (%)	33	42	25	91
No change (%)	67	58	75	9

[a]SO = sphincter of Oddi.
[b]ES = endoscopic sphincterotomy.

conclusion that patients with significant sphincter of Oddi dysfunction as characterized by an elevated basal pressure (stenosis) should be treated by division of the sphincter of Oddi.

In many patients with idiopathic recurrent pancreatitis, manometry reveals sphincter stenosis. Pancreatic duct stenosis may also be found in patients who have had a biliary sphincterotomy for the treatment of recurrent pancreatitis. Thus endoscopic sphincterotomy is often ineffective for recurrent pancreatitis, and treatment must include division of the pancreatic sphincter. This result is achieved via a transduodenal approach at open operation with division of the septum between the bile duct and pancreatic duct, which creates a wide opening for both ducts.

The results of this operation in producing symptomatic relief in patients with recurrent pancreatitis depend on the selection of patients. Approximately 70% of patients with an abnormally elevated basal pressure are improved by sphincteroplasty and pancreatic septoplasty. Lack of improvement may relate to the fact that many of these patients have been treated for many years with a variety of analgesics, including opiates, and that some have developed a dependence on medication.

Recently, an attempt has been made to provide temporary drainage from the pancreatic duct in patients with stenosis of the pancreatic sphincter and idiopathic recurrent pancreatitis by endoscopically introducing a 5 French stent into the pancreatic duct. Relief from recurrent symptoms has been reported, after which patients may proceed to sphincteroplasty and pancreatic duct septoplasty to achieve permanent drainage. Thus this temporary insertion of a stent may further assist in the selection of patients who will benefit from sphincteroplasty and pancreatic duct septoplasty.

The role of pharmacotherapy in sphincter of Oddi dysfunction is limited because no drugs exist which are specific, long-acting, and free of side effects. Buscopan may be helpful for acute episodes of pain. However, its action is short-lived and cannot be taken prophylactically. The calcium channel blocker nifedipine has also been used with some success in relieving pain, but may be associated with cardiovascular side effects.

The authors' approach to patients with sphincter of Oddi dysfunction, either biliary or pancreatic in type, is to determine whether a manometrically defined stenosis is present. Most of the patients with stenosis proceed to division of the sphincter. For patients with biliary-type symptoms, this division is achieved via the endoscopic approach, whereas in patients with pancreatic symptoms, division is achieved via open operation.

Conclusions

Motility disorders of the gallbladder and sphincter of Oddi are now recognized as real clinical entities. Little is known about the etiology of these rare disorders. Diagnosis of gallbladder dysmotility is best made by calculating the gallbladder ejection fraction from cholescintigraphy with cholecystokinin octapeptide infusion. Diagnosis of sphincter of Oddi stenosis or dysfunction is best achieved by sphincter manometry. Laparoscopic cholecystectomy is recommended for patients with typical biliary symptoms and documented abnormal gallbladder emptying. Endoscopic sphincterotomy is preferred for biliary sphincter stenosis, whereas pancreatic sphincter dysfunction often requires surgical sphincteroplasty.

Selected Readings

Bar-Meir S. Frequency of papillary dysfunction among cholecystectomized patients. *Hepatology* 1984; 4: 328–330.

Bobba VR, et al. Gallbladder dynamics induced by a fatty meal in normal subjects and patients with gallstones: Concise communication. *J Nucl Med* 1984; 25: 21–24.

Geenen JE, et al. The efficacy of endoscopic sphincterotomy in post-cholecystectomy patients with sphincter of Oddi dysfunction. *N Engl J Med* 1989; 320: 82–87.

Hunt DR, Scott AJ. Changes in bile duct diameter after cholecystectomy: A 5 year perioperative study. *Gastroenterology* 1989; 97:1485–1488.

Nardi GL, Acosta JM. Papillitis as a cause of pancreatitis and abdominal pain: Role of evocative test operative pancreatography and histologic evaluation. *Ann Surg* 1966; 164:611–621.

Rhodes M, et al. Cholecystokinin (CCK) "provocation test": Longterm followup after cholecystectomy. *Br J Surg* 1988; 75:951–953.

Thune A, et al. Reproducibility of endoscopic sphincter of Oddi manometry. *Dig Dis Sci* 1991; 36:1401–1405.

Toouli J, et al. Manometric disorders in patients with suspected sphincter of Oddi dysfunction. *Gastroenterology* 1985; 88:1243–1250.

Toouli J, et al. Sphincter of Oddi manometric disorders in patients with idiopathic recurrent pancreatitis. *Br J Surg* 1985; 72:859–863.

Yap L, et al. Gallbladder ejection fraction for acalculous gallbladder pain. *Gastroenterology* 1991; 101: 786–793.

27

Gallbladder Cancer

Xabier de Aretxabala Urquiza
Ricardo L. Rossi
Richard A. Oberfield
Glenn A. Healey

Etiology and Pathogenesis

Although the exact pathogenesis of carcinoma of the gallbladder remains controversial, several causative factors can be related to the development of this tumor.

Cholelithiasis

The presence of gallstones is the most common associated factor. This relationship, suggested by Mayo in 1903, has been confirmed by multiple studies, with an incidence of gallstones of more than 80% in most reported series (Table 27-1). This incidence is considerably greater than that of a control population with similar characteristics of age and sex. The mechanisms of how gallstones relate to the development of carcinoma remain controversial. Chronic inflammation, favoring the sequence of hyperplasia-dysplasia-carcinoma, has been suggested.

Reports of patients with gallstones in countries with a high incidence of carcinoma of the gallbladder and in countries with a low incidence of carcinoma of the gallbladder have been analyzed. The composition of both the bile and gallstones in countries with a high incidence of carcinoma of the gallbladder was different from that of bile and gallstones in countries with a low incidence.

The role of gallstones in the development of carcinoma has also been suggested in studies that have reviewed the relationship between the frequency of cholecystectomy and the incidence of carcinoma. As the frequency of cholecystectomy increases per 100,000 inhabitants, a decrease in the incidence of carcinoma of the gallbladder has been observed.

Analysis of gallstones in patients with cystic conditions of the biliary tree has demonstrated that they have increased mutagenic activity. Other causative factors identified in the development of carcinoma of the gallbladder include the association of an abnormal junction between the common duct and the pancreatic duct, a carrier state of the typhoid bacillus, race, the presence of a porcelain gallbladder, and the presence of gallbladder polyps.

Anomalous Junction of the Common Duct and Pancreatic Duct

The incidence of neoplasia in these patients varies between 12% and 67%. The anomalous junction is also seen in as many as 75% of patients with choledochal cysts. Choledochal cysts are also associated with a high incidence of bile duct carcinoma; the incidence is about 9% in different series. The Lahey Clinic experience in adults showed that synchronous or metachronous tumors developed in 18% of patients. Reflux of pancreatic juice into the biliary tree is thought to cause chronic inflammation and metaplasia of the bile duct epithelium. These changes could be precursors of the development of carcinoma of the bile duct.

Table 27-1. Presence of Gallstones
in Gallbladder Carcinoma

Author	Percent
de Aretxabala et al[a]	99
Nevin et al[b]	93
Morrow et al[c]	92
Donohue et al[d]	82
Tsuchiya[e]	63

[a]Data from de Aretxabala X, et al. Gallbladder cancer in Chile. *Cancer* 1992;69:60–65.
[b]Data from Nevin JE, et al. Carcinoma of the gallbladder: Staging, treatment, and prognosis. *Cancer* 1976;37:141–148.
[c]Data from Morrow CE, et al. Primary gallbladder carcinoma: Significance of subserosal lesions and results of aggressive surgical treatment and adjuvant chemotherapy. *Surgery* 1983;94:709–714.
[d]Data from Donohue JH, et al. Carcinoma of the gallbladder: Does radical resection improve outcome? *Arch Surg* 1990;125:237–241.
[e]Data from Tsuchiya Y. Early carcinoma of the gallbladder: Macroscopic features and US findings. *Radiology* 1991;179:171–175.

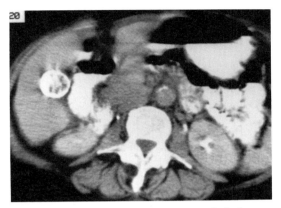

Figure 27-1. CT scan demonstrating a calcified "porcelain" gallbladder.

Carrier of Typhoid Bacillus

The relationship between carriers of the typhoid bacillus and carcinoma of the gallbladder has been reported in different areas of the world. In one study, carriers of typhoid bacillus had a mortality rate associated with hepatobiliary carcinoma of 5.7%, a figure significantly higher than the 1.0% of the control group. It has been suggested the typhoid bacillus could alter the bile, making it more carcinogenic.

Race

An unequal distribution of gallbladder carcinoma in the world suggests a relationship between racial factor or an environmental factor and a major predisposition to the development of such a carcinoma. Carcinoma of the gallbladder is more common in certain Latin American countries, whereas it is uncommon in the black population.

Porcelain Gallbladder

A porcelain gallbladder is a gallbladder in the end stage of inflammatory changes secondary to gallstone disease (Fig. 27-1). It is unknown whether calcification of the gallbladder wall per se or the fact that it represents a late stage of inflammatory changes in the wall of the gallbladder in patients with gallstones is the determining factor causing the high risk of the development of carcinoma of the gallbladder. In general, the incidence of carcinoma of the gallbladder in patients with porcelain gallbladder varies between 13% and 61%.

Gallbladder Polyps

Gallbladder polyps are found in 0.004% to 13.000% of gallbladders removed. The presence of a polyp has been associated with an increased incidence of neoplasia in up to 8% of patients. Most polypoid lesions of the gallbladder are pseudotumors, such as cholesterol polyps or hyperplastic polyps. Large polyp size, gallstones that have been present for a

Table 27-2. Relation Between the Size of the Polyp and the Presence of Carcinoma*

	< 5 mm	5–10 mm	10–20 mm	20–30 mm	30–50 mm	> 50 mm
Cholesterol polyp	12	9	—	—	—	—
Adenomyomatous hyperplasia	3	1	—	—	—	—
Adenoma	—	—	1	—	—	—
Adenomatous hyperplasia	1	—	—	—	—	—
Inflammatory polyp	1	3	—	—	—	—
Other	—	—	1	—	—	—
Adenocarcinoma	—	1	2	1	2	2

Source: Adapted from Koga A, et al. Diagnosis and operative indications for polypoid lesions of the gallbladder. *Arch Surg* 1988;123:28.

long time, and single polyps appear to be more frequently associated with carcinoma of the gallbladder. The incidence of carcinoma developing in a polyp increases appreciably when the polyp is larger than 5 mm (Table 27-2).

Diagnosis

Early diagnosis is of major importance in improving the prognosis of patients with carcinoma of the gallbladder. However, the presence of symptoms is usually related to infiltration of other organs or to obstruction of the gallbladder and biliary tree and portends an advanced stage of the disease. The only possibility of a long-term survival is to discover the tumor before it invades the serosa of the gallbladder and surrounding soft tissue.

Of the imaging techniques available for early detection, ultrasonography is less expensive, less invasive, and easier to apply to a larger number of patients than other modalities. Computerized tomography (CT), magnetic resonance imaging (MRI), endoscopic retrograde cholangiopancreatography, percutaneous transhepatic cholangiography, and endoscopic ultrasonography are not performed for early diagnosis but are used to stage the disease (Fig. 27-2).

Ultrasonography is diagnostic in about 75% to 80% of patients with advanced carcinoma of the

Figure 27-2. MRI (T-2) demonstrating a carcinoma of the gallbladder invading the portal hepatis.

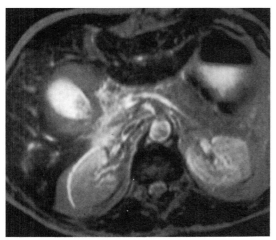

gallbladder. Findings include thickening of the gallbladder wall and the presence of a mass in the gallbladder. Only patients who do not have serosal invasion can be treated successfully by operation, but early diagnosis is still infrequent. Studies dealing with early carcinoma of the gallbladder were able to establish the diagnosis of carcinoma in no more than a third of patients. Polypoid lesions and mass lesions are commonly diagnosed, whereas flat and infiltrating lesions are less likely to be identified. Often the differential diagnosis of a thickened gallbladder wall in the presence of gallstones increases the difficulty of making an accurate diagnosis. Despite these limitations, the frequent use of ultrasonography as a diagnostic tool has made it possible to diagnose an increasing number of early tumors.

In view of the difficulties in establishing an early diagnosis preoperatively, it is easy to understand why so many early gallbladder carcinomas are identified at the time of cholecystectomy for gallstone disease or on pathologic examination of the gallbladder specimen after its routine removal. It is important, therefore, that the gallbladder is examined carefully at the time of operation. Immediately after the gallbladder is removed, it should be emptied and placed in 10% formalin for 10 minutes while the mucosa and wall of the gallbladder are being examined. This step facilitates visualization of the mucosal surface. Any abnormality of the mucosa should be studied with frozen section analysis before the procedure is concluded. Similarly, in geographic areas where the incidence of carcinoma of the gallbladder is high, random areas of the gallbladder wall should be sampled and studied pathologically. The gallbladder wall and cystic duct should be tagged for the presence of carcinoma.

Management and Results

Surgical Treatment

The resectability rates associated with gallbladder carcinoma vary between 10% and 30%, with a 5-year survival rate that does not exceed 5%. The basic treatment for patients with carcinoma of the gallbladder is resection of the primary tumor and the most common areas of metastases. Although metastatic disease can occur, primary dissemination of disease is by local extension. The routes of spread are primarily venous, lymphatic, and in continuity. Additional pathways of dissemination are peritoneal spread and involvement of the primary biliary tree. The latter pathway tends to occur more often with papillary types of tumor.

The veins of the serosa of the gallbladder wall drain directly to veins of the liver parenchyma and to branches of the portal vein of segments V and VIII. The gallbladder lymphatics drain into the cystic duct node and into the lymphatics around the extrahepatic biliary tree. They can spread to the lymphatics of the retropancreatic area and the celiac trunk and thereafter to the periaortic lymph nodes. Based on these routes of dissemination, the surgical treatment theoretically includes resection of the gallbladder bed and the lymphatics of the porta hepatis and retropancreatic area.

Because prognosis is primarily related to depth of invasion of the gallbladder wall, therapy is best tailored to the degree of wall involvement. In patients with tumors limited to the mucosa, simple cholecystectomy appears to suffice. The presence of local dissemination or metastatic disease in these patients is rare, and a different surgical approach is not justified.

For patients with serosal invasion and extension of tumor to adjacent organs, surgical therapy with curative intent is controversial because survival is unlikely to be affected significantly. Only a few patients with advanced disease are treated aggressively, and therefore, it is difficult to assess the therapeutic value of these procedures in this situation. In some patients with advanced disease, palliative procedures, such as endoscopic or percutaneous stenting, may be preferable. A more aggressive surgical approach could perhaps affect outcome in patients with an intermediate stage of disease, that is, tumor infiltrating the muscular or subserosal layer.

When the diagnosis is suspected preoperatively, CT may be of help in identifying the stage of disease. When the diagnosis is suspected during an operation for gallstone disease, the diagnosis should be confirmed histologically, and the degree of infiltration of the wall by tumor should be as-

sessed. The surgeon should evaluate the extent of disease to the parenchyma and the status of the cystic duct node, hepatic hilar nodes, and retropancreatic and periaortic nodes. Nodal metastatic disease is associated with poor survival and in most instances precludes surgery with curative intent.

In general, for the treatment of carcinoma of the gallbladder, the surgical technique consists of resection of segment V and the anterior portion of segment IV (Fig. 27-3). The nodes of the hilum of the liver and the retropancreatic area are dissected (Fig. 27-4). The extrahepatic biliary tree may be resected to achieve a more complete lymph node dissection and to ensure prolonged patency of the biliary tree.

The identification of carcinoma in lymph nodes or in the parenchyma of the liver in resected specimens is directly related to the extent of invasion of the wall of the gallbladder (Table 27-3). When infiltration is limited to the muscular layer, identifying additional tumor is unlikely. When the tumor extends to the subserosa, about a third of patients will have either lymphatic or hepatic parenchymal disease. This percentage increases to more than 80% in patients in whom invasion extends to the serosa or the periserosal fat of the gallbladder bed.

When cholecystectomy has been performed for benign gallstone disease and several days later the pathologic report indicates carcinoma of the gallbladder, the therapy chosen should also be based on the degree of infiltration of the gallbladder wall. Patients with mucosal lesions do not require additional surgery. With invasion of the muscularis and subserosa, operative reintervention is indicated for resection of the gallbladder bed and hilar lymph nodes. With extension of tumor to the serosa or periserosal structures or perilymphatic involvement, the decision should be individualized and discussed with each patient, keeping in mind the poor results of extensive surgery in this group of patients.

It is important to discuss the relation of laparoscopic surgery and carcinoma of the gallbladder. According to some reports, the routine use of laparoscopic cholecystectomy has resulted in a delayed diagnosis of carcinoma of the gallbladder. The implantation of tumor at trocar sites has been described. The authors have also been referred to a patient who became jaundiced several months after

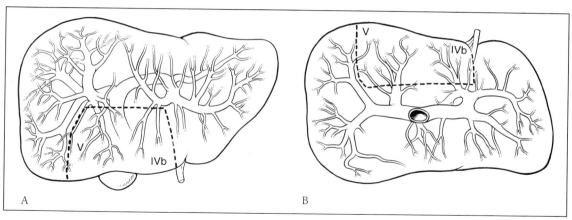

Figure 27-3. En bloc resection of the gallbladder with adjacent liver segments IVb and V. Illustration of the portal venous system of the liver from original corrosion casts. A. Frontal superior view. B. Dorsal inferior view. (Reproduced by permission of Lahey Clinic.)

uneventful laparoscopic cholecystectomy. The patient was referred for a possible benign bile duct stricture. At operation, biliary carcinoma with peritoneal metastases and tumor invasion of the trocar sites was found. The authors believe that the lack of suspicion of carcinoma results in the dissemination of tumor cells to the peritoneum and incisions at the time of laparoscopic cholecystectomy. Therefore, when carcinoma is suspected preoperatively

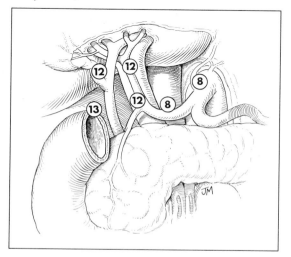

Figure 27-4. Lymph node nomenclature according to the Japanese Society of Biliary Surgery rules for carcinoma of the biliary tract. (Reproduced by permission of Lahey Clinic.)

or at the time of laparoscopy, conversion to an open procedure is indicated. In geographic areas where carcinoma of the gallbladder is frequent, a high index of suspicion is required, and the gallbladder should be removed and placed in a plastic bag.

Controversial Issues

A major problem with regard to results of surgical therapy of carcinoma of the gallbladder is the small number of patients in many of the reported series. The Mayo Clinic series accumulated only 111 patients over a 12-year period, whereas the experience of the Roswell Park group accumulated 71 patients over a 22-year period. In addition, most patients had advanced stages of disease, and any surgical therapy would produce limited results. In addition, aggressive surgical therapy is associated with a significant operative mortality rate of about 5% or 6%.

Different surgical treatment options fluctuate between simple cholecystectomy and radical procedures that include resection of the liver and pan-

Table 27-3. Findings in Reoperations

	Muscular Layer	Subserosa	Fatty Tissue	Serosa
Liver (+)	1	4	3	4
Liver (−)	9	18	0	2
Nodes (+)	0	3	5	5
Nodes (−)	10	17	1	1

creatoduodenectomy. The lack of consensus in the surgical management of this disease became evident from a poll conducted of North American hepatobiliary surgeons. The authors evaluated the choice of operation of different surgeons for different stages of invasion of the disease.

Most groups agree that simple cholecystectomy suffices in patients with involvement of the mucosa only. The suggested effectiveness of radical surgery compared with simple cholecystectomy for patients with tumors involving the muscularis or the subserosa is confirmed in only a limited number of publications. Most of these reports are retrospective and combine different time periods, which makes analysis of results difficult. However, a more radical approach is preferred in selected patients.

The controversy concerning the surgical management of patients with infiltration of the muscularis is summarized in Table 27-4. Although some authors believe that radical surgery is of no benefit in these patients, other authors favor extensive surgery in an attempt to improve the 20% to 40% 5-year mortality rate of these patients.

When the tumor infiltrates the subserosa but does not extend to it or beyond it, the consensus is that radical surgery is beneficial. Some surgeons add resection of the extrahepatic biliary tree.

Table 27-4. Radical Surgery for Patients with Involvement of Muscular Wall

Tsunoda et al[a]	Yes
Ouchi et al[b]	Yes
Matsumoto et al[c]	Yes
Nevin et al[d]	No
Yamaguchi & Tsuneyoshi[e]	No
Gall et al[f]	No

[a]Tsunoda T, et al. The surgical treatment for carcinoma of the gallbladder: Rationale of the second-look operation for inapparent carcinoma. *Jap J Surg* 1987; 17:478–486.
[b]Ouchi K, et al. Prognostic factors in the surgical treatment of gallbladder carcinoma. *Surgery* 101:731–737, 1987.
[c]Matsumoto Y, et al. Surgical treatment of primary carcinoma of the gallbladder based on the histologic analysis of 48 surgical specimens. *Am J Surg* 1992; 163:239–245.
[d]Nevin JE, et al. Carcinoma of the gallbladder: Staging, treatment, and prognosis. *Cancer* 1976; 37:141–148.
[e]Yamaguchi K, Tsuneyoski M. Subclinical gallbladder carcinoma. *Am J Surg* 1992; 163:382–386.
[f]Gall FP, et al. Radical operations for carcinoma of the gallbladder: Present status in Germany. *World J Surg* 1991; 15:328–336.

When tumor infiltrates the serosa, Morrow et al. did not find any benefit to radical surgery when all layers of the gallbladder wall were involved with or without involvement of the cystic duct node. On the other hand, Donohue et al. suggested a benefit in such a group of patients. With regard to the Japanese experience, Ouchi et al. confirmed the poor prognosis in patients with these tumors. In 17 patients treated with simple cholecystectomy, no patient survived 2 years, whereas the 3-year survival rate for patients treated with radical surgery was 17%. This difference was not statistically significant, and no patient survived 5 years. A series reported by de Aretxabala showed no difference between patients with serosal extension treated by cholecystectomy compared with radical surgery, confirming that serosal involvement is fatal in almost all patients.

Reports of more aggressive surgery, including pancreatoduodenectomy and extensive hepatic resection, are associated with a higher morbidity and mortality, and they usually represent few cases. Benefits, if any, are limited.

The controversy with regard to the surgical therapy of patients with a delayed diagnosis of carcinoma of the gallbladder after cholecystectomy for gallstone disease suggests that patients who benefit most from reoperation and a more radical procedure are those with infiltration limited to the subserosa. Unfortunately, this difference in survival in favor of a radical approach was only significant in the first few years of the follow-up study from Chile. Later on, this difference ceased to be of statistical significance.

The selection of surgical therapy based on age, tumor differentiation, histologic type, or DNA needs further study before conclusions can be reached.

Based on the limited results of surgical therapy, a prospective trial has been started by de Aretxabala using chemoradiation with 5-fluorouracil administered for 5 weeks before operation. This study was undertaken because of reported benefits of chemoradiation in patients with other types of gastrointestinal tumors. Although no results are available yet with regard to survival advantage, the addition of chemoradiation has not increased the morbidity and mortality associated with subsequent operations.

Chemotherapy

Over the years, chemotherapy and radiation therapy have been employed separately or in combination both as adjuvant therapy after operation and for palliation of locally advanced and metastatic disease in the hope of improving survival and providing palliation. Many of the studies reported over the past 20 years have been small series of patients that combined patients with biliary carcinoma and gallbladder carcinoma, making results difficult to evaluate. Such studies have usually included median survival time, occasionally objective response rates, and, finally, palliation of symptoms.

SYSTEMIC CHEMOTHERAPY

Systemic chemotherapy has been employed over the past 20 years for palliation of symptoms. Ten studies from 1976 to 1981 involved about 216 patients with carcinoma of the gallbladder and employed predominantly 5-fluorouracil but included mitomycin C, adriamycin, and methyl-CCNU. About 70% of patients experienced clinical benefit, with 30% showing no improvement or progression. In many of these reports, objective measurements for the evaluation of results were infrequently used, but extension of median survival with statistical significance was obtained. Authors often concluded that "benefit accrued through these patients." Therefore, it is difficult to assess the scientific validity of many of these studies, but we must use these trials to decide recommendations for chemotherapy.

The time-honored drug has been 5-fluorouracil; overall response rates vary from 10% to 20%, with conflicting reports of increase in survival. Other single agents used have been mitomycin C, with increased activity, and drug combinations employing 5-fluorouracil, mitomycin C, and adriamycin, known as the FAM program, have been used frequently for patients with biliary carcinoma. Attempts have been made to employ drug sensitivity testing of carcinoma of the gallbladder in human tumor cloning assays, but no correlations could be made between results of cloning and the chemotherapy administered.

ADJUVANT CHEMOTHERAPY

Improved survival has been reported in three clinical trials from 1984 to 1991 that employed chemotherapy as an adjunct to total surgical removal of the gallbladder and lymph nodes. No studies have ever been performed in an adjuvant setting employing a randomized trial. In 1976, Treadwell and Hardin reported slightly increased survival with adjuvant chemotherapy in 15 patients. In 1984, Buskirk et al. also reported on a few patients treated after cholecystectomy with radiation in combination with 5-fluorouracil during the first and last 3 days of radiation therapy, with indeterminate results. They also employed a transcatheter boost with iridium 192. An excellent review of Wanebo and Vezeridis in 1993 recommended adjuvant treatment after resection of the gallbladder bed and lymph node dissection. In high-risk patients with stage II lesions invading all layers, radiation therapy plus chemotherapy should be used. For patients with positive nodes, stage III disease, positive margins, or extension into the liver, postoperative radiation therapy and chemotherapy would be indicated in addition to placement of radiopaque clips to facilitate treatment.

COMBINED CHEMOTHERAPY AND RADIATION THERAPY

Four studies between 1984 and 1991 involved 27 patients using chemotherapy and radiation therapy with additional administration of radioactive iodine 125 intraoperatively or iridium 192 by transcatheter. Clinical benefit was reported in 75% of the studies. The most recent study in 1991 by Minsky et al. reported their experience with mitomycin C, 5-fluorouracil, and radiation therapy in patients undergoing subtotal resection and in patients with unresectable disease. Their data showed that this approach was possible and that survival might be improved. In addition, they employed iridium 192 for brachytherapy.

REGIONAL CHEMOTHERAPY

Carcinoma of the gallbladder is often confined to a regional site, the gallbladder bed, adjacent liver, and regional nodes and would logically provide the basis for regional chemotherapy in view of these anatomic considerations. Six studies from 1974 to

1988 involving about 36 patients reported the use of intra-arterial chemotherapy for the treatment of patients with carcinoma of the gallbladder. Increased survival was described in 50% of these studies. In 1979, von Eyben et al. reported slight improvement in survival. In 1984, Smith et al. reported the use of 5-fluorouracil and mitomycin C intra-arterially. The authors of this chapter employed hepatic artery infusion treatment for many years in patients with carcinoma of the biliary tract and in infrequent numbers of patients having carcinoma of the gallbladder, and the results were inconclusive. Kairaluoma et al. and Shieh et al. found no benefit with regional infusion treatment. However, it must be realized that the numbers of patients are small, various methods of hepatic artery infusion are used, and results are often inconclusive. In 1983, Morrow et al. employed intra-arterial therapy for adjuvant treatment and suggested a slightly improved survival time.

COMMENT

From reviewing these studies, it can be concluded that the use of chemotherapy and radiation therapy after cholecystectomy and lymphadenectomy with minimal tumor burden remaining will promote the best survival with potential cure of these patients. No carefully designed studies have been performed that stage patients similarly and use all three modalities of treatment, that is, surgery, radiation therapy, and chemotherapy intravenously or intra-arterially. If the toxicity of regional infusion could be minimized, this approach should offer the best opportunity for survival or cure of patients with advanced disease. Combinations of radiation therapy with single-agent chemotherapy, such as 5-fluorouracil, or combinations of 5-fluorouracil and mitomycin C might be of benefit. The recent enhancement of 5-fluorouracil activity employing leucovorin should also be employed in the hope of improving response rates. Despite the discouraging results over the years, we should continue to pursue aggressive multimodality therapy for better control of carcinoma of the gallbladder.

Radiation Therapy

In the multidisciplinary management of carcinoma of the gallbladder, the role of radiation therapy is limited. Local recurrence is among the causes of death in patients whose disease relapses after cholecystectomy. In the literature review of Kopelson et al., local recurrence was present or was the cause of death of 95 of 110 patients (86%) who died within 5 years after simple cholecystectomy. Of the 25 patients who survived beyond 5 years, 11 (44%) experienced local recurrence. Among 16 patients selected for radical cholecystectomy, 12 (75%) died with or as a consequence of local recurrence. The rationale for radiotherapy is the high incidence of local-regional failure after operation and the documented ability of adjuvant irradiation to control microscopic residual carcinoma of other gastrointestinal tract sites.

One controversy surrounding the role of adjuvant radiotherapy is that the subset of patients with carcinoma of the gallbladder at high risk for local failure in the absence of peritoneal seeding or distant metastases has not been defined. In one series, 12 patients were treated for carcinoma of the gallbladder with radical cholecystectomy alone. Among the 11 postoperative survivors, 7 (63%) had failure to control disease in local-regional sites, and 4 of these 7 patients also had failure to control disease at distant sites. In a series of 4 patients who underwent radiation therapy for residual disease after simple cholecystectomy, diffuse peritoneal carcinomatosis developed in 3 patients. Randomized trials are needed to demonstrate the best populations of patients who may benefit from postoperative irradiation.

TECHNIQUE

The region at risk for local-regional failure includes the operative bed and the drainage nodal basin. The tumor bed is outlined at the time of operation with judiciously placed clips. The radiation oncologist should be present in the operating room to evaluate placement of the clips. In addition to direct vision during the operation, radiologic studies, operative notes, and histopathologic findings provide information for determining the radiation treatment volume. When possible, the surgeon should be present at the time that radiation treatment is simulated to evaluate the simulation films. External beam therapy is the preferred irradiation modality in that the entire volume at risk is rarely accessible to interstitial and intracavitary brachytherapy. Intraoperative radiation therapy has been used in the management of patients with unresectable carcinoma of the gallbladder. A potential role for intraoperative radiation therapy as adjuvant therapy has been suggested.

Patients found to have carcinoma in situ or invasive carcinoma limited to the muscularis propria in general do not require adjuvant local-regional therapy after complete resection. Patients who have microscopic residual disease, such as a close or involved margin of resection, are treated to an initial dose of 45 Gy in 25 fractions followed by a reduced-field–size boost. The initial target consists of the tumor bed with a 3- to 5-cm margin around the surgically clipped region as well as the regional nodal drainage system of the cystic duct, the hepatic duct, the common bile duct, and the pancreaticoduodenal and celiac axis nodes. A three-field or four-field technique is used. Custom beam-shaping devices limit the dose to uninvolved adjacent structures. The margin around the tumor bed in the reduced field takes into consideration the tolerance doses of the tissues of the spinal cord, the kidneys, the liver, the small bowel, and the stomach. The reduced field is treated to a dose of 5.4 to 9.0 Gy in 3 to 5 fractions for a cumulative dose to the region at risk of 50.4 to 54.0 Gy over 5.5 to 6.0 weeks.

For residual disease after maximal surgical resection, higher doses are needed for local control. In some circumstances, a carefully defined boost volume can be carried to 60+ Gy. Such high boost doses can also be considered in the setting of brachytherapy or intraoperative radiotherapy. For patients with massive unresectable carcinoma, palliative treatment is considered for relief of symptoms, such as pain or bleeding from local tumor or nodal metastasis. A dose of 40 Gy in 20 fractions with a split-course technique is adequate. However, aggressive therapy with curative intent does not substantially alter the natural history of patients with unresectable tumors.

RESULTS

The literature is scant on adjuvant irradiation for patients with carcinoma of the gallbladder. Bosset and colleagues described the management of seven patients treated to 54 Gy (45 Gy to the tumor bed and regional nodes plus a 9 Gy reduced-field boost)

after complete resection. In two patients, disease recurred in the abdomen, and these patients died. Five patients are alive at 5 to 58 months. This prospective study complements several other small, single-institution retrospective studies indicating a role for adjuvant therapy. In other retrospective studies, adjuvant treatment for carcinoma of the gallbladder produced poor results. In the absence of confirming randomized trials, careful patient selection is indicated.

For residual or unresectable disease, intraoperative radiotherapy produced hopeful results in one study, yet this was not confirmed by other authors. Busse and colleagues suggested that intraoperative radiotherapy may be of value to maximize local control in patients at high risk for local failure after total resection. However, the use of intraoperative radiotherapy as a surgical adjuvant has not been documented, and the patient population at risk for local failure in the absence of recurrent disease in the peritoneum or distant metastasis has not been defined adequately.

Conclusions

Several factors have been associated with an increased incidence of gallbladder cancer. These factors include cholelithiasis, an anomalous junction of the common duct and pancreatic ducts, typhoid carriers, race, a porcelain gallbladder, and gallbladder polyps. Ideally, ultrasonography should be sufficient for diagnosis. However, with more advanced tumors, CT, MRI, cholangiography, or angiography may be required to adequately stage the patient. Cholecystectomy alone may be sufficient for stage I tumors confined to the mucosa. Controversy persists regarding the role of extended operations which include liver or pancreatic resection for more advanced tumors. Similarly, no controlled data have demonstrated increased survival with chemotherapy or radiation therapy.

Selected Readings

Busse PM, et al. Intraoperative radiation therapy for carcinoma of the gallbladder. *World J Surg* 1991; 15: 352–356.

Clair DG, Lautz DB, Brooks DC. Rapid development of umbilical metastases after laparoscopic cholecystec-

tomy for unsuspected carcinoma. *Surgery* 1993;
113:355–358.

de Aretxabala X, et al. Gallbladder cancer in Chile. *Cancer*
1992; 69:60–65.

Gagner M, Rossi RL. Radical operations for carcinoma of
the gallbladder: Present status in North America.
World J Surg 1991; 15:344–347.

Koga A, et al. Diagnosis and operative indications for
polypoid lesions of the gallbladder. *Arch Surg* 1988;
123:26–29.

Oberfield RA, Rossi RL. The role of chemotherapy in the
treatment of bile duct cancer. *World J Surg* 1988;
12:105–108.

Ouchi K, et al. Do recent advances in diagnosis and
operative management improve the outcome of gallbladder carcinoma? *Surgery* 1993; 113:324–329.

Tanaka K, et al. Cancer of the gallbladder associated with
anomalous junction of the pancreatobiliary duct system without bile duct dilatation. *Br J Surg* 1993;
80:622–624.

Todoroki T, et al. Resection combined with intraoperative
radiation therapy (IORT) for stage IV (TNM) gallbladder carcinoma. *World J Surg* 1991; 15:357–366.

Wanebo HJ, Vezeridis MP. Carcinoma of the gallbladder.
J Surg Oncol Suppl 1993; 3:134–139.

28

Cholangiocarcinoma

CHARLES J. YEO
ANTHONY C. VENBRUX
PAUL J. THULUVATH

This chapter is devoted to the management of patients with cholangiocarcinoma, focusing upon intrahepatic (peripheral) tumors and tumors of the hepatic hilus. Cholangiocarcinomas arising in the distal common bile duct that lie within the pancreatic parenchyma are best considered in discussions of periampullary (Chapter 41) or pancreatic (Chapter 42) malignancy.

Etiology and Pathogenesis

Several etiologic factors have been linked to cholangiocarcinoma (Table 28-1). Cholangiocarcinoma is clearly associated with cystic dilatation of the bile duct, including both choledochal cyst disease and Caroli's disease. This association has been recognized for over 50 years, with a 2.5% to 28% incidence of cholangiocarcinoma being seen in such patients. Patients with choledochal cyst–associated cholangiocarcinoma are typically diagnosed in the fourth decade of life, 20 to 30 years prior to the mean age of diagnosis of patients with cholangiocarcinoma without choledochal cysts. Factors that may account for the association between choledochal cysts and subsequent formation of cholangiocarcinoma include (1) the finding of an anomalous pancreatic–bile duct junction (APBDJ), which suggests a causative role for the reflux of pancreatic exocrine secretions into the bile duct lumen; (2) stone formation within the choledochal cyst; (3) bile stasis; and (4) chronic inflammation within the cyst.

A clear association is also recognized between infection with the liver fluke Clonorchis sinensis and cholangiocarcinoma. Clonorchiasis is common in Asia, where the ingestion of raw fish allows the parasite to gain entry via the host's duodenum. The adult trematodes prefer the intrahepatic, and less commonly the extrahepatic, biliary ducts as their habitats. In these sites the trematodes can obstruct the flow of bile and cause periductal fibrosis and hyperplasia, which are putative causative factors in the subsequent production of cholangiocarcinoma. Another liver fluke, Opisthorchis viverrini, is endemic in Thailand and has also been proposed as a risk factor for cholangiocarcinoma.

Cholelithiasis has been seen in up to one third of patients with cholangiocarcinoma. However, although there is a strong association between gallstones and gallbladder carcinoma, a definite cause-and-effect relationship has not been established for cholangiocarcinoma.

Hepatolithiasis is prevalent in East Asia, being seen in up to 50% of patients undergoing cholecystectomy in endemic regions. Recent studies suggest a 5% to 10% risk of cholangiocarcinoma in patients with hepatolithiasis. In these patients, bile stasis, bactibilia, and cystic dilatation of the intrahepatic biliary tree all may be risk factors for the development of cholangiocarcinoma.

An extremely strong association exists between the use of the radiocontrast agent thorium dioxide (Thorotrast) and the subsequent development of cholangiocarcinoma. Thorium dioxide as a 25% colloidal solution was used from the late 1920s until the 1940s as a contrast agent for radiography. Thorium dioxide emits energy as alpha particles;

Table 28-1. Cholangiocarcinoma: Etiologic Factors

Strongly Associated	Weakly Associated
Cystic dilatation of the bile duct	Asbestos
Choledochal cyst	Dioxin (Agent Orange)
Caroli's disease	Gallstones
Clonorchis sinensis	Isoniazid
Hepatolithiasis	Methyldopa
Sclerosing cholangitis	Nitrosamines
Thorium dioxide (Thorotrast)	*Opisthorchis viverrini*
Ulcerative colitis	Oral contraceptives
	Polychlorinated biphenyls

Source: Modified from Yeo CJ, Pitt HA, Cameron JL. Cholangiocarcinoma. *Surg Clin North Am* 1990;70:1429–1447.

when it is injected intravenously, it is retained within the reticuloendothelial system for life. Thorium-related cholangiocarcinomas have been diagnosed on the average of 35 years after exposure, occurring at least one decade earlier than non–thorium-related cases.

Cholangiocarcinoma has been observed to develop in many patients with sclerosing cholangitis. Unrecognized cholangiocarcinoma has been found at autopsy in up to 40% of patients dying with sclerosing cholangitis and in 9% of patients undergoing orthotopic liver transplantation for sclerosing cholangitis. An association between ulcerative colitis and cholangiocarcinoma is also well established, although not as strongly as the association between sclerosing cholangitis and cholangiocarcinoma. Cholangiocarcinoma is found in 0.4% to 1.4% of patients with ulcerative colitis, thus representing a manyfold increased risk over the general population. Ulcerative colitis patients who develop cholangiocarcinoma typically have had pancolonic involvement with inflammatory bowel disease, as well as a long duration of colitis.

In addition to the above-mentioned etiologic factors, exposure to several other drugs and carcinogens is associated with cholangiocarcinoma (see Table 28-1): asbestos, dioxin (Agent Orange), isoniazid, methyldopa, nitrosamines, oral contraceptives, and polychlorinated biphenyls.

Diagnosis

The average age at the diagnosis of cholangiocarcinoma ranges between 60 and 65 years. Patients who develop cholangiocarcinoma in association with choledochal cyst disease, clonorchiasis, hepatolithiasis, thorium dioxide exposure, sclerosing cholangitis, or ulcerative colitis tend to present at younger ages. The male-female ratio approximates 1.3:1.0. The most common finding at clinical presentation is jaundice, which is present in over 90% of patients. Pruritus, weight loss, anorexia, mild abdominal pain, and fatigue may be present in one half to two thirds of patients. Hepatomegaly or a palpable gallbladder may be seen occasionally, whereas cachexia and ascites are less frequent findings. Cholangitis is not a common presenting feature, although it may be seen following biliary manipulation by endoscopic or percutaneous techniques.

In most patients, serum chemistry abnormalities are limited to elevations in the levels of bilirubin and of markers of bile duct epithelial cell injury (alkaline phosphatase and gamma-glutamyl transferase), with only mild elevations of the markers of hepatocellular injury (alanine aminotransferase and aspartate aminotransferase). Other serum chemistries are typically normal, as are routine hematologic parameters. In patients with long-standing jaundice, prolongation of the prothrombin time may be noted, reflecting a diminution in hepatic synthetic function. Serum tumor markers such as carcinoembryonic antigen (CEA), alpha-fetoprotein (AFP), or carbohydrate antigen 19-9 (CA 19-9) are typically normal. At present, no screening blood test is specific for cholangiocarcinoma.

In patients with peripheral cholangiocarcinoma (originating above the hepatic duct bifurcation), the intrahepatic biliary tree may become obstructed in a unilobar fashion. These patients typically present with mild upper abdominal pain, unilobular hepatic enlargement, and elevations in the levels of alkaline phosphatase and gamma-glutamyl transferase, without elevations of serum bilirubin and without clinical jaundice.

The goals of imaging studies in patients with presumed cholangiocarcinoma include the delineation of the level and extent of the biliary obstruction, the search for metastatic disease, and the evaluation of local extension that might preclude curative resection. An ordered use of imaging tests is typically successful in imaging the obstructing lesion and defining the biliary anatomy. Initial radiographic studies (Fig. 28-1) consist of either abdominal ultrasound or computerized tomography (CT). Findings suggestive of **hilar** bile duct carcinoma include a dilated intrahepatic biliary tree associated with a normal gallbladder, extrahepatic biliary tree, and pancreas. In contrast, the findings suggestive of a **distal** cholangiocarcinoma involving the intrapancreatic portion of the common bile duct include a dilated intrahepatic and extrahepatic biliary tree with a distended gallbladder. The primary tumor mass is visualized by CT or ultrasound in only a minority of patients. Early experience suggests that magnetic resonance imaging (MRI) may be a more sensitive modality for visualizing the primary tumor.

After ultrasound or CT scan document bile duct dilatation, the biliary anatomy is studied cholangiographically via either percutaneous transhepatic cholangiography (PTC; Fig. 28-2) or endoscopic retrograde cholangiopancreatography (ERCP; Figs. 28-3, 28-4). For tumors of the distal common bile duct that are partially obstructing, ERCP may allow visualization of the uppermost extent of the tumor within the extrahepatic biliary tree, and decompression of the obstructed biliary tree can be performed via placement of a biliary endoprosthesis (Fig. 28-5). Percutaneous transhepatic placement

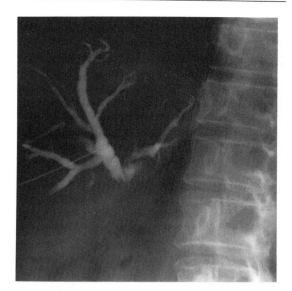

Figure 28-2. PTC of a patient with hilar cholangiocarcinoma showing intrahepatic ductal dilatation and no flow of contrast into the extrahepatic biliary tree.

Figure 28-1. CT scan of a patient with hilar cholangiocarcinoma predominantly involving the left hepatic ducts, revealing dilated ducts on the left side of the liver.

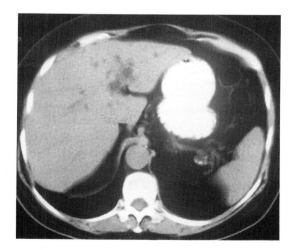

of a biliary stent is also possible for tumors in this location.

When the cholangiocarcinoma involves the more proximal biliary tree, PTC is favored because it defines the extent of the proximal tumor involvement of the hepatic hilus and allows for the preoperative placement of percutaneous transhepatic catheters. In cases of hilar obstruction of both the right and left hepatic ducts, transhepatic catheters may be placed into both the right and left hepatic lobes and through the obstructing tumor. The advantages of transhepatic catheter placement in patients undergoing surgical exploration for hilar cholangiocarcinoma are that it (1) assists in the technical aspects of hilar dissection and (2) facilitates intraoperative placement of polymeric silicone (Silastic) transhepatic stents. Currently available data do not support the practice of placing preoperative transhepatic catheters solely in an effort to reduce operative or perioperative mortality.

Establishing a tissue diagnosis prior to surgery in cases of suspected cholangiocarcinoma can employ techniques such as percutaneous fine-needle aspiration, scrape and brush biopsy, and cytologic examination of bile. Although these techniques are

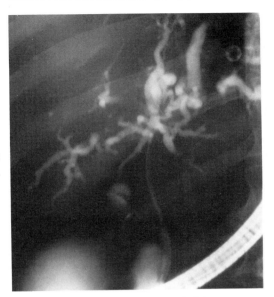

Figure 28-3. ERCP of a patient with hilar cholangiocarcinoma. The intrahepatic ducts are dilated and the extrahepatic biliary tree is normal.

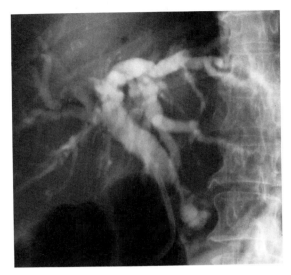

Figure 28-5. A patient with a distal cholangiocarcinoma after ERCP and endoscopic placement of a plastic biliary endoprosthesis.

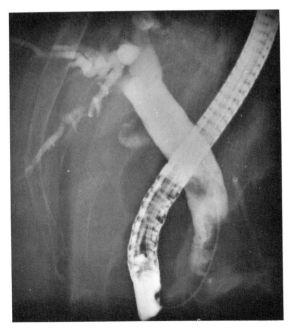

Figure 28-4. ERCP of a patient with distal cholangiocarcinoma showing a dilated extrahepatic biliary tree and an irregular tumor mass at the level of the intrapancreatic portion of the common bile duct.

available, they are not essential in the management of most patients. Prolonged efforts at obtaining a preoperative tissue diagnosis are not indicated unless the patient is not an operative candidate. Negative results from such attempts should not delay further assessment of tumor resectability and management.

A multitude of diseases can mimic cholangiocarcinoma (Table 28-2). In many cases, the distinction between cholangiocarcinoma and these other disease processes can be made on the basis of the clinical presentation, the past medical history, and the results of imaging studies such as CT scan and cholangiography.

Management

Following the diagnosis of cholangiocarcinoma, management issues commence with an assessment of the general medical condition of the patient. The overall performance status is judged, as are factors such as cardiac function, respiratory status, and renal function. Obstructive jaundice alters multiple hepatic functions, including mitochondrial respiratory function, protein synthesis, and reticuloendothelial function, as well as cell-mediated immunity,

Table 28-2. Differential Diagnosis
of Cholangiocarcinoma

Congenital dilatation of the bile duct
  Choledochal cyst
  Caroli's disease
Nonneoplastic strictures
  Chronic pancreatitis
  Sclerosing cholangitis
  Inflammatory strictures (typically secondary to calculus
    disease)
  Postoperative strictures (typically secondary to
    cholecystectomy)
  Postradiation strictures
  Chemotherapy-induced strictures
  Mirizzi's syndrome
  Strictures secondary to external trauma
  Retroperitoneal fibrosis
  Strictures related to AIDS
Neoplastic lesions
  Benign tumors of the bile duct
    Leiomyomas
    Carcinoid tumors
    Neuromas
    Hemangiomas
    Papillomas
    Adenomas
    Cystic hepatobiliary neoplasms
    Granular cell myoblastomas
  Malignant tumors in proximity to the bile duct
    Periampullary tumors
      Pancreatic
      Ampullary
      Duodenal
    Islet cell tumors
    Gallbladder carcinomas
    Lymphomas
    Lymphosarcomas
    Metastases to porta hepatis or hepatic parenchyma
    Hepatocellular carcinomas
Infestations
  Ascaris lumbricoides
  Clonorchis sinensis
  Opisthorchis viverrini

Source: Modified from Yeo CJ, Pitt HA, Cameron JL. Bile duct carcinoma:
Diagnosis. In John Terblanche (ed), *Hepatobiliary Malignancy: Its Multidisciplinary Management.* Edward Arnold, London, 1994.

the coagulation system, and wound healing. Therapies directed at cholangitis should include appropriate intravenous antibiotics and drainage of
obstructed biliary radicals via endoscopic or percutaneous approaches. Coagulopathy related to
prolongation of the prothrombin time is corrected
by the administration of vitamin K and fresh-frozen plasma.

Patients with the diagnosis of cholangiocarcinoma should undergo an assessment of tumor resectability prior to therapeutic intervention. Such
an assessment is accomplished using a combination
of CT scan, cholangiography, and visceral angiography. Findings on CT scan such as bilobar peripheral
hepatic metastases or extrahepatic disease preclude
curative resection. Cholangiographic findings such
as peripheral bilobar hepatic parenchymal involvement indicate unresectability. Visceral angiography
with portal venous phase studies may reveal encasement or occlusion of the common hepatic artery
or main portal vein, findings that suggest unresectability. Endosonography has recently been reported
to be of additional benefit in staging patients with
cholangiocarcinoma, although the benefits of this
technique remain unproven at present.

A recent study from The Johns Hopkins Hospital compared the results of cholangiography and
angiography over a 12-year period in 97 patients
with pathologically proven perihilar cholangiocarcinoma. Overall, 62% of the patients were resected,
and 38% underwent palliation via operative or nonoperative techniques. Cholangiographic involvement of four or more segmental ductal systems by
tumor was observed in 19 patients (20%), and none
of these patients were resectable. In contrast, those
78 patients (80%) with three or fewer hepatic segments cholangiographically involved with tumor
had a 50% resectability rate, and those 12 patients
(12%) with only one segment involved had a resectability rate of 83%. Angiographic findings of arterial
or venous encasement were observed in 33% of
patients, and major arterial anatomic variants were
identified in 13% of patients. The positive predictive value of cholangiography alone was 60%,
the positive predictive value for angiography alone
was 71%, and the positive predictive value for the
combination of cholangiography and angiography
was 79%. Thus the authors' current practice is to
stage patients with both cholangiography and visceral arteriography as a means of determining if
surgical exploration will be undertaken.

Palliative Therapy

Palliative therapy in patients with cholangiocarcinoma may include nonoperative or operative ap-

proaches. A nonoperative approach to palliation may be undertaken because the tumor is considered unresectable by preoperative staging studies, or because the patient is considered unfit for surgery. Criteria that exclude patients from surgery include poor general medical condition, refusal of surgery, distant metastases, extensive tumor extension into both the right and left lobes of the liver, and portal vein or main hepatic artery occlusion. Patients undergoing nonoperative palliation may have their biliary decompression performed using either percutaneously or endoscopically placed drainage catheters.

PERCUTANEOUS TRANSHEPATIC PALLIATION

Percutaneous transhepatic cholangiography with percutaneous biliary drainage can serve to palliate jaundice in those patients who are not surgical candidates. Attempts at obtaining a definitive tissue diagnosis can utilize these percutaneous catheters. Percutaneous fine-needle aspiration of the region of suspected malignancy under fluoroscopic guidance may be accomplished using the biliary drainage catheters as radiopaque markers. Overall, the sensitivity of percutaneous fine-needle aspiration for malignant biliary obstruction ranges between 50% and 90%. Additionally, the transhepatic tube tracts can be used as a direct route for endoluminal biopsy of the bile ducts using a flexible bioptome under fluoroscopic guidance, a forceps via the transhepatic tract, or choledochoscopy to biopsy lesions under direct vision.

At the authors' institution, percutaneous palliation using transhepatic stents typically involves the ultimate placement of 12 to 16 French soft polymeric silicone catheters into both the right and left hepatic ductal systems, with the tubes advanced through the tumor and into the duodenum (Fig. 28-6). This intubation allows the biliary drainage to be "internalized," resulting in bile being delivered to the duodenum and small intestine. In most cases these percutaneous stents are exchanged over guidewires as an outpatient procedure every 3 to 4 months to avoid the complications of side hole occlusion, biliary obstruction, and cholangitis. Intravenous antibiotics are generally administered as a single dose before the cholangiogram and biliary catheter exchange as prophylaxis against procedure-related cholangitis.

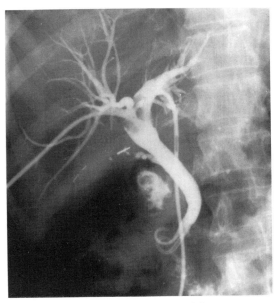

Figure 28-6. PTC of a patient with a hilar cholangiocarcinoma revealing a filling defect at the hepatic duct bifurcation. Right- and left-sided transhepatic catheters traverse the tumor and the entire extrahepatic biliary tree to enter the duodenum via the ampulla of Vater.

A further percutaneous palliative option is the transhepatic placement of a biliary endoprosthesis. Such a biliary endoprosthesis has the advantage of allowing the patient to be free of a tube exiting the skin. These devices allow internal drainage of bile but have the disadvantage of eliminating percutaneous access to the biliary tree. Metallic devices include (a) the Wallstent (Schneider, Inc., Minneapolis, Minn.), (b) the Gianturco Z-stent (Cook, Inc., Bloomington, Ind.), and (c) the Palmaz stent (Johnson & Johnson Interventional Systems Co., Warren, NJ). The Wallstent and Z-stent are self-expanding stents, whereas the Palmaz stent is a balloon-expandable metallic stent. The Wallstent may be introduced through a 7 French introducer; the Gianturco Z-stent and Palmaz stents require a larger delivery sheath (10 to 13 French). The Wallstent may be placed in a single-step procedure if there is no significant bleeding during the initial percutaneous biliary drainage. The other metallic stents, which require larger delivery sheaths, may require a two-step procedure: initial biliary drainage and tract maturation followed by tract dilatation and stent placement. Complications associated with endoprosthesis include occlusion, dislodgement, and migration, all of which may require intervention to reachieve palliation.

ENDOSCOPIC PALLIATION

Plastic biliary endoprostheses varying in diameter from 7.0 to 11.5 French can be successfully inserted into the obstructed biliary tree via the endoscopic approach in patients with cholangiocarcinoma. Proper endoprosthesis placement requires considerable endoscopic skill and correct assessment of the biliary anatomy with respect to the site of tumor obstruction. Plastic endoprostheses have been shown to have a high occlusion rate, since the walls of the endoprosthesis become covered with biliary sludge and bacterial biofilm, leading to recurrent jaundice, pruritus, and cholangitis. One solution to this occlusion problem is to endoscopically exchange the endoprostheses at short (2- to 3-month) intervals. The use of self-expanding metal stents has improved the results of endoscopic palliation of obstructive jaundice (Fig. 28-7).

Several randomized, controlled studies have shown that self-expanding metal stents (Wallstent) are superior to 10 French plastic stents for palliation of jaundice in malignant bile duct obstruction, mainly dealing with distal bile duct obstruction. A study by Davids et al. from Amsterdam randomized 105 patients with distal strictures to plastic versus metal stents. The success of the initial drainage was equal (95%) with both treatments, but the median patency was significantly longer for the metal stent than for the plastic stent (273 vs. 126 days), with fewer endoscopic reinterventions needed for the metal stent. Overall, there appeared to be a considerable cost savings in the metal stent group, despite the higher initial cost of the stent. Unfortunately, the number of patients with hilar tumors treated via endoscopic approaches is much smaller than those with distal tumors, and the results have not been as well established.

When an endoscopist may be unable to pass a guidewire from below through the cholangiocarcinoma into the dilated proximal biliary tree, the percutaneous transhepatic placement of a guidewire may allow the endoscopist to proceed with endoprosthesis placement. Such a multidisciplinary

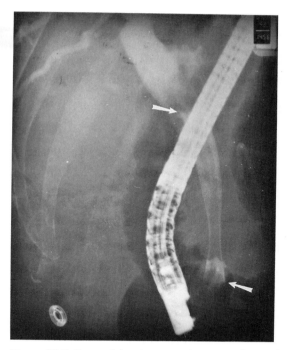

Figure 28-7. Successful endoscopic placement of a metal endoprosthesis (Wallstent) in a patient with distal cholangiocarcinoma. Stent shown from arrow to arrow.

approach to the management of the patients with cholangiocarcinoma is often essential to obtain optimal results.

SURGICAL PALLIATION

In low-risk patients without evidence of metastatic or locally unresectable disease, surgical exploration is appropriate. In a small number of patients, exploration will reveal intraperitoneal tumor dissemination or extensive tumor involvement of the porta hepatis, precluding resection or operative palliation. Patients with such extensive tumor should undergo minimal operative intervention. Preoperatively placed transhepatic catheters can be left in place for palliation of the biliary obstruction. The gallbladder should be removed, if possible, to prevent the subsequent development of acute cholecystitis from cystic duct obstruction related to tumor growth or to the presence of the catheters. Postoperatively, the transhepatic catheters can be exchanged fluoroscopically over guidewires for larger-diameter, softer, polymeric silicone transhepatic catheters, which can be used for long-term palliation.

In patients with unresectable tumor at the porta hepatis, two standard operative approaches for palliation exist. These include (1) choledochojejunostomy to a Roux-en-Y limb of jejunum, with intraoperative placement of polymeric silicone transhepatic stents and (2) segment III bypass to decompress the left biliary tree.

Roux-en-Y choledochojejunostomy with polymeric silicone transhepatic stents commences with cholecystectomy and isolation of the distal extrahepatic biliary tree. The common bile duct distal to the tumor mass is isolated and divided, and the distal bile duct stump is oversewn. The proximal extrahepatic biliary tree can then be examined using intraoperative choledochoscopy, and biopsies of the malignant stricture can be obtained to establish a tissue diagnosis. Next, the bile duct can be dilated using dilators and progressively larger catheters, coudés, and the previously placed percutaneous transhepatic catheters can be exchanged for larger polymeric silicone transhepatic stents. The procedure is completed with a choledochojejunostomy, using a Roux-en-Y jejunal limb. The advantages of this approach over nonoperative palliation alone include the performance of cholecystectomy, the placement of larger stents, and the positioning of the stents into a defunctionalized Roux-en-Y limb of jejunum. Although it is difficult to document, larger stents that drain into a defunctionalized limb of jejunum appear to reduce the incidence of subsequent cholangitis, as compared to stents passed through the tumor and into the duodenum.

Segment III bypass is appropriate when the hilar tumor is unresectable and undilatable from below and when the tumor predominates on the right side of the liver. Using this technique, the liver is decompressed via the segment III branch of the left hepatic duct above the tumor. The duct of segment III is identified by following the falciform ligament into the recess of Rex in the umbilical fissure. The duct can be intubated using a polymeric silicone transhepatic stent brought out via the lateral segment of the left lobe of the liver, and a biliary-enteric anastomosis is performed to a Roux-en-Y jejunal limb. A similar, although somewhat more difficult, procedure can be performed through the gallbladder fossa on the right side (segment V

bypass) if the tumor is unresectable and nondilatable and extensively involves the left side of the hepatic hilum.

The morbidity and mortality rates of nonoperative and operative palliation for cholangiocarcinoma are difficult to compare. These differences may largely reflect selection bias and enrollment differences for the patients entered into the two different treatment groups. In a recent series from The Johns Hopkins Hospital treating biliary obstruction in 65 patients with hilar cholangiocarcinoma, 21 patients were managed completely nonoperatively, and 44 patients were palliated surgically. The mean survival was 5 months in the nonoperative group and 8 months in the operative group. There was a significant difference in survival rate at 6 months, with the nonoperative group having a 30% survival rate and the operated group having a 64% survival rate. The incidence of cholangitis following initial treatment was 50% in each of the two groups. No overall differences were observed between the two groups in the number of readmissions to the hospital; however, there were fewer unscheduled emergency stent changes in the operated group than in the nonoperated group.

Surgical Resection

RESECTION OF HILAR CHOLANGIOCARCINOMA WITH BILATERAL HEPATICOJEJUNOSTOMY

The first step is exploration of the entire abdomen for evidence of tumor dissemination. In typical cases, the gallbladder and extrahepatic biliary tree appear normal, and the tumor is palpated by feeling for the divergence of the preoperatively placed percutaneous transhepatic catheters at the level of the hepatic duct bifurcation. Exposure and dissection of the hepatic duct bifurcation are facilitated by early mobilization of the gallbladder and early division of the distal common bile duct (Fig. 28-8). Once the common bile duct has been divided distally, the dissection continues cephalad, posterior to the bile duct, until the hepatic duct bifurcation is reached. The right and left hepatic ducts are divided above the tumor, and the specimen is removed; the right and left hepatic ducts and the distal common bile duct margin are marked to help the pathologist check the microscopic margin status (Fig. 28-9). At this point the preoperatively placed

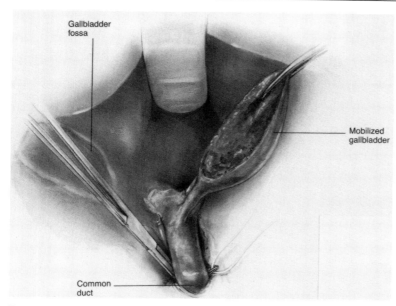

Figure 28-8. Exposure and dissection of the hepatic duct bifurcation are facilitated by two maneuvers: early mobilization of the gallbladder and early dissection and subsequent division of the common bile duct. (From Cameron JL. *Atlas of Surgery,* vol. 1. Philadelphia: BC Decker, 1990. Used with permission.)

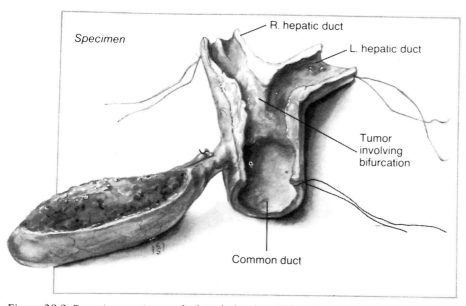

Figure 28-9. Resection specimen, which includes the gallbladder, upper common bile duct, entire common hepatic duct, tumor at the level of the bifurcation, and portions of the right and left hepatic ducts above the tumor. (From Cameron JL. *Atlas of Surgery,* vol. 1. Philadelphia: BC Decker, 1990. Used with permission.)

transhepatic catheters are exchanged for polymeric silicone transhepatic biliary stents, and biliary reconstruction is completed by creating a 60-cm-long Roux-en-Y jejunal limb in a retrocolic position and performing bilateral hepaticojejunal anastomoses. Each polymeric silicone transhepatic stent is brought out through a separate stab wound in the right or left upper quadrant and sutured to the skin (Fig. 28-10).

RESECTION OF HILAR CHOLANGIOCARCINOMA INCLUDING HEPATIC LOBECTOMY WITH RECONSTRUCTION VIA HEPATICOJEJUNOSTOMY

A minority of patients with proximal cholangiocarcinoma will have extensive tumor involvement of one hepatic lobe, with sparing of the opposite lobe. In such cases the lobe involved with tumor may also have evidence of tumor involvement of the

Figure 28-10. The completed operative procedure following resection of the hepatic duct bifurcation, showing bilateral hepaticojejunostomies to a retrocolic Roux-en-Y jejunal limb. (From Cameron JL. *Atlas of Surgery*, vol. 1. Philadelphia: BC Decker, 1990. Used with permission.)

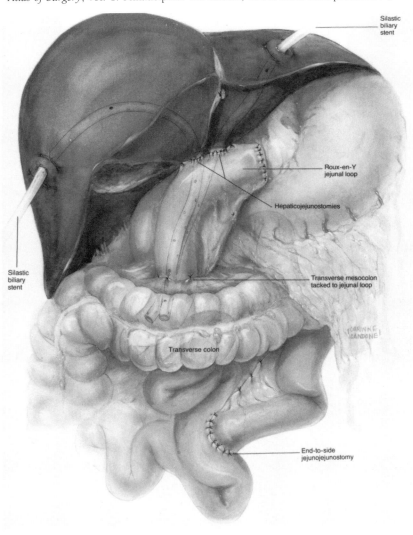

Silastic biliary stent

Roux-en-Y jejunal loop

Hepaticojejunostomies

Silastic biliary stent

Transverse mesocolon tacked to jejunal loop

Transverse colon

End-to-side jejunojejunostomy

ipsilateral hepatic artery or portal venous branch. Such patients can undergo complete surgical resection if hepatic lobectomy is added to the resection of the hepatic duct bifurcation. The operative procedure commences as discussed above. Once the hepatic duct bifurcation has been mobilized and the tumor is verified to extend into one lobe of the liver, then the hepatic duct on the opposite side is divided above the tumor, and an en bloc resection of the hepatic duct bifurcation and involved hepatic lobe is performed. Following resection, a biliary-enteric anastomosis to the retained lobar hepatic duct is performed (Fig. 28-11).

RESECTION OF PROXIMAL CHOLANGIOCARCINOMA WITH CAUDATE LOBECTOMY AND BILATERAL HEPATICOJEJUNOSTOMIES

Because of the anatomic proximity of the caudate lobe to the hepatic duct bifurcation, the caudate lobe can be involved with proximal cholangiocarcinoma in a variable proportion of patients. In such circumstances, resection of the hepatic duct bifurcation combined with some form of hepatic lobectomy plus caudate lobectomy has been advocated by some groups. In the most typical circumstances, these resections involve either right or left triseg-

Figure 28-11. The completed operative procedure following resection of the hepatic duct bifurcation and left hepatic lobectomy in a patient with hilar cholangiocarcinoma involving the hepatic duct bifurcation and left hepatic lobe. Shown is the right-sided hepaticojejunostomy to a Roux-en-Y jejunal limb and the final position of a right-sided polymeric silicone (Silastic) transhepatic biliary stent. (From Cameron JL. *Atlas of Surgery*, vol. 1. Philadelphia: BC Decker, 1990. Used with permission.)

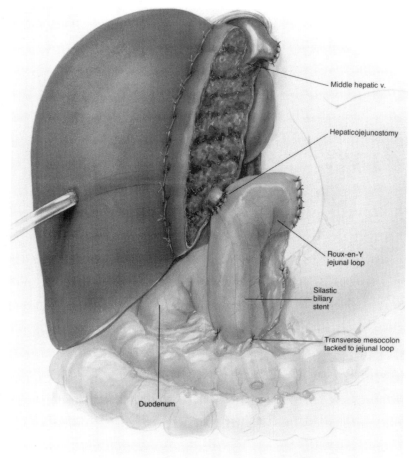

mentectomy or extended right or left lobectomy. In rare cases, central liver resections have been performed, without the addition of right or left hepatic lobectomy.

HEPATIC RESECTION FOR PERIPHERAL CHOLANGIOCARCINOMA

In contrast to patients with hilar cholangiocarcinoma, patients with peripheral cholangiocarcinoma have different clinical presentations and radiographic findings, and they require different operative treatment. Peripheral cholangiocarcinoma is approached surgically in a fashion similar to hepatocellular carcinoma, with treatment typically involving hepatic lobectomy or segmentectomy, without resection of the hepatic duct bifurcation and without biliary-enteric anastomosis.

Controversies

The palliation of jaundice can be achieved in the majority of patients with cholangiocarcinoma by endoscopic stenting, transhepatic stenting, surgical bypass, or, rarely, by a combination of these techniques. The choice depends to some extent on the local expertise. Several randomized, controlled studies have compared these different modes of palliation in patients with malignant bile duct obstruction. Bornman et al. compared percutaneous stenting with surgery in 50 patients with distal bile duct obstruction. Technical success was achieved in 84% of the patients in the percutaneously stented group and in 76% of the patients in the surgery group. The procedure-related complications (28% and 32%, respectively) and 30-day mortality rate (8% and 20%) were similar. Although the initial hospital stay was significantly shorter in the stented group (18 vs. 24 days), this difference was not maintained when readmissions for obstructed endoprostheses and duodenal obstruction were also considered.

Several other studies have compared surgery with endoscopic stenting for distal bile duct obstruction, and the findings have been similar. For example, one study by Dowsett et al. included 127 patients with unresectable malignancy obstructing the distal bile duct. Sixty-five patients were treated via endoscopic stenting, and 62 had surgical palliation. Successful biliary drainage was achieved in 94% of patients using both techniques, with the 30-day mortality rate being 6% after endoscopy and 15% after surgery. No procedure-related complications were observed in the endoscopic group, whereas 10% of patients treated surgically had complications. Recurrent jaundice (17% vs. 3%) and late duodenal obstruction (14% vs. 3%) were seen more commonly in the endoprosthesis group than in the surgery group. The median survival was comparable between the two groups (16 weeks vs. 22 weeks). Unfortunately, no prospective randomized studies comparing surgical to nonsurgical palliation of hilar cholangiocarcinoma have been reported.

In a randomized study comparing endoscopic stenting with percutaneous stenting in patients with obstructive jaundice, Speer and colleagues found that the endoscopic method had a significantly higher success rate for relief of jaundice (81% vs. 61%), even though there were more hilar tumors in the endoscopically stented group (49% vs. 28%). The procedure-related complications (19% vs. 67%) and 30-day mortality rate (15% vs. 33%) were significantly lower in the endoscopically stented group than in the percutaneously stented group, with the morbidity related to percutaneous stenting being mainly due to bleeding and bile leak at the liver puncture site. In this study, as in others, distal bile duct obstruction predominated. Data are more limited when comparing the efficacy of endoscopic versus percutaneous stenting in patients with hilar tumors.

Preferred Approach

The team approach is imperative in the management of patients with cholangiocarcinoma. A multidisciplinary team should include a surgeon, an interventional radiologist, an endoscopist, an oncologist, and appropriate support staff, including nurse specialists. All have important roles to play in the evaluation and management of these patients. Currently, the longest survivals are reported following complete surgical resection of these biliary malignancies. Palliative options include surgery, percutaneous approaches, or endoscopic approaches, and must take into consideration the expertise of the treating physician, patient performance status, biliary anatomy and tumor extent, and quality of life after the intervention.

Chemotherapy

The use of chemotherapeutic agents such as 5-fluorouracil, alone or in combination with other drugs, has not been demonstrated to improve survival in patients with either resected or unresected cholangiocarcinoma. Treatments using hormonal manipulations (antiestrogens and luteinizing hormone–releasing hormone (LHRH) inhibitors) and cholecystokinin receptor antagonists have some rationale, and merit investigation.

Radiation Therapy

Many studies have investigated the effect of ionizing radiation in patients with cholangiocarcinoma, using techniques which include external beam radiotherapy, intraoperative radiotherapy, internal radiotherapy, radioimmunotherapy, and charged particle radiation. To date, no prospective randomized trials have reported on the use of radiotherapy in patients with cholangiocarcinoma. Some retrospective studies have suggested that radiotherapy may prolong survival in both resected and unresected patients, although conflicting data exist and the issue remains unsettled.

Results

Hilar Cholangiocarcinoma

Survival rates in patients with bilar cholangiocarcinoma are highly correlated with whether the patient can be rendered grossly disease-free at the time of surgical resection. The overall resectability rates for hilar cholangiocarcinoma are as high as 50% to 60% in some series, and are largely dependent upon the completeness of preoperative staging studies. In those patients who undergo surgical therapy, factors which influence survival include the performance status at diagnosis, the completeness of resection, the histologic grade of the tumor, the status of nodal metastases, the extent of liver invasion, and the presence or absence of perineural tumor invasion.

Table 28-3 presents the data from selected recent series reporting patients undergoing potentially curative resection of hilar cholangiocarcinoma. The data from the 596 patients tabulated indicate an average mean survival of 21.9 months

Table 28-3. Selected Recent Results After Curative Resection of Hilar Cholangiocarcinoma

Author	Number of Patients	Mean Survival (mo)	% Patients Alive at		
			1 yr	3 yr	5 yr
Baer	20	34	73	—	—
Boerma	295	21	67	24	13
Cameron	39	21	70	27	11
Childs	17	21	—	—	—
Fortner	14	38	100	60	21
Hadjis	24	25	70	26	22
Iida	22	26	85	36	—
Langer	12	28	—	25	17
Reding	82	24	70	28	12
Tompkins	47	9	45	15	0
Tsuzuki	24	24	80	28	19
Total	596	21.9 (average)			

Source: Modified from Yeo CJ, Pitt HA, Cameron JL. Bile duct carcinoma: Outcome, prognosis and follow-up. In John Terblanche (ed), *Hepatobiliary Malignancy: Its Multidisciplinary Management.* Edward Arnold, London, 1994.

following resection. The percentages of patients alive at 1 year, 3 years, and 5 years following potentially curative resection of hilar cholangiocarcinoma approximate 70%, 30%, and 15%, respectively.

A recent collective review of patients with resected hilar cholangiocarcinoma analyzing only cases since 1980 was reported by Boerma. In this review, outcomes in patients undergoing local hilar resection alone versus hilar resection plus major liver resection were compared. In 201 patients undergoing local hilar resection alone, the operative mortality rate was 8%, the mean survival was 21 months, and the percentages of patients alive at 1, 3, and 5 years were 76%, 21%, and 7%, respectively. In contrast, in 188 patients undergoing hilar resection plus major liver resection, the operative mortality rate was doubled (15%), the median survival was 24 months, and the percentages of patients alive at 1, 3, and 5 years were 61%, 28%, and 17%, respectively. These results indicate that mean survival was not notably improved by the addition of major liver resection in patients with hilar cholangiocarcinoma, but the pathologic stage of the tumors in these patients was not a controlled variable. Although the addition of major liver resection was associated with nearly a doubling of the operative mortality rate, it was also followed by an improvement in the 5-year survival rate. However, the data presented in this review were retrospective and nonrandomized. Hence, a definitive answer to the question of whether routine hepatic resection improves survival in patients with hilar cholangiocarcinoma has not been adequately addressed.

Peripheral Cholangiocarcinoma

The outcome of treatment for peripheral cholangiocarcinoma has been the subject of fewer reports. This entity is much less common than hilar cholangiocarcinoma, and the clinical presentation, radiographic findings, and operative treatment differ. The long-term prognosis for resectable peripheral cholangiocarcinoma appears to be somewhat more favorable than for hilar cholangiocarcinoma, with 1-year survival rates approaching 70% and 5-year survival rates varying between 20% and 50%.

Conclusions

Cholangiocarcinoma is a rare tumor which occurs in approximately 3000 people annually in the United States. Cholangiocarcinoma is strongly associated with several etiologic factors: cystic dilatation of the bile duct, clonorchiasis, hepatolithiasis, thorium dioxide exposure, sclerosing cholangitis, and ulcerative colitis. In the proper clinical setting the radiographic diagnosis of cholangiocarcinoma can be suspected using CT scan and cholangiography. Tumor staging involves the combination of CT scan, cholangiography, and visceral arteriography. Patients with distant metastases, bilobar peripheral liver metastases, or involvement of the hepatic artery or main portal vein are considered unresectable and are best palliated nonoperatively using either endoscopic or percutaneous approaches. Patients with staging studies revealing tumors confined to the extrahepatic biliary tree or to one side of the liver may be resectable, and they should be con-

sidered candidates for exploration with curative intent.

In the future it can be anticipated that better studies of the risk factors associated with cholangiocarcinoma will be reported, leading to a better understanding of the pathogenesis of these tumors. Continued evolution of imaging techniques may provide assistance in earlier diagnosis and simplify staging. Approaches to the palliation of jaundice will continue to improve, and newer delivery systems for innovative types of biliary prostheses will be found. In addition, treatments beyond currently employed surgery, radiotherapy, and chemotherapy require investigation. Novel therapeutic strategies should be tested for tumor responsiveness in the hope of improving the overall patient survival in this disease.

Selected Readings

Becker CD, et al. Percutaneous palliation of malignant obstructive jaundice with the Wallstent endoprostheses: Follow-up and reintervention in patients with hilar and non-hilar obstruction. *JVIR* 1993; 4: 597–604.

Bengmark S, et al. Major liver resection for hilar cholangiocarcinoma. *Ann Surg* 1988; 207:120–125.

Boerma EJ. Research into the results of resection of hilar bile duct cancer. *Surgery* 1990; 108:572–580.

Cameron JL, et al. Management of proximal cholangiocarcinoma by surgical resection and radiography. *Am J Surg* 1990; 159:91–98.

Davids PHP, et al. Randomized trial of self-expanding metal stents versus polyethylene stents for distal malignant biliary obstruction. *Lancet* 1992; 340: 1488–1492.

Lammer J. Biliary endoprostheses: Plastic versus metal stents. *Radiol Clin North Am* 1990; 28:1211–1221.

Nagorney DM, et al. Outcomes after curative resection of cholangiocarcinoma. *Arch Surg* 1993; 128:871–879.

Nordback IH, et al. Unresectable hilar cholangiocarcinoma: Percutaneous versus operative palliation. *Surgery* 1994; 115:597–603.

Venbrux AC, et al. Endoscopy as an adjuvant to biliary radiologic intervention. *Radiology* 1991; 180:355–361.

Yeo CJ, Pitt HA, Cameron JL. Cholangiocarcinoma. *Surg Clin North Am* 1990; 70:1429–1447.

29

Acute Pancreatitis

PETER A. BANKS

JAMES M. BECKER

GREGORY T. SICA

Etiology and Pathogenesis

Most episodes of acute pancreatitis are caused by either alcohol or biliary calculi. A multitude of additional factors can also cause pancreatitis. Of particular concern is the high incidence of pancreatitis following endoscopic retrograde cholangiopancreatography (ERCP), endoscopic sphincterotomy, and particularly sphincter of Oddi manometric studies.

The pathophysiology has not been clearly established and is not necessarily the same for each etiology. In several experimental models of acute pancreatitis, the initial abnormality is blockage of the secretion of pancreatic enzymes, causing zymogen granules to accumulate within acinar cells. The next step appears to be colocalization of zymogens with lysosomes within large vacuoles. Following colocalization, trypsinogen may be activated to trypsin by cathepsin B (a lysosomal hydrolase). Trypsin then activates other proteases and phospholipase A_2, which are released into the cytoplasm, causing intracellular injury. It remains unclear whether the initial steps of acute pancreatitis in man resemble these abnormalities in the experimental animal.

Diagnosis

Initial Detection

Acute pancreatitis should be suspected when upper abdominal pain and tenderness persist for many hours. Serum amylase and lipase are usually elevated at least three times the normal levels. Neither the clinical presentation nor laboratory tests are specific for acute pancreatitis. The diagnosis of acute pancreatitis can be confirmed if abdominal ultrasound or computerized tomography (CT) show convincing evidence of pancreatic and peripancreatic inflammatory changes. As originally described by Hill et al. in 1982 and further explored by Balthazar et al., several image-based criteria were reported to stage acute pancreatitis. Under this system, acute pancreatitis was graded A through E as follows: grade A, normal-appearing pancreas; grade B, focal or diffuse enlargement, nonhomogeneous gland, pancreatic duct dilatation but without peripancreatic changes; grade C, intrinsic pancreatic abnormalities with inflammatory changes in the peripancreatic fat; grade D, single, ill-defined fluid collection; and grade E, two or more fluid collections or the presence of gas in or adjacent to the pancreas. Later, evaluation for the presence of pancreatic necrosis was added. Using this system, a severity index score was obtained and shown to correlate well with both clinical staging and morbidity and mortality.

The ability of CT to detect pancreatitis is related to the severity of disease. Overall, CT has been reported to have a sensitivity between 77% and 92% with a very high specificity. More recently, the development of spiral CT with the single-breathhold technique has shown promise for imaging the pancreas. The role of magnetic resonance imaging (MRI) is under exploration, and its future awaits the outcome of these studies.

Prognostic Indicators

It is particularly important to determine as early as possible whether an episode of pancreatitis is severe. A recent international symposium has updated and revised the terminology of acute pancreatitis and the criteria that should be used to gauge severity. Regarding terminology (Table 29-1), the major emphasis is the distinction between interstitial and necrotizing pancreatitis. This differentiation can be achieved by incremental dynamic bolus computerized tomography. Without intravenous contrast, it is virtually impossible to determine whether an inflamed, enlarged pancreas has undergone necrosis. The use of intravenous contrast with the bolus technique, however, is helpful. If the microcirculation of the swollen pancreas is intact, the pancreatic parenchyma is uniformly enhanced following intravenous contrast, and the process is defined as interstitial pancreatitis. If enhancement is patchy, and particularly if large areas do not enhance at all, the microcirculation is clearly disrupted, and the process is defined as necrotizing pancreatitis. The terms *phlegmon* and *infected pseudocyst* are no longer used. In accordance with the new terminology, the term *pancreatic abscess* should be used in describing infection within a pseudocyst or a localized collection of purulent material.

Although it is recognized that most patients with interstitial pancreatitis have mild illness (that is, they do not experience organ failure), and many patients with necrotizing pancreatitis have severe disease (that is, they may have evidence of organ failure that lasts for several days and even weeks), the consensus of the conference was that the difference between mild and severe pancreatitis should be established on clinical rather than morphologic evidence. Accordingly, the conference established

the principle that the most important feature that defines severity is the presence or absence of organ failure (Table 29-2). A secondary feature of severe acute pancreatitis is the presence of local complications, including pancreatic necrosis, abscess, or pseudocyst.

It was further recognized that there were early prognostic signs that can help in assessing severity, such as the presence of three or more Ranson's signs (Table 29-3) and eight or more APACHE II points (Table 29-4) within the first 48 hours. Although organ failure may be defined in a variety of ways, most individuals considered shock, pulmonary insufficiency, renal failure, and gastrointestinal (GI) bleeding as four important criteria (Table 29-5). Other investigators have included coagulopathy and a general septic picture manifested by leukocytosis and temperature as two additional markers of systemic complications or organ failure.

The importance of organ failure is the fact that patients who do not experience organ failure can be expected to survive, whereas those who have significant and persisting organ failure have a high

Table 29-1. Terminology of Acute Pancreatitis

Interstitial pancreatitis
Necrotizing pancreatitis
  Sterile necrosis
  Infected necrosis
Pancreatic fluid collection
  Sterile
  Infected
Pancreatic pseudocyst, sterile
Pancreatic abscess

Table 29-2. Severe Acute Pancreatitis

Organ failure
and/or
Local complications
  Necrosis
  Abscess
  Pseudocyst
Prognostic signs
  ≥ 3 Ranson's signs
  ≥ 8 APACHE II points

Table 29-3. Ranson's Criteria of Severity

At admission
  Age > 55 years
  WBC $> 16,000/mm^3$
  Glucose > 200 mg/dl
  LDH[a] > 350 IU/liter
  AST > 250 U/liter
During initial 48 hours
  HCT[b] decrease of > 10
  BUN increase of > 5 mg/dl
  $CA^{++} < 8$ mg/dl
  $Pao_2 < 60$ mm Hg
  Base deficit > 4 mEq/liter
  Fluid sequestration > 6 liter

[a]LDH = lactate dehydrogenase.
[b]HCT = hematocrit.

Table 29-4. Apache II Severity of Disease Classification System

Physiologic Variable	High Abnormal Range				0	Low Abnormal Range			
	+4	+3	+2	+1		+1	+2	+3	+4
Temperature, rectal (°C)	≥ 41°	39.0°–40.9°		38.5°–38.9°	36.0°–38.4°	34.0°–35.9°	32.0°–33.9°	30.0°–31.9°	≤ 29.9°
Mean arterial pressure (mm Hg)	≥ 160	130–159	110–129		70–109		50–69		≤ 49
Heart rate (ventricular response)	≥ 180	140–179	110–139		70–109		55–69	40–54	≤ 39
Respiratory rate (nonventilated or ventilated)	≥ 50	35–49		25–34	12–24	10–11	6–9		≤ 5
Oxygenation: A-aDO$_1$ or Pao$_1$ (mm Hg)									
a. Fio$_1$ ≥ 0.5 record A-aDo$_1$	≥ 500	350–499	200–349		< 200				
b. Fio$_1$ < 0.5 record only Pao$_1$					PO$_1$ > 70	PO$_1$ 61–70		PO$_1$ 55–60	PO$_1$, < 55
Arterial pH	≥ 7.7	7.60–7.69		7.50–7.59	7.33–7.49		7.25–7.32	7.15–7.24	< 7.15
Serum sodium (mmol/liter)	≥ 180	160–179	155–159	150–154	130–149		120–129	111–119	< 110
Serum potassium (mmol/liter)	≥ 7	6.0–6.9		5.5–5.9	3.5–5.4	3.0–3.4	2.5–2.9		< 2.5
Serum creatinine (mg/dl) (double point score for acute renal failure)	> 3.5	2.0–3.4	1.5–1.9		0.6–1.4		< 0.6		
Hematocrit (%)	≥ 60		50.0–59.9	46.0–49.9	30.0–45.9		20.0–29.9		< 20
White blood count (total/mm³) (in 1000s)	≥ 40		20.0–39.9	15.0–19.9	3.0–14.9		1.0–2.9		< 1
Glasgow Coma Score (GCS): score = 15 minus actual GCS									
A. Total acute Physiology Score (APS): sum of the 12 individual variable points									
Serum HCO$_2$ (venous-mmol/liter) (not preferred, use if no ABGs)	≥ 52	41.0–51.9		32.0–40.9	22.0–31.9		18.0–21.9	15.0–17.9	< 15

B. Age points
Assign points to age as follows:

AGE (yrs)	POINTS
≤ 44	0
45–54	2
55–64	3
65–74	5
≥ 75	6

C. Chronic health points
If the patient has a history of severe organ system insufficiency or is immunocompromised, assign points as follows:
a. For nonoperative or emergency postoperative patients—5 points or
b. for elective postoperative patients—2 points.

Definitions: Organ insufficiency or immunocompromised state must have been evident prior to this hospital admission and conforms to the following criteria:

Liver: Biopsy-proven cirrhosis and documented portal hypertension; episodes of past upper GI bleeding attributed to portal hypertension; or prior episodes of hepatic failure/encephalopathy/coma.

Cardiovascular: Heart Association Class IV.

Respiratory: Chronic restrictive, obstructive, or vascular disease resulting in severe exercise restriction, i.e., unable to climb stairs or perform household duties; or documented chronic hypoxia, hypercapnia, secondary polycythemia, severe pulmonary hypertension (> 40 mm Hg), or respirator dependency.

Renal: Recurring chronic dialysis.

Immunocompromised: The patient has received therapy that suppresses resistance to infection (e.g., immunosuppression, chemotherapy, radiation, long-term or recent high-dose steroids) or has a disease that is sufficiently advanced to suppress resistance to infection (e.g., leukemia, lymphoma, AIDS).

APACHE II SCORE
Sum of A + B + C

A   APS points   _____
B   Age points   _____
C   Chronic Health points   _____
Total APACHE II SCORE   _____

Table 29-5. Organ Failure

Shock: systolic BP < 90 mm Hg
Pulmonary insufficiency: Pao₂ ≤ 60 mm Hg
Renal failure: creatinine > 2 mg/dl
GI bleeding: > 500 ml/24 hr

mortality rate. The importance of local complications is the fact that most patients with interstitial pancreatitis either do not experience organ failure or have self-limited organ failure, whereas many patients with necrotizing pancreatitis have significant organ failure that may be sustained over many days. Furthermore, pancreatic infection is distinctly uncommon in interstitial pancreatitis, whereas at least 30% of patients with necrotizing pancreatitis experience secondary infection. The likelihood of infection appears to be greatest among patients with subtotal or total pancreatic necrosis. The mortality rate of interstitial pancreatitis is approximately 1% to 2%. The mortality rates of sterile necrosis of the pancreas and infected necrosis are approximately 10% and 30%, respectively.

Management and Results

Principles of Management

Mild pancreatitis can usually be managed on an open floor with appropriate fluid replacement and careful monitoring. Severe pancreatitis invariably requires treatment in an intensive care unit, with emphasis on fluid resuscitation and respiratory care and with careful surveillance from a multidisciplinary team that includes gastroenterology, surgery, and radiology. If the patient has interstitial pancreatitis, aggressive treatment invariably leads to a successful outcome. If the patient has necrotizing pancreatitis, three clinical settings can ensue (Fig. 29-1).

First, toxicity as evidenced by organ failure may improve rapidly. Under these circumstances, medical treatment should be continued, and there is no need to consider radiologic or surgical maneuvers. Clinical judgment will determine whether total parenteral nutrition is required.

Second, organ failure may persist and may also be associated with a pronounced leukocytosis (> 18,000) and a higher fever (Fig. 29-2). A patient

with these characteristics has either infected necrosis or severe sterile necrosis. The best way to make this distinction is by CT-guided percutaneous aspiration (GPA) for Gram's stain and culture. This technique has been shown to be safe and accurate. In almost all instances of infection, Gram's stain and culture reveal organisms. In the presence of bacteria, the preferred approach is surgical debridement. The role of percutaneous catheter drainage for definitive treatment of infected necrosis remains controversial. On occasion, prolonged percutaneous catheter drainage using very large catheters has eradicated infected necrosis without surgery. In these instances, it is possible that most of the necrosis had already undergone liquefaction so that thick infected fluid could be removed through large catheters. However, in most instances, the necrotic infected slough has a consistency that does not permit ready egress through catheters. Since a delay in surgical debridement may lead to an increased mortality, the preferred approach to infected necrosis is surgical debridement.

Third, increasing organ failure in association with pancreatic necrosis may develop (see Fig. 29-1). If GPA reveals bacteria, surgical debridement should be carried out. If aspiration is negative, the choices would be continuation of medical therapy in an intensive care unit or debridement of the sterile necrosis. The factors that influence survival in sterile necrosis remain unclear. Patients who experience systemic complications appear to have an increased mortality. Karimgani et al. recently identified prognostic factors associated with mortality in sterile pancreatic necrosis. The overall mortality rate in patients with necrosis and at least one systemic complication was 38%. Factors that correlated with a fatal outcome were high Ranson's scores during the first 48 hours, high APACHE II scores at admission and at 48 hours, shock, renal insufficiency, multiple systemic complications, and high body mass index. Logistic regression analysis showed that shock was the best predictor of a fatal outcome. Patients with favorable prognostic factors survived whether treated medically or surgically, whereas those with unfavorable factors had a fatal outcome whether treated medically or surgically. It is not known whether earlier surgical debridement among patients with unfavorable factors would have been beneficial.

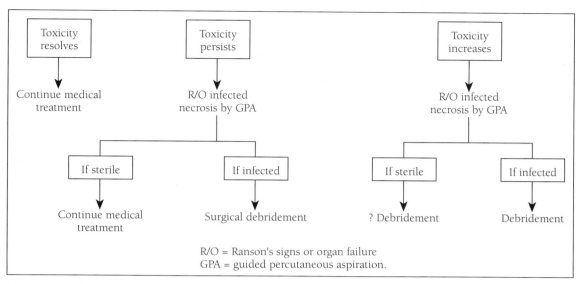

Figure 29-1. Clinical settings for necrotizing pancreatitis.

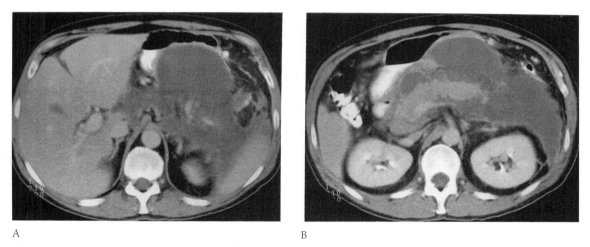

A   B

Figure 29-2. A. Incremental dynamic bolus CT scan of a patient with severe necrotizing pancreatitis. Scan shows a considerable amount of loculated fluid in the lesser sac and fluid in the anterior pararenal space. Serial CT scans at levels above and below the scan failed to reveal enhancement of the tail of the pancreas, indicating that the tail of the pancreas has undergone necrosis. B. CT scan at a lower level reveals normal enhancement of the head and body of the pancreas. There are considerable peripancreatic inflammatory changes. Because the patient became febrile and developed a leukocytosis, CT-guided percutaneous aspiration was performed and was negative by Gram's stain and culture. The patient was treated medically and made an uneventful clinical recovery.

Surgical Management of Necrotizing Pancreatitis

STERILE NECROSIS

The treatment of patients with sterile necrosis is extremely controversial. Operative mortality is rare in patients with sterile necrosis operated on after the first week. However, postoperative complications such as fistula and abscess are frequent, occurring in up to 25% of patients, leading some to question whether sterile necrosis should be operated on at all. Bradley and Allen reported successful nonoperative treatment of 11 patients with sterile necrosis despite the presence of renal or respiratory failure in 6 of 11 patients. However, no controlled series comparing operative and observational therapy exist for this group of patients.

If sterile necrotic areas are small, they may resolve nonoperatively. Larger necrotic areas without infection remain a major concern. If large collections are truly asymptomatic, they can be managed nonoperatively, with the realization that a small percentage will become infected and require debridement and drainage. However, many sterile collections produce symptoms by mass effect or local inflammation. Patients who are systemically ill, significantly anorexic, febrile, or in intractable pain should not be denied a laparotomy simply because a necrotic collection is sterile.

INFECTED NECROSIS

Secondary pancreatic infections occur in only 1% to 9% of all cases of pancreatitis. However, sepsis is the major cause of death in acute pancreatitis. It has been estimated that 80% of all deaths from acute pancreatitis are the result of sepsis. Death associated with pancreatic infection treated nonsurgically has proved to be inevitable, and even surgical drainage is associated with a perioperative death rate ranging between 11% and 61% in various series. Several recent studies have reported a mortality rate of closer to 10% to 15%.

It has become increasingly clear that *pancreatic infection* is a term that includes several disease entities and lacks the precision needed for scientific evaluation and comparison. Beger et al. presented the first clinical series demonstrating that infected pancreatic necrosis was a much more virulent form of infection than a well-localized pancreatic abscess. Lumsden and Bradley have proposed a list of defini-

tions to more precisely characterize the different forms of secondary pancreatic infection. This system differentiates infected pseudocyst, pancreatic abscess, sterile pancreatic necrosis, and infected pancreatic necrosis. (The reader should bear in mind that, in accordance with the new terminology, *infected pseudocyst* as well as *localized purulent collections* are now termed **pancreatic abscess**.)

Fedorak et al. recently evaluated these different categories of secondary pancreatic infection and found that, although they had similar bacteriologic findings, infected pseudocysts, pancreatic abscesses, and infected pancreatic necrosis had significantly different clinical presentations, clinical courses, and outcomes. Patients with infected pseudocysts generally presented with abdominal pain or mass without accompanying signs of sepsis, whereas patients with either pancreatic abscesses or infected pancreatic necrosis presented clinically with sepsis. Patients with infected pseudocysts were effectively treated with either percutaneous drainage or internal drainage. Patients in the latter two groups required either operative drainage or open packing. Morbidity and mortality rates were relatively low in the infected pseudocyst group: 26% and 9%, respectively. In contrast, the morbidity rate was 40% in the pancreatic abscess group, and the mortality rate was 25%. In those patients with infected pancreatic necrosis, the morbidity rate was 90% and the mortality rate approached 50%. In a prospective but nonrandomized study, Davidson and Bradley reported a dramatic improvement in survival of patients with infected necrosis treated by "marsupialization" or open packing.

Patients with either sterile or infected pancreatic necrosis and postnecrotic processes have significantly different presentations, clinical courses, and outcomes. These distinctions are important when treating modalities and therapeutic outcomes are compared. Among patients with necrotizing pancreatitis, approximately 30% to 70% develop infected necrosis. Approximately one half of pancreatic infections occur within the first 2 weeks. Almost all infections can be documented by guided percutaneous aspiration within the first 3 weeks. Hence, pancreatic infection takes place early in necrotizing pancreatitis.

The development of infected necrosis is an absolute indication for debridement. However, it is not necessarily infection alone that creates the toxic state. Beger et al. have shown that the hemodynamic consequences of pancreatic necrosis are virtually identical whether the necrosis is infected or sterile. Infected necrosis can at times be indolent, and sterile necrosis can produce severe hemodynamic consequences.

Three main surgical approaches exist for debridement of pancreatic necrosis: (1) aggressive initial debridement with external drainage; (2) necrosectomy with continuous local lavage; and (3) open packing. It is very difficult to compare the results of these three techniques because published series contain patients with differing severities of illness, differing indications for surgery, and differing levels of paramedical and ancillary support. When more than 100 g of necrotic tissue is removed, when there is poor delineation of viable from nonviable tissue, or when there is extensive peripancreatic necrosis with extension into the root of the mesentery, pararenal spaces, and lateral gutters, often more than one debridement is necessary. If there is concern that the initial debridement is likely to be incomplete, greater consideration should be given to open packing or continuous postoperative lavage.

Treatment of Pancreatic Pseudocysts

Extrapancreatic fluid collections commonly occur after severe pancreatitis. Many regress spontaneously. A fluid collection that persists for at least 4 weeks and becomes encased by a wall of fibrous tissue is then properly termed a pancreatic pseudocyst (Fig. 29-3). Options for pancreatic pseudocyst include watchful waiting and decompression. Whereas it was once thought that all pancreatic pseudocysts over 5 cm in size should be decompressed if they persisted for more than 6 weeks, more recent studies indicate that an asymptomatic pseudocyst may not require therapy. Accordingly, the authors' preferred approach for an asymptomatic pseudocyst following acute pancreatitis is to observe medically.

Options for a symptomatic pseudocyst include radiologic decompression by pigtail catheter, endoscopic decompression, and surgical decompression (see Fig. 29-3). To date, no randomized prospective trials have compared these modalities of therapy.

Radiologic decompression by a pigtail catheter has been shown to be safe and effective as long as it can be determined by ERCP that the pseudocyst is in continuity with the downstream portion of the main pancreatic duct. If it is not, and if a pigtail catheter is inserted into the pseudocyst, it will continue to fill from the upstream pancreatic ducts and will not close. Because of these considerations, radiologic decompression should not be offered unless there is continuity between the main pancreatic duct downstream and the pseudocyst itself.

Complications from the use of a pigtail catheter include secondary infection and bleeding. A radiologist should be available at all times to exchange a pigtail catheter that becomes inspissated with material and rendered nonfunctional. A clinician experienced with the use of a pigtail catheter should also be available to the patient. A rapid decrease in drainage associated with fever and abdominal pain should signal the strong probability of either a blockage within the pigtail catheter or possibly dislodgement of the catheter so that it is no longer within the pseudocyst.

Increasingly, endoscopic cystogastroscopy or cystoduodenoscopy has been used as an alternative to radiologic decompression. This technique requires the pseudocyst to be impacted against the wall of the stomach (or duodenum) in order to permit a safe decompression. The most important complication is bleeding. Once an endoscopic window has been created, a double-pigtail stent is usually inserted to provide continued drainage from the pseudocyst into the stomach (see Fig. 29-3). If the stent becomes blocked, infection within the pseudocyst is likely.

An additional endoscopic method of decompressing a pancreatic pseudocyst is the transpapillary approach of inserting a stent within the pancreatic duct. Although the tip of the stent can be advanced into the pseudocyst itself, it is possible that insertion of a short stent into the pancreatic duct to a location just beyond the sphincter of Oddi may suffice, since reduction of sphincteric pressure itself may facilitate the outflow of fluid from the pseudocyst. Endoscopic stent placement will not be helpful unless it has been ascertained that the pseudocyst is in continuity with the main pancreatic duct. These endoscopic techniques should be re-

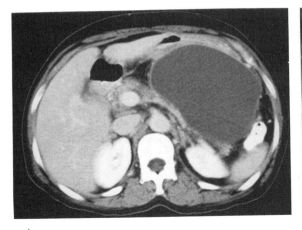

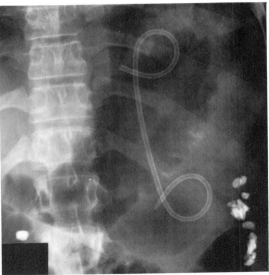

A

B

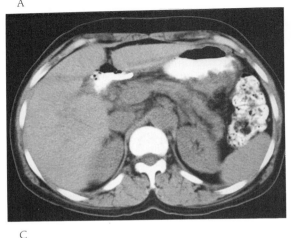

C

Figure 29-3. A. Large pancreatic pseudocyst with encroachment on the posterior wall of the stomach following an episode of acute pancreatitis. B. The patient underwent endoscopic cystogastrostomy with insertion of a double-pigtail catheter. C. Six weeks later, the pancreatic pseudocyst had resolved, and the double-pigtail catheter was removed. The patient remained well 3 months later.

stricted to centers that specialize in therapeutic endoscopy.

The time-honored treatment for pseudocyst drainage is surgical. Several general principles of surgical management of pancreatic pseudocysts have emerged (Fig. 29-4). Frankly infected pseudocysts should be drained externally. External drainage should also be selected if the wall of the pseudocyst is immature or friable and in the face of difficult anatomic problems. A persistent fistula or pancreatic ascites may be anticipated in 10% to 20% of patients. More than 90% of these fistulas close within 3 to 4 months, a process that may be hastened by the administration of a somatostatin analog.

Small, easily accessible pseudocysts may be excised, especially if they are located in the distal pancreas. If the wall of the pseudocyst consists partly of adjacent viscera, it will probably be impossible to resect the cyst itself, and internal drainage will be necessary.

A well-matured pseudocyst membrane is necessary for safe internal drainage. The pseudocyst wall must be firmly attached to the duodenum or stomach before either a cystogastrostomy or cystoduodenostomy is performed. If pseudocyst excision or drainage into the stomach or duodenum is not technically possible, a Roux-en-Y cystojejunostomy should be performed if the cyst is not grossly infected and has a sufficiently matured capsule. In patients with chronic pancreatitis and a dilated pancreatic duct, combined drainage of the pseudocyst and pancreatic duct may be performed.

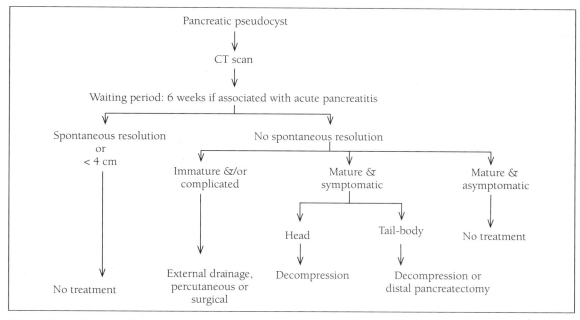

Figure 29-4. Schematic for the management of pancreatic pseudocysts.

The hospital mortality rate following drainage of pancreatic pseudocysts ranges from 2% to 12% (Table 29-6). Although external drainage is reported to have a higher mortality rate, this rate may partly reflect the type of patients who are operated on early in the course of severe pancreatitis. The lowest recurrence rates have been reported for excision (0% to 2%), followed by internal drainage (3% to 5%) and external drainage (5% to 25%).

In summary, in the absence of randomized prospective trials, surgical therapy should be considered as the gold standard. In a hospital that specializes in either international radiology or therapeutic endoscopy, radiologic or endoscopic methods can be attempted.

Role of Endoscopic Sphincterotomy in Gallstone Pancreatitis

Two recent reports have proposed a role of endoscopic sphincterotomy in gallstone pancreatitis. In one report, marked improvement in systemic complications and shorter hospitalization among patients with severe gallstone pancreatitis was observed in patients who underwent urgent endoscopic sphincterotomy, as compared to controls

Table 29-6. Results of Surgical Drainage of 1020 Pseudocysts

Procedure	Number of Patients	Mortality (%)	Recurrence (%)
Excision	126	10.3	2.6
External drainage	443	6.3	22.2
Cystogastrostomy	220	3.6	2.3
Cystoduodenostomy	40	5.0	5.2
Cystojejunostomy	191	7.3	4.5
Total	1,020	6.4	11.5

Source: Becker WF, Pratt HS, Ganju H. Pseudocysts of the pancreas. *Surg Gynecol Obstet* 1968;127:744. Reprinted by permission from Surgery, Gynecology & Obstetrics.

who did not. However, there was no significant improvement in mortality rate. In the other report, urgent endoscopic sphincterotomy reduced biliary sepsis in both mild and severe gallstone pancreatitis but also did not improve mortality. Clearly, the development of biliary sepsis in association with acute pancreatitis warrants urgent decompression of the biliary system. Among the possible choices, endoscopic decompression would be preferred to either radiologic (transhepatic) or surgical decompression.

In the absence of overt biliary sepsis, the role of urgent endoscopic sphincterotomy is more difficult to state definitively. Since neither study provided CT scans, it is not clear to what extent elimination of biliary tract stones improved the natural history of pancreatitis.

The authors' preferred approach is not to perform endoscopic sphincterotomy in mild gallstone pancreatitis. In severe gallstone pancreatitis, if there is suspicion of biliary obstruction or sepsis, or if there is intensification of organ dysfunction, immediate ERCP should be performed, assuming an experienced therapeutic endoscopist is available.

Conclusions

The distinction between mild and severe pancreatitis is best made by the presence or absence of organ failure. A secondary marker of severity is the presence of local complications, in particular pancreatic necrosis. The distinction between sterile and infected necrosis can be made accurately, safely, and promptly by CT-guided percutaneous aspiration. Infected necrosis requires surgical debridement. The role of debridement of sterile necrosis remains controversial. In the authors' institution, surgical debridement is strongly considered for patients who exhibit increased evidence of organ failure despite maximal medical therapy and for patients who exhibit a prolonged need for assisted ventilation for more than 1 month. Asymptomatic pseudocysts require no therapy. The definitive time-honored method of treatment of a symptomatic pseudocyst is surgical decompression. In centers with experienced interventional radiologists, percutaneous catheter drainage can be attempted if it can be ascertained that there is no obstruction of flow in

the pancreatic duct downstream from the pseudocyst. Alternatively, in institutions with experienced therapeutic endoscopists who are conducting clinical research, endoscopic decompression of a pseudocyst can be attempted in selected instances by a cystogastrostomy (or cystoduodenostomy) or by the insertion of a pancreatic stent.

Selected Readings

Balthazar EJ, Robinson DL, Megibow AJ. Acute pancreatitis: Value of CT in establishing prognosis. *Radiology* 1990; 174:331–336.

Bradley EL III. A clinically based classification system for acute pancreatitis. *Arch Surg* 1993; 128:586–590.

Bradley EL III, Allen K. A prospective longitudinal study of observation versus surgical intervention in the management of necrotizing pancreatitis. *Am J Surg* 1991; 161:19–24.

Fan S-T, et al. Early treatment of acute biliary pancreatitis by endoscopic papillotomy. *N Engl J Med* 1993; 328: 228–232.

Freeny PC. Incremental dynamic bolus computed tomography of acute pancreatitis. *Int J Pancreatol* 1993; 13:147–158.

Gerzof SG, et al. Early diagnosis of pancreatic infection by computed tomography-guided aspiration. *Gastroenterology* 1987; 93:1315–1320.

Karimgani I, et al. Prognostic factors in sterile pancreatic necrosis. *Gastroenterology* 1992; 103:1636–1640.

Neoptolemos JP, et al. Controlled trial of urgent endoscopic retrograde cholangiopancreatography and endoscopic sphincterotomy versus conservative treatment for acute pancreatitis due to gallstones. *Lancet* 1988; 2:979–983.

Rao R, Fedorak I, Prinz RA. Effect of failed computed tomographic-guided and endoscopic drainage on pancreatic pseudocyst management. *Surgery* 1993; 114:843–847.

Rattner DW, et al. Early surgical debridement of pancreatic necrosis is beneficial irrespective of infection. *Am J Surg* 1992; 162:137–143.

30

Gallstone Pancreatitis

JOHN SEKIJIMA
MICHAEL KIMMEY
CARLOS A. PELLEGRINI
SUM P. LEE

Our understanding of inflammatory diseases affecting the pancreas has suffered because of confusion over the terms *acute* and *chronic pancreatitis*. These terms are not meant to be used to define the rapidity of onset or resolution of the disease. Instead, they define the reversibility of structural as well as functional changes of the gland. The current concept regards acute pancreatitis as an inflammatory disease affecting a pancreas that had been morphologically and functionally normal and returns to normal when the provoking factors have been corrected. On the other hand, chronic pancreatitis is an inflammatory disease involving a gland which had been morphologically and/or functionally abnormal before the onset of symptoms. These changes also persist after the precipitating factors are corrected. Defined this way, alcoholism is the most common cause of chronic pancreatitis, and gallstone disease is the most common cause of acute pancreatitis.

Etiology and Pathogenesis

The etiology of acute pancreatitis is summarized in Table 30-1. On the basis of early reports, for example, that of Opie in 1901, gallstone impaction in the common duct has been recognized as a cause of acute pancreatitis. Since then, many documentations have been made of this association from operative findings, imaging techniques such as CT, and endoscopic retrograde cholangiopancreatography (ERCP). In patients with acute pancreatitis who require urgent surgery, the incidence of common bile duct stone has been reported to be as high as 63% to 78%. Small pieces of gallstones can be recovered from the feces of 85% to 95% of patients with gallstones who are recovering from acute pancreatitis, compared with a 10% recovery rate in patients who have symptomatic cholelithiasis without pancreatitis. Stone impaction in the majority of patients is a transient event. Most stones will pass spontaneously into the duodenum in a matter of hours. Stones which are too small to be detected by oral cholecystography may appear as gallbladder sludge on biliary microscopy of gallbladder bile drainage or on ultrasonography. Increasing evidence implicates gallbladder sludge (microlithiasis, microcrystalline disease) as part of the spectrum of gallstone disease which can cause symptoms of biliary pain and cholecystitis as well as acute pancreatitis. Biliary sludge–induced acute pancreatitis may also account for acute pancreatitis occurring after extracorporeal lithotripsy, in patients on total parenteral nutrition, after a major operation, during pregnancy, in patients with rapid weight loss, or in patients on treatment with ceftriaxone—all conditions associated with a high incidence of gallbladder sludge. It has also been suggested that gallstone pancreatitis is more likely to occur in patients with multiple small stones and not in those with large stones. This observation probably reflects the fact that small stones or sludge is more likely to migrate to the terminal biliopancreatic ductal system.

Table 30-1. Etiologic Factors in Acute Pancreatitis

Common causes (80% or more)
   Cholelithiasis*
   Ethanol
Others (20% or less)*
   Endoscopic retrograde cholangiopancreatography
   Familial or hereditary
   Hypercalcemia
   Hyperlipoproteinemia
   Infections
      Intraductal parasites
      Mycoplasma pneumoniae
      Viral: coxsackie, mumps
   Medications
      Ceftriaxone*
      Chlorothiazides
      Estrogens
      Furosemide
      L-asparaginase
      Pentamidine
      Sulfonamides
      Tetracyclines
      Valproic acid
   Pancreas divisum
   Pancreatic duct obstruction
      Choledochocele
      Stricture
      Tumor
   Post–extracorporeal shock wave lithotripsy*
   Postoperative*
   Pregnancy*
   Total parenteral nutrition*
   Scorpion bite
   Trauma
   Vascular disease
      Arteritis
      Embolic
   Rapid weight loss*

*Includes the possibility of biliary sludge (microlithiasis) as a cause of acute pancreatitis.

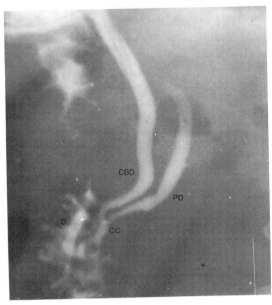

Figure 30-1. Cholangiopancreatogram demonstrating a common channel. CBD, common bile duct; PD, pancreatic duct; CC, common channel; D, duodenum.

The pathogenesis of gallstone pancreatitis remains controversial. The obstructive theory reasons, as Opie did in 1901, that a stone can be small enough to lodge in the common channel of the common bile duct and pancreatic duct. This obstruction will allow the reflux of bile into the pancreatic duct, triggering an attack of pancreatitis. Operative cholangiograms have shown reflux of contrast into the pancreatic duct in approximately 60% of patients with a history of acute pancreatitis, compared with 15% in controls. A common channel (Fig. 30-1) has been found in 72% of patients, compared with only 20% in controls. The duodenal reflux theory involves transient sphincter of Oddi dysfunction when a stone passes through it, allowing the reflux of duodenal contents into the pancreatic duct. Activating enzymes such as enterokinases as well as membrane toxins such as lysolecithin may then precipitate pancreatitis. The passage of a gallstone may sometimes be identified at ERCP as a patulous, incompetent papilla. These two pathogenetic mechanisms are not mutually exclusive, and may indeed both contribute to the creation of pancreatic duct hypertension and the activation of intracellular lysosomal enzymes as well as zymogen granules.

Diagnosis

Typical symptoms of acute pancreatitis are central upper abdominal pain, nausea, and vomiting. Pain is usually sharp and constant, often radiating to the back. Vomiting does not relieve the pain. The clinical features vary greatly with the severity and extent of the pancreatitis. Most patients will have mild distention or the feeling of fullness or a mass at the epigastrium with direct and sometimes rebound tenderness. Bowel sounds are usually diminished. Chest examination will often disclose basilar atelactasis from abdominal distention and splinting of diaphragmatic excursion. Pleural effusion, also not infrequently seen, occurs more often on the left side. Patients with severe hemorrhagic pancreatitis may have ecchymosis seen in the periumbilical or flank regions, referred to as Cullen's and Grey Turner's signs.

Elevation of the serum amylase level is useful in establishing inflammation of the pancreatic gland. However, other nonpancreatic causes of abdominal pain are also associated with the elevation of amylase levels, and even severe cases of pancreatitis may occur with a normal serum amylase level. An increase in the serum lipase level (more than three times normal) has been shown to be more specific as well as more sensitive. Elevations of the serum lipase level persist longer than amylase after an attack of pancreatitis.

Several different systems or sets of criteria have been proposed as indicators of gallstone pancreatitis. Specific cutoff levels of alanine and aspartate aminotransferases, alkaline phosphatase, and bilirubin have been examined, as have the variables of sex, age, and absolute amylase values. The approximate sensitivities of such predictive systems have been reported to be in the range of 70% to 85%. In one prospective study, the mere finding of ALT and AST values greater than 60 U/liter was calculated to have a specificity and sensitivity of around 75%. Similarly, an admission bilirubin level of over 3 mg/dl has been reported to have a sensitivity of over 80% for common duct stones.

Organ imaging can be very helpful in establishing the diagnosis of acute pancreatitis. CT features include a swelling of the pancreas, obliteration of the tissue planes between the pancreas and neighboring structures, and edema of fat surrounding the pancreas. Moreover, CT is helpful in defining the severity and extent of inflammation and necrosis and the presence of complications such as pancreatic ascites, fluid collections, phlegmon, and pseudocysts. Abscesses can be differentiated from pancreatic necrosis using contrast enhancement, and infected necrosis or abscess can be distinguished from sterile inflammatory processes via directed needle aspirations and culture. CT and ultrasound also yield information on the etiology of acute pancreatitis. Gallstones in the gallbladder are seen with high sensitivity with ultrasound and, to a lesser degree, with CT. However, with either modality, small stones in the common bile duct are often missed. The absence of gallbladder sludge and stones and a normal common bile duct on imaging studies do not eliminate gallstones as the etiology of an episode of pancreatitis; many patients have a single gallstone that may have passed through the ampulla or that may be missed on imaging studies.

Management

Options

Advances in the techniques of laparoscopic surgery, endoscopic retrograde cholangiopancreatography (ERCP), and endoscopic sphincterotomy (ES) have led to major changes in the management of biliary pancreatitis. Clinical decisions are often arrived at in multidisciplinary fashion, and whether the care involves primarily conservative, surgical, or endoscopic treatment, a close working relationship between the surgeon, gastroenterologist, and other care providers is essential.

With conservative management, most patients with acute biliary pancreatitis will recover within 7 to 10 days after the onset of symptoms. The treatment consists of general supportive measures, which include giving the patient nothing by mouth, ensuring adequate pain control, and vigorously maintaining fluid and electrolyte balances. It is also imperative to make frequent interval laboratory and physical evaluations to look for signs and symptoms of clinical deterioration or complications. In addition, because of the threat of biliary sepsis associated with gallstone pancreatitis, many clinicians routinely administer empiric antibiotic coverage. However, given the lack of proven benefit to support this practice, the use of antibiotics should be reserved for documented infections, signs of cholangitis, or for prophylactic coverage immediately prior to ERCP/ES.

SURGICAL MANAGEMENT

As mentioned previously, biliary pancreatitis is thought to be triggered by the passage of stones or sludge through the distal common duct and ampullary mechanism. With the goal of ameliorating the severity of the pancreatitis, some observers have advocated urgent biliary tract surgery in the hope of relieving any residual obstruction of the common bile duct or pancreatic duct. Others, however, have claimed that the offending stone will probably pass into the duodenum shortly after the onset of symptoms and that early intervention will not change the course of pancreatitis once it has been initiated. In contrast to this debate, there is little disagreement that concomitant cholangitis should be urgently treated and that underlying gallstone disease must eventually be addressed if repeated bouts of biliary pancreatitis (a risk of up to 50% within 3 months) are to be prevented. Therefore, the majority of patients is best served by having their gallbladders removed and their common bile duct cleared of stones prior to discharge. Laparoscopic cholecystectomy has rapidly been adopted as the procedure of choice in the treatment of symptomatic cholelithiasis. Some reports suggest that this procedure can be performed safely as soon as the symptoms of pancreatitis resolve. How to manage intraoperatively discovered choledocholithiasis is controversial and will be discussed in later sections.

ENDOSCOPIC MANAGEMENT

The early reports on the use of ERCP and ES in the management of biliary pancreatitis were either isolated case studies or retrospective analyses. Initially, fears and concerns existed not only over the usual complications of bleeding and perforation but also over the possibility of exacerbating the ongoing pancreatitis. Additional studies have allayed those concerns, and ERCP and ES have been shown to be safe in the acute setting and also to be of significant benefit in a defined group of patients with gallstone pancreatitis.

Controversies

Controversy in treatment strategies surfaces whenever alternative therapies are introduced and whenever there are conflicting or discrepant reports in the literature. Some of the common dilemmas that confront the attending physician are raised in the following questions: Which patients should be observed and which patients require a more aggressive stance? When, in the clinical course of gallstone pancreatitis, should we intervene, and should this

intervention be endoscopic or surgical? Is it appropriate for a greater number of patients to undergo early ERCP examinations irrespective of the severity of the presenting pancreatitis? What about the role of ERCP and ES in relation to laparoscopic cholecystectomy? How should biliary sludge be managed, and should we be more aggressive in looking for it (as with bile sampling, etc.)? What is the best management for patients who are elderly or poor operative candidates? These issues will be addressed more fully in succeeding sections.

Preferred Approach

Whereas alcoholic acute pancreatitis (or acute relapsing pancreatitis) carries a mortality rate of over 2%, biliary pancreatitis has been reported to have a mortality rate of 10% or more. Because of this fact, investigators have attempted to identify those patients who are at the highest risk to suffer from a serious or prolonged hospital course. A number of established criteria are currently used to assist in making this prognosis (e.g., Ranson, modified Glasgow, Apache II; Tables 30-2, 30-3). Categorizing patients as having either mild or severe pancreatitis has enabled clinicians to more accurately target those individuals who may benefit the most from aggressive treatment. This practice also facilitates a more meaningful comparison of patient outcome results as they are peer-reviewed in the literature.

Table 30-2. Prognostic Factors in Acute Pancreatitis (Ranson)[a]

At admission or diagnosis
Age over 50
WBC 16,000/mm^3 or more
Blood glucose 100 mg/dl or more
Serum LDH[b] 500 IU/liter or more
Serum ALT 250 IU/liter or more
During initial 48 hours
Hematocrit fall of 10% or more
BUN rise of 5 mg/dl or more
Serum calcium 8 mg/dl or less
PaO$_2$ 60 mm Hg or less
Base deficit 4 mEq/liter or more
Fluid sequestration 6 liters or more

[a]Two or fewer factors is considered to be a mild attack; three or more factors, a severe attack.
[b] LDH = lactate dehydrogenase.

Table 30-3. Modified Glasgow System*

Age 55 or more
WBC 15,000/mm³ or more
Serum glucose 180 mg/dl or more (no previous history
  of diabetes)
Serum urea 96 mg/dl or more (no response to IV fluids)
Pao₂ 60 mm Hg or less (no O₂ by mask for 15 min)
Serum CA 8 mg/dl
Serum albumin 3.2 g/dl or less

*Two or fewer factors constitutes a mild attack; three or more, a
severe attack.

The preferred approach to the management of acute biliary pancreatitis (Fig. 30-2) should therefore begin with an initial attempt to assign the degree of clinical severity. Those patients who are thought to have mild pancreatitis (the majority) are best treated with conservative measures. If they fail to improve or have evidence of persistent choledocholithiasis on the basis of elevated serum liver tests or imaging studies, then an ERCP and ES should be performed to clear the common bile duct. A laparoscopic cholecystectomy should then be performed when the symptoms subside. On the other hand, if the patient's symptoms rapidly resolve and the liver tests return to normal, the gallbladder can be removed laparoscopically without doing an ERCP beforehand. It is imperative under these circumstances, however, to obtain a high-quality intraoperative cholangiogram. If stones are found at that time, then the options for the surgeon are to remove them laparoscopically via the cystic duct, to convert to an open procedure, or to pursue subsequent endoscopic retrieval. Though some investigators are reporting good success with laparoscopic common duct exploration, this technique has not yet been widely employed in the average clinical setting and awaits further development.

In contrast to the above, those patients demonstrating either severe disease or evidence of cholangitis should undergo urgent ERCP by an experienced endoscopist. Endoscopic sphincterotomy (ES) and stone extraction should be performed if stones are found. Cholecystectomy is delayed until the patient recovers from the pancreatitis. ERCP and ES would also seem to be ideal for patients who may be elderly or poor operative candidates

for a cholecystectomy. In these patients, since interval cholecystectomy is not anticipated, endoscopic sphincterotomy may be performed even when stones are not found on cholangiography. Previous published studies have suggested that after successful ES has been performed, only approximately 7% to 10% of these high-risk patients eventually require a cholecystectomy. Furthermore, future attacks of gallstone pancreatitis appear to be averted in the small numbers of patients followed thus far. Performing a sphincterotomy to adequately open up the ampullary mechanism is probably crucial to allowing other stones to pass without significant consequence. Thus, if the common bile duct has been cleared endoscopically and if there is no evidence of acute cholecystitis in a poor operative candidate, the gallbladder should be left in situ. Surgery can be reconsidered or the alternative of percutaneous cholecystostomy can be proposed in the future if necessary.

With regard to urgent biliary surgery, the authors believe that the risks are hazardous and should be respected in the seriously ill. Operative intervention (e.g., cholecystectomy with or without common duct exploration) should be avoided or delayed until after the patient has recovered.

Results

Biliary Sludge

Interest has been growing in the underestimated role that biliary sludge appears to play in the etiology of acute pancreatitis. Lee et al. and Ros et al. in separate prospective studies found microscopic evidence of biliary sludge in two thirds of patients with idiopathic pancreatitis. Evidence exists to indicate that both biliary sludge and gallstones impose a high risk of recurrent pancreatitis. These observations were consistent with the fact that biliary sludge patients who had their gallbladders removed were virtually cured of further attacks or episodes of pancreatitis. Moreover, ultrasonography frequently failed to detect small stones in patients with sludge who eventually underwent a cholecystectomy. Taking these findings into account, an argument can now be made to treat biliary sludge and stone patients similarly with respect to prognosis stratifica-

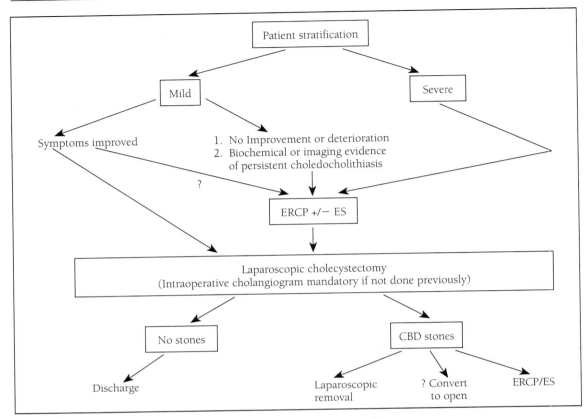

Figure 30-2. Approach to biliary pancreatitis. ERCP, endoscopic retrograde cholangiopancreatography; ES, endoscopic sphincterotomy; CBD, common bile duct.

tion, interventional strategies, and recommendations for a laparoscopic cholecystectomy during the same hospital admission.

Whether bile sampling should be pursued more aggressively in patients with idiopathic pancreatitis without overt ultrasonographic evidence of biliary sludge is another matter. Many of these individuals should be observed and have follow-up ultrasound evaluations as well as possible bile analysis (if available) only if recurrent episodes become apparent. The basic technique of bile sampling involves the placement of a duodenal tube under either fluoroscopic or endoscopic guidance. Intravenous cholecystokinin (CCK) is given, and the fluid is aspirated through the tube over 30 minutes. The sample is then centrifuged for 10 minutes at 4000 G, and the residual sediment is examined under a polarizing microscope at 200×. A diagnosis of microscopic sludge may be made

when five or more birefringent cholesterol crystals or reddish brown clumps of calcium bilirubinate granules are present per slide (Fig. 30-3). If the patient is fit for surgery, then a cholecystectomy can be recommended. However, either ES or a trial of ursodeoxycholic acid (if cholesterol crystals predominate) would be appropriate for the high-risk patient.

Early Surgical Intervention

It is somewhat difficult to interpret and compare the surgical literature for gallstone pancreatitis. Many of the studies failed to stratify patients according to the severity of their pancreatitis. Moreover, historical controls were often used and at times different operative techniques were employed. However, two frequently cited, randomized, prospective trials have

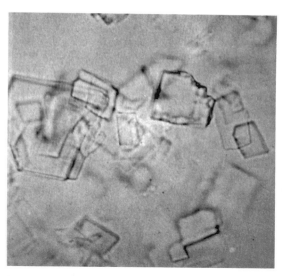

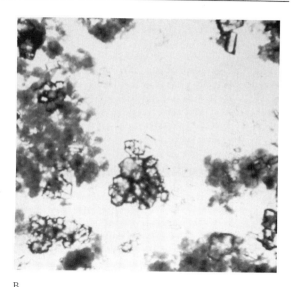

A   B

Figure 30-3. Microscopic features (×200) of biliary sludge containing predominantly cholesterol crystals (A) and predominantly calcium bilirubinate granules (B). (From Lee SP, Nichols JF, Park HZ. Biliary sludge as a cause of acute pancreatitis. *N Engl J Med* 1992;326:589–593. Reproduced with permission.)

been published. Stone et al. randomized 36 patients to early surgery (< 73 hours) and 29 patients to late surgery (> 3 months). They reported mortality rates of 2.9% for the early group and 6.8% for the late group. Though their results appeared to support the notion of early surgery, the study was somewhat weakened by the fact that their patients were not classified in terms of mild or severe disease.

In contrast, Kelly and Wagner examined a larger group of patients. Eighty-three patients underwent early surgery (< 48 hours), and 82 patients underwent delayed surgery (> 48 hours). Overall, the mortality rates were 15% and 2.4%, respectively. In addition, Ranson's prognostic criteria were used to differentiate mild pancreatitis (fewer than three positive signs) from severe pancreatitis (more than three positive signs). In patients with mild disease no demonstrable increase was observed in either morbidity or mortality with urgent surgery. In contradistinction, those undergoing early surgery with severe disease showed a striking mortality rate of 48% compared to the rate of 11% in the delayed group (Table 30-4). It should be noted that these two trials differed not only in study design and size,

Table 30-4. Biliary Surgery in Severe Pancreatitis

	No. of Severe Pts.	Morbidity (%)	Mortality (%)
Surgery > 48 hrs	23	18	11
Surgery < 48 hrs	17	83	48

Source: Kelly TR, Wagner DS. Gallstone pancreatitis: A prospective randomized trial of the timing of surgery. *Surgery* 1988; 104:600–605. Used with permission.

but also in the operative approach to the biliary tree. Stone et al. routinely performed transduodenal sphincteroplasty, whereas Kelly and Wagner most often explored the common duct directly and placed a T tube for drainage. Nevertheless, the balance of the evidence on the whole points away from urgent biliary surgery in acute pancreatitis.

With regard to the role of ERCP and laparoscopic cholecystectomy, a review of the available data reveals that the incidence of choledocholithiasis diminishes the longer one waits to surgically explore. The relative rates vary from 60% to 80% in the first 3 days to 3% to 33% in 3 days to a few months later. These data are in general agreement with the results obtained in the endoscopic literature. Since most patients will have passed their stone by the time of cholecystectomy, a strong argument can be made against the routine use of preoperative ERCP. This policy makes sense not only because it is more cost-effective but also because it decreases the number of patients exposed to potential complications.

Early Endoscopic Intervention

Currently, two randomized prospective studies have examined urgent ERCP and ES in acute gallstone pancreatitis. Neoptolemos et al. randomly assigned 121 patients to either nonoperative, conservative treatment or to urgent endoscopic intervention. Fifty-nine patients underwent ERCP within 72 hours. Patients had ES performed if common duct stones were found. The other 62 patients were followed conservatively. Overall, a significant reduction in the morbidity rate (12%) was observed in the endoscopically treated group as compared to the control group (24%). The patients were also stratified according to the modified Glasgow criteria. The severe pancreatitis patients had the most marked response to ERCP/ES, with a morbidity rate of 24% versus 61% and a mortality rate of 4% versus 18%. Patients with severe pancreatitis were more likely to have common bile duct stones on ERCP than those with mild pancreatitis (63% vs. 25%). Notably, patients undergoing early ERCP also had a shorter hospital stay (9.5 vs. 17.0 days). Much like in the results reported in the surgical literature, those patients with mild pancreatitis did not appear to benefit from early intervention.

Fan et al. from Hong Kong recently reported 195 patients with acute pancreatitis who were randomized to either ERCP and possible ES or conservative treatment and selective ERCP if they deteriorated clinically. Of these, 127 patients were later shown to have common duct stones. Those patients judged to have severe disease on the basis of their admission BUN and glucose levels had a lower morbidity rate (13%) if they had urgent ERCP (i.e., within 24 hours) than the conservative control group (54%). Thus, despite obvious study design variances as well as different environmental and ethnic factors, there appears to be growing support for urgent ERCP in at least the select group of patients with severe gallstone-induced pancreatitis

Table 30-5. Urgent Endoscopic Sphincterotomy in Severe Pancreatitis

	No. of Severe Pts.	Morbidity (%)	Mortality (%)
Neoptolemos et al.[a]			
ERCP/ES < 72 hrs	25	21	4
Conservative	28	64	18
Fan et al.			
ERCP/ES < 24 hrs	41	23	12
Conservative	40	58	23

[a]Data from Neoptolemos JP, et al. Controlled trial of urgent endoscopic retrograde cholangiopancreatography and endoscopic sphincterotomy versus conservative treatment for acute pancreatitis due to gallstones. *Lancet* 1988; 2:979–983. Used with permission.
[b]Data from Fan ST, et al. Early treatment of acute biliary pancreatitis by endoscopic papillotomy. *N Engl J Med* 1993; 32:228–232. Used with permission.

(Table 30-5). It also now appears that, despite earlier concerns regarding the potential complications of endoscopic intervention, ERCP can be performed safely in the acute setting. The authors go one step further and suggest that early ERCP in almost all patients with acute pancreatitis, irrespective of the predicted severity or suspected etiology, is reasonable. Certainly, this contention is debatable and reflects, in part, the high incidence of common duct stones noted in their study and the particular geographic location in which they practice.

Conclusions

Some general conclusions can now be proposed. Urgent surgery on the gallbladder and bile ducts is associated with unacceptably high morbidity and mortality rates and should, if possible, be avoided in the patient with severe gallstone pancreatitis. Surgery should be reserved for complications such as infected necrosis or abscess formation. This situation does not hold true for urgent endoscopic intervention, which in expert hands has been shown to be a safe and efficacious therapy for selected patients. The routine use of ERCP and ES can now be supported in the following clinical scenarios involving gallstone pancreatitis: (1) patients with severe pancreatitis on initial assessment using a validated grading system, (2) patients presenting with mild pancreatitis who subsequently fail to improve or show signs of clinical deterioration, (3) patients with evidence of cholangitis, significant biliary obstruction, or previous cholecystectomy, and (4) patients who are elderly or deemed to have prohibitive operative risks for cholecystectomy.

With respect to the management of patients with mild gallstone pancreatitis, the vast majority will respond to conservative treatment, and neither urgent endoscopic nor operative intervention can be shown to improve the clinical outcome. Any patient with persistent elevations in liver biochemical tests or evidence of biliary obstruction on the basis of imaging modalities should undergo preoperative ERCP. If, on the other hand, liver tests have normalized and symptoms have resolved, the gallbladder can be removed laparoscopically. An intraoperative cholangiogram is mandatory in this setting; if stones are found, the options are to laparoscopically remove them, convert to an open procedure, or proceed with an ERCP and ES. The ultimate choice will depend upon the surgeon's laparoscopic expertise, the availability of an expert endoscopist, and the clinical experiences of those involved. Further advancements in laparoscopic surgery and endoscopic techniques are awaited, and, as they continue to evolve, corresponding changes in recommendations are sure to follow.

Selected Readings

Davidson BR, Neoptolemos TL, Carr-Locke DL. Biochemical production of gallstones in acute pancreatitis: A prospective study of three systems. *Br J Surg* 1988; 75:213–215.

Davidson BR, Neoptolemos TL, Carr-Locke DL. Endoscopic sphincterotomy for common bile duct calculi in patients with gallbladder in situ, considered unfit for surgery. *Gut* 1988; 29:114–120.

Fan ST, et al. Early treatment of acute biliary pancreatitis by endoscopic papillotomy. *N Engl J Med* 1993; 32:228–232.

Kelly TR, Wagner DS. Gallstone pancreatitis: A prospective randomized trial of the timing of surgery. *Surgery* 1988; 104:600–605.

Lee SP, Nichols JF, Park HZ. Biliary sludge as a cause of acute pancreatitis. *N Engl J Med* 1992; 326:589–593.

Neoptolemos JP, et al. Controlled trial of urgent endoscopic retrograde cholangiopancreatography and endoscopic sphincterotomy versus conservative treatment for acute pancreatitis due to gallstones. *Lancet* 1988; 2:979–983.

31

Pseudocysts

Daniel J. Deziel
Richard A. Prinz
Michael F. Uzer
Terence A. S. Matalon

Etiology and Pathogenesis

A pancreatic pseudocyst is a nonepithelial lined collection of pancreatic secretions and debris resulting from disruption of the glandular integrity. Leakage of activated pancreatic enzymes into the parenchyma and the peripancreatic tissue produces a variable degree of necrosis and consequent fibrosis. This intra- and extraglandular collection of fluid and necrotic debris is isolated and walled off by adjacent retroperitoneal and visceral structures. Histologically, the wall of a developed pseudocyst is composed of an inflammatory cellular infiltrate and fibrosis in the surrounding tissues.

Pancreatic pseudocysts occur in fewer than 10% of patients with acute pancreatitis but in as many as 40% of patients with chronic pancreatitis. Elevated pancreatic ductal pressure in chronic pancreatitis may increase the risk of rupture and subsequent cyst formation. In adults, approximately 75% of pseudocysts are related to alcoholic pancreatitis, and 10% follow biliary pancreatitis. This difference is due to the high incidence of pseudocysts in chronic pancreatitis, which is predominantly caused by alcohol. Trauma accounts for an additional 5% to 10% of pseudocysts, and the remainder are attributed to pancreatitis from various etiologies, including hyperlipidemia, pancreatic cancer, drugs, and operative injury. Abdominal trauma is the cause of most pseudocysts in children. Epidemiologically, pseudocysts are twice as common in males as in females and have a peak incidence in the fourth to sixth decades, as might be anticipated from the etiologic prevalence of alcohol.

Pseudocysts typically are located in the lesser sac and develop on the anterior surface of the gland with variable retroperitoneal extension. Tracking behind the mesocolon is common; occasionally pseudocysts extend inferiorly into the pelvis or superiorly into the chest and mediastinum. Most pseudocysts are single and unilocular; 10% to 15% are multiple. Cysts contain a high concentration of pancreatic enzymes and variable amounts of necrotic and inflammatory debris. This situation produces a content of variable viscosity, which affects the expected efficacy of various drainage techniques.

It is critical to distinguish between pseudocysts occurring in association with acute pancreatitis and those diagnosed in the clinical setting of chronic pancreatitis. Pseudocysts that have well-developed fibrous walls sufficient to tolerate suturing are referred to as "mature" pseudocysts. The process of fibrous thickening and maturation takes 4 to 6 weeks. Immature cysts that develop during an episode of acute pancreatitis are not suitable for internal drainage by gastrointestinal anastomosis if surgical intervention should be necessary. Furthermore, a substantial proportion of acute peripancreatic fluid collections will resolve spontaneously. This process probably occurs most commonly by resorption of the extracellular fluid. Pseudocysts can also resolve by spontaneous decompression into the gastrointestinal tract or by drainage of cyst contents back into the pancreatic duct.

Pseudocysts detected in patients with chronic pancreatitis are invariably mature unless a recent episode of acute pancreatitis has occurred. Moreover, spontaneous resolution of pseudocysts associated with chronic pancreatitis occurs less frequently. Additional considerations with important therapeutic implications in patients with pseudocysts and chronic pancreatitis include the presence of associated obstruction or dilatation of the main pancreatic duct that may warrant concomitant drainage. Complications that influence the timing and choice of therapy include infection, bleeding, rupture, and obstruction. The risk of these complications seems to increase as the cyst endures. Clinically infected pseudocysts are treated by external drainage. Bleeding from pseudoaneurysms of the gastroduodenal, pancreaticoduodenal, or splenic vessels along the cyst wall necessitates emergent intervention. Rupture is most frequently manifested as pancreatic ascites and occasionally as fistulization into the gastrointestinal or genitourinary tract. Obstruction may involve the biliary tract, duodenum, transverse colon, or splenic vein. Obstruction or thrombosis of the splenic vein causes left-sided portal hypertension with resulting varices.

Diagnosis

Computerized tomography (CT) is the most valuable imaging modality for diagnosing pancreatic pseudocysts. CT accurately depicts the size, number, and location of the cysts, provides information on chronicity, detects associated pancreatic or bile duct dilatation, and delineates the surrounding normal and abnormal anatomy (Fig. 31-1). Dynamic contrast-enhanced CT will demonstrate the presence of associated pancreatic necrosis as well as splenic vein thrombosis with secondary varices. Ultrasonography (US) is also a highly accurate technique for identifying pseudocysts. Since US is less expensive than CT, its primary value is for serial imaging of a pseudocyst that is being expectantly managed in order to detect resolution or enlargement.

Endoscopic retrograde cholangiopancreatography (ERCP) can delineate pancreatic and bile duct

Figure 31-1. CT scan demonstrating two large pancreatic pseudocysts following acute alcoholic pancreatitis. Note extension of lateral cyst into splenic hilum.

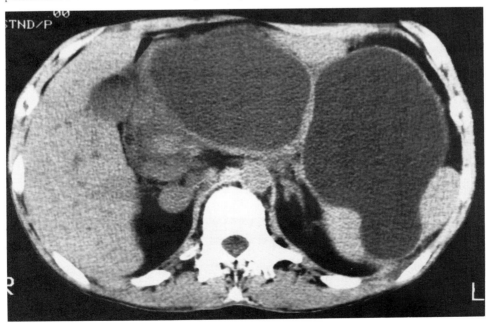

anatomy, and in one half to two thirds of cases ERCP will demonstrate communication of the cyst with the pancreatic duct (Fig. 31-2). Some have advocated routine preoperative ERCP as a means of detecting ductal abnormalities indicative of chronic pancreatitis. In most instances, however, this information is provided by CT. ERCP is an invasive procedure that should be used only if it will influence management. Chronic pancreatitis can generally be suspected on the basis of a history of excessive alcohol use, recurrent pain, evidence of exocrine or endocrine insufficiency, or pancreatic calcifications. CT will not detect communication between the pseudocyst and the pancreatic duct, but preoperative demonstration of this does not alter operative strategy.

Selective celiac and mesenteric angiography is required in the less than 5% of patients who manifest significant bleeding complications. Pseudoaneurysms and splenic vein thrombosis can be detected and bleeding sites can be embolized.

Dynamic CT scanning can definitely detect splenic vein obstruction and may help to identify pseudoaneurysms before they are clinically evident from bleeding.

Prior to the wide availability of the direct imaging techniques of CT and US, the diagnosis of pancreatic pseudocyst was based on symptoms of abdominal pain, nausea, and vomiting, physical findings of an abdominal mass or fullness, and indirect evidence provided by displacement of adjacent organs on plain abdominal films or contrast studies. Laboratory studies are still frequently nonspecific. Persistent elevations of serum or urinary amylase levels are the most consistent findings and may be diagnostic. Amylase isoenzyme patterns demonstrating an increased proportion of deaminated amylase ("old amylase") in the serum support the diagnosis.

It is critical to differentiate inflammatory cysts from cystic pancreatic neoplasms. A reliable distinction can usually be made based on clinical history and presentation and recognition of CT appearance.

Figure 31-2. Endoscopic retrograde pancreatogram demonstrating communication of the pancreatic duct with a large pseudocyst in the tail (small arrows) and small pseudocysts in body (curved arrow) and head (straight arrow).

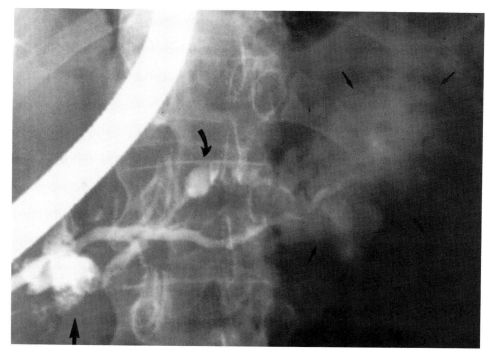

Cystic neoplasms characteristically occur in middle-aged women and present with vague abdominal pain, an abdominal mass, and weight loss. Symptoms are indolent and may have been present for years. In contrast to those with pseudocysts, patients with cystic neoplasms have no history of an attack of acute pancreatitis or its precipitating factors of alcoholism or gallstone disease. CT usually demonstrates a large multiloculated lesion with cystic areas of varying size and internal septations. A solid component or internal tumor excrescences may be identified. Occasionally, central stellate or peripheral calcifications are found, but the remaining pancreas is normal. Inflammatory pseudocysts are most commonly single and unilocular; pancreatic duct dilatation and calcifications of chronic pancreatitis may be observed. Analysis of cyst fluid obtained by percutaneous aspiration may be helpful if this differentiation is not clear with clinical evaluation. Inflammatory lesions typically contain high amylase and lipase concentrations as well as deaminated amylase, whereas the enzyme content of neoplastic cysts is variable and often low. A distinction between pseudocysts and mucinous cystic neoplasms can be made by a consideration of fluid cytology, viscosity, and the concentration of certain tumor markers such as carcinoembryonic antigen (CEA), carbohydrate antigen 125 (CA 125), CA 72-4, and CA 15-3.

Management

The traditional management concept that most pancreatic pseudocysts should be treated operatively has evolved to a more selective strategy based on a better understanding of their natural history and on the availability of alternative nonoperative methods for drainage. Which patients require invasive therapy and what the best method of drainage is for any given situation remain controversial. Current therapeutic decisions are influenced by multiple factors, including pseudocyst size, age, location, number, etiology, and the presence of symptoms or complications. Associated pancreatic ductal abnormalities and the general physiologic status of the patient are also important considerations.

Expectant Management

Peripancreatic fluid collections occur in 20% of patients with acute pancreatitis. Most of these are not true pseudocysts and many will resolve spontaneously, particularly if they are small (< 4–5 cm). Any form of intervention is unnecessary for these collections that will regress naturally. The likelihood of spontaneous resolution is directly related to cyst size and is adversely affected by subsequent increase in size, the presence of multiple cysts, and the presence of chronic pancreatitis.

The classic teaching has been that pseudocysts that are larger than 5 to 6 cm in size and that are present longer than 6 weeks are associated with a low rate of spontaneous resolution and a high rate of complications and therefore require drainage. Aranha and coworkers documented ultrasonographic resolution in only 15% of pseudocysts larger than 6 cm. Bradley and associates found that pseudocysts present for under 6 weeks had a 40% resolution rate and a 20% complication rate, whereas those followed longer had a 4% resolution rate and a 60% risk of life-threatening complications. These findings have been challenged by more recent data indicating that expectant management of asymptomatic pseudocysts is usually safe and results in a high rate of cyst resolution.

Yeo and colleagues reported that expectant management was successful in approximately one half of 75 patients with pseudocysts. At a mean follow-up of 1 year, 60% of cysts in the nonoperative group had completely resolved. Pseudocyst size correlated with the need for operative management in that 67% of those over 6 cm required intervention as compared to 40% of those under 6 cm. Pseudocyst-related complications occurred in 11% of all patients but in only 1 of 36 patients being observed.

In a similar report of 114 pseudocyst patients, Vitas and Sarr found that noninterventional management was sufficient for nearly 40% of patients. Among 24 patients managed nonoperatively with adequate radiologic follow-up, cyst resolution occurred in 57%. Resolution was observed at much later times than in previous studies. Thirty-eight percent of cysts that resolved did so after 6 months. Operative intervention was eventually necessary in 36% of the expectantly managed group; 9% of these patients developed serious complications of hemorrhage, pancreatic infection, or cyst perforation. Pseudocyst complications occurred in 10% of all patients and were most frequent within the first 8 weeks of diagnosis. Serious morbidity occurred in 67% of patients requiring emergent intervention, as compared to only 10% of patients undergoing elective operations.

Neither pseudocyst size nor duration is the sole determinant of the need for intervention. Expectant management is appropriate for a substantial proportion of patients with pseudocysts diagnosed during an episode of acute pancreatitis. Persistent symptoms, development of a pseudocyst-related complication, pseudocyst enlargement, and pseudocyst recurrence are indications for intervention.

Unlike pseudocysts diagnosed during acute pancreatitis, most investigators agree that those occurring in the setting of chronic pancreatitis are unlikely to resolve. Nonetheless, if the cyst is stable, asymptomatic, and uncomplicated, no intervention is indicated, and follow-up with interval imaging is appropriate. If treatment is required, these lesions are generally amenable to internal drainage at the time of diagnosis. Concomitant drainage of the pancreatic duct or bile duct may be indicated.

Some groups have favored percutaneous catheter drainage as an alternative to either mandatory operation or to long-term expectant management for larger, asymptomatic pseudocysts. Proponents of operative therapy argue that percutaneous therapy is often not curative and imposes unnecessary risks, such as the development of infection or a pancreatic fistula. Advocates of expectant management feel that any form of intervention is unnecessary in the absence of specific indications because many asymptomatic pseudocysts will resolve.

Percutaneous Catheter Drainage

External pseudocyst drainage by percutaneous catheter placement can be an effective method of management that avoids the morbidity of operative intervention or that allows stabilization of critically ill patients prior to surgery. Percutaneous intervention is generally reserved for acute pancreatic pseudocysts in symptomatic patients with collections that are enlarging or that demonstrate evidence of

a complication. Unilocular or bilobar collections are particularly well suited to percutaneous catheter drainage, providing that a safe percutaneous route can be established. Some institutions advocate percutaneous catheter drainage as the initial intervention for nearly all pancreatic fluid collections. Surgical therapy is then reserved for failures of percutaneous treatment or when a catheter cannot safely be introduced. The authors believe that pancreatic fluid collections should be managed expectantly and that the same criteria for operative intervention should be used for other forms of drainage, including percutaneous drainage.

Technically, either ultrasonography or CT can be used to guide catheter placement. Most interventional radiologists prefer the more complete anatomic detail that CT provides. Percutaneous catheter drainage of a pseudocyst requires a thorough knowledge of peritoneal anatomy and of the proximity of the large and small bowel. Transperitoneal or retroperitoneal approaches have been most frequently used. Transenteric catheter placement has been advocated by some groups on the basis of the alleged similarity to traditional surgical cyst enterostomies (Fig. 31-3). No published series has documented superior results using this method. Catheter placement with this technique is decidedly more demanding, particularly when a large catheter needs to be placed initially.

Figure 31-3. Percutaneous catheter drainage of pseudocysts from patient in Fig. 31-1. Catheter on patient's right is transperitoneal. Catheter on patient's left is transgastric.

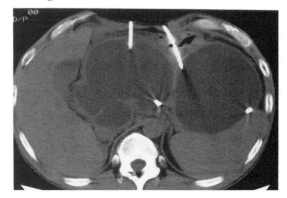

Large anterior collections with no anticipated intervening structures may be approached using a trocar technique. More commonly, however, catheter placement is preceded by CT-directed needle placement, coiling of a guidewire, tract dilatation, and finally catheter placement through a peel-away sheath. The entire cavity should be aspirated.

Findings of viscous, particulate, or solid material dictate replacement of the initial catheter with a larger sump drain. Adjunctive use of fibrinolytic enzymes may prevent catheter occlusions in patients with viscous cyst contents. Initial catheter manipulation must be minimized in patients with evidence of sepsis. Frequent irrigation will hasten complete evacuation of the cavity. The initial irrigation volume should be about 50% of the volume aspirated during the drainage procedure. Irrigation volumes are reduced by one half at regular intervals. Contrast injections through the catheter monitor the size of the cavity and communication with either the pancreatic duct or bowel. Decreasing output from the catheter signals cavity closure, which permits a gradual removal of the catheter. The mean duration of catheter drainage ranges from 20 to 60 days. Communication with the pancreatic duct prolongs the duration of drainage. Persistent pancreaticocutaneous fistula has not been a major problem in several large experiences.

Endoscopic Management

Since the mid-1980s endoscopists have sought alternatives to operative and percutaneous drainage of pancreatic pseudocysts. Endoscopic drainage procedures attempt to create a communication between the pseudocyst cavity and the intestinal lumen much as in surgical cyst enterostomy. The establishment of this communication allows the cyst fluid to drain internally until resolution is achieved. Endoscopic methods of pseudocyst drainage include endoscopic cystogastrostomy, cystoduodenostomy, and transpapillary drainage. The primary clinical indications for endoscopic therapy have been to relieve cyst-related pain or associated biliary obstruction caused by the pseudocyst. Although endoscopic drainage was initially introduced as treatment for patients deemed too ill to undergo surgery, some centers with endoscopic ex-

pertise feel that it can be considered a primary therapeutic modality.

Before attempting endoscopic drainage of pancreatic pseudocysts, one must be certain that the cyst bulges into the intestinal lumen and that it adheres to the intestinal wall. The luminal bulge can be seen endoscopically. Adherence to the gut wall can usually be identified by CT scanning, but this method has limitations. Generally, endoscopic drainage should not be attempted if the distance between the cyst cavity and intestinal lumen exceeds 10 mm or if the cyst cannot clearly be seen bulging into the gut lumen. Transendoscopic ultrasonography (EUS) may be useful for measuring the distance between the lumen and the cyst and for identifying vascular structures which may interfere with cystotomy. EUS requires an end-viewing scope, and cyst puncture is performed with a side-viewing scope. If EUS is performed, the cystotomy site can be injected with colored dye to mark it for subsequent endoscopic drainage. The cystotomy site, either the stomach or the duodenum, is chosen endoscopically at the point of maximal bulging of the pseudocyst into the intestinal lumen. ERCP is not essential but may be useful in documenting communication between the pancreatic ductal system and the cyst. This situation may be amenable to transpapillary drainage of the cyst.

Once the proper drainage site has been chosen, the initial step is to create an opening between the intestinal lumen and the cyst. This step can usually be accomplished with a diathermy needle. Alternatively, a Nd:YAG laser contact probe may be used to perform cystotomy. The puncture must be made perpendicular to the bulge. When the needle reaches the cyst cavity, fluid escapes into the digestive tract lumen, and the catheter must quickly be advanced into the cavity to maintain access. A double-channel fistulatome, which allows for removal of the diathermy needle while maintaining cyst access with the outer sheath, has been developed to eliminate the need to recannulate the fistula. At this point, radiographic dye can be injected into the cyst to precisely identify its size, location, and communication with the main ductal system. An Erlangen papillotome is then inserted, and the opening is enlarged to a size of 8 to 20 mm using alternating cutting and coagulation currents. Once the cystotomy is completed, the endoscopist may terminate the procedure or may insert a double-pigtail prosthesis between the cyst cavity and gut lumen to keep the cystotomy open long enough for the cyst to adequately drain. The prostheses are generally left in place 1 to 2 months. They are probably more essential in maintaining patency when draining larger, low-pressure, retrogastric cysts. Paraduodenal cysts may be managed with cystotomy alone.

Transpapillary endoscopic drainage is a technique reserved for cysts that communicate with the main pancreatic ductal system. Endoscopic sphincterotomy is usually performed, and selective cannulization of the pancreatic duct is achieved. The major hurdle is gaining access to the cyst cavity via the pancreatic duct. This step is best accomplished with the aid of hydrophilic guidewires that become slippery when wet and traverse narrow passages with minimal trauma to the ductal system. Once access is achieved, cyst fluid can be aspirated, and a transpapillary prosthesis can be inserted using the same technique as for biliary stenting. The feasibility of this approach is dictated by the pancreatic ductal anatomy. Generally, pseudocysts in the head of the pancreas are more amenable to transpapillary drainage than are caudal lesions.

Objections to Nonoperative Drainage

When one should use percutaneous or endoscopic drainage rather than traditional operative intervention remains one of the most controversial issues in pseudocyst management. Despite the impressive success rates and the relative safety that some groups have achieved using nonoperative techniques, most surgeons are concerned by several aspects of these approaches. In some reports, rates of treatment failure and of cyst recurrence have been higher than those anticipated following definitive operative management. The inability of small catheters to effectively drain cysts containing thick fluid or solid necrotic residue is easily appreciated by the surgeon who evacuates this material during open drainage procedures. It is unclear whether ERCP demonstration of pancreatic duct obstruction or of communication between the duct and the pseudocyst should dictate operative therapy or whether

percutaneous drainage may be sufficient. Most authorities have observed a higher rate of recurrence and fistula formation if percutaneous drainage is used in this setting. Others have not found that ductal disruption is predictive of the success of nonoperative therapy. Nonetheless, nonoperative drainage cannot treat associated pancreatic ductal obstruction in patients with chronic pancreatitis and a pseudocyst. Similarly, biliary obstruction, which is most commonly due to distal bile duct stenosis rather than extrinsic compression from the pseudocyst, will usually not be relieved by nonoperative decompression of the pseudocyst.

Percutaneous drainage may contribute to the risk of secondary infection of the pseudocyst, thereby complicating the patient's subsequent course and operative management. Rao and associates demonstrated that the morbidity of operative intervention following failed percutaneous or endoscopic drainage was twice that of initial operative management. In particular, intra-abdominal abscess occurred four times more frequently in the group that had undergone nonoperative drainage. Failed nonoperative intervention significantly prolonged the time between cyst diagnosis and resolution.

Histologic examination may be important to differentiate neoplastic from inflammatory cystic lesions. Percutaneous techniques allow aspiration of cyst fluid for cytological analysis and needle biopsy of the cyst wall. However, sampling error is a recognized problem in the diagnosis of cystic neoplasms. More adequate histologic material may be obtained by excising a portion of the cyst wall at the time of operation.

Transenteric routes for percutaneous or endoscopic drainage rely on adherence between the pseudocyst and the adjacent stomach or duodenum. Occasionally, such adherence does not exist. Furthermore, the reliability of CT imaging in assessing adherence is not established.

Nonoperative pseudocyst decompression requires the expertise of specially skilled endoscopists or interventional radiologists. No randomized prospective studies demonstrate an advantage of nonoperative drainage over conventional surgical therapy. A critical need exists for such studies to resolve the role of these alternative therapeutic modalities. Surgeons and nonsurgeons must cooperate to establish accepted parameters by which complication rates and outcomes can be legitimately and equitably assessed.

Surgical Management

Operative management of a pancreatic pseudocyst may be indicated for persistent symptoms, cyst enlargement, or development of complications such as hemorrhage, secondary infection, rupture, or obstruction of the gastrointestinal or biliary tracts. The choice of operation depends upon several factors, such as cyst size, maturity, location, and multiplicity, the status of the pancreatic duct, and the presence of specific complications.

Internal drainage by anastomosis of the pseudocyst to a portion of the gastrointestinal tract is the preferred procedure for most pseudocysts. A mature fibrous wall is a prerequisite for successful internal drainage. The site of anastomosis is determined by cyst location, adherence, and in part by the surgeon's choice. The anastomosis most commonly involves the stomach or a Roux-en-Y limb of proximal jejunum, but occasionally the duodenum can be used.

CYSTOGASTROSTOMY

Internal drainage by anastomosis of the pseudocyst to the posterior gastric wall is suitable for large cysts in the body of the pancreas that are adherent to the stomach (Fig. 31-4). An anterior gastrotomy is made, and the cyst is localized by needle aspiration of some of the cyst contents through the posterior gastric wall. Entry into the cyst is established by making an opening at least 3 cm in size; an ellipse of tissue can be excised to ensure a better stoma. A portion of the cyst wall is sent for frozen section histology to exclude a cystic neoplasm. Any bleeding from the cyst gastric anastomosis is controlled with sutures.

Postoperative upper gastrointestinal tract hemorrhage occurs more frequently after cystogastrostomy than after cystojejunostomy. Potential sites of hemorrhage include the cystogastrostomy, the anterior gastrotomy, and pseudoaneurysms along the wall of the cyst. A sufficient opening into the cyst should be made to evacuate the contents and to be sure that there is no evidence of bleeding. Postoperative bleeding should be aggressively in-

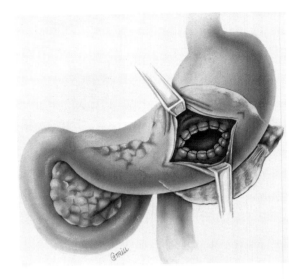

Figure 31-4. Cystogastrostomy.

vestigated to identify the source. Bleeding from pseudoaneurysms is best controlled by emergent angiographic embolization. Prompt reoperation is advised if embolization is unsuccessful or unavailable.

ROUX-EN-Y CYSTOJEJUNOSTOMY

Cystojejunostomy is indicated for cysts that are not adherent to the stomach or duodenum. Roux-en-Y cystojejunostomy is also particularly useful for drainage of multiple pseudocysts which can separately be incorporated into the jejunal limb and for concomitant pancreatic duct drainage in patients requiring lateral pancreaticojejunostomy for chronic pancreatitis (Figs. 31-5, 31-6). After conclusive identification of the pseudocyst's location by needle aspiration, a 50- to 60-cm Roux-en-Y loop is constructed. The pseudocyst is entered, its contents are evacuated, and a portion of the wall is sent for frozen section. A wide anastomosis is created, usually to the side but occasionally to the end of the jejunal limb, in one or two layers. This formal enteric anastomosis dictates caution in utilizing cystojejunostomy for a potentially infected cyst. Intraabdominal sepsis has been a more common postoperative problem with cystojejunostomy than with cystogastrostomy, presumably as the result of anastomotic leakage.

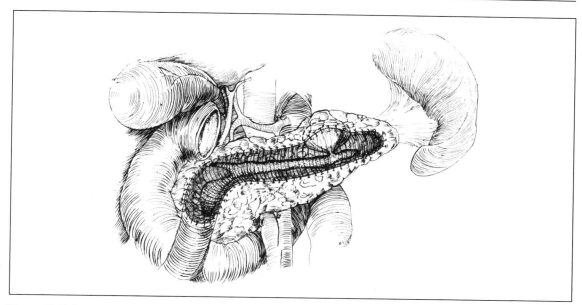

Figure 31-5. Intrapancreatic pseudocyst drained by extending pancreatic ductal incision into pseudocyst and incorporating opening into overlying jejunal limb. (From Munn JS, et al. Simultaneous treatment of chronic pancreatitis and pancreatic pseudocyst. *Arch Surg* 1987; 122:664. Copyright 1987 American Medical Association.)

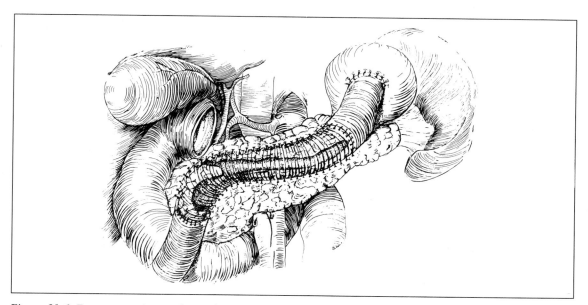

Figure 31-6. Extrapancreatic pseudocyst drained by anastomosing free end of Roux-en-Y loop of jejunum to dependent portion of cyst. (From Munn JS, et al. Simultaneous treatment of chronic pancreatitis and pancreatic pseudocyst. *Arch Surg* 1987; 122:664. Copyright 1987 American Medical Association.)

CYSTODUODENOSTOMY

Drainage into the duodenum is appropriate for pseudocysts in the head of the pancreas that are adherent or adjacent to the duodenum (Fig. 31-7). Transduodenal cystoduodenostomy is preferred over laterolateral anastomosis because of a high rate of anastomotic disruption and potential fatality with the latter procedure. The duodenum is mobilized by a wide Kocher maneuver and the site of closest proximity between the pseudocyst and the duodenum is identified. A lateral longitudinal duodenotomy is made, and the pseudocyst is entered through the medial wall of the duodenum with an opening of at least 2 cm. If the medial opening is in the second portion of the duodenum, injury to the ampulla of Vater and bile duct must be avoided. It may be necessary to cannulate the common bile duct to conclusively identify its site of entry into the duodenum. Sutures are placed to control bleeding, and the lateral duodenotomy is closed. The gastroduodenal and pancreaticoduodenal vessels are potential sites of bleeding during cystoduodenostomy. In the first portion of the duodenum, the opening in the medial wall should be several centimeters distal to the pylorus. In the second and third portions, entering the cyst bluntly rather than sharply and staying in the midplane of the duodenum may avoid excessive bleeding.

CONCOMITANT LATERAL PANCREATICOJEJUNOSTOMY

As many as 40% of patients with chronic pancreatitis undergoing lateral pancreaticojejunostomy have associated pancreatic pseudocysts. Higher rates of pseudocyst recurrence and of reoperation for pain have been observed among patients with chronic pancreatitis undergoing pseudocyst drainage alone. Combined drainage of the pseudocyst and the dilated pancreatic duct is the most effective method for treating patients with these coexisting conditions. Simultaneous drainage into a Roux-en-Y jejunal limb is not associated with a higher rate of operative complications than pseudocyst drainage alone. For patients undergoing lateral pancreaticojejunostomy, intrapancreatic pseudocysts can be drained by extending the ductal incision into the pseudocyst and incorporating the opening into the jejunal limb (see Fig. 31-5). Extrapancreatic pseudocysts can likewise be managed by anastomosis to either the side or the end of the jejunal limb, depending upon their location (see Fig. 31-6).

RECOMMENDED METHOD OF OPERATIVE INTERNAL DRAINAGE

In certain situations, either cystogastrostomy or Roux-en-Y cystojejunostomy may be a technically feasible operation for internal pseudocyst drainage. Overall, outcomes appear to be roughly compara-

Figure 31-7. Transduodenal cystoduodenostomy.

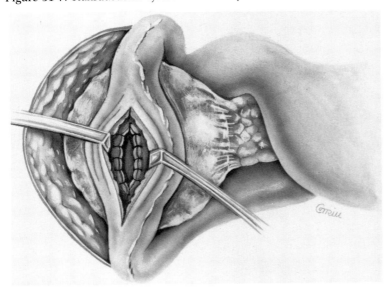

ble, although a few distinctions have been noted. Cystogastrostomy has generally been associated with a greater risk of postoperative gastrointestinal hemorrhage, whereas Roux-en-Y cystojejunostomy may be complicated more frequently by intra-abdominal infection. Some have found cystogastrostomy to be more expeditious and to result in less intraoperative blood loss than cystojejunostomy. Some advocate cystojejunostomy for large pseudocysts that extend inferiorly behind the transverse mesocolon, since a cystogastrostomy may not provide adequate dependent drainage. This situation does not seem to be a common problem.

PANCREATIC RESECTION

Resection is generally reserved for small pseudocysts in the caudal portion of the pancreas. Since the cyst or associated inflammatory changes typically extend into the splenic hilum, en bloc splenectomy is usually required. Concomitant lateral pancreaticojejunostomy is appropriate if the patient has chronic pancreatitis and a dilated pancreatic duct. Excisional therapy may be necessary for pseudocysts complicated by hemorrhage from rupture of pseudoaneurysms that cannot be adequately controlled by other modalities. Resection of pseudocysts in the head by pancreaticoduodenectomy is rarely necessary. Pancreatic resection for pseudocysts can be a technically demanding and difficult procedure because of the amount of fibrosis and inflammation.

EXTERNAL DRAINAGE

Operative external drainage is indicated for immature pseudocysts that lack an adequate wall for suturing and for grossly infected pseudocysts. Drainage is currently accomplished by placement of soft sump tubes rather than by marsupialization, as was formerly practiced. Dependent drainage of well-localized upper retroperitoneal collections may be achieved by a posterior extraperitoneal approach through the bed of the resected twelfth rib. Disadvantages of external drainage are a higher rate of recurrence and of development of a pancreaticocutaneous fistula. Most fistulas will close spontaneously in 6 to 10 weeks, and closure may be facilitated by administrating the synthetic somatostatin analog octreotide. The high associated operative morbidity and mortality of external drainage reflects the fact that this operation is typically used in poor-risk patients with complicated pseudocysts. External drainage can be a life-saving procedure in critically ill patients.

LAPAROSCOPIC MANAGEMENT

Surgical options for the management of pancreatic pseudocysts have been expanded by developments in laparoscopic technology. Early experiences with limited numbers of patients have been reported. Both laparoscopic cystogastrostomy and laparoscopically assisted cystojejunostomy have been accomplished. An innovative technique of intraluminal laparoscopic pseudocyst drainage may be one of the most promising approaches. This technique uses specially designed trocars that are placed through the anterior gastric wall to provide intraluminal access for the laparoscope and the laparoscopic instruments. The trocars consist of an 18-gauge needle wrapped by an elastic sheath with a balloon on the tip. The balloon secures the trocar in the stomach and maintains gastric insufflation. The unique design of this device allows for radial dilatation of the gastrotomy site by the passage of an obturator and sleeve through the sheath. Radial dilatation prevents tearing of the gastric wall. Following dilatation, a 5-mm laparoscope can be introduced into the stomach via the sheath. Two additional gastrotomies are similarly established for the laparoscopic instruments. The pseudocyst is located visually by a bulge in the posterior gastric wall or by laparoscopic ultrasonography. A 3- to 6-cm cystotomy is created with electrocautery, and the cyst contents are evacuated. A single suture suffices to close each gastrotomy site.

Way and colleagues attempted this approach in nine patients with pancreatic pseudocysts. One cyst was not adherent and one cyst had spontaneously resolved, so they were able to perform it in seven patients. The pseudocyst resolved in six of these seven. One cyst persisted, which they attributed to too small a cystotomy. Advantages of this technique over endoscopic drainage are that a large opening can be made, the cyst can be completely evacuated, and bleeding can be directly controlled.

MANAGEMENT OF INFECTED PSEUDOCYSTS

Differing recommendations as to whether infected pseudocysts require external drainage or can be selectively handled by internal drainage hinge on the definition of *infection*. External drainage is clearly necessary for infected pancreatic fluid collections in acutely ill patients or when the cyst wall is thin and inadequate for safe suturing. Up to 30% of pseudocysts may contain bacteria even though the patient may be free of systemic manifestations. These cysts are perhaps better considered "colonized" rather than "infected." Internal pseudocyst drainage has been safely accomplished in these patients. A higher threshold for performing cystojejunostomy rather than cystogastrostomy has been recommended when bacterial contamination exists because a formal anastomosis of the jejunum to the cyst is considered at higher risk for breakdown. Since postoperative wound infection and intraabdominal abscess are more common in patients with pseudocysts harboring bacteria, prophylactic antibiotics have been recommended. Antibiotics may have to be continued for 5 to 7 days if bacterial contamination is confirmed.

Preferred Approach

A rational approach to the treatment of pancreatic pseudocysts is one of selective intervention based upon the specific clinical situation and the availability of local expertise. Uncomplicated fluid collections diagnosed in a patient with acute pancreatitis are managed expectantly. Expectant management consists of initial hospitalization with supportive care and withholding of oral nutrition until the patient's acute symptoms resolve. If the patient can subsequently tolerate adequate oral intake without pain and does not develop complications, he or she can be discharged with serial ultrasound or CT follow-up at monthly intervals to assess pseudocyst resolution or enlargement. If the patient has persistent symptoms and is unable to eat but does not have a complication, parenteral nutrition may be instituted for 4 to 6 weeks to allow resolution or cyst maturation. The use of octreotide, a synthetic somatostatin analog, will decrease pancreatic secretions, but its role in the management of patients with pancreatic pseudocyst has not been clearly established.

Intervention is indicated if the pseudocyst becomes symptomatic or increases in size or if complications develop. Internal drainage by cystogastrostomy, Roux-en-Y cystojejunostomy, or cystoduodenostomy is the preferred method of operative management. Pseudocysts that are discovered to be immature or infected are drained externally. Adjuvant use of sandostatin to prevent pancreatic fistula is unsubstantiated, although it may have benefit in expediting closure of established fistulas. The presence of bacteria in cyst contents does not alone mandate external drainage. Internal drainage is appropriate for selected patients whose cysts harbor bacteria, providing that the patient is not clinically toxic, the cyst wall is mature, and no local signs of infection are present. When bacteria are present, antibiotics are continued postoperatively. Small cysts located in the distal pancreas can be managed by distal pancreatectomy.

Hemorrhage from associated pseudoaneurysms is potentially life-threatening and must be handled emergently. Bleeding is best detected angiographically and is controlled by embolization. Pseudocyst rupture most commonly manifests as pancreatic ascites, with or without pleural effusion, and is managed by initial paracentesis and/or thoracentesis, and by parenteral hyperalimentation. Administration of sandostatin may be beneficial in these patients. If leakage of pancreatic secretions continues, operative internal drainage of the pseudocyst or the resulting pancreatic fistula is undertaken.

Pseudocysts in patients with chronic pancreatitis can be followed expectantly if the patient is asymptomatic. Frequently, however, these patients are symptomatic, although it may not be possible to discern whether the symptoms are related primarily to the pseudocyst or to the underlying chronic pancreatitis. Symptomatic pseudocysts in chronic pancreatitis are managed by operative internal drainage. CT is usually sufficient to detect dilatation of the pancreatic duct or bile duct that would be managed by concomitant anastomosis. ERCP is reserved for unclear cases when chronic pancreatitis is suspected but calcifications or ductal dilatation are not seen on CT.

Direct percutaneous or transenteric catheter drainage is the most widely performed method of nonoperative drainage. In acute pancreatitis with immature collections, it is best to avoid intervention whenever possible. Premature or injudicious use of any intervention risks secondary infection and serious attendant morbidity. Percutaneous drainage may be useful as definitive therapy if the patient is symptomatic and if the cyst contains primarily fluid and little or no debris. Large acute pseudocysts imply a substantial episode of pancreatitis, and some degree of necrosis is invariably present. Percutaneous drainage is not appropriate for patients with suspected infected pancreatic necrosis as determined by dynamic CT pancreatography. Percutaneous drainage is not commonly performed in patients with chronic pancreatitis. Occasionally, percutaneous management may benefit high-risk symptomatic patients such as those with portal hypertension or a prohibitive anesthetic risk.

Endoscopic pseudocyst drainage at the present time is reserved for patients with mature, noninfected symptomatic cysts who are considered at high risk for operative internal drainage. The availability of a skilled and experienced interventional endoscopist broadens the application of endoscopic drainage. A team approach is needed at all points in the diagnostic evaluation and therapeutic management of the patient with a pancreatic pseudocyst. Appropriate surgical consultation and backup are advised when nonoperative drainage is undertaken.

Results

Surgery

The outcomes of various operative approaches to pancreatic pseudocysts are summarized in Table 31-1. In current series, the overall operative mortality rate is less than 5%. Internal drainage procedures generally have the lowest mortality and overall morbidity rates. External drainage is associated with the highest morbidity rate since patients undergoing external drainage are commonly critically ill. The majority of postoperative deaths occurs in patients

with severe pancreatitis complicated by pancreatic necrosis and sepsis. Hemorrhage and sepsis with multiple organ failure are common causes of postoperative death and are not uncommonly related. Pseudocyst recurrence is seen in 5% to 10% of patients and is more frequent following external drainage. Pseudocyst recurrence after internal drainage is most likely due to missed multiple cysts or inadequate pancreatic ductal drainage rather than to premature anastomotic closure or inadequacy of the drainage procedure itself.

Percutaneous Catheter Drainage

Percutaneous aspiration of a pancreatic pseudocyst can be useful for the diagnosis of infection. Aspiration alone has been associated with a high recurrence rate. Percutaneous drainage via an indwelling catheter has been more successful, as demonstrated by several representative series in Table 31-2. Success, although variably defined, generally means cyst evacuation without operative intervention. Complications occur in 12% of patients from combined series, with an overall reported mortality rate of less than 1%. Secondary infection and pancreaticocutaneous fistula are the most frequent complications. Other problems include catheter dislodgement or occlusion, gastrointestinal fistulization, and hemorrhage. Most reports give only short-term results, so long-term follow-up is needed to ascertain the eventual outcome of patients treated with percutaneous drainage.

A crucial need exists to establish standard definitions so that techniques of nonoperative treatment such as percutaneous drainage can be reasonably compared to conventional surgical management. Patient characteristics and the type of collection being treated must be adequately described to permit a distinction between acute peripancreatic fluid

Table 31-1. Operative Treatment of Pancreatic Pseudocysts

Procedure	Mortality (%)	Morbidity (%)	Recurrence (%)
Internal drainage			
Cystogastrostomy	0–10	10–36	7–10
Cystojejunostomy	0–6	5–15	0–7
Cystoduodenostomy	0–8	8–20	0–6
Cystojejunostomy & pancreaticojejunostomy	0–8	10–20	0
External drainage	0–25	33–67	8–33
Excision	0–15	14–50	0–3

Table 31-2. Percutaneous Catheter Drainage of Pancreatic Pseudocysts

Author	Number of patients	Success (%)	Morbidity (%)	Mortality (%)	Recurrence (%)
vanSonnenberg, 1989[a]	77	90	13	0	5
Stanley, 1988[b]	25	72	32	16	4
Grosso, 1989[c]	40	72	5	0	23
Freeny, 1988[d]	23	70	13	0	9

[a]Data from vanSonnenberg E, et al. Percutaneous drainage of infected and noninfected pancreatic pseudocysts: Experience of 101 cases. *Radiology* 1989; 170(3):757–761.
[b]Data from Stanley JH, et al. Percutaneous drainage of pancreatic and peripancreatic fluid collections. *Cardiovasc Interven Radiol* 1988; 11:21–5.
[c]Data from Grosso M, et al. Percutaneous treatment of 74 pancreatic pseudocysts. *Radiology* 1989; 173:493–7.
[d]Data from Freeny PC, et al. Infected pancreatic fluid collections: Percutaneous catheter drainage. *Radiology*, 1988; 167:435–441.

collections and pseudocysts associated with chronic pancreatitis. Infection must be defined and documented. Morbidity and mortality and long-term outcome must be evaluated by similar criteria. Without such standardization, accumulating reports attesting to the high rate of "technical success" or the low rate of "procedure-related" adverse outcomes do little to advance patient care.

Endoscopic Drainage

Cumulative results of 114 patients undergoing endoscopic pseudocyst drainage demonstrate a procedure-related mortality rate of 3% and a morbidity rate of 9%, with overall successful treatment in 80% to 90% of patients (Table 31-3). Notable complications include retroperitoneal and free intestinal perforation, bleeding from the cystotomy site or pseudocyst itself, and secondary infection of the pseudocyst cavity. Cumulative morbidity rates related to subsequent therapy and disease-related 30-day or hospital mortality rates are generally not reported.

Cremer and associates performed endoscopic drainage in 33 patients with chronic pseudocysts, of which 22 were cystoduodenostomies (ECD) and 11 were cystogastrostomies (ECG). Technical success rates were 96% for ECDs and 100% for ECGs. Complication rates were 0% for ECDs and 18% (one hemorrhage, one secondary cyst infection) for ECGs. Clinical relief of pain was achieved in 20 of 21 ECD patients and in 8 of 11 ECG patients. Endoscopic treatment was considered definitive therapy in 19 of 22 patients undergoing cystoduodenostomy and in 8 of 11 patients undergoing cys-

togastrostomy, for an overall success rate of 82%. Complications occurred in only 6% of patients, and there was no mortality. These results reflect considerable technical expertise and care in patient selection.

Sahel and associates have reported another large series of endoscopic pseudocyst drainage operations consisting of 20 cystoduodenostomies in 19 patients. ECD was successfully accomplished in 18 of 20 patients. Both failures occurred in patients whose cyst caused no endoluminal bulge into the duodenum. Of the five major complications reported in this series, two perforations occurred in patients where no bulge could be seen. These data emphasize the importance of close adherence of the cyst to the intestinal wall in the performance of an endoscopic drainage procedure.

Comparative Studies

Adams and Anderson retrospectively reviewed 42 patients with pancreatic pseudocysts with internal operative drainage and 52 patients treated by percutaneous catheter drainage. Use of percutaneous catheter drainage was limited to the latter portion of the 27-year study period, and two thirds of the operated patients were managed prior to the availability of percutaneous drainage. The mortality rate of 7% in the surgical group was significantly greater than the zero mortality observed in percutaneously drained patients. Major complications occurred in 17% of operated patients and in 8% of percutaneous catheter drainage patients. The frequency of reoperation for chronic pancreatitis–related complications was 10% in the surgical group and 20% in the

Table 31-3. Endoscopic Treatment of Pancreatic Pseudocysts

Author	Number of patients	Number of procedures	Transpapillary prostheses	ECD[a]		ECG[b]		Morbidity	Mortality
				ATT[c]	SUC[d]	ATT	SUC		
Cremer, 1989[e]	33	33	0	22	21	11	11	3	0
Sahel, 1991[f]	37	43	0	30	28	3	1	5	1
Dohmoto, 1992[g]	17	NR[k]	7	2	2	8	8	1	0
Huibregtse, 1988[h]	7	7	6	1	1	0	0	1	0
Kozarek, 1985[i]	4	4	0	1	1	3	3	2	1
Grimm, 1989[j]	16	18	9	8	8	1	1	0	1
TOTAL	114	105	22	64	61	26	24	12	3

[a]ECD = endoscopic cystoduodenostomy.
[b] ECG = endoscopic cystogastrostomy.
[c]ATT = attempted.
[d]SUC = succeeded.
[e]Data from Cremer M, Deviere J, Engelholm L. Endoscopic management of cysts and pseudocysts in chronic pancreatitis: Long term follow-up after 7 years of experience. *Gastrointest Endosc* 1989; 35(7):1–9.
[f]Data from Sahel J. Endoscopic drainage of pancreatic cysts. *Endoscopy* 1991; 23:181–4.
[g]Data from Dohmoto M, Rupp KD. Endoscopic drainage of pancreatic pseudocysts. *Surg Endosc* 1992; 6:118–24.
[h]Data from Huibregtse K, Schneider B, Vrij AA, Tytgat GNJ. Endoscopic pancreatic drainage in chronic pancreatitis. *Gastrointest Endosc* 1988; 34:9–15.
[i]Data from Kozarek RA et al. Endoscopic drainage of pancreatic pseudocysts. *Gastrointest Endosc* 1985; 31:322–8.
[j]Data from Grimm H, Meyer V, Soehendra N, Nam Vch. New modalities for treating chronic pancreatitis. *Endoscopy* 1989; 21:70–4.

percutaneous group. None of these complication rates or reoperation rates were statistically different. However, catheter-related infections and pancreaticocutaneous fistulas were not considered as complications in this series.

One half of patients with percutaneous catheters became clinically infected with fever or leukocytosis and required systemic antibiotics. The mean duration of catheter drainage was 61 days for secondarily infected patients compared to 24 days for noninfected patients ($P < 0.05$). All percutaneously drained patients developed a pancreaticocutaneous fistula which closed after a mean duration of 6 weeks. Much of the 40-day mean hospital stay for percutaneously drained patients was necessary for management of drain-related infections or the resulting pancreatic fistula. The authors concluded that percutaneous catheter drainage is preferred for the initial treatment of large pseudocysts. Since none of the infected patients had documented bacteremia or required operative drainage and since all of the fistulas eventually closed, the drawbacks of percutaneous drainage were considered surmountable. Current operative mortality and morbidity may be considerably less than that reported for patients in this study, the majority of which was operated on prior to 1982.

Lang et al. reported a prospective study of 52 patients with infected and noninfected acute pseudocysts; initially 26 patients were treated with percutaneous catheter drainage and 26 were treated surgically. Eventual success was achieved in 77% of percutaneously treated patients and in 88% of operated patients. Fifteen percent of patients in each group required a subsequent operation, and 8% of surgically treated patients later had percutaneous catheter drainage. The indications for reoperation in the two groups differed. Reintervention following initial surgical management was primarily required because of recurrent pancreatitis and not because of failure of the initial operation to resolve the pseudocyst. Reoperation in the percutaneous catheter drainage group was necessary to provide resolution after initial palliation. A 6-month follow-up documented recurrence in 12% of percutaneously drained patients and in 19% of those surgically treated. Massive gastric bleeding occurred in 2 of 16 patients treated by transgastric percutaneous catheter drainage. The authors concluded that percutaneous catheter drainage is highly effective in the initial stabilization of critically ill patients.

Although this study alternately assigned patients to operative or percutaneous treatment, it does not provide sufficient information for a valid assessment of percutaneous drainage or operative outcome. Neither the specific operative procedures nor the interval between symptom onset and intervention was reported. The rate of reintervention following operation and the rate of cyst recurrence are not representative of most surgical series, particularly for internal drainage procedures (see Table 31-1). Operating too early in the course of the disease necessitates external drainage, which is suboptimal as definitive therapy. Moreover, there was no control arm of expectantly managed patients to assess whether intervention was necessary at all.

Conclusions

Pancreatic pseudocysts are an important cause of morbidity and mortality for patients with pancreatitis. They pose a wide array of challenging problems to the physicians and surgeons charged with the care of these patients. CT is highly accurate in the diagnosis and characterization of cystic pancreatic lesions. Modern imaging modalities have also better defined the natural history of inflammatory pseudocysts.

Spontaneous resolution of acute pseudocysts is not uncommon, and the risk of secondary complications may be lower than previously observed. The therapeutic approach to acute pseudocysts has therefore evolved toward expectant management with selective intervention based on persistent symptoms, cyst enlargement, or the development of complications. Stable, asymptomatic pseudocysts do not require any form of intervention. Intervention for immature cysts is best avoided unless necessitated by complications.

Mature pseudocysts may be managed by operative or percutaneous drainage if circumstances permit. Pseudocysts in patients with chronic pancreatitis are more likely to require intervention, and operative drainage is usually preferred. Concomitant lateral pancreaticojejunostomy and/or choledochoenterostomy may also be indicated in chronic pancreatitis. Early experience with laparoscopic treatment of pseudocysts has been encouraging. Pseudocyst drainage by endoscopic techniques can also be useful when intervention is required. This approach should only be attempted by endoscopists with considerable technical expertise, and skilled surgical support must be available to deal with problems such as bleeding. As yet, nonoperative drainage has not been confirmed to be superior to conventional surgical techniques.

It is imperative that surgeons, endoscopists, and interventional radiologists cooperate in a critical evaluation of various therapeutic options. Only well-designed prospective studies will establish the proper role of nonoperative intervention in relation to both conventional surgical techniques and newly emerging laparoscopic alternatives.

Selected Readings

Adams DB, Anderson MC. Percutaneous catheter drainage compared with internal drainage in the management of pancreatic pseudocyst. Ann Surg 1992; 215(6):571–578.

Bradley EL III, Clements JL Jr, Gonzalez AC. The natural history of pancreatic pseudocysts: A unified concept of management. Am J Surg 1979; 137:135–141.

Cremer M, Deviere J, Engelholm L. Endoscopic management of cysts and pseudocysts in chronic pancreatitis: Long term follow-up after 7 years of experience. Gastrointest Endosc 1989; 35(7):1–9.

Lang EK, Paolini RM, Pottmeyer A. The efficacy of palliative and definitive percutaneous versus surgical drainage of pancreatic abscesses and pseudocysts: A prospective study of 85 patients. South Med J 1991; 84(1):55–64.

Munn JS, et al. Simultaneous treatment of chronic pancreatitis and pancreatic pseudocyst. Arch Surg 1987; 122:662–667.

Newell KA, et al. Are cystgastrostomy and cystjejunostomy equivalent operations for pancreatic pseudocysts? Surgery 1990; 108(4):635–640.

Rao R, Fedorak I, Prinz RA. Effect of failed computed tomography-guided and endoscopic drainage on pancreatic pseudocyst management. Surgery 1993; 114(4):843–849.

vanSonnenberg E, et al. Percutaneous drainage of infected and noninfected pancreatic pseudocysts: Experience in 101 cases. Radiology 1989; 170(3):757–761.

Vitas GJ, Sarr MG. Selected management of pancreatic pseudocysts: Operative versus expectant management. Surgery 1992; 111(2):123–130.

Yeo CJ, et al. The natural history of pancreatic pseudocysts documented by computed tomography. Surg Gynecol Obstet 1990; 170:411–417.

32

Pancreatic Abscesses

GREGORY J. SLATER

DAVID W. RATTNER

PETER R. MUELLER

The infectious complications of acute pancreatitis are still a major medical challenge, trying the skill and patience of health care providers and the budgets of hospitals and insurance carriers. Sepsis has been estimated to cause 80% of all deaths from acute pancreatitis.

The literature on the infectious complications of acute pancreatitis has been troubled by the lack of widely accepted definitions of terminology. Papers and trials on the subject have rarely described the same clinical entity. This chapter uses the terminology of the International Symposium on Acute Pancreatitis held in Atlanta in September 1992, which defined a pancreatic abscess as a circumscribed intra-abdominal collection of pus, usually in proximity to the pancreas, containing little or no pancreatic necrosis and arising as a consequence of acute pancreatitis or pancreatic trauma.

Other complications of acute pancreatitis should be distinguished from pancreatic abscess. In contrast to abscesses, acute fluid collections occur early in the course of severe pancreatitis and lack a discrete wall. Pseudocysts and pancreatic abscesses both occur later, usually requiring 4 or more weeks for their walls to develop, but pseudocysts contain pancreatic juice whereas abscesses contain pus. Infected pancreatic necrosis is defined by the dominant presence of semisolid material rather than pus. Despite some overlap in what is in reality a spectrum of disease, these categories are of clinical relevance because each is a discrete entity with a different prognosis and management. When

reviewing the literature it is important to realize that most papers on pancreatic abscess include cases of infected necrosis in the cohort.

Etiology and Pathogenesis

Pancreatic abscess occurs as a complication of acute pancreatitis, with an incidence usually reported as 1% to 4%. Reported incidences of up to 28% in the literature of the last 30 years most likely reflect differences in diagnostic methods, terminology, and patient selection. Rarely, abscesses complicate chronic pancreatitis, particularly after surgery.

Etiology

The etiology of the preceding episode of acute pancreatitis includes the wide spectrum of insults described in the literature. Chronic alcohol abuse and gallstones are associated with the large majority of cases, and surgery, endoscopic retrograde cholangiopancreatography, trauma, hyperlipidemia, pancreas divisum, and idiopathic and hereditary causes make up most of the remainder. Less commonly reported causes include pancreatic carcinoma, certain drugs, vasculitis, AIDS, and pancreatic transplantation. The proportion of patients who proceed to septic complications is a function of the severity of the pancreatitis, but the distribution between abscess and infected necrosis remains the same whatever the etiology.

355

Pathogenesis

The pathogenesis of acute pancreatitis remains obscure, but whatever the etiology, the final common pathway is autodigestive tissue destruction. In mild pancreatitis only multiple small peripancreatic necroses are found, with or without interstitial edema. In severe pancreatitis large peripancreatic necroses are accompanied by pancreatic parenchymal necrosis which develops in the interlobular fatty tissue and which may also involve small veins and venules, resulting in thrombosis and hemorrhage. Destruction of interlobular ducts and peripheral acinar cells may accompany expanding fat necrosis. Arterial thrombosis results in panlobular ischemic necrosis, and these areas are demarcated by granulocytes and macrophages.

The fate of necrotic areas is controversial. The small areas of fat necrosis (< 1 cm) seen on the surface of the gland in mild pancreatitis resolve completely. The areas of fat necrosis 2 to 4 cm in diameter that characterize severe fat necrosis become demarcated by macrophages and may be slowly reabsorbed. In larger necrotic areas sponta-

neous resolution may not occur, and the lining macrophages are replaced by a layer of granulation tissue which thickens to form a fibrotic, grossly visible wall after 20 to 30 days.

If fat necrosis becomes infected, this process usually takes place early at around 4 to 20 days, when the liquefied areas of necrosis are demarcated only by a rim of macrophages or a thin rim of granulation tissue (Fig. 32-1). The mechanism of bacterial colonization remains speculative, but its origin is obviously enteric because these organisms predominate in microbial isolates, with skin flora making up the remainder (Table 32-1). Polymicrobial infections are present in 48% of patients. The incidence of infection of pancreatic necrosis increases with time, rising from 24% during the first week to 71% during the third week. The importance of necrosis is that it is the antecedent of secondary infection.

Clinical Course

The course of pancreatic abscess occupies the middle ground between pancreatic necrosis, represent-

Figure 32-1. Consecutive CT examinations in a patient who developed gallstone pancreatitis and over a period of 4 weeks demonstrated progressive changes on CT examination. A. Initial CT scan demonstrating a slightly swollen pancreas with inflammatory changes along the body and tail. B. CT scan 10 days later demonstrating further changes with evidence of liquefaction in the head and body of the pancreas posterior to the stomach. It is difficult to say by the scan whether this is infected material or not. Needle aspiration or surgical expiration would be necessary to determine infection.

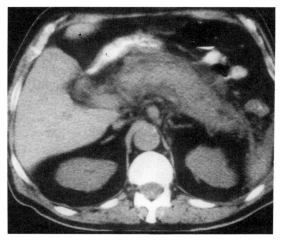
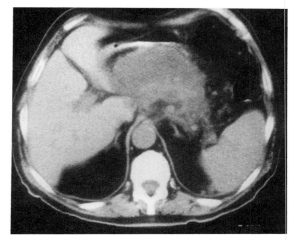

A   B

Table 32-1. Bacteriology of Pancreatic Abscess

Organism	Patients/total	Percentage	Range (%)
Escherichia coli	164/494	33	11–49
Enterobacter	60/284	21	7–43
Klebsiella	26/189	14	7–42
Proteus	50/430	12	5–21
Serratia	8/162	5	2–11
Pseudomonas	16/386	4	3–29
Enterococcus	57/260	22	6–48
Staphylococcus	58/323	18	4–36
Streptococcus	69/499	14	0–38
Bacteroides	31/285	11	5–29
Candida/yeast	15/158	9	2–9
Polymicrobial	140/380	37	21–57
Monomicrobial	207/380	54	29–78

Source: Witt MD, Edwards JE. Pancreatic abscess and infected pancreatic pseudocyst. *Curr Clin Top Infect Dis* 1992; 12:111–137. Reproduced by permission.

ing the most fulminant course of acute pancreatitis, and a colonized pseudocyst, which is the most benign. Infected necrosis develops in the inflammatory phase of acute pancreatitis, and in these patients surgery is usually required within 14 days of the onset of symptoms of severe unrelenting pancreatitis leading rapidly to sepsis. In these patients vasoactive substances produced by autodigestion as well as bacteria and toxins enter the bloodstream freely and result in a high incidence of pulmonary and renal insufficiency.

In pancreatic abscess the host defenses have been better able to confine the infection. Signs of sepsis are fewer, and a well-developed abscess wall is usually present. The clinical course has not been as fulminant as in infected necrosis, and treatment has been conservative until the presentation of the abscess. As a rule, abscesses do not become evident before the fifth week after the onset of symptoms, after the acute phase of the disease has subsided, and they may not present for months. Indeed, the presentation of pancreatic abscess is commonly indolent, with some patients presenting with fewer than three Ranson's signs and no fever. In some the presentation is subtle, with malaise, anorexia, persistent hyperamalasemia, or leukocytosis. Occasionally, however, in the presence of highly virulent microorganisms, the abscess capsule may be incom-

plete or may rupture, allowing sudden entry of bacteria and toxins into the circulation, resulting in septic shock. In practice, infected necrosis and pancreatic abscess may coexist.

The clinical presentation of pancreatic sepsis reflects the severity of the illness in the respective groups. APACHE II scores are highest in the infected necrosis group, with three quarters of the patients in one study having scores of 15 and an equal fraction suffering multiple organ failure. Morbidity and mortality are also considerably higher with infected pancreatic necrosis than with abscess, whereas colonized pseudocyst patients as a group have the lowest morbidity, mortality, and APACHE II scores during their illness.

In a large combined series, abdominal pain, abdominal tenderness, and a palpable mass were the most common findings (Table 32-2) but were nonspecific, occurring frequently also in pancreatic necrosis and colonized pseudocysts. Laboratory investigations (Table 32-3) are similarly unhelpful, and more specific diagnostic tests are required once an infective complication is suspected.

Pancreatic abscess should be considered in any patient with acute pancreatitis and persisting fever, abdominal pain, leukocytosis, or failure to improve. The single most important factor leading to a poor outcome in pancreatic abscess patients is late diagnosis. A very high index of suspicion should be maintained for this complication of acute pancreatitis.

Table 32-2. Signs and Symptoms of Pancreatic Abscess

	Patients/total	Percentage	Range (%)
Abdominal pain	308/331	81	35–100
Anorexia	131/274	48	27–93
Nausea, vomiting	164/312	53	19–100
Fever	364/432	84	76–100
Weight loss	123/305	40	22–100
Abdominal mass	166/366	45	33–86
Abdominal tenderness	238/283	84	58–100
Shock	83/273	30	7–88
Jaundice	47/247	19	7–22

Source: Witt MD, Edwards JE. Pancreatic abscess and infected pancreatic pseudocyst. *Curr Clin Top Infect Dis* 1992; 12:111–137. Reproduced by permission.

Table 32-3. Laboratory Abnormalities in Patients with Pancreatic Abscess

	Patients/total	Percentage	Range (%)
Leukocytosis	367/473	80	54–100
Elevated amylase	139/362	38	8–83
Hypocalcemia	90/340	27	11–63
Elevated LDH*	88/136	65	56–86
Elevated bilirubin	79/171	46	38–51
Elevated SGOT	66/146	45	15–54
Hyperglycemia	51/114	45	34–69
Hypoalbuminemia	151/251	61	44–83

*LDH = lactate dehydrogenase.
Source: Witt MD, Edwards JE. Pancreatic abscess and infected pancreatic pseudocyst. *Curr Clin Top Infect Dis* 1992; 12:111–137. Reproduced by permission.

Diagnosis

Necrosis

Since the recognition of pancreatic or peripancreatic necrosis as the principal risk factor for pancreatic infection, attention has been directed toward identification of necrosis. Efforts have been concentrated in three areas: clinical parameters, serum tests, and imaging techniques.

No clinical parameters have been found that correlate with the presence or extent of pancreatic or peripancreatic necrosis. The severity of an episode of acute pancreatitis is commonly underjudged clinically, and no clinical parameters reliably predict the later complications of acute pancreatitis.

A number of circulating compounds, including ribonuclease, C-reactive protein, alpha$_2$-macroglobulin, pancreas-specific protein (PASP), phospholipase A$_2$, alpha$_1$-protease inhibitor and complements C3 and C4, fibronectin, plasma-free fatty acid concentration, trypsinogen activation peptide, DNase 11, and carbolic ester hydrolase (CAH), have been shown to have predictive value for pancreatic necrosis. They fail to differentiate between microscopic and clinically significant necrosis, and none has been shown to correlate with the infective complications of pancreatic necrosis and the necessity for intervention.

Modified imaging techniques have become the "gold standard" for the detection of pancreatic necrosis. Neither sonography nor computerized tomography (CT) without intravenous contrast possesses this ability. However, Kivisaari demonstrated

in 1984 that necrotic pancreatic parenchyma failed to enhance normally at CT performed immediately after the administration of a large-volume intravenous bolus of iodinated contrast agent (incremental dynamic bolus pancreatography) (Fig. 32-2). This finding has been confirmed prospectively by others who have also shown that dynamic CT pancreatography can markedly assist in differentiating between acute pseudocyst, pancreatic abscess, and infected necrosis. The accuracy of dynamic CT in demonstrating parenchymal pancreatic necrosis is greater than 90%. The similar CT attenuation coefficients of necrotic fat, hemorrhagic fluid, and fibrinous debris mean that CT is unable to reliably detect peripancreatic fat necrosis.

Ranson and Balthazar evaluated the relationship of CT findings in the first 10 days of acute pancreatitis to the subsequent development of pancreatic infection. The CT scans were graded A to E depending on the presence of pancreatic enlargement, on peripancreatic changes, and on the presence of fluid collections. No patient with a scan graded A or B developed pancreatic infection, but abscesses or infected necrosis developed in 11.9% of patients with grade C scans, in 16.7% with grade D, and in 60.9% with grade E. Mortality was restricted to patients with grade D or E scans. The authors subsequently described a CT severity index which combined this grading system with the results of dynamic CT pancreatography. All deaths and most complications developed in patients with necrosis, but a smaller incidence of complications ensued in patients with grade D or grade E pancreatitis and a normally enhancing pancreas. Ransom had previously described a positive correlation between the number of a group of laboratory signs, pancreatic sepsis, duration of hospital stay, and death. At present, APACHE II is considered the best clinical scoring system for stratifying patients with severe acute pancreatitis.

Nuutinen has shown that the lack of contrast enhancement in necrotizing pancreatitis is due to microcirculatory thrombosis, not pancreatic hypoperfusion. The underlying microangiopathy is directly related to the severity of the pancreatitis. Foitzik et al. have recently shown that, in a rodent model, administration of intravenous iodinated contrast in an equivalent dose to that used in humans causes significant worsening of severe pancre-

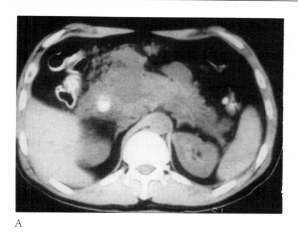
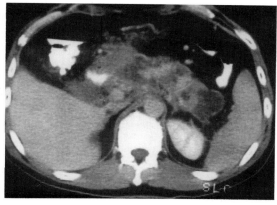

A   B

Figure 32-2. Use of intravenous contrast to demonstrate pancreatic necrosis. A. CT scan obtained on a patient 20 days after onset of pancreatitis. There is obvious swelling of the pancreas, but specific definition of areas of necrosis is difficult in this noncontrast study. B. Same patient with intravenous contrast. Multiple low-density areas (pancreatic necrosis) are well demonstrated.

atitis when given within the first 3 days of the disease, but not when given later. Although this result awaits verification by others, it would seem prudent to delay the prognostic administration of intravenous contrast in humans with clinically severe pancreatitis until after the third day, particularly since necrosis may not occur until the second week.

Prediction of necrosis, or documentation of its presence early in acute pancreatitis, does not presently alter treatment because there is no specific therapy for prevention of necrosis, and because debridement is rarely indicated in the first week. Dynamic CT pancreatography remains the single most valuable investigation later in the disease. By this time, areas of necrosis are well established and are less likely to evolve further, and CT can have a real impact on the management strategy and prognosis. Delaying the CT scan until the second week will limit its application to those with severe pancreatitis, since those with mild disease will all have recovered.

Infection

Plain radiography may suggest pancreatic inflammation through the presence of calcified gallstones or a sentinel loop of dilated bowel, but the findings are not specific. Abnormal gas collections in the

pancreatic region which may indicate pancreatic abscess are very difficult to interpret on plain radiographs in view of the proximity of bowel and the frequent occurrence of ileus in acute pancreatitis. Gastrointestinal barium studies are similarly unable to distinguish between pancreatic enlargement, pseudocyst, and abscess.

Ultrasound (US) offers the advantages of ready availability, low cost, portability, and reliability in the identification of fluid collections. The sensitivity of US in detecting intra-abdominal abscesses in various published series ranges from 60% to 100%, and its specificity ranges from 55% to 100%. In acute pancreatitis its role is limited by the frequent occurrence of ileus and the presence of wounds and dressings, both of which limit the identification of an acoustic window. US is highly accurate in the diagnosis of pancreatic pseudocyst, but frequently cannot differentiate between necrosis and abscess. Ultrasound may not detect multiple abscesses or those remote from the pancreas.

CT is invaluable in diagnosing pancreatic abscesses and in differentiating them from the other infectious complications of acute pancreatitis. CT provides excellent visualization of the entire abdomen and pelvis, including the subphrenic spaces, interloop areas, and retroperitoneum, where abscesses may be difficult to visualize with ultrasound (Fig. 32-3). The disadvantages of CT are that it

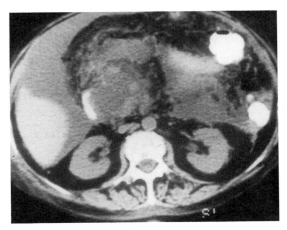

Figure 32-3. CT demonstration of complicated grade E pancreatitis. Although ultrasound might show the superficial collection around the liver, the deeper collection in the retroperitoneum would be difficult to delineate with ultrasound.

Proteinaceous debris, blood, and necrotic tissue may have similar nonspecific attenuation values on CT. To distinguish infection from sterile inflammation, CT-guided needle aspiration should be performed. This simple procedure has a sensitivity of 90% to 100% and a specificity of 100% in the diagnosis of pancreatic sepsis and deserves its current status as the diagnostic procedure of choice when an abscess is suspected on CT (Fig. 32-4). Complications are rare, with only a few cases of hemorrhage or contamination of previously sterile pseudocysts reported. Many unnecessary diagnostic laparotomies may thus be avoided, and definitive therapy of infectious complications may be instituted early. Delay in diagnosis has been identified as a major factor resulting in a poor outcome, and mortality in pancreatic abscess is reduced by early drainage.

On the other hand, it deserves to be emphasized that infection is not the only determinant of

is more expensive than ultrasound, requires good bowel opacification with oral contrast, necessitates transporting the patient to the radiology department, and carries a significant radiation burden, which should be kept in mind in those patients requiring multiple follow-up examinations. Nevertheless, the advantages are such that CT is usually the **only** radiological test that should be performed to localize a suspected intra-abdominal abscess following acute pancreatitis.

In the demonstration of intra-abdominal abscesses the sensitivity of CT is 90% to 100% and the specificity 85% to 100%. In acute pancreatitis the specificity of CT is lower than this because necrosis, sterile fluid collections, and even pseudocysts may have an identical appearance to abscesses. In a retrospective study of 45 patients with pancreatic abscess, Warshaw and Jin showed that CT demonstrated changes specific for abscess in 74%, compared with only 35% for ultrasound. The presence of gas bubbles within the collection is highly suggestive of an abscess, occurring in 22% to 88% of abscesses. However, these gas bubbles may also be seen in uninfected patients with a fistula between the pancreas or pseudocyst and an adjacent viscus, in postoperative patients, and in those with a perforated duodenal ulcer.

Figure 32-4. Scan of a 62-year-old man with clinical evidence of gallstone pancreatitis, including high fever and white blood cell count. The surgeon was concerned about a pancreatic infection. A 20-gauge needle was inserted through the stomach into the body of the pancreas. A small amount of yellowish fluid was withdrawn which showed no evidence of white blood cells or bacteria on Gram's stain. No growth was seen on culture. The patient was treated without surgical intervention.

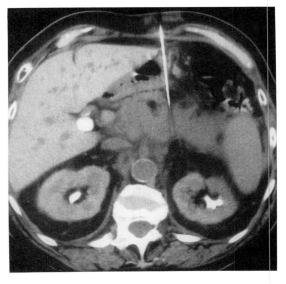

outcome, and the severity of the underlying pancreatitis may be equally important. Symptomatic collections should therefore be drained regardless of their bacterial status.

Management and Results

The mortality of an untreated pancreatic abscess approaches 100%. The basic principles of management are as follows:

Early diagnosis
Accurate anatomical localization
Early and complete evacuation of pus
Imaging follow-up to document resolution or detect complications

Supportive care must be rendered before definitive therapy is instituted. Patients presenting in shock require urgent fluid resuscitation with hemodynamic monitoring. Patients may require very large volumes of intravenous fluid over the initial 24 hours to maintain adequate cardiac output and filling pressures. Cardiac output and oxygen consumption should be maximized by serial Swan-Ganz determination because this measurement correlates with improved outcome. Mechanical ventilation should be instituted early when indicated.

Pancreatic abscess should be diagnosed by abdominal CT, and the presence of infection should be confirmed by CT-guided percutaneous fine-needle aspiration. The therapeutic options available are medical therapy, surgical drainage, and percutaneous drainage. The decisions to be made are what patients to drain, when to drain, and how to drain.

Options

ANTIBIOTIC THERAPY

Sepsis is the main cause of death in severe pancreatitis. Antibiotics alone have not been demonstrated to reduce mortality in this disease, but their empirical use is almost universal. Concern remains that antibiotic treatment alone will not eradicate infection that is complicating acute pancreatitis and will only promote the selection of resistant organisms.

Variation in the penetration of antibiotics into the pancreas has been demonstrated, suggesting the existence of a "blood-pancreas barrier." This barrier may be disrupted in acute pancreatitis. Although it has been shown that antibiotics which are secreted into pancreatic juice are also present in similar concentrations in viable pancreatic parenchyma, this correlation has not been demonstrated in pancreatic necrosis and pancreatic abscess, which parenteral antibiotics may not reach.

Appropriate antibiotic therapy depends on following the identification of the causative organism(s) with sensitivity testing. Randomized clinical trials are required before definitive statements can be made regarding the choice of antibiotic before sensitivity results are available. Bradley has recently recommended the combination of ceftazidime and clindamycin, which covers all common pancreatic pathogens except enterococcus. Imipenem has an extremely broad spectrum of activity and may be the best single agent. A recent study showed that imipenem and quinolines achieve higher relative concentrations in the pancreas than aminoglycosides and cephalosporins. Ciprofloxacin penetrates well into the pancreas, is active against eight of the nine most common pancreatic pathogens, and is now available in intravenous form. Particular attention must be paid to central venous catheter hygiene to minimize the risk of contamination of pancreatic necrosis by organisms such as *Staphylococcus epidermidis* or *Candida* arising from this source.

SURGERY

Sterile fluid collections may resolve spontaneously, although approximately half of all such collections will go on to form pseudocysts or abscesses. Untreated pancreatic abscesses do not resolve spontaneously. Altemeier and Alexander stressed the necessity for early intervention when they demonstrated in 1963 that the mortality for pancreatic abscess was reduced from 100% in patients treated medically to 15% with incision and drainage. Other workers have confirmed these findings, and consensus now exists that early diagnosis and drainage of pancreatic abscess lower mortality compared with delayed diagnosis and drainage. On the other hand, aggressive, very early surgical intervention within the first week, before the necrotic tissues and abscess are well defined, carries higher morbidity and mortality rates than surgery performed after 10 days, and carries a particular danger of severe hemorrhage.

Surgical treatment of pancreatic abscess is straightforward in principle, consisting of drainage of the pus, removal of any necrotic component, and placement of one or more drains. Surgical options include the site of the incision, the route of access to the pancreas if an anterior approach is chosen, the type of drainage instituted, and the nature and timing of follow-up operations where these are deemed necessary. The traditional surgical treatment of pancreatic abscess has involved anterior laparotomy for debridement, sequestrectomy, and lavage, followed by either multiple drainage with wound closure or open packing. The thoroughness of the initial debridement is the most important factor affecting survival and the need for reexploration.

Although drainage of simple pancreatic abscess, which by definition contains little or no necrosis, is straightforward, the picture is often complicated by the coexistence of necrosis. The presence and extent of peripancreatic fat necrosis cannot be determined by dynamic CT. It is often impossible to distinguish preoperatively the relative proportions of pus and necrosis within an infected collection because of their similar appearances on CT or ultrasound. The nature and timing of inter-vention in the individual case will be determined by estimating the extent and relative proportions of pus and necrosis in combination with the patient's clinical status.

RADIOLOGIC DRAINAGE

Imaging-guided percutaneous drainage of abscesses is now widely accepted as a safe and effective technique. In uncomplicated unilocular abdominal and pelvic abscesses percutaneous drainage is highly effective, and cure is achieved in 90% to 100% of cases. Cure rates for these abscesses when complicated by such factors as recent surgery, multiloculation, or enteric communication are somewhat lower, at 65% to 95% (Fig. 32-5, 32-6). However, reported cure rates for primary percutaneous drainage of pancreatic abscesses are significantly lower than for other intra-abdominal abscesses and range from 14% (Rotman et al.) to 69% (vanSonnenberg). Although liquid pus will be satisfactorily drained by a well-situated and patent catheter, particulate necrotic matter will remain undrained, and the patient will not be cured.

It is tempting to speculate that patients selected by CT criteria as having collections with the appearance of liquid pus without necrosis will respond to percutaneous drainage, but this situation is not the case. Rotman et al. selected 12 patients with limited,

Figure 32-5. Drainage of pancreatic abscess after partial pancreatectomy. A. A large, low-density collection is seen in the left upper quadrant anterior to the spleen that displaces the stomach anteriorly and laterally. B. Under CT guidance, a 14 French catheter was placed within the collection and 650 cc of purulent material was removed. The catheter remained in place for 3 weeks. The patient was discharged after drainage was completed.

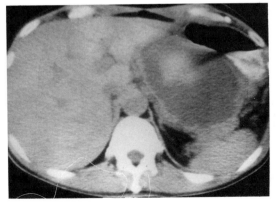

A

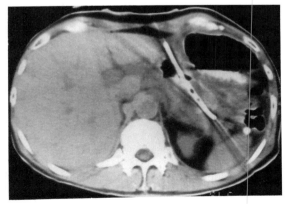

B

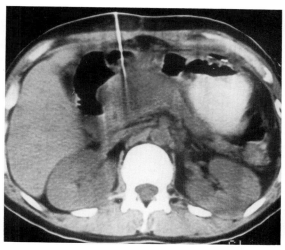 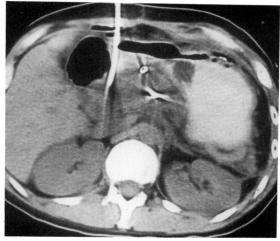

A   B

Figure 32-6. Successful drainage of pancreatic head abscess. A. CT scan demonstrates a low-density abnormality in the head of the pancreas. An 18-gauge needle was inserted under CT guidance through the antrum of the stomach and yielded purulent material. B. A 12 French catheter was inserted via trocar technique. The postinsertion image demonstrates no evidence of residual collection. The patient recovered uneventfully.

low-density pancreatic abscesses and normal pancreatic parenchymal enhancement on dynamic CT for percutaneous drainage. The cure rate was only 14.3%, and at surgery performed in those patients not cured, significant peripancreatic necrosis was found. Similar operative findings were found by Steiner et al. and by Brolin and associates in cases of failed percutaneous drainage. Many patients with pancreatic abscess undergoing primary percutaneous drainage will not be cured, will not improve, and will eventually deteriorate, progressing to multiorgan failure and death if surgical drainage is not performed.

The use of percutaneous abscess drainage as a "temporizing" measure to allow correction of abnormal physiological and laboratory criteria in critically ill patients has been described by vanSonnenberg and others. Although useful in a variety of settings, this approach was not found to be beneficial by Steiner et al. in patients with pancreatic sepsis, most likely because of the presence of concomitant infected necrosis. In view of the frequent coexistence of necrosis with pancreatic abscess, primary treatment of pancreatic abscess should usually be by surgical means, not radiological.

Percutaneous pancreatic abscess drainage finds its widest application in the treatment of residual or recurrent abscesses following surgical debridement and drainage. In these instances the necrotic material has usually been removed, and there is no hindrance to catheter drainage. Steiner et al. reported that percutaneous drainage was curative of six of six patients with residual abscesses following surgical drainage of pancreatic sepsis, and similar results have been obtained by others. Abscesses remote from the pancreas, such as in the interloop region or pelvis, are less likely than pancreatic abscesses to contain significant necrotic material, and are usually drained successfully by the percutaneous route.

Treatment of pancreatic abscess by whatever means is difficult, and percutaneous treatment requires a large commitment of time by the radiologist. Even those patients who are successfully drained will frequently require multiple catheters, multiple catheter manipulations, and a long duration of catheter drainage. In the study by Steiner et al., patients in whom percutaneous drainage was attempted required an average of 1.7 catheters, 2.3 catheter manipulations, and an average duration of drainage of 25 days (range 7 to 97 days). Daily ward rounds by the interventional radiologist while the drainage catheter is in place will forestall problems with catheter management and facilitate communication with the other members of the caregiving team regarding ongoing management.

The technical aspects of percutaneous abscess drainage are now well understood. After infiltration of local anesthetic, diagnostic needle aspiration is performed under imaging guidance. CT guidance will be necessary for deep collections or those with complicated anatomical relations, such as those in the lesser sac or subphrenic space. Ultrasound is used when the collection is more superficial, such as in the left anterior pararenal space. The authors perform initial aspiration with a 22-gauge needle, taking care not to transgress bowel to avoid contaminating a sterile field. If no fluid is aspirated, an 18-gauge needle may be used. Lack of freeflowing fluid aspirate through an 18-gauge needle usually indicates that a drainable fluid collection is not present. A Gram's stain should be performed immediately if the fluid aspirated is not frankly purulent.

The authors usually place catheters by the trocar technique because of its speed and simplicity. The catheter is placed in tandem with the aspiration needle, which is left in place for reference. Care is taken to avoid transgressing small and large bowel. Drainage through the liver or stomach is sometimes necessary when no other access route exists, and has been shown to be safe. The Seldinger technique may be used if the abscess is small or located immediately adjacent to a vital organ, and is probably a safer technique in inexperienced hands. The authors prefer 12 to 14 French double-lumen sump catheters such as the vanSonnenberg, or 12 to 16 French single-lumen Cope or nephrostomy catheters for pancreatic abscess drainage. The efficacy of sump catheters has been shown to be two to four times that of single-lumen catheters of the same external diameter. If the drainage catheters become repeatedly blocked by necrotic debris, larger catheters such as the 24 French or 30 French Saratoga may later be placed over a guidewire.

The abscess is completely aspirated, and follow-up imaging is performed to rule out any undrained locules which would require a further drainage catheter. Irrigation with multiple aliquots of normal saline is performed in the radiology department until the irrigant is clear. The catheter is securely fixed to the skin, preferably by anchoring it to the plastic rim of a stomal wafer with adhesive tape and sutures. This system avoids skin problems and is well tolerated. Continuous suction has not been shown to increase success rates over gravity drainage alone. Instillation of intracavitary antibiotics has been unrewarding, but intracavitary urokinase may be useful in cases otherwise resistant to drainage with multiple large-bore catheters.

The patient's temperature, white blood cell count, and general clinical status are all excellent indicators of the success or failure of the procedure. Catheters may be withdrawn when output is less than 10 cc per day and follow-up imaging shows resolution of the abscess.

Controversies

The role of intravenous iodinated contrast in diagnosis and management decisions remains to be clearly established. Animal evidence indicates that contrast given early in acute pancreatitis may adversely affect the outcome. Dynamic CT has been enthusiastically accepted because of its ability to define parenchymal necrosis, but CT is unable to reliably detect peripancreatic necrosis, which is the usual morphological pattern in severe pancreatitis. CT also cannot distinguish between liquid pus and infected necrosis. The contribution of intravenous contrast to management decision making can also be questioned. The decision to operate is made almost completely on clinical grounds. Although the administration of intravenous contrast for follow-up CT scans is almost routine, recent evidence from Boland indicates that it may provide little or no useful information which would affect patient management and therefore may be unnecessary.

MRI may prove to be more accurate than CT in defining peripancreatic necrosis and in discriminating between pus and infected necrosis, but this possibility is unproved. The advent of fast echo sequences is rapidly overcoming the disadvantage of long scan times and associated movement artifacts in MRI, but monitoring of critically ill patients inside the MRI scanner remains more of a problem than for CT.

Surgical controversies are many. Although exploration of all patients with pancreatic necrosis has been advocated by some, many patients with necrosis never become infected and do not require surgery. Most surgeons now agree that a very aggressive approach with early debridement is not indicated in these patients and that surgery is in fact detrimental because it will result in infected pancreatitis. On the other hand, a small percentage of patients with necrosis but no infection deteriorate hemodynamically to develop multiple organ failure, and most agree that these patients require surgery. Laparotomy for suspected abdominal sepsis is usually a futile endeavor once multiple organ failure is established. Therefore, the challenge is to detect clinical deterioration early and respond aggressively in those patients with a worsening clinical status.

Additional incisions may be required to give adequate access to retroperitoneal necrosis, particularly when it extends posterior to the colon. Flank incisions, subcostal incisions, or rib-resecting incisions have variously been used. Open drainage is probably not necessary in all patients and has its major benefit in those patients with an extensive component of necrosis accompanying the abscess. Patients with little necrosis may be treated simply and effectively with multiple sump drains. If persistent or recurrent sepsis develops after closed drainage, the options are re-exploration, which should be performed early and often, commencement of open drainage, or percutaneous drainage of any secondary collections.

The place of a feeding jejunostomy is also controversial. Although evidence exists that prevention of translocation of enteric pathogens requires preservation of gut mucosal integrity by enteral feeding, no improvement in survival has been demonstrated in septic hypermetabolic patients treated with enteral versus parenteral nutrition. Moreover, an increased incidence of abdominal complications was noted in the enterally fed group, possibly resulting from stimulation of pancreatic secretion. Although it may be tempting to consider jejunostomy tube placement at the time of the initial laparotomy to allow a transition from parenteral to enteral nutrition early in the recovery phase, this procedure should probably not be routine and should not be performed in patients with extensive peritonitis involving the small bowel wall.

Conclusions

Acute pancreatitis is mild in 85% of patients, who recover rapidly with nonoperative management and require no imaging evaluation. Patients who are suspected of harboring a pancreatic abscess should undergo diagnostic CT, which will rarely provide information affecting management before the second week. Good bowel opacification with oral contrast is essential for the assessment of abdominal fluid collections versus loops of bowel.

A high index of suspicion for pancreatic abscess should be maintained because it may present late and in an indolent fashion. The presence of infection may be confirmed by imaging-guided fine-needle aspiration, which is safe and accurate. Guided aspiration should be used selectively and is indicated in those patients who are neither well nor so ill as to unequivocally require operation. In these patients management is determined by the bacteriological status.

The best results are obtained following early diagnosis and prompt aggressive surgical drainage. In some severely ill patients early debridement is beneficial regardless of infection. Recurrent abscesses and persisting infected fluid collections extending beyond the margins of surgical debridement are effectively treated by percutaneous drainage. Postoperative morbidity is high, and patients who deteriorate or fail to improve following drainage should undergo early follow-up CT with fine-needle aspiration, repeat debridement, or drainage as clinically indicated.

Adjunctive care includes intravenous antibiotics and may require early vigorous fluid resuscitation and total parenteral nutrition. The hospital course may be protracted, and complications are common and frequently severe. Optimal management of pancreatic abscess requires the skills of multiple specialties, and in no other disease is it more important to patient outcome to make use of a dedicated team approach.

Selected Readings

Bradley EL, Olson RA. Current management of pancreatic abscess. *Adv Surg* 1992; 24:361–388.
Brolin RE, et al. Limitations of percutaneous catheter drainage of abdominal abscesses. *Surg Gynecol Obstet* 1991; 173:203–210.

Fernandez-del Castillo C, Rattner DW, Warshaw AL. Acute pancreatitis. *Lancet* 1993; 342:475–479.

Foitzik TH, et al. Intravenous contrast medium impairs oxygenation of the pancreas in acute necrotizing pancreatitis in the rat. *Arch Surg* (in press).

Lee MJ, et al. Acute complicated pancreatitis: Redefining the role and cost-effectiveness of radiology. *Radiology* 1992; 183:171–174.

Rattner DW, et al. Early surgical debridement of pancreatic necrosis is beneficial irrespective of infection. *Am J Surg* 1992; 163:105–110.

Rotman N, et al. Failure of percutaneous drainage of pancreatic abscesses complicating severe acute pancreatitis. *Surg Gynecol Obstet* 1992; 174:141–144.

Stanten R, Frey CF. Comprehensive management of acute necrotizing pancreatitis and pancreatic abscess. *Arch Surg* 1990; 125:1269–1275.

Steiner E, et al. Complicated pancreatic abscess: Problems in interventional management. *Radiology* 1988; 167:443–446.

Witt MD, Edwards JE. Pancreatic abscess and infected pancreatic pseudocyst. *Curr Clin Top Infect Dis* 1992; 12:111–137.

33

Pancreatic Necrosis

EDWARD L. BRADLEY III
EMIL J. BALTHAZAR

For every four patients requiring hospital admission for acute pancreatitis, three will recover uneventfully with judicious supportive management. However, the fourth patient will suffer a complication and will stand a 1 in 3 chance of dying. Accordingly, the optimum management of patients with acute pancreatitis clearly involves considerable patient selection. At the very least, this selection process requires determining those factor(s) that are responsible for the more severe episodes. Recently, as a result of extensive clinicopathologic correlations conducted in European surgical centers, it has been shown that the development of pancreatic necrosis, to a very great extent, determines both the severity and the overall survival from acute pancreatitis.

Etiology and Pathogenesis

Although the precise intracellular and extracellular events responsible for the initiation of acute pancreatitis are unknown, clinical and experimental studies clearly demonstrate that the necrotizing form of acute pancreatitis involves obstruction of the pancreatic microcirculation. Total pancreatic necrosis is rare; however, patchy necrosis is the rule, a finding which suggests regional intraglandular involvement of the lobular end-arteries. Peripancreatic and intrapancreatic fat necrosis are additional constant features accompanying necrotizing pancreatitis. The relative contributions of fat necrosis and parenchymal necrosis to the local and systemic sequelae of necrotizing pancreatitis are equally unknown. Attempts at modifying the natural course of necrotizing pancreatitis will nec-

essarily remain empiric until a clearer understanding of the underlying pathophysiology has been achieved.

Similar data from several natural history studies show that pancreatic necrosis develops in approximately 20% of patients admitted with acute pancreatitis. In half of the patients with necrotizing pancreatitis, secondary bacterial infection of the necrotic tissues will occur. Mortality rates for conservative treatment of pancreatic necrosis which remains sterile are in the range of 10% to 15%; in contrast, infected pancreatic necrosis is uniformly fatal without drainage. Therapeutic options must be judged against these data.

Diagnosis

Given the importance of the development of pancreatic necrosis to the clinical course of acute pancreatitis, recognition becomes the first step in therapy. Previous attempts at stratifying the severity of acute pancreatitis have centered around systems requiring specific constellations of clinical data (Ranson, Imrie, Bank, Agarwal). Although such systems were acceptable in describing severity in large numbers of patients (overall accuracies approaching 70%), the demonstrated 30% predictive error essentially invalidated these systems for the clinical management of individual cases. Moreover, these prognostic systems were subsequently found to correlate poorly with the presence and extent of pancreatic necrosis. Today, these clinical parameter prognostic systems have their principal value in comparisons of institutional data.

In 1983, Kivisaari and her associates observed that normal enhancement of the pancreatic parenchyma following the administration of an intravenous bolus of contrast material failed to occur in areas of pancreatic necrosis which developed in patients with severe acute pancreatitis. Subsequent extensive animal and human data established that the observed failure of enhancement was due to widespread microvascular thrombosis in the pancreatic parenchyma. Currently, this technique, known as dynamic contrast-enhanced computerized tomography, has been adopted throughout the world as the "gold standard" for the detection of pancreatic necrosis (Fig. 33-1). Overall accuracy rates exceeding 90% are commonly reported.

The CT diagnosis of pancreatic necrosis is based on the evaluation of the appearance and density of the pancreatic gland following the administration of intravenous contrast material. To obtain an adequate study, a bolus administration of contrast material, using a power injector, is essential. Images of the pancreas are obtained during the arterial phase of enhancement by using fast scans (1–2 sec acquisition time) and acquiring thin (5 mm) collimation.

Pancreatic necrosis is diagnosed when there is lack of enhancement of a portion or of the entire gland. The process is often focal and only rarely diffuse. The process appears initially as poorly marginated zones of nonenhanced parenchyma which are almost always associated with peripancreatic inflammation or fluid collections. The extent of pancreatic necrosis is better diagnosed on a follow-up CT examination when the necrotic zones are better defined, being sharply marginated and liquefied (Fig. 33-2). Minor areas of pancreatic necrosis can be missed on the initial CT examination. An overall CT sensitivity of 85% with 100% sensitivity for extended necrosis and 50% for minor necrotic areas has been reported. For descriptive purposes, the CT findings are reported as a normally enhanced gland (lack of necrosis), necrosis affecting less than 30% of the gland, affecting approximately 50%, or affecting more than 50% of the pancreas. A good correlation between the presence and degree of necrosis and the development of complications (abscess, pseudocyst) and mortality has been documented.

Peripancreatic fat necrosis and infected necrosis are more difficult to diagnose on CT. The presence of bubbles of air in areas of necrotic parenchymal tissue is a reliable indicator of infection. In the absence of extraluminal gas collections, infected necrosis cannot be diagnosed or ruled out. When the clinical situation is appropriate, percutaneous needle aspiration is indicated. This diagnostic procedure has acquired wide acceptance as the best and most reliable modality to diagnose infected necrosis.

More recently, efforts have intensified to develop a serum test capable of identifying some circulating product(s) of necrotizing pancreatitis (Table 33-1). The impetus for this approach has been the expense and restricted availability of computerized tomography. Despite early promise, as yet none of these putative "serum necrosis markers" have been validated for accurate clinical use. Considerable current attention is being focused on determination of trypsinogen activation peptide (TAP), a compound released into various body fluids when trypsinogen is activated to trypsin. However, more data are required.

Although few would disagree that accurate diagnosis is imperative for effective therapy, the practical implications of this principle to acute inflammatory conditions of the pancreas have been difficult to determine because there is no accepted

Figure 33-1. Dynamic CT pancreatogram in a patient with necrotizing pancreatitis. Note enhancement of the tail of the pancreas (arrows) with almost complete absence of enhancement in proximal areas of the gland. Pancreatic necrosis involving the head and body was found at surgery.

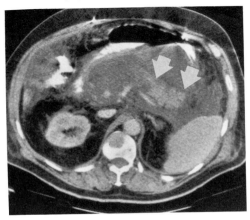

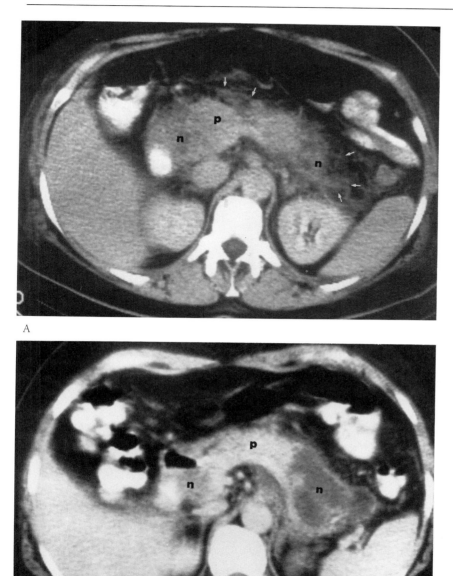

Figure 33-2. Pancreatic necrosis affecting the tail and the head of the pancreas. A. Initial CT examination reveals peripancreatic inflammation (arrows) and zones of decreased attenuation with alteration of glandular texture suggestive of necrosis (n) in the tail and head of the pancreas. B. Twenty days later the residual pancreatic gland (p) is sharply delineated, and liquefaction necrosis is present in the head and tail of the pancreas (n). Despite surgical drainage and debridement, the patient went on to develop pseudocysts in the head and tail of the pancreas.

Table 33-1. "Markers" for Pancreatic Necrosis

Methemalbumin
Fibrinogen
$PaO_2 < 60$ mm Hg
Hypocalcemia
Ribonuclease I
Deoxyribonuclease
Alpha$_1$-antitrypsin
Alpha$_2$-macroglobulin
Complements C3 and C4
C-reactive protein
Pancreas-specific protein
Phospholipase A$_2$
Trypsinogen activation peptide
Free fatty acids
Carbolic ester hydrolase
Fibronectin
Absolute lymphocyte count

series of definitions for clinical use. As a case in point, pancreatic abscess differs from infected pancreatic necrosis in terms of clinical presentation, mortality, morbidity, and therapy, yet precise clinical definitions of these conditions have previously been unavailable. This situation has led to considerable confusion in the literature. Hopefully, the clinically based classification system for acute pancreatitis recently adopted at the Atlanta International Symposium will provide an accurate definitional framework for future communications (Table 33-2).

Management and Results

Historical Perspective

The role of surgery in the management of patients with pancreatic necrosis continues to evolve. From a historical perspective, surgical intervention in severe acute pancreatitis was proposed at the turn of the century, enjoyed a brief acceptance, but because of high mortality, became discredited in the 1920s. For the next 30 years, surgical exploration was considered contraindicated in patients with acute pancreatitis. In the mid 1950s, the pendulum reversed, and several groups reported the survival of small numbers of patients with necrotizing pancreatitis who underwent extensive pancreatic resections.

The rationale was logical: removal of necrotic pancreatic tissue might eliminate the source of the circulating vasoactive and cytotoxic materials responsible for the systemic complications of acute pancreatitis.

This theory was enthusiastically adopted by many continental surgeons, and various clinical indicators were proposed to identify the necrotizing subgroup of patients with acute pancreatitis (surgical) from those with edematous pancreatitis (nonsurgical). In practice, however, mortality rates were often in excess of 50%, and viable pancreatic tissue was removed more often than not. Despite persistent efforts to refine the patient group and the clinical indicators for surgery, it became apparent that clinical indicators alone were not sufficiently reliable in detecting pancreatic necrosis to act as reasons for surgical intervention. Patients with self-limiting edematous pancreatitis continued to undergo unnecessary surgical exploration and resection.

Uninfected Necrosis

With the arrival in the 1980s of dynamic computerized tomography of the pancreas, a reliable indicator for pancreatic necrosis was found, and the surgical experience with pancreatic necrosis grew rapidly. Several groups reported mortality rates of 15% to 20% with surgical debridement of pancreatic necrosis, and this apparent "improvement" in mortality was attributed solely to surgical intervention. However, a control group of patients with necrotizing pancreatitis who did *not* undergo surgical debridement was conspicuously absent in all of these early reports.

Several retrospective reports then appeared which challenged the basis of surgical intervention in necrotizing pancreatitis by failing to demonstrate that removal of necrotic pancreatic tissues either improved patient survival or ameliorated the course of organ failure. It was then reasoned that, in the absence of any convincing data, it was equally possible that surgical debridement of pancreatic necrosis under certain conditions might not be beneficial and could even be harmful, particularly if surgical debridement actually resulted in bacterial contamination of sterile pancreatic necrosis. Examples of tissue necrosis for which excision of necrotic tissue

Table 33-2. Distinctions Between Pancreatic Necrosis and Pancreatic Abscess[a]

	Pancreatic Necrosis	Pancreatic Abscess
Definition:	Diffuse or focal area(s) of nonviable pancreatic parenchyma, usually associated with fat necrosis	A circumscribed parapancreatic collection of pus, with little or no associated pancreatic necrosis, which arises as a consequence of acute pancreatitis or trauma
Clinical:	Recognized by CECT[b] lack of enhancement < 40 HU[c] > 3 cm in size or > 30% of area of pancreas	Occurs later in the course of acute pancreatitis, often 4 or more weeks after onset
Pathology:	Macroscopically devitalized areas of pancreatic parenchyma and peripancreatic fat necrosis; microscopically interstitial fat necrosis with necrosis of acinar, islet, and ductal cells	Pus and a positive culture in the absence of pancreatic necrosis (due to limited pancreatic necrosis which liquefies?)
Discussion:	Differentiating between sterile and infected pancreatic necrosis by NAB[d] is critical for appropriate management	Term previously incorrectly used for all forms of pancreatic infection

[a]Definitions proposed by International Symposium on Acute Pancreatitis
[b]CECT = contrast-enhanced CT.
[c]HU = Hounsfield units.
[d]NAB = needle aspiration bacteriology.

represents increased risk over observation include cerebral, pulmonary, and myocardial infarctions. Was it possible that pancreatic necrosis, when it remained sterile, might be another such example? A prospective study was clearly necessary to address this problem.

In a 2-year prospective longitudinal study of 194 patients admitted with acute pancreatitis, the authors found that 38 exhibited unequivocal CT evidence of pancreatic necrosis. All 38 were assigned to continuous nonsurgical management. Twenty-seven of the 38 patients developed infected pancreatic necrosis during the period of observation and were reassigned to surgical debridement and drainage. The 11 patients with persistently sterile pancreatic necrosis (including 6 with pulmonary or renal failure) were all successfully managed without surgery. These observations suggested several things: (1) sterile pancreatic necrosis per se is not an absolute indication for surgery and (2) organ failure in sterile pancreatic necrosis is not an absolute indication for surgery.

A continuation of this study in patients with sterile pancreatic necrosis exceeding 50% of the gland (as shown by CT) has demonstrated that a conservative approach is equally successful in patients with extensive sterile pancreatic necrosis, again even in those cases associated with organ failure (Fig. 33-3). In this analysis, only 2 of 22 patients (9%) with extensive sterile necrosis died. From the latter observations, the authors concluded that the extent of pancreatic necrosis per se is also not an indication for surgery, and that "failure to improve after 48 to 72 hours of intensive care" should not be considered an absolute indication for surgery. Currently, the authors believe that surgical intervention in patients with sterile pancreatic necrosis is indicated for the late complications of necrosis, that is, pancreatic duct or bile duct obstruction, persistent pseudocysts, and so on. Whether surgical debridement of sterile pancreatic necrosis might be indicated in a patient who continues to deteriorate despite full supportive measures is not known. No convincing evidence suggests that such an approach either is or is not justified.

Infected Necrosis

In contrast to sterile pancreatic necrosis, secondary infection which develops in the necrotic tissues injured by the inflammatory process is an ominous development. Mortality rates increase sixfold when sterile pancreatic necrosis becomes converted to infected necrosis (Table 33-3). The bacteria commonly responsible for secondary pancreatic infections are listed in Table 33-4. The marked pre-

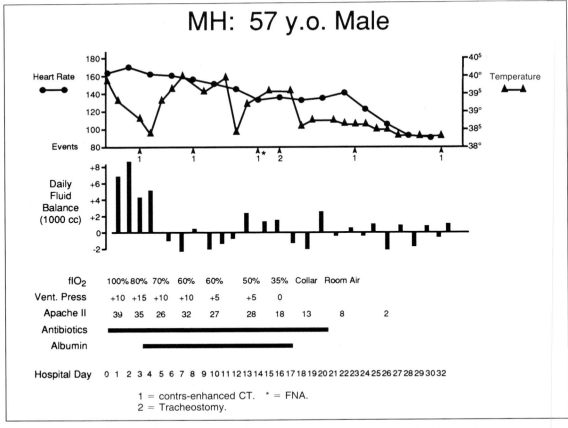

Figure 33-3. Hospital course of a patient with sterile pancreatic necrosis involving 80% of the gland. Despite a stormy course, the patient recovered without pancreatic debridement.

Table 33-3. Importance of Infection in Necrotizing Pancreatitis

	SPN[a]	Deaths	IPN[b]	Deaths
Beger et al (1986)[c]	97	7	72	17
Machado et al (1986)	8	0	47	14
Allardyce (1987)	26	0	17	14
Bradley and Allen (1991)[d]	11	0	27	4
Gillaumes et al (1992)	27	2	17	5
TOTALS (Mortality)	169	9(5.2%)	180	54(30.0%)

[a]SPN = sterile pancreatic necrosis.
[b]IPN = infected pancreatic necrosis.
[c]Data from Beger HG, et al. Results of surgical treatment of necrotizing pancreatitis. *World J Surg* 1985; 9:972–979. Used with permission.
[d]Prospective study. Data from Bradley EL III, Allen KA. A prospective longitudinal study of observation versus surgical intervention in the management of necrotizing pancreatitis. *Am J Surg* 1991; 161:19–24. Used with permission.

ponderance of gram-negative bacteria has been explained by transcolonic migration of coliforms to the injured tissues. Routes of enteric bacterial migration have been shown to be via the blood, lymph, bile, and peritoneal fluid. Recently, several groups have shown that administration of an appropriate antibiotic which crosses the "blood-pancreas barrier" can significantly decrease the number of patients with sterile pancreatic necrosis who are subsequently converted to infected necrosis. Both ciprofloxacin and imipenem-cilastin have resulted in significant reductions of secondary pancreatic infection when compared to placebo controls.

Since secondary infection of sterile pancreatic necrosis represents a significant escalation in morbidity and mortality risk, early recognition is desirable. However, because necrotic pancreas tissue releases the same inflammatory cytokine cascade as

Table 33-4. Bacteriology of Secondary Pancreatic Infections (1300 collected cases 1966 to 1987)

Escherichia coli
Klebsiella pneumoniae
Enterococcus
Staphylococcus aureus
Pseudomonas aeruginosa
Proteus mirabilis
Streptococcus spp.
Enterobacter aerogenes
Bacteroides fragilis

does actual infection, it is not possible by clinical means alone to distinguish between systemic inflammation from sterile necrosis and the clinical response to infected necrosis. Currently, this distinction is best determined by CT-guided transcutaneous fine-needle aspiration of the demonstrated areas of necrosis for smear and culture. This technique is safe and reliable, with overall accuracies for detecting infection exceeding 90% in many centers.

Several reports have documented the universal mortality associated with untreated infected pancreatic necrosis. Moreover, current techniques for nonsurgical drainage using CT-guided drainage catheters have also resulted in unacceptable mortality risk, perhaps because of the relatively small caliber of the drainage tubes. Accordingly, surgical debridement and drainage are widely accepted as the standard of care for infected pancreatic necrosis. Unfortunately, although almost everyone agrees that surgical debridement of infected pancreatic necrosis is beneficial, controversy continues to exist regarding the optimal form of surgical drainage.

CLOSED DRAINAGE

Debridement of the pancreas followed by closed abdominal drainage has been the traditional surgi-

cal approach. Postoperative mortality rates of 30% to 50% were commonly seen. Despite the necessity for re-exploration for sepsis in almost half of the patients treated in this manner, postoperative deaths continued to be caused by recurrent or persistent infection in more than 75% of cases. The traditional form of surgical drainage demands an expertise with re-exploration and redebridement that apparently few surgeons possess. If this approach is chosen, an extremely low threshold for re-exploration must be accepted.

OPEN PACKING

In 1976, the authors began to employ a technique involving debridement, gauze packing, partial abdominal closure, and re-exploration every 2 days (open packing). That periodic redebridement of infected pancreatic necrosis was necessary was demonstrated not only by the high recurrent infection rates after traditional drainage, but also by the finding of continuing retroperitoneal necrosis upon re-exploration (Table 33-5). Using this approach, the authors were able to reduce mortality rates for patients with infected pancreatic necrosis to 15%. This favorable mortality experience was attributed, in part, to the mandatory removal of reaccumulated retroperitoneal infection and necrosis, thereby obviating any delay in removal caused by indecision over the necessity and the timing of re-exploration.

An alternative approach to drainage after debridement has been to place large-bore drainage tubes into the lesser sac and to perform debridement by high-volume continuous lavage. This technique of drainage by lesser sac lavage has been employed successfully by several European surgical groups (Table 33-6). Re-exploration for recurrent or persistent sepsis continues to be necessary in 30% to 40% of cases treated in this fashion, however. Claims that drainage by lesser sac lavage alone pro-

Table 33-5. Weight of Necrotic Tissue Removed at Initial and Subsequent Re-explorations

	Number of patients*	Average weight (g)	Weight range (g)
Initial exploration	16	156 ± 20	54–261
First re-exploration	16	67 ± 31	33–101
Second re-exploration	16	29 ± 23	7–64
Third re-exploration	14	15 ± 12	0–38
Fourth re-exploration	13	9 ± 7	0–19

*Three patients had undergone secondary closure by the fourth re-exploration.

Table 33-6. Results of Lesser SAC Lavage for Infected Pancreatic Necrosis

	Number of patients	Reoperations (%)	Mortality (%)
Beger et al (1988)[a]	46	23	15
Larvin et al (1989)[b]	14	21	21
Nicholson et al (1989)[c]	11	10	27
Teerenhovi et al (1989)[d]	12	66	36
Pederzoli et al (1990)[e]	93	NS	29
TOTAL (Average)	176	30	(25.6)

[a]Data from Beger HG, et al. Necrosectomy and postopoerative local lavage in patients with nectrotizing pancreatitis. *World J Surg* 1988;12:255–262.
[b]Data from Larvin M, et al. Debridement and closed cavity irrigation for the treatment of pancreatic necrosis. *Br J Surg* 1989;76:465–471.
[c]Data from Nicholson ML, et al. Pancreatic abscess: Results of prolonged irrigation of the pancreatic bed after surgery. *Br J Surg* 1988;75:88–91.
[d]Data from Teerenhovi O, et al. High volume lesser sac lavage in acute necrotizing pancreatitis. *Br J Surg* 1989;76:370–373.
[e]Data from Pederzoli P, et al. Retroperitoneal and peritoneal drainage and lavage in the treatment of severe necrotizing pancreatitis. *Surg Gynecol Obstet* 1990;170:197–203.

Table 33-7. Worldwide Experience with Open Drainage for Infected Pancreatic Necrosis

	Year	Number of patients	Mortality (%)
Bradley et al (Atlanta)	1993	71	14
Levy et al (Paris)	1984	26	23
Pemberton et al[a] (Rochester)	1986	17	18
Wertheimer and Norris[b] (Massachusetts)	1986	19	16
Vogel (unpublished) (Gainesville)	1987	11	0
Garcia-Sabrido et al[c] (Madrid)	1988	9	22
Stanten and Frey[d] (Sacramento)	1990	36	14
Eckhauser et al[c] (Ann Arbor)	1991	18	22
TOTALS		219	16

[a]Data from Pemberton JH, et al. Controlled open lesser sac drainage for pancreatic abscess. *Ann Surg* 1986;203:600–604.
[b]Data from Wertheimer MD, Norris CS. Surgical management of necrotizing pancreatitis. *Arch Surg* 1986;121:484–487.
[c]Data from Garcia-Sabrido JL, Tallado JM, Christou NV, et al. Treatment of severe intra-abdominal sepsis and/or necrotic foci by an "open-abdomen" approach. *Arch Surg* 1988;123:152–156.
[d]Data from Stanten R, Frey CF. Comprehensive management of acute necrotizing pancreatitis and pancreatic abscess. *Arch Surg* 1990;125:1269–1275.
[e]Data from Personal communication.

Table 33-8. Results of Open Drainage for Infected Pancreatic Necrosis in 71 Patients

	Number of points
Mortality	
Sepsis	3
Hepatic failure	2
Myocardial infarction	1
Massive aspiration	1
Air embolism	1
Adrenal hemorrhage	1
Unknown	1
Morbidity	
Pancreatic fistula	33
Incisional hernia	23
Gastric outlet obstruction	12
Major venous hemorrhage	5
Intestinal fistula	5

duces mortality results equivalent to those obtained by open packing may be premature.

More recently, the authors have modified original technique of open packing, which requireu healing of the abdominal cavity entirely by second-ary intention, to one in which the abdomen is closed whenever repeated re-explorations have led to the formation of retroperitoneal granulation tissue. Lesser sac lavage is begun simultaneously with secondary abdominal closure. When compared to the original procedure of persistent open packing, this variation has significantly reduced hospital length of stay, while at the same time producing survival figures similar to the authors' original approach.

The results of the open packing technique for infected pancreatic necrosis as experienced around the world are shown in Table 33-7. In brief, the technique is not operator-dependent, nor are favorable experiences geographically limited. Considerable morbidity and the expense of resources and time attend the care of patients with infected pancreatic necrosis (Table 33-8), making relegation of these cases to specialized centers desirable.

Conclusions

The experienced pancreatic surgeon is aware that an appropriate place exists for each of the three drainage techniques for pancreatic infections. Traditional closed drainage is best suited for walled-off purulent collections without significant necrosis (pancreatic abscesses); lesser sac lavage is ideal for relatively minor amounts of infected necrosis (< 100 g); and open packing works best for extensive infected pancreatic necrosis. The dynamic CT scan is often helpful in deciding on the method of surgical drainage, since the presence and extent of necrosis can be gauged. Close cooperation between the surgeon and the radiologist is imperative. In this regard, open packing should be chosen whenever infected necrosis extends posterior to the colic flexures, since the flexures must be taken down for adequate debridement, and the confines of the lesser sac are subsequently destroyed. If the open packing technique is indicated, careful attention to the details of performance is necessary to prevent intestinal fistulization. The authors have also become convinced of the value of enteral alimentation in these patients, and recommend that a feeding jejunostomy be placed at the first exploration.

Although the indications for surgical intervention in patients with sterile pancreatic necrosis are still evolving, it seems increasingly certain that future patients with sterile pancreatic necrosis will receive longer trials of medical management before a surgical option is offered.

Selected Readings

Banks PA, et al. Diagnosis of pancreatic infection by CT guided aspiration. *Pancreas* 1988; 3:590–596.

Beger HG, et al. Results of surgical treatment of necrotizing pancreatitis. *World J Surg* 1985; 9:972–979.

Bradley EL III. A clinically based classification system for acute pancreatitis: Summary of the International Symposium on Acute Pancreatitis, Atlanta, Georgia, September 11th–13th, 1992. *Arch Surg* 1993; 128:586–590.

Bradley EL III. A fifteen year experience with open drainage for infected pancreatic necrosis. *Surg Gynecol Obstet* 1993; 177:215–222.

Bradley EL III, Allen KA. A prospective longitudinal study of observation versus surgical intervention in the management of necrotizing pancreatitis. *Am J Surg* 1991; 161:19–24.

Bradley EL III, Murphy F, Ferguson C. Prediction of pancreatic necrosis by dynamic pancreatography. *Ann Surg* 1989; 210:495–504.

Kloppel G. Pathology of severe acute pancreatitis. In Bradley EL III (ed), *Acute Pancreatitis: Diagnosis and Therapy*. New York: Raven, 1993.

Pederzoli P, et al. A randomized multicenter clinical trial of antibiotic prophylaxis of septic complications in acute necrotizing pancreatitis with imipenem. *Surg Gynecol Obstet* 1993; 176:480–483.

Steiner E, et al. Complicated pancreatic abscesses. Problems in interventional management. *Radiology* 1988; 167:443–446.

Pancreatic Hemorrhage

JOHN A. KAUFMAN
ARTHUR C. WALTMAN
CARLOS FERNANDEZ-DEL CASTILLO

Pancreatic hemorrhage is an uncommon but potentially lethal complication of acute and chronic pancreatic diseases. Arterial pseudoaneurysms have been described in 10% of patients with a history of severe pancreatitis, and in 15% to 20% of patients with pseudocysts. Bleeding from these lesions occurs in only 1% to 2% of all patients with pancreatitis, but with catastrophic results. Untreated, the mortality rate of hemorrhage related to pseudocysts and secondary arterial pseudoaneurysms exceeds 90%. The diagnosis and treatment of this complex clinical entity are well suited to the multidisciplinary approach.

Etiology and Pathogenesis

Pancreatic hemorrhage occurs most commonly in association with pancreatitis, both acute and chronic. The presumed mechanism is proteolytic digestion (principally elastase) of the arterial walls. This digestion leads to the formation of pseudoaneurysms, focal arterial defects that are contained by two or fewer layers of the arterial wall. The arterial structures most frequently involved are the splenic, gastroduodenal, pancreaticoduodenal, hepatic, and intrinsic pancreatic arteries. However, the tendency of pseudocysts to extend beyond the expected confines of the pancreas can lead to pseudoaneurysms of other visceral and retroperitoneal vessels (Table 34-1). Multiple lesions are present in 10% of patients. Less common etiologies of pancreatic bleeding include trauma, cystic or vascular neoplasms,

and congenital or acquired arteriovenous fistulas and malformations.

Pseudoaneurysms have a tendency to increase in size with time because the walls of the lesions are relatively weak in comparison to those of normal arteries. Alternatively, a large pseudoaneurysm can form quickly if a communication is established between a pseudocyst and an arterial structure. As pseudoaneurysms enlarge, they may erode into adjacent structures, create a mass effect, or rupture into a free or potential space. Rupture can occur spontaneously or following trauma or manipulation.

The clinical presentation of rupture varies depending on the structures surrounding the pseudoaneurysm and the rate of bleeding. If the aneurysm communicates with a hollow viscus, the patient may present with GI hemorrhage, as opposed to a contained hematoma in a solid viscus or the retroperitoneum. Rupture into a portal venous structure can lead to high-flow portal hypertension and variceal hemorrhage. Communication with a pancreatic duct results in hemosuccus pancreaticus, whereas involvement of the bile ducts will lead to hemobilia. The pseudoaneurysm may bleed slowly and intermittently, or torrentially. The location of the aneurysm does not help to predict the likelihood or severity of the hemorrhage.

Diagnosis

No single "classic" presentation exists for pancreatic hemorrhage. The most common symptoms, ab-

Table 34-1. Vessels Associated with Hemorrhage
Due to Pancreatitis

Splenic artery
Gastroduodenal artery
Pancreaticoduodenal arteries
Dorsal pancreatic artery
Pancreatica magna
Transverse pancreatic artery
Hepatic artery
Left gastric artery
Right gastric artery
Gastroepiploic artery
Superior mesenteric artery
Middle colic artery
Left inferior phrenic artery
Left renal artery
Aorta
Portal vein
Superior mesenteric vein
Splenic vein

dominal pain, nausea, and vomiting, are non-specific complaints that may have many possible explanations in a patient with pancreatic disease. Abdominal pain with a new or rapidly enlarging pancreatic mass or evidence of active blood loss should suggest the diagnosis. Approximately 50% of patients present with GI bleeding, manifested as hematemesis, hematochezia, or melena. The bleeding may be episodic and slow or massive with hemodynamic collapse. The diagnosis should be suspected in patients with spontaneous retroperitoneal, intrasplenic, or intrahepatic hematomas in the setting of pancreatitis. Hemoperitoneum, hemorrhage through abdominal fistulas, and bleeding from retroperitoneal drains after pancreatic surgery have also been reported. Bleeding may occur simultaneously from more than one arterial site, resulting in confusing clinical presentations, such as melena combined with retroperitoneal bleeding. Jaundice has also been described in association with hemorrhage into the bile ducts and subsequent ductal obstruction by thrombus.

Examination of the patient with pancreatic hemorrhage may reveal a tender, enlarging, pulsatile mass, an abdominal bruit, or bleeding from peripancreatic surgical drains. Most often, the findings are nonspecific. A plain film of the abdomen is of limited value but may depict a soft tissue mass

in the abdomen with displacement of bowel loops and the stomach. In the absence of overt GI bleeding, cross-sectional imaging with either ultrasound (US) or, preferably, computerized tomography (CT) is recommended. US may reveal a peripancreatic hematoma or may identify the actual pseudoaneurysm with duplex or color flow imaging. Because the point of bleeding may be surrounded by thrombus, the pseudoaneurysm may appear as an anechoic structure in the center of a larger cystic mass.

Although US has the advantage of speed and portability, the abdominal CT scan affords a more comprehensive evaluation of the abdomen in these typically complex patients. Intravenous contrast should be administered, with the aim of identifying the pseudoaneurysm as an enhancing mass with surrounding low-attenuation thrombus. The pseudocyst itself may enhance centrally if it communicates with the aneurysm (Fig. 34-1). In practice, the CT findings are usually nonspecific, such as extra- or intraperitoneal blood, or a splenic hematoma. The appearance of fresh blood in any abdominal structure or space in a patient with pancreatic pathology should suggest an arterial pseudoaneurysm. Oral contrast should be avoided because it may interfere with later angiography.

In stable patients with overt GI bleeding, endoscopy is the procedure of choice. The aim of endoscopy is to exclude other, more likely causes of GI bleeding. Varices, ulcers, mucosal erosions, Mal-

Figure 34-1. Contrast-enhanced CT scan of the abdomen in a patient with a known pancreatic pseudocyst. A focal area of enhancement is present within the pseudocyst (arrow), consistent with a pseudoaneurysm.

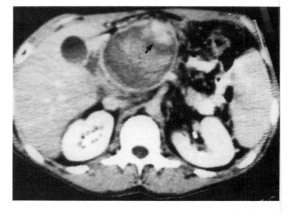

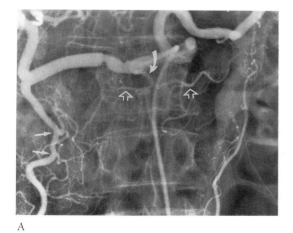

A

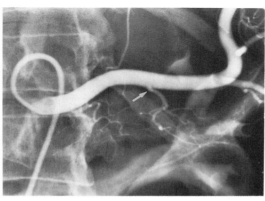

B

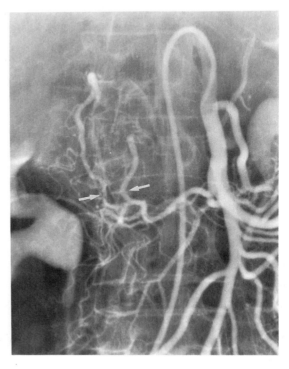

Figure 34-2. Normal angiographic anatomy of the pancreas. A. Celiac artery injection. The dorsal pancreatic artery (curved arrow) arises from the proximal splenic artery and supplies the transverse pancreatic artery (open arrows). Superior pancreaticoduodenal arteries (straight arrows) are visualized arising from the gastroduodenal artery. A focal area of spasm can be seen in the proximal common hepatic artery, caused by catheter manipulation. B. Splenic artery injection, magnification view. Multiple pancreatic arteries can be seem arising from the inferior margin of the splenic artery. The largest, most distal artery is the pancreatica magna artery (arrow). C. Superior mesenteric artery (SMA) injection. The inferior pancreaticoduodenal arteries (arrows) arise as the second branch of the SMA in this patient.

lory-Weiss tears, gastritis, vascular malformations, or a mass may be identified at upper endoscopy, and diverticulosis, ulcers, and erosions at colonoscopy. A clinical dilemma arises when one or more of these lesions are visualized but do not appear to be actively bleeding. Conversely, blood may be present but without an apparent source. In these cases, the suspicion for a pancreatic etiology should remain high. Rarely, blood is seen emanating from the ampulla, indicating rupture of a pseudoaneu-

rysm into either the biliary tree or the pancreatic duct. Endoscopic retrograde cholangiopancreatography (ERCP) may reveal thrombus in the ductal system, but is typically noncontributory.

Nuclear medicine bleeding scans have little role in the evaluation of the patient with suspected pancreatic hemorrhage. Accumulation of technetium Tc 99m–labeled sulfur colloid and red blood cells in large pancreatic pseudoaneurysms has been reported in patients studied for presumed GI

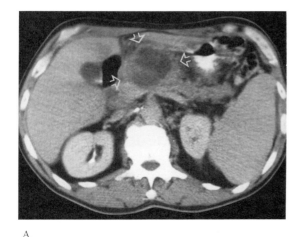

A

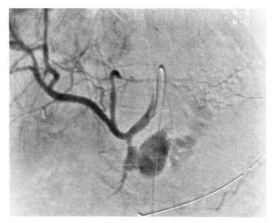

B

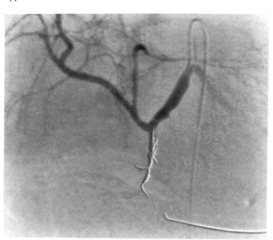

C

Figure 34-3. Rupture of a gastroduodenal artery pseudoaneurysm into a pancreatic pseudocyst.
A. Contrast-enhanced abdominal CT scan depicting a pseudocyst (open arrows) in the head of the pancreas of a patient with a history of acute and chronic pancreatitis. B. Two days later the patient became hypotensive. A digital subtraction angiogram of the common hepatic artery revealed massive extravasation of contrast from the gastroduodenal artery into the pseudocyst. C. The gastroduodenal artery distal and proximal to the pseudoaneurysm was embolized with multiple coils and gelatin sponge. The arterial supply of the liver was preserved.

bleeding. In most instances, these studies will add only time delays, since patients will require further evaluation regardless of a positive or negative result.

Angiography should be obtained in all patients with suspected pancreatic hemorrhage: as the first study in unstable patients, and after cross-sectional imaging or endoscopy in stable patients. Selective celiac and superior mesenteric artery (SMA) angiography is necessary (Fig. 34-2). Supraselective gastroduodenal (GDA), splenic, pancreaticoduodenal, and dorsal pancreatic artery injections are rarely required for diagnosis. Intravenous digital subtraction angiography (IVDSA) or flush intra-arterial aortograms do not opacify the pancreatic vasculature

sufficiently to allow adequate evaluation. Ideally, free extravasation of contrast will confirm the location of the bleeding site, but this is only seen in the presence of active bleeding (Fig. 34-3). The extravasation may be focal or from multiple sites along the course of a vessel. Extravasation from the same point may be seen after injection into both the celiac artery and the SMA if the lesion arises from a vessel that can be supplied by both arteries, such as the GDA.

In stable patients, the most common finding is one or more pseudoaneurysms (Fig. 34-4). These should not be confused with true atherosclerotic visceral artery aneurysms, in which all three walls of the artery are intact. The typical locations, calcified

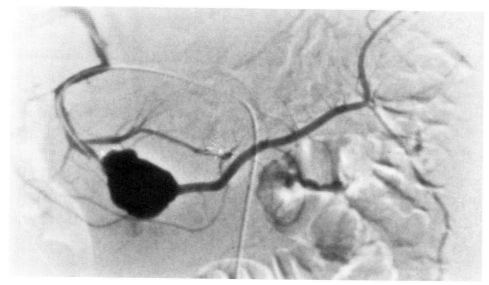

A

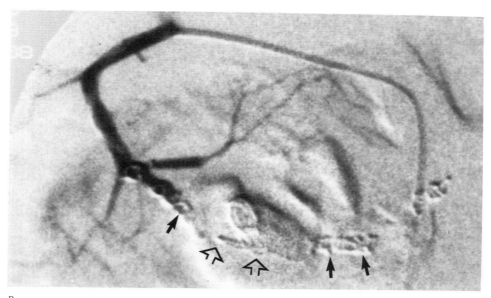

B

Figure 34-4. Pseudoaneurysm of the gastroepiploic artery. A. Digital subtraction angiogram of a selective gastroduodenal artery injection demonstrating a large pseudoaneurysm arising from the gastroepiploic artery. B. Postembolization digital subtraction angiogram of the same vessel. Coils and gelatin sponge have been deposited in the gastroepiploic artery on both sides of the pseudoaneurysm (solid arrows) and within the aneurysm itself (open arrows).

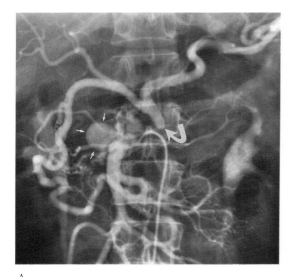

A

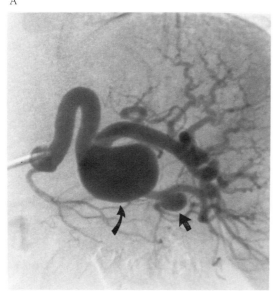

C

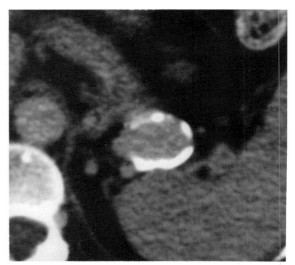

B

Figure 34-5. Visceral artery aneurysms not due to pancreatitis. A. True aneurysms of the inferior pancreaticoduodenal arteries (small arrows) in a patient with an occluded celiac artery origin (curved arrow) and retrograde flow through an enlarged pancreatic head arcade. Note that the hepatic and splenic arteries fill from an SMA injection. These aneurysms are the result of the increased flow through the small pancreatic arteries that serve as collateral pathways for the hepatic and splenic circulation. B. Atherosclerotic aneurysm of the splenic artery in a 54-year-old woman with no history of pancreatic disease. An enhancing lesion with calcified walls is present in the splenic hilum on a magnification view of a contrast-enhanced abdominal CT scan. C. Digital subtraction angiogram of the same patient depicting the large aneurysm (curved arrow) seen on CT, plus a smaller aneurysm (straight arrow) in the hilum of the spleen.

walls, and lack of associated pancreatic disease should help identify these lesions (Fig. 34-5). Rare lesions include arterioportal fistulas and arteriovenous malformations. Identifying vascular variants, such as replacement of the middle colic artery to the dorsal pancreatic artery, is as important as finding the bleeding site (Table 34-2). The angiographer must have knowledge of prior surgery and the ana-

tomic location of the pancreatic lesion to ensure that the appropriate vessels are studied.

Management and Results

The initial steps in the management of a patient with pancreatic hemorrhage are, as in all forms of GI bleeding, initiation of appropriate resuscitative

Table 34-2. Important Anatomic Variants of the Pancreatic Arterial Supply

Variant	Incidence (%)
Dorsal pancreatic artery from the common hepatic or celiac arteries	40
Dorsal pancreatic artery from the superior mesenteric artery or aorta	14
Transverse pancreatic artery from the superior mesenteric artery	10
Middle colic or jejunal branches from the dorsal pancreatic artery	4

therapy. Next, the choice of diagnostic modality will be determined by the clinical presentation and status of the patient. With the exception of the most critically ill patients, angiography will ultimately be required to define the vascular anatomy and to identify the source of bleeding. Once this information has been obtained, several therapeutic options are available.

Transcatheter Embolotherapy

Transcatheter embolotherapy may be performed at the time of the angiogram as a primary method of treatment or as an adjunct to a subsequent surgical procedure. Prophylactic antibiotics should be begun if the patient is not already receiving antibacterial therapy. After the vascular lesion is identified, supraselective catheterization is performed. This step may be achieved with a 5 French catheter, or with a 3 French catheter inserted coaxially through a 5 French or larger guiding catheter. The ready availability of specialized wires and 3 French embolization catheters has made cannulation of small intrinsic pancreatic arteries feasible in most patients. When a discrete bleeding point can be identified, occlusion of the actual hole in the wall of the artery may be possible, such as placement of a coil in the neck of a pseudoaneurysm. More commonly, the feeding vessel is angiographically "ligated" by first occluding the vessel just distal to the lesion to eliminate backflow, and then occluding the vessel proximally to stop inflow (see Figs. 34-3C; 34-4B). Multiple small points of extravasation can be

occluded with large embolic particles. However, some lesions may not be suitable for angiographic embolization, either because they are inaccessible or because the risk of embolization of nontarget structures is unacceptably high (Fig. 34-6). A critical final step in this procedure is completion angiography to exclude either incomplete embolization or collateral reconstitution of the bleeding vessel.

Permanent embolic materials should be used, such as stainless steel or platinum coils, polyvinyl alcohol particles, or tissue adhesive ("glue") (Table 34-3). Gelatin sponge (Gelfoam, Upjohn, Kalamazoo, Mich.) is useful in conjunction with permanent agents to promote thrombosis but should not be

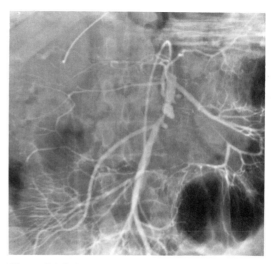

Figure 34-6. SMA angiogram in a patient with multiple episodes of pancreatitis. Several pseudoaneurysms of the proximal SMA are present, as well as occlusion of many of the jejunal arteries. These pseudoaneurysms are not amenable to embolotherapy because of the high risk of occlusion of the SMA. Surgical repair would be similarly difficult.

Table 34-3. Embolic Materials Suitable for Pancreatic Hemorrhage

Coils
Polyvinyl alcohol particles
Gelatin sponge
Thrombin
Tissue adhesive
Detachable balloon occlusion devices

employed as a sole form of therapy because it is resorbed after 4 to 6 weeks. Pitressin infusions have proven ineffective in the pancreatic bed, and absolute alcohol is contraindicated because of the risk of necrosis of surrounding tissues. Autologous clot is not recommended because it is rapidly recanalized.

The overall complication rate of transcatheter embolization in pancreatic hemorrhage is approximately 3% to 18%, with a mortality rate that increases from 0% to 16% with the severity of the patient's pre-existing clinical status. The risks of embolization include occlusion of nontarget vessels, pancreatitis, pancreatic necrosis, splenic infarction, bowel infarction, contrast-induced renal failure, and infection. Careful attenuation to anatomic variants, supraselective catheterization prior to embolization, and selection of appropriate embolic materials are all measures that will reduce the morbidity of the procedure.

Direct Puncture Embolization

An alternative, less widely practiced radiologic approach is direct puncture and embolization of large pseudoaneurysms. The technique has been described as both a percutaneous and intraoperative procedure. After a 21- or 18-gauge needle is inserted into the lesion, correct positioning is confirmed by either injection of contrast or imaging with US or CT. Embolization coils, gelatin sponge, and thrombin can then be injected directly into the pseudoaneurysm until occlusion occurs. Although this method does not permit the same degree of procedural control as intravascular embolization, it is a useful adjunct when large pseudoaneurysms are inadvertently punctured during attempted percutaneous pancreatic drainage.

Surgery

Patients may proceed directly to surgery after angiographic localization of the bleeding, without embolization. The operative strategy will depend upon the location of the pseudoaneurysm or extravasation as well as on the underlying pathology. Hemorrhage of the body and tail of the pancreas associated with chronic pancreatitis or neoplasms is best treated with distal pancreatectomy (Fig. 34-7). In this setting, early ligature of the splenic artery is extremely useful to diminish intraoperative blood loss. Unless the spleen is also involved in the inflammatory process, it does not necessarily have to be

Figure 34-7. Celiac artery angiogram demonstrating a splenic artery pseudoaneurysm with extravasation of contrast into the transverse colon (arrow) in a patient with chronic pancreatitis and lower gastrointestinal bleeding. The splenic artery proximal to the pseudoaneurysm is narrowed and has an irregular contour, consistent with postinflammatory changes. The inferior mesenteric artery and superior mesenteric artery injections were normal.

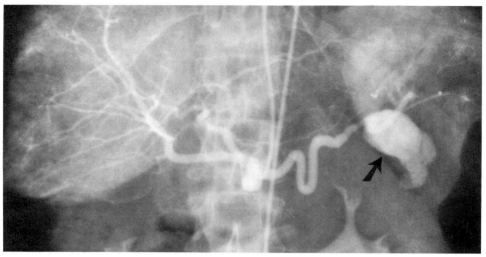

resected, because arterial inflow through the short gastric vessels is enough to maintain its viability in most cases. Pancreatic resection in acute necrotizing pancreatitis has prohibitive morbidity and mortality rates, which are even greater when bleeding is the indication for surgery. Typically, these patients have multiple bleeding points, and suture ligation coupled with either closed packing (using Penrose drains stuffed with gauze) or an open packing technique is the preferred method of treatment.

When bleeding is associated with a pseudocyst which is not amenable to resection or is located in the head of the pancreas, the pseudocyst should be unroofed to provide ample exposure and to permit suture ligature of the bleeding vessel. This step is then followed by external drainage and, only rarely, by anastamosis to an internal viscus. Free intraperitoneal hemorrhage secondary to a cystic or vascular tumor in the head of the pancreas requires pancreatoduodenectomy. However, if the patient is unstable or if the surgical team does not have experience with this surgical procedure, it is better to control the bleeding with suture ligation and reoperate on the patient at a later stage for resection. In pancreatic trauma, significant bleeding is usually from concomitant injury to neighboring major vessels and not the pancreatic parenchyma.

Surgery for pancreatic hemorrhage without preoperative angiography is associated with a 29% overall mortality rate: a 43% rate for lesions in the pancreatic head, and a 16% rate for those localized to the body and tail. These figures may be derived in part from the most unstable group of patients, those who bleed at rates that preclude diagnostic studies. The difficulty encountered in precisely locating the site (or sites) of bleeding at the time of surgery, even in stable patients, also contributes to the high surgical mortality. The technical challenge of operating upon the relatively inaccessible pancreas, with its complex arterial supply, is compounded by the surrounding inflammation in cases of acute and chronic pancreatitis. Furthermore, patients with pancreatitis may not be bleeding from the pancreas itself or its surrounding tissue, but as a consequence of segmentary portal hypertension with bleeding gastric varices. Overall, the prognosis for bleeding in association with a pseudocyst or a neoplasm is better than that for acute necrotizing pancreatitis.

Preferred Approach

The preferred therapeutic approach to pancreatic hemorrhage at the authors' institution is early angiographic localization and embolization of the bleeding, followed by an appropriate surgical procedure. In stable patients, occlusion of the pseudoaneurysm provides complete therapy in up to 80% of cases. When surgery is required, prior embolization of the lesion may prevent intraoperative or postoperative rupture and massive hemorrhage. The friable nature of the surrounding vessels can make intraoperative control of bleeding in the pancreatic bed difficult. Postoperative hemorrhage after internal or external surgical drainage procedures has a 60% mortality rate.

In unstable patients, angiographic control of bleeding may allow for resuscitation and a more controlled surgical approach. These patients have a poorer outcome in general, with an overall mortality rate of 40% for bleeding in the setting of acute pancreatitis despite combined angiographic and surgical efforts. However, these results compare favorably with a mortality rate that exceeds 80% for the same group of patients treated with surgery alone. Transcatheter embolization of bleeding may permit an acute inflammatory process to mature into a stable chronic pancreatic lesion prior to surgery, with the attendant decreased operative risks.

Conclusions

The rapid diagnosis and treatment of hemorrhage due to pancreatic disease require a high clinical awareness of the entity and the coordinated efforts of the surgeon, endoscopist, and radiologist. When hemorrhage presents as GI bleeding, exclusion of other gastrointestinal lesions, such as varices or ulcers, by the endoscopist, or visualization of blood issuing from the ampulla, should suggest the correct diagnosis. Intraperitoneal or retroperitoneal hemorrhage on an abdominal CT scan in these patients should be considered pancreatic in origin until proven otherwise. Selective celiac and SMA angiography is the primary mode of identification of the site of bleeding, with supraselective catheterization and embolization performed as part of the same procedure. Surgery can then occur on a more elective basis, or perhaps not at all. The strategy of diagnostic angiography with transcatheter embolization prior to operative intervention for pancreatic hemorrhage results in diminished morbidity and mortality from this potentially catastrophic event.

Selected Readings

Boudghene F, L'Hermine C, Bigot JM. Arterial complications of pancreatitis: Diagnostic and therapeutic aspects in 104 cases. *JVIR* 1993; 4:551–558.

Lee MJ, et al. Pancreatitis with pseudoaneurysm formation: A pitfall for the interventional radiologist. *AJR* 1991; 156:97–98.

Mauro MA, Jaques P. Transcatheter management of pseudoaneurysms complicating pancreatitis. *JVIR* 1991; 2:527–532.

Stabile BE, Wilson SE, Debas HT. Reduced mortality from bleeding pseudocysts and pseudoaneurysms caused by pancreatitis. *Arch Surg* 1983; 118:45–51.

Stanley JC, et al. Major arterial hemorrhage: A complication of pancreatic pseudocysts and chronic pancreatitis. *Arch Surg* 1976; 111:435–440.

Stroud WH, Cullom JW, Anderson MC. Hemorrhagic complications of severe pancreatitis. *Surgery* 1981; 90:657–663.

Waltman AC, et al. Massive arterial hemorrhage in patients with pancreatitis: Complementary roles of surgery and transcatheter occlusive techniques. *Arch Surg* 1986; 121:439–443.

White AF, Baum S, Buranasiri S. Aneurysms secondary to pancreatitis. *AJR* 1976; 127:393–396.

35

Pancreas Divisum

ROBERT H. SCHAPIRO
ANDREW L. WARSHAW

Etiology and Pathogenesis

Strictly defined, the term *pancreas divisum* describes those situations in which the ducts from the dorsal and ventral portions of the pancreas fail to fuse, usually during the fifth and sixth week of embryonic life. As a result, each portion may drain through a separate orifice: the ventral pancreas through the ampulla of Vater or "major" ampulla, and the dorsal portion through the accessory or "minor" papilla. The duct draining through the major papilla is referred to as the duct of Wirsung, and that through the accessory papilla as the duct of Santorini. With normal fusion, the pancreatic secretions, up to 2 liters/d, drain through the major ampulla or, if the duct of Santorini is preserved, through either ampulla.

Many variants of the normal anatomical situation occur, pictured in Fig. 35-1 as variants A through E. These variants include absence (regression) of the duct of Santorini (variant B), absence of the duct of Wirsung (variant D), or the presence of a filamentous connection between the ducts of Wirsung and Santorini which is functionally inadequate to handle pancreatic duct flow (variant E). The frequencies of these anatomical variations are estimated as follows: 30% of patients have equal drainage from Wirsung and Santorini (variant A), 52% have complete or near-complete regression of the duct of Santorini (variant B), 5% have complete nonunion of dorsal and ventral ducts (variant C), 4% have an absent duct of Wirsung (variant D), and probably less than 1% have incomplete pancreas divisum (variant E). In variants C, D, and E, the

vast majority of pancreatic secretions exit the pancreas into the duodenum through the duct of Santorini or dorsal duct. Thus a more appropriate term for this condition would be a *dominant dorsal duct*. In Western populations, epidemiological studies have shown that a dominant dorsal duct may occur in as many as 10% of the general population, without any predisposition as to gender. Other studies have suggested that this anomaly is much less common in Japan.

Many have questioned how an anatomical variation that is so common could be disease-producing. Moreover, this putative disease often presents as recurrent pancreatitis without any chronic dilatation of the dorsal duct, or as obstructive-type pain suggestive of pancreatitis unaccompanied by elevations in the levels of serum amylase or lipase. It is important to recognize that the dominant dorsal duct by itself does not cause pancreatic disease as long as drainage from the dorsal duct is unimpeded. However, if, in addition, the accessory papillary orifice is of insufficient size, the combination of accessory papillary stenosis and a dominant dorsal duct can lead to obstructive consequences such as pain, pancreatitis, or even fibrosis. If accessory papillary stenosis were unusual, the combination of this problem with a dominant dorsal duct would be even rarer, and one would need statistical studies of extraordinary size to demonstrate that a dominant dorsal duct predisposes to an obstructive pancreatopathy. Alternatively, a cause-and-effect relationship could be established if affected symptomatic individuals with the hypothetical disease could be followed to see if enlargement of the acces-

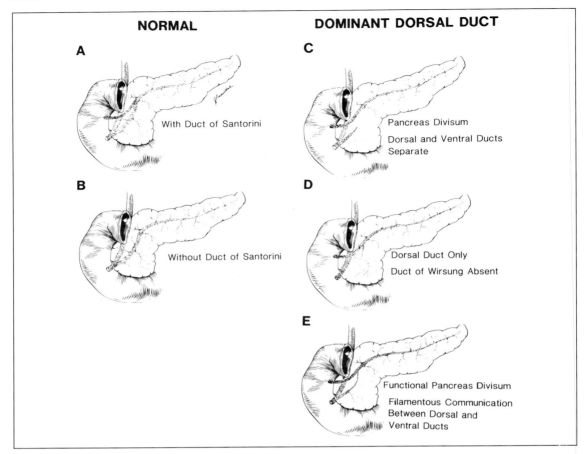

Figure 35-1. Common variations of pancreatic duct anatomy. Those variations (C, D, E) characterized by a dominant dorsal duct are found in about 10% of normal Western populations.

sory papillary orifice relieved their symptoms. Ideally, one would want some reproducible objective technique for demonstrating that the accessory papilla was indeed stenotic.

Diagnosis

Pancreas divisum, or a dominant dorsal duct, should be suspected whenever endoscopic retrograde pancreatography (ERP) done through the ampulla of Vater fails to demonstrate a pancreatic duct that fills beyond the head of the gland. The typical foreshortened ventral duct of pancreas divisum is shown in Fig. 35-2A. When the bile duct fills repeatedly without the pancreatic duct being visualized at all, complete absence of the ventral duct

must be suspected. Nevertheless, the proof that this anomaly is present requires cannulation through the accessory ampulla with demonstration of a main pancretic duct that fills only by that route, as in Fig. 35-3. As viewed through the endoscope, the accessory ampulla is generally found 1 to 2 cm to the right (anterior) and 1 to 3 cm cephalad to the main ampulla. The accessory ampulla may be represented by a tiny and barely discernible mound, or by a prominent ampullary structure that may be easily mistaken for the major ampulla. The size of the accessory ampulla does not reliably predict whether it is stenotic. The ampullary orifice can often not be identified until pancreatic flow has been stimulated, usually by the intravenous injection of 1 U/kg of secretin. This test should be done

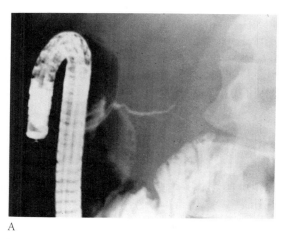

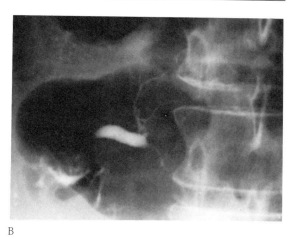

A

B

Figure 35-2. True and false pancreas divisum. A. The typical foreshortened ventral duct of pancreas divisum. Note the relatively small diameter of the main duct and the arborizing branches at its termination. B. Malignant obstruction of the ventral duct mimicking pancreas divisum. The duct diameter is generous in size and terminates abruptly. Although side ducts are visible, there is no arborization.

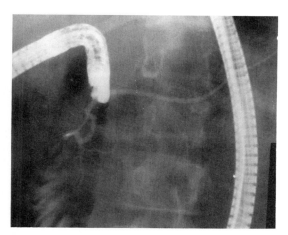

Figure 35-3. Dominant dorsal duct. A needle-tipped catheter has been used to fill the dorsal duct through the accessory ampulla. A small tributary of this duct supplies the uncinate lobe but does not communicate with the duct of Wirsung or the ampulla of Vater.

ber (23- or 25-gauge), blunt, metal-tipped endoscopic cannulas; thus experienced endoscopists should be able to identify and cannulate the accessory ampulla in at least 90% of cases of pancreas divisum. Other techniques include the use of soft-tipped 0.018- or 0.021-in.–diameter guidewires through a tapered-tip catheter. In a common interpretive error, some patients with obstruction of the duct of Wirsung in the head of the gland, either by tumor or occasionally by benign disease, may be misinterpreted as having pancreas divisum. This "false" pancreas divisum can be suspected by the appearance of a normal-caliber pancreatic duct in the periampullary portion, by a longer-than-usual ventral duct (> 3 cm) up to the point of termination, and by a lack of arborization of secondary ducts in the proximal, cutoff end. In true pancreas divisum, the duct of Wirsung is often quite narrow in diameter and branches extensively at its proximal termination (see Fig. 35-2).

Considerable disagreement exists as to what may constitute a reliable means of demonstrating accessory papilla stenosis in association with the dominant dorsal duct. Dilatation of the dorsal duct is rare when the duct is visualized in the resting state during endoscopic cannulation. Endoscopic manometry of the accessory ampulla is technically very difficult, and the reproducible documentation

in anyone being investigated for recurrent pancreatitis or pancreaticlike pain in whom the main pancreatic duct cannot be visualized through the ampulla of Vater and in whom a ductal orifice is not readily visible in the accessory ampulla.

Cannulation of the accessory ampulla has been greatly facilitated by the introduction of small-cali-

of elevated ampullary pressures is beyond the expertise of almost all centers. It has been suggested that the endoscopic placement of a drainage tube or stent through the accessory papillary orifice with the aid of a guidewire might help in predicting those patients with functional obstruction by demonstrating relief of symptoms through improved drainage. This hypothesis needs further testing and clinical experience. The authors have serious concerns about the safety of this approach because of the potential for duct injury and stenosis produced by long-term endoscopic stenting, as discussed later.

The authors' approach has been to try to demonstrate physiologically significant stenosis of the accessory pancreatic duct orifice by simulating food ingestion, through administration of intravenous secretin and measuring its effect on the size of the dorsal pancreatic duct as determined by ultrasonography. Intravenous secretin (1 U/kg) is given over 1 minute, and duct size is measured at baseline and at 1, 5, 15, and 30 minutes after injection. Prolonged dilation, for 15 to 30 minutes after administration, is considered an index of abnormal resistance to the emptying of the duct (Fig. 35-4). Transient dilation of the pancreatic duct for up to

5 minutes is seen in normal glands with normal emptying dynamics. When there is chronic fibrotic pancreatitis, the duct may not dilate at all, the result both of restriction by fibrosis and of secretory failure. Other investigators have approached this same phenomenon with serial CT scans or have studied it with the morphine-prostigmine tests or an attempt at intraductal manometry.

Management and Results

As noted, considerable concern still exists that pancreas divisum may be an incidental anomaly unrelated to pancreatic pain or pancreatitis. In this school of thought, any management directed at the anatomical aspects of this condition would be inappropriate. Proponents of this argument point out the difficulty of demonstrating an increased statistical association between pancreatitis and pancreas divisum in epidemiological studies, imply that endoscopic retrograde cholangiopancreatography (ERCP) series with a positive association reflect populations with inherent referral bias, and observe that dorsal pancreatic duct changes on ERP are not the rule and that the response to endoscopic or surgical management is variable. Con-

Figure 35-4. Secretin ultrasound provocative test. A. A normal-sized pancreatic duct (presecretin). The normal duct is best seen in the pancreatic body and has a diameter of 1 mm or less. The markers (+) indicate the pancreatic duct lumen. B. After intravenous secretin administration, dilation of the duct to 3 mm is seen in the same patient at 30 minutes. A short period of dilation is normal, but prolonged dilation (15 to 30 minutes) is seen in patients with impaired outflow of pancreatic secretions.

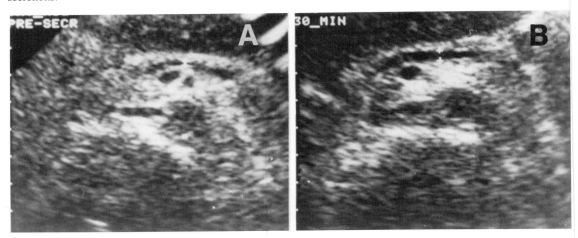

versely, in favor of an association is the aforementioned increased incidence of pancreas divisum in a number of ERCP series of acute relapsing pancreatitis. Histological studies of resected specimens in a few cases have shown changes consistent with chronic pancreatitis confined to the dorsal pancreas.

Several series have shown a symptomatic response in selected patients when therapy is directed at the accessory papillary orifice. Most authors agree that successful therapy is most likely to occur in patients with a dominant dorsal duct who present with documented acute recurrent pancreatitis with documented amylase level elevations. Therapy is less successful in patients with recurrent pain but without amylase level elevations. Therapy directed at the ampullary orifice is least successful in patients with established endoscopic criteria of chronic pancreatitis, including dilated ducts, pancreatic duct stones, chain of lakes, marked strictures, or markedly dilated secondary ducts. When gross ductal abnormalities of chronic pancreatitis are present in the body of the pancreas, it is unlikely that anything done to the ampullary orifice is going to radically change the patient's symptoms.

Endoscopic Therapy

Relief of putative stenosis of the accessory ampulla can be effected by surgical sphincteroplasty, by endoscopic papillotomy and stent placement, or by a combination of the two methods. Lehman et al. in 1993 reported on the results of endoscopic therapy in 52 patients with pancreas divisum. Of these, 17 had recurrent pancreatitis, 24 had disabling pancreatic-type pain without significant enzyme elevations, and 11 had endoscopic changes of chronic pancreatitis. Their technique involved performing a papillotomy of the accessory ampulla using a needle-knife papillotome over a previously inserted pancreatic duct stent. The stent was subsequently removed after a period of several weeks. Patients had been symptomatic for a mean of 5.1 years and had failed to respond to conservative therapy. In patients with previous acute pancreatitis, 76.5% benefited, whereas only approximately 25% of patients with chronic pancreatitis or chronic pain were helped. Improvement was assessed by scoring the symptoms and by comparing the number of hospi-

tal days and admissions for pancreatitis or pain for a comparable period before and after therapy. The latter measurement has the tendency to bias the results in favor of therapy, since intervention is usually considered in highly symptomatic patients with frequent hospital admissions. Complications, primarily mild pancreatitis, occurred in 15% of the procedures. Changes in the dorsal duct that were thought to be stent-induced were found to be present in 50% of patients evaluated endoscopically at the time of stent removal.

A somewhat different approach to endoscopic therapy was proposed by Lans et al. They proposed to treat symptomatic patients with prolonged endoscopic stenting of the accessory papilla. Their controlled, prospective, but unblinded series included 19 patients with pancreas divisum and "idiopathic" pancreatitis, as documented by at least two episodes of amylase elevations twice the normal range. Nine patients served as controls and 10 received stents after catheter dilation of the lesser ampulla. To avoid bias secondary to technical factors, patients were not subject to randomization until a guidewire was successfully placed in the duct of Santorini. Follow-up, usually with stent exchange, was performed at 4-month intervals for a year. Statistically significant improvement ($P < 0.05$) occurred in the stented group, both in terms of the episodes of pain requiring emergency ward or hospital admission and in terms of the number of episodes of documented pancreatitis (0 and 1, respectively, in the stented group). The mean follow-up was close to 2.5 years. Nine of 10 treated patients and only 1 of 10 untreated patients reported a 50% or greater improvement in symptoms. The nature of the study prevented "blinding" of the patients to the therapy they received.

Of particular importance, no inflammatory strictures of the dorsal duct were noted by Lans et al., either during or after stent therapy. This observation is in contrast to other studies, in which stent-induced damage to the pancreatic duct has been a major concern. In a series of 34 patients reported by Cotton's group, 36% of all patients and 72% of those with normal initial pancreatograms developed diffuse duct enlargement or side branch ectasia or occlusion, although there was a tendency of these changes to improve with time. Experimental studies in dogs have similarly shown a high incidence of duct injury after stent placement. The authors have been struck, both in their own treated patients and in referrals initially treated in other programs, by the frequency of ductal changes either at the proximal end of the stent or at the approximate level of the retaining "barbs."

Equally disturbing from the standpoint of long-term stent placement is the very high rate of occlusion of pancreatic duct stents. Lehman's group tested all pancreatic duct stents for patency when they were removed and found that 50% of all 5 to 7 French stents were occluded by 5 to 6 weeks, and 100% by 9 weeks.

Surgical Therapy

Because of concerns abut the patency and potential hazard of long-term stenting, the authors' more traditional approach has involved definitive treatment by means of surgical transduodenal sphincteroplasty of the accessory papilla in patients with pain or pancreatitis associated with pancreas divisum. Surgery was offered to 100 such patients referred to one surgeon; these patients did not have evidence of alcoholism or chronic pancreatitis. Eighty-eight agreed to undergo surgery, of whom 66 were felt to have clear ductal stenosis on the basis of their inability to accept a no. 1 (0.75-mm) lacrimal probe. At mean follow-up of 53 months, 85% of those operated on were improved if the duct was stenotic, whereas only 27% were improved if it was not (Table 35-1). Of those with documented recurrent pancreatitis, 82% were improved versus 56% with only chronic pain. Of those with a preoperatively abnormal ultrasonography secretin test, 92% were improved versus only 40% if the test was negative (Table 35-2). Of those with negative tests, 64% were improved if they presented with attacks of pancreatitis, whereas only 21% were helped if they presented with chronic pain. Seven percent of patients were documented to have restenosis (and recurrent pain) in long-term follow-up. The authors' current experience has now grown to 140 patients who have had an accessory papilla sphincteroplasty, and the outcomes have remained similar.

An important provision in selecting patients for management by therapy directed at the accessory papilla is the observation that once endoscopic changes of chronic pancreatitis have occurred (stricture, irregular dilation, ectasia of secondary ducts, pseudocysts), surgical intervention, if warranted, should be directed at resection of maximally involved segments, drainage of pseudocysts, or performance of pancreatic duct jejunal anastomosis if the duct is sufficiently capacious (Fig. 35-5).

Table 35-1. Postoperative Outcome and Ultrasound Secretin Test Correlated with Surgical Assessment of Stenosis of the Accessory Papilla

| | Postoperative Outcome | | | | | |
Stenosis	Good (n)	Fair (n)	Poor (n)	Total (n)	Negative Test	Positive Test
No	6	0	16	22	15	1
Yes*	46	10	10	66	10	36

*$P < 0.0001$ for patients with stenosis versus those without stenosis.

Table 35-2. Ultrasound Secretin Test Results Versus Postoperative Outcome

| | Ultrasound Secretin Test Scores (n) | | | | Mean Score | Negative Tests (%) | Positive Tests (%) |
Outcome	0	1	2	3			
Good	10	9	12	5	1.4	40	70
Fair	0	1	7	0	1.9	0	22
Poor	15	2	1	0	0.2	60	8

*$P < 0.0001$ both for mean scores and for distribution of positive and negative tests versus outcome.

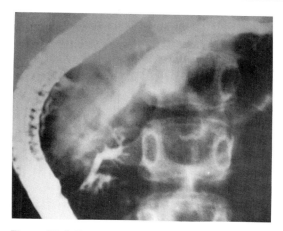

Figure 35-5. Pancreatogram in a 9-year-old child with recurrent attacks of pancreatitis. The dorsal and ventral ducts are unfused (pancreas divisum), but both ducts are abnormally dilated, suggesting chronic pancreatitis. Improvement in ductal drainage is unlikely to be helpful in such a patient.

Combined Approach

A reasonable synthesis of the endoscopic and surgical approaches to this problem has been suggested by Siegel et al., although their series does not provide sufficient detail to draw any firm conclusions. They have suggested that a trial of endoscopic stenting, with or without endoscopic papillotomy, may predict the subsequent response to transduodenal surgery. Fifteen of 17 patients submitted to surgery are said to have derived long-term benefits and improvements which directly correlated with their response to stenting. Although this seems a logical corollary, more prospectively controlled experience is needed to validate these results. Similarly, although the experience of Lans et al. is encouraging, additional long-term follow-up will be needed to see whether endoscopic sphincterotomy of the lesser ampulla is equally or more effective and safe when compared with surgical sphincterotomy, and whether continued patency of the ampullary orifice is maintained. It should be re-emphasized that the endoscopic series included only patients whose duct had been satisfactorily cannulated with a guidewire. There will always be cases of severe accessory ampullary stenosis where cannulation will not be possible and only a sugical intervention is feasible. Moreover, the specialized endoscopic skills needed for deep cannulation of the accessory ampulla are available in only a minority of institutions.

Conclusions

Pancreas divisum (dominant dorsal duct syndrome) is a common anomaly of pancreatic duct development which the authors believe can predispose to pancreatitis and pancreatic pain in that small minority of patients in whom it occurs in association with stenosis of the accessory ampullary orifice. Confirmation of such accessory ampullary stenosis is difficult, but the authors have found a functional assessment of dorsal duct emptying, the ultrasound secretin test, to be helpful. In such patients, and especially in those with recurrent pancreatitis, a sphincteroplasty of the accessory ampulla often brings improvement. Recent evidence suggests that in many patients the sphincter may be effectively divided endoscopically (or bypassed by indwelling stents). The potential for ductal injury from such indwelling stents is of concern, especially when they are placed for a protracted period, but stenting may prove to have a valid role in the identification of patients who, by their short-term improvement with stenting, are likely to obtain long-term relief from surgical sphincteroplasty. The authors believe that therapy directed at the accessory ampulla is not indicated if there are other obvious causes of pancreatitis, such as alcohol abuse, and will probably be ineffective if there are already established ductal changes of chronic pancreatitis in the body of the gland.

Selected Readings

Benage D, et al. Minor papilla cannulation and dorsal ductography in pancreas divisum. *Gastrointest Endosc* 1990; 36:553–557.

Bernard JP, et al. Pancreas divisum is a probable cause of acute pancreatitis: A report of 137 cases. *Pancreas* 1990; 5:248–254.

Ikenberry S, et al. Pancreatic stent occlusion rate. *Gastrointest Endosc* 1993; 39:318. (Abstract)

Kozarek RA. Pancreatic stents can induce ductal changes consistent with chronic pancreatitis. *Gastrointest Endosc* 1990; 36:93–95.

Lans JI, et al. Endoscopic therapy in patients with pancreas divisum and acute pancreatitis: A prospective randomized controlled clinical trial. *Gastrointest Endosc* 1992; 38:430–434.

Lehman GA, et al. Pancreas divisum: Results of minor papilla sphincterotomy. *Gastrointest Endosc* 1993; 39:1–8.

Lindstrom E, Ihse I. Dynamic CT scanning of pancreatic duct after secretin provocation in pancreas divisum. *Dig Dis Sci* 1990; 35:1371–1376.

Siegel JH, et al. Effectiveness of endoscopic drainage for pancreas divisum: Endoscopic and surgical results in 31 patients. *Endoscopy* 1990; 22:129–133.

Warshaw AL, et al. Evaluation and treatment of the dominant dorsal duct syndrome (pancreas divisum redefined). *Am J Surg* 1990; 159:59–66.

Warshaw AL, et al. Objective evaluation of ampullary stenosis with ultrasonography and pancreatic stimulation. *Am J Surg* 1985; 149:65–72.

36

Chronic Pancreatitis

Frederic E. Eckhauser
Lisa M. Colletti
Grace H. Elta
James A. Knol

Prior to the early 1960s attempts to classify pancreatitis were mainly descriptive and based on clinical observations and surgical and/or pathologic findings at operation or autopsy. More recently, acute and chronic forms of pancreatitis are defined by whether restitution of normal pancreatic anatomy and function will occur once primary causes or factors are eliminated. The two forms are morphologically distinct, and it is unusual for acute pancreatitis to develop into chronic pancreatitis. In addition, chronic pancreatitis may manifest as chronic disease from the onset. The prevalence of chronic pancreatitis in autopsy studies varies from 0.04% to 5.00%, but little prospective epidemiologic data are available to ascertain the true incidence of this disease worldwide.

Etiology and Pathogenesis

The most common cause of chronic pancreatitis in temperate areas of the world is alcohol. No uniform threshold for alcohol toxicity exists, but clearly the quantity and duration of alcohol consumption correlate with the risk of developing chronic pancreatitis. In contrast, the type of alcohol consumed and the pattern of consumption do not appreciably alter the risk of chronic pancreatitis. It has been suggested that genetic susceptibility and diet may be important because nutritional factors such as high-fat, high-protein diets and alcohol consumption are additive risks.

An unusual variant of chronic pancreatitis occurs in tropical areas of the world. This form of the disease occurs with equal frequency in men and women and is not associated with known etiologic factors such as alcohol, hypercalcemia, heredity, or trauma. Typically, young individuals are affected, with a mean age at onset of 12 to 15 years. Pain is less prominent than with the alcoholic form, and endocrine insufficiency (diabetes mellitus) is common. Radiological evidence of pancreatic stones is present in a significant percentage of patients.

Hereditary pancreatitis affects familial aggregates involving small numbers of related individuals, and the more typical form is inherited as an autosomal dominant disease with variable penetrance. Many of these patients exhibit a decreased concentration in their pancreatic juice of pancreatic stone protein (PSP), which may play an important role in calcium precipitation and stone formation. PSP, recently renamed lithostatine, is an intermediate-size glycoprotein (molecular weight 13,500) that is secreted by acinar cells and has no enzymatic or immunological cross-reactivity with pancreatic enzymes. Lithostatine acts as a calcium stabilizer in pancreatic juice, which is normally supersaturated. Evidence suggests that the relative concentration of PSP to total pancreatic juice protein is constantly decreased in patients with chronic pancreatitis. Furthermore, PSP levels may be determined genetically and thereby contribute to the pathogenesis of several forms of chronic pancreatitis. Characteristically, hereditary disease presents at an early age (10–12 years) with recurrent attacks of abdominal pain. Diabetes develops in 20% of patients after a variable latency period.

Obstructive chronic pancreatitis is associated with obstruction of the pancreatic duct secondary to benign or malignant tumors or strictures related to pancreatic inflammation or biliary pathology. Sphincter of Oddi dysfunction involving either the ampullary or pancreatic portion of the sphincter is thought to be one cause. This form of disease can usually be differentiated from other forms of chronic pancreatitis on the basis of specific pathological findings, including infrequent or absent intraductal calculi or plugs, uniform dilatation of the pancreatic duct distal to the site of obstruction, and relative preservation of pancreatic duct morphology and epithelium. Experimental studies have shown regression of pathology after duct decompression, but it is not known whether the same response occurs in humans.

Pancreatitis also occurs in a small percentage of patients with hyperparathyroidism. Hypercalcemia is implicated in the pathogenesis of this condition. In experimental animals hypercalcemia causes excessive stimulation of the acinar cell, increased secretion of calcium into pancreatic juice, and alteration in the diffusion barrier between the pancreatic duct lumen and the interstitial compartment.

Diagnosis

Clinical Presentation

Pain is the major presenting symptom in the majority of patients with chronic pancreatitis. Pain is epigastric in location, is variable but often severe in intensity, and frequently has a prominent back component. In contrast to biliary or peptic ulcer disease, the pain of chronic pancreatitis is aggravated by ingestion of food. Absence of pain is uncommon but does occur in 15% of patients, especially those with idiopathic pancreatitis. The pathogenesis of pain is multifactorial, but increased pancreatic ductal pressure and perineural inflammation and scarring are important contributing factors. Elevated ductal pressure has been documented at the time of surgical duct decompression in several clinical studies. In addition, pain in patients with

radiographic evidence of ductal obstruction frequently decreases with the onset of pancreatic insufficiency and decreased pancreatic secretion. Many of the current medical, endoscopic, and surgical efforts to treat the pain of chronic pancreatitis are directed toward decreasing pancreatic ductal pressure.

Nausea, vomiting, and weight loss are common in patients with chronic pancreatitis. In this setting weight loss is usually due to food avoidance rather than true pancreatic insufficiency. Malabsorption presenting with diarrhea, steatorrhea, and weight loss does occur but not until enzyme secretion is reduced to less than 10% of normal. Diabetes due to endocrine insufficiency usually occurs late in the course of chronic pancreatitis.

The diagnosis of chronic pancreatitis can frequently be made on the basis of a comprehensive history and several simple diagnostic tests. Plain radiographs of the abdomen show pancreatic calcification in up to 30% to 40% of patients. Serum levels of pancreatic enzymes (amylase, lipase) vary with the stage and severity of pancreatitis but may be mildly elevated during periods of exacerbation in patients with pancreatic exocrine reserve. Progressive inflammation and scarring in the head region of the pancreas may entrap the intrapancreatic portion of the common bile duct and lead to biochemical evidence of cholestasis or frank jaundice.

Pancreatic Function Tests

Several tests of pancreatic exocrine function are available, but their utility is limited by relatively low sensitivity, especially in patients with mild chronic pancreatitis. Table 36-1 is a summary of currently available tests of pancreatic function. Direct measurement of pancreatic enzymes or bicarbonate in duodenal aspirates after combined secretin-cholecystokinin or secretin-cerulein simulation is the most valuable pancreatic function test for confirming the diagnosis of chronic pancreatitis but is not widely available. All measured parameters will be decreased in patients with advanced disease, whereas only one or two parameters will be decreased in patients with mild to moderate disease. Although direct pancreatic function tests are accurate and reproducible, they are also invasive, time-consuming, and expensive.

Table 36-1. Sensitivity of Various Pancreatic Function Tests for Detecting Chronic Pancreatitis

Test	Range (%)	Overall Sensitivity	
		Mild Chronic Pancreatitis	Severe Chronic Pancreatitis
Secretin + CCK[a]	74–90+		
Lundh test meal	66–94		
Bentiromide (NBT-PABA)[b]	37–90 (mean 71)	46% (57/123)[c]	71% (103/146)
Fluorescein dilaurate	46–93 (mean 74)	39% (32/82)	79% (93/118)
Fecal chymotrypsin	45–100	49% (54/111)	85% (179/211)
Trypsinlike immunoreactivity	33–65 (mean 48)		

[a]CCK = Cholecystokinin.
[b]NBT-PABA = N-benzoyl-L-tyrosyl-P-aminobenzoic acid
[c]The numerator indicates the number of patients with positive tests and the denominator indicates the number of patients tested.
Source: Reprinted by permission of the publisher from Diagnosis of chronic pancreatitis, by Niederan C, Grendell JH, *Gastroenterology* 88:1973–1995. Copyright 1985 by the American Gastroenterological Association.

Oral function tests such as the bentiromide test are capable of detecting moderate and severe pancreatic insufficiency, require less technical support, and are more widely used because they cause less patient discomfort. These studies provide indirect information regarding pancreatic exocrine function and consist of administering a complex substrate containing a marker that is liberated after hydrolysis by pancreatic enzymes. The recovery rate of the altered marker measured in urine or serum is related to the specific amount of enzyme released by the pancreas. In general, pancreatic function tests are used as a complement to imaging studies for evaluating the presence and severity of chronic pancreatitis.

Imaging Studies

Imaging of the pancreas with ultrasonography (US), computerized tomography (CT), and endoscopic retrograde cholangiopancreatography (ERCP) may be useful to evaluate morphological abnormalities associated with chronic pancreatitis and to document the presence of complications such as splenic vein thrombosis, biliary strictures, or pseudocysts. CT is relatively insensitive for detecting subtle changes

in early stages of chronic pancreatitis, but diagnostic accuracy increases in patients with advanced disease. Pathognomonic CT findings such as marked duct dilation and pancreatic calcification are evident in the majority of patients with severe chronic pancreatitis (Fig. 36-1). In patients with advanced disease there is generally a good correlation between the severity of parenchymal changes noted on CT and the degree of exocrine dysfunction.

Pancreatography may be extremely useful in patients with chronic pancreatitis, but one must keep in mind that radiologic changes may correlate poorly with the clinical or pathological features of the disease. In patients with chronic pancreatitis, ERCP is indicated to establish a diagnosis and to

Figure 36-1. CT scan of chronic pancreatitis showing macrocalcifications (A) and dilatation of both the main pancreatic duct and the common bile duct (B).

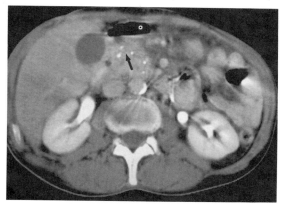

A

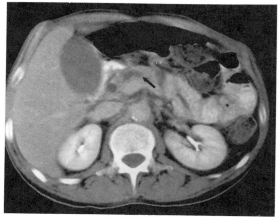

B

assess pancreatic ductal anatomy prior to surgical or endoscopic therapy. A normal pancreatogram is defined by the presence of a completely normal main pancreatic duct and side branches. Typical changes of chronic pancreatitis include obstruction of the main pancreatic duct with diffuse or segmental distal duct dilation and the presence of cavities or calculi. In an effort to standardized reporting, a morphologic classification system was developed to grade the degree of chronic pancreatitis (Table 36-2). The sensitivity of ERCP for detecting chronic pancreatitis is comparable to that of other imaging techniques and is generally better than that of pancreatic function tests, which may be nondiagnostic until considerable pancreatic damage has occurred.

Pancreatography has certain limitations in patients with presumed chronic pancreatitis. In patients with mild or moderate chronic pancreatitis, a significant discrepancy may exist between morphologic (ERCP) and functional studies. In this setting both ERCP and pancreatic function tests should be obtained to detect or confirm the slight abnormalities identified by either study alone. Ductal changes may be minimal or absent in a variable percentage of patients with documented chronic pancreatitis, and the interpretation of subtle side branch changes may be difficult in patients with early disease. Furthermore, ERCP is not suitable for distinguishing between the various etiologies of chronic pancreatitis. ERCP may be most valuable in patients with known chronic pancreatitis, for whom information pertaining to ductal anatomy

Table 36-2. Morphologic Classification of Chronic Pancreatitis

Normal
  Main duct is normal, as are side branches. Side branches show no sacculations.
Equivocal
  Main duct is normal and fewer than three side branches are abnormal. Some sacculations occur in side branches, but changes are minimal.
Moderate
  Main duct is abnormal and there are more than three abnormal side branches.
Marked
  Significant abnormalities appear in the main duct and there are usually more than three abnormal side branches. Typically, the duct is dilated, segmented, and obstructed.

Source: Sarner M, Cotton PB. Classification of pancreatitis. *Gut* 1984; 75:756–759. Used with permission.

will be used to assess the feasibility of surgical or endoscopic intervention and to detect associated pathology (biliary strictures, pseudocysts, splenic vein thrombosis, etc.) that might alter the therapeutic approach.

Management and Results

Treatment objectives in patients with chronic pancreatitis include relief of pain, correction of problems related to pancreatic exocrine and endocrine insufficiency, and correction of associated pathology involving the biliary tract or the gastrointestinal tract.

Pain Control

Elimination of factors known to exacerbate pancreatitis is an important cornerstone of therapy. In patients with an alcoholic etiology, abstinence is recommended. Although the relationship between alcohol and pain is controversial, most authorities believe that eliminating pancreatic secretagogues such as alcohol decreases pancreatic secretion and thereby may relieve pain. Simple analgesics such as aspirin or acetaminophen supplemented with codeine should be used initially whenever possible. Ultimately, many patients may become dependent on narcotic analgesics. When this situation develops, single or combination drug programs that are least likely to interfere with the patient's lifestyle should be used.

Many authorities have advocated pharmacologic doses of pancreatic extracts to inhibit pancreatic secretion and decrease intraductal pressure, thereby relieving pain. These clinical observations support animal studies showing that the presence of serine proteases (trypsin, chymotrypsin, and elastase) in the duodenal lumen reduces pancreatic secretion via a negative feedback mechanism. Feedback regulation appears to be mediated through the inhibition of cholecystokinin (CCK) by serine proteases. Controlled trials have demonstrated that large doses of conventional pancreatic enzymes decrease abdominal pain in patients with chronic pancreatitis. Patients most likely to respond have mild to moderate exocrine insufficiency and minimal radiographic findings on ERCP. The administration of pancreatic extracts in uncontrolled trials has also been shown to reduce the frequency of attacks of recurrent acute pancreatitis.

After extrapancreatic causes of pain have been excluded, a CT scan of the upper abdomen should be obtained. If no pancreatic abnormality is identified, a direct test of pancreatic function such as secretin-CCK stimulation should be performed. Alternatively, an ERCP may be obtained at this time to establish the radiological presence of "early" disease. If the pancreatic function test is abnormal, a trial of pancreatic extract therapy for 1 or 2 months should be recommended. An H_2 receptor antagonist should be added if satisfactory pain relief is not achieved. The combination of pancreatic extracts and H_2 blockers will provide satisfactory pain relief in the majority of patients with idiopathic chronic pancreatitis and in many patients with alcoholic pancreatitis. If results are unsatisfactory, an ERCP should then be performed to identify an anatomical lesion that might be amenable to endoscopic or surgical treatment. Nonsurgical interventions such as celiac plexus block and complete bowel rest with hyperalimentation have been used with varied success, but these measures are only temporary at best. Figure 36-2 illustrates the approach to pain management outlined above.

Pancreatic Insufficiency

Several treatment options are available once the diagnosis of steatorrhea has been confirmed (Fig. 36-3). Fecal fat losses not exceeding 10 g/d usually require no treatment unless diarrhea becomes troublesome. Larger fecal fat losses invariably require treatment with pancreatic extracts and dietary restriction of fat. Treatment may be unsuccessful because most available commercial preparations contain too few enzymes and may be inactivated by the acid environment of the stomach and duodenum. In this setting the addition of an aluminum-based antacid or H_2 receptor antagonist may be useful. If all of these treatments are unsuccessful, the patient should be further evaluated for the possibility of bacterial overgrowth or mucosal disease. Individuals receiving adequate enzyme replacement should not have azotorrhea or protein malabsorption. If hypoproteinemia or edema develops in this setting, other factors such as protein-losing enteropathy, cirrhosis, or pancreatic ascites should be considered.

Diabetes is common in patients with chronic pancreatitis, and the incidence increases over time with disease progression. Overall, 45% of patients

Figure 36-2. Schematic for management of chronic pancreatitis and pain. (Reprinted with permission from Rowell WG, Toskes PP. Pain of chronic pancreatitis. In Barkin J and Rogers A [eds], *Different Decisions in Digestive Diseases.* Copyright © 1989 by Year Book Medical Publishers, Inc., Chicago.)

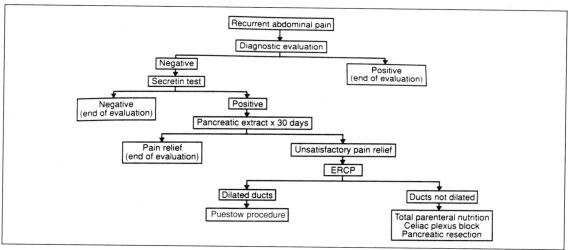

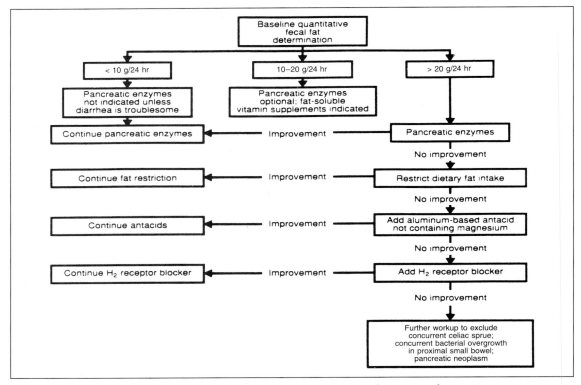

Figure 36-3. Treatment of steatorrhea associated with chronic pancreatitis. (From Greenberger NJ. Chronic pancreatitis and exocrine insufficiency. *Hosp Pract* 1985; 20[1A]:33–45. Used with permission.)

with chronic pancreatitis will develop overt diabetes. The pancreatic form of diabetes is usually mild, and ketoacidosis is extremely rare. Vascular complications of diabetes, including retinopathy, nephropathy, and vasculopathy, are uncommon in patients with chronic pancreatitis. However, neuropathic complications are common because of the additive risks of continued alcohol abuse and malnutrition. Since many patients with alcoholic pancreatitis are noncompliant and unreliable, undertreatment of the diabetic state is preferable to avoid severe hypoglycemic reactions.

Endoscopic Treatment

Patients with debilitating pain that is unresponsive to treatment with pancreatic extracts and a stable dose of narcotic analgesics should undergo ERCP to delineate pancreatic ductal anatomy. Preferably,

this procedure should be done at a center with expertise in therapeutic ERCP. Patients with idiopathic pancreatitis should also undergo sphincter of Oddi manometry. Although the clinical significance of elevated sphincter pressures in the pathogenesis of pancreatitis is unclear, elevated baseline pressures limited solely to the pancreatic portion of the sphincter of Oddi have been demonstrated in selected patients with idiopathic pancreatitis. Most of these reports involve patients with a relapsing clinical course. In patients with pancreas divisum for whom endoscopic ablation of the minor sphincter is performed to improve duct drainage, the likelihood of a favorable outcome correlates with the severity of pancreatic duct pathology at the time of the sphincterotomy. If these data are extrapolated to patients with idiopathic chronic pancreatitis secondary to obstruction at the level of the sphincter of Oddi, endoscopic sphincterotomy would be most likely to benefit patients with radiographic evidence of mild to moderate disease. Since results of endoscopic sphincter ablation may be highly variable in patients with markedly abnormal pancreatograms, these procedures should be referred to centers conducting prospective, randomized trials.

Several endoscopic treatment options are available for patients with chronic pancreatitis. In patients with a normal or minimally abnormal pancreatogram and elevated sphincter of Oddi pressures, endoscopic sphincterotomy of only the biliary portion of the sphincter may yield satisfactory pain relief. If this treatment fails, repeat cannulation of the pancreatic duct, ablation of the pancreatic portion of the sphincter, and placement of a short 5 or 7 French endoprosthesis should be attempted. The stent should remain in place for approximately 2 weeks to ensure adequate pancreatic duct drainage while the sphincterotomy is healing and then should be removed. If the site of the sphincterotomy becomes stenotic over time, surgical sphincteroplasty should be considered.

Stones obstructing the main pancreatic duct can also be treated by endoscopic extraction alone or combined with extracorporeal shock wave lithotripsy (Fig. 36-4). Anatomical factors such as a narrow or tortuous proximal pancreatic duct may complicate access to a pancreatic duct stone and thereby preclude successful extraction. Extracorporeal lithotripsy has been used successfully to clear the biliary tract of retained stones and may be applicable in selected patients with pancreatic duct stones. In one recent series, complete stone clearance was achieved in four of eight patients, all of whom experienced partial relief of pain. In the remaining four patients partial stone clearance was achieved. Unfortunately, relief of symptoms did not always correlate with successful stone extraction. This observation is not surprising, since the pain of chronic pancreatitis is multifactorial and not related solely to pancreatic ductal hypertension.

Endoscopic placement of prosthetic stents across strictures involving the main pancreatic duct is technically feasible in the majority of patients (Fig. 36-5). Some patients require sphincterotomy to facilitate insertion of the endoprosthesis. Although the number of patients treated with this technique is small, preliminary reports suggest that patients presenting with pain and biochemical evidence of pancreatic exocrine reserve (e.g., elevated serum levels of amylase and lipase) respond better than patients presenting with pain alone. It also appears that patients with strictures and distal duct dilatation respond better than patients with strictures alone. Overall, relief of symptoms is achieved

Figure 36-4. Endoscopic retrograde pancreatogram (ERP) in a patient with chronic pancreatitis showing obstruction of the main pancreatic duct by a single, large stone (arrow) and marked distal duct dilatation.

Figure 36-5. Placement of a pancreatic duct stent in a patient with an obstructing pancreatic duct stone resulted in complete amelioration of pain and resolution of hyperamylasemia and hyperlipasemia.

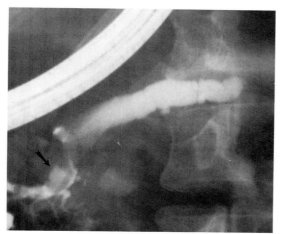

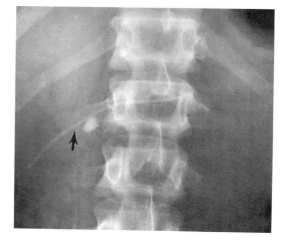

in 60% to 70% of patients. In practice, pancreatic stents are left in place for 3 to 12 months.

Although stent placement unequivocally improves pancreatic duct drainage in properly selected patients, the presence of a stiff endoprosthesis in the pancreatic duct for extended periods of time may lead to ductal abnormalities and even strictures. Follow-up pancreatograms usually show resolution of stent-induced ductal abnormalities, but incomplete resolution of these radiologic findings persists in up to one third of patients. In addition, the relatively narrow caliber of currently available pancreatic duct stents (5 or 7 French) leads to a 50% occlusion rate at 1 month and, in patients with persistent or recurrent symptoms, often necessitates the placement of a new stent. Successful balloon dilation of pancreatic duct strictures has been reported in small series of patients, but long-term results have been disappointing because of restenosis of the pancreatic duct.

Endoscopic therapy of pancreaticobiliary disease is relatively safe, but complication rates of 7% to 10% have been reported. Successful intervention can be achieved in patients with either benign or malignant disease, but complications appear to be more common among patients with underlying malignancy. Acute complications of endoscopic retrograde sphincterotomy include bleeding and pancreatitis, which occur with almost equal frequency, cholangitis, perforation, and entrapment of devices used for stone extraction. The overall mortality rate reported from Europe, the United States, and the United Kingdom is approximately 1.4%.

Treatment of complications is usually successful and does not require surgical intervention. Bleeding can usually be managed by observation or transfusion. Only 15% of patients with bleeding require surgical intervention, and the mortality rate among these patients approaches 60%. Inflammatory or infectious complications can be treated expectantly with bowel rest and antibiotics. When necessary, an endobiliary stent can be inserted to improve biliary drainage in patients with cholangitis. The incidence of perforation approaches 15% in some series and is associated with a mortality rate of 2% to 3%. Up to 50% of patients with perforation require surgical intervention. Patients with a confined perforation limited to the retroperitoneum and no evidence of sepsis can be treated with observation, bowel rest, and antibiotics. However, patients with free intraperitoneal air should undergo surgical exploration along with repair and drainage of the site of perforation.

Endoscopic interventions involving the pancreatic portion of the sphincter of Oddi, the minor pancreatic sphincter, or the pancreatic duct inevitably create unique and interesting problems. Complications reported thus far include stent migration, procedure-induced pancreatitis, duodenal perforation, and occasionally death. Moreover, no incontrovertible evidence suggests that these procedures are beneficial in treating chronic pancreatitis. Endoscopic therapy is reasonable in referral centers with necessary expertise and ancillary support and for patients enrolled in prospective, comparative trials. Clearly, endoscopic and surgical therapy should be reserved for patients with medically intractable pain. Patients with inaccessible strictures, normal-caliber pancreatic ducts, and failed attempts at endoscopic treatment should be referred for surgical management.

Surgical Treatment

The course of chronic pancreatitis is erratic but typically progresses to intractable abdominal pain, inanition, chronic depression, and in many cases chemical dependency. The major metabolic complications of chronic pancreatitis, malabsorption and diabetes mellitus, can usually be treated successfully with medical therapy. Intractable pain ultimately develops in up to 95% of patients and serves as the major indication for surgical intervention in up to one third of patients. Pancreatic pain is frequently difficult to treat, partly because the pathogenesis is not completely understood. For example, among patients with an alcoholic etiology, cessation of alcohol intake may improve the clinical course of the disease by reducing the frequency and severity of painful attacks. However, despite improved symptoms, functional changes persist and progress, albeit at a slower rate. Once established, morphological changes such as duct obstruction, calculi, and fibrosis appear to perpetuate parenchymal damage, regardless of whether the etiologic agents have been withdrawn.

Many medical and endoscopic or surgical treatments are based on the hypothesis that increased pancreatic intraductal pressure leads to pain. Medical efforts are directed at reducing pancreatic secretion, whereas the goal of endoscopic and surgical intervention is to decompress the pancreatic duct. Surgical intervention in chronic pancreatitis is usually reserved for managing complications of the disease (Table 36-3). However, the role and timing of surgery to relieve pain and to preserve pancreatic function are controversial. On the basis of observations that the lesions of chronic pancreatitis are both persistent and progressive, some authorities advocate early intervention to prevent irreversible functional impairment of the pancreas. Others recommend expectant therapy, on the basis of observations by Amman et al. that pain relief is a fairly predictable outcome in patients with progressive disease that ultimately leads to severe pancreatic insufficiency.

SURGICAL OPTIONS

No single surgical procedure is uniformly appropriate for all patients with chronic pancreatitis. The operative strategy should take into account specific alterations in pancreatic morphology and ductal anatomy. Preoperative evaluation should include routine computerized tomography (CT) of the abdomen with fine cuts through the pancreaticobiliary axis and endoscopic retrograde cholangiopancreatography (ERCP). These studies provide different information and should be viewed as complementary. For example, CT may be useful in demonstrating unsuspected complications (e.g., pseudocyst or splenic vein thrombosis) or extrapancreatic pathology that might alter surgical strategy. ERCP clearly demonstrates the main pancreatic duct and its side branches and therefore is indispensable, since the operative approach is frequently dictated by pancreatic ductal anatomy.

Table 36-3. Indications for Surgical Treatment in Chronic Pancreatitis

Pseudocyst
Biliary obstruction
Duodenal obstruction
Pain
Pancreatic fistula
Pancreatic ascites or pleural effusion
Inability to exclude carcinoma

The principal goal of surgical intervention for chronic pancreatitis is to relieve incapacitating pain while preserving pancreatic endocrine and exocrine function whenever possible. Over the past several decades, two surgical strategies have proved most useful for relieving the pain of chronic pancreatitis: duct drainage or decompression and pancreatic resection. As mentioned previously, the choice of procedure is influenced by pancreatic ductal anatomy, the presence or absence of extrapancreatic pathology (duodenal or bile duct obstruction), and the patient's overall condition.

DRAINAGE PROCEDURES

The prototypic drainage procedure is the longitudinal pancreaticojejunostomy, or modified Puestow procedure (Fig. 36-6). This procedure is generally restricted to patients with "large-duct" pancreatitis characterized by marked dilatation (> 7–8 mm) of the main pancreatic duct. The operation consists of unroofing a segment of pancreatic duct and creating an anastomosis to a defunctionalized Roux-en-Y limb of jejunum. To achieve optimal results, one must adhere to several important technical details. Adequate drainage requires unroofing a long (8- to 10-cm) segment of duct and removing intraductal concretions to eliminate foci of smoldering pancreatitis. Failure to establish adequate duct drainage, especially in the head and tail of the pancreas, may lead to an unacceptably high incidence of persistent or recurrent pain. Probe patency of the proximal pancreatic duct should also be demonstrated to improve antegrade drainage of pancreatic secretions. Finally, the intestinal and pancreatic duct mucosa should be carefully apposed to ensure long-term patency of the anastomosis and to reduce the likelihood of late stricture formation.

Duct drainage can be accomplished with low mortality and morbidity and is technically less formidable than extensive pancreatic resection. If adequate drainage is established, significant relief of pain can be anticipated in approximately 80% of patients. Duct drainage preserves islet cell mass and reduces the likelihood of postoperative insulin-requiring diabetes more effectively than extensive distal pancreatic resection, and should be used preferentially when feasible. This goal is especially important in alcoholics, who are not likely to carefully monitor their diet and insulin requirements. De-

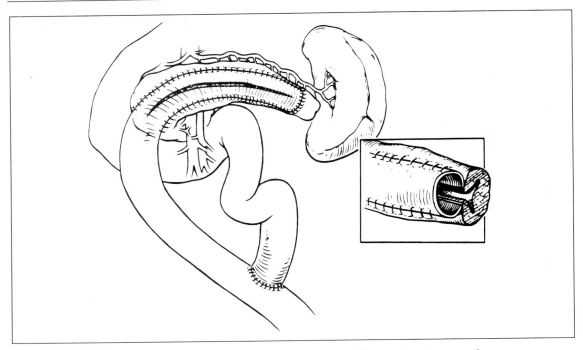

Figure 36-6. Side-to-side pancreaticojejunostomy (Puestow procedure) for complete drainage of
the main pancreatic duct. (From Eckhauser FE, Turcotte JG. Current trends and new developments
in the management of chronic pancreatitis. In Zuidema GD [ed], *Shackleford's Surgery of the Alimentary
Tract.* Philadelphia: Saunders, 1991. P. 38. Used with permission.)

spite acceptable mortality and morbidity and satisfactory pain relief, the progression of pancreatic
endocrine and exocrine insufficiency after pancreaticojejunostomy and a reoperation rate approaching
20% suggest that duct drainage does not appreciably alter the natural history of chronic pancreatitis.

A significant proportion of patients with
chronic pancreatitis who undergo duct drainage
have associated pathology that requires surgical intervention. Clinical, radiological, and biochemical
evidence of biliary tract or duodenal obstruction as
well as unsuspected pseudocysts can be demonstrated in 30%, 15%, and 40% of these patients,
respectively. Inflammation involving the head of
the pancreas typically leads to the development of
a long (2- to 4-cm), tapered stricture involving the
intrapancreatic portion of the common bile duct. In
patients with evidence of fixed obstruction, biliary
drainage can be achieved by creating a choledochoduodenostomy or by extending the Roux-en-Y limb
used to drain the pancreatic duct to create a choledochojejunostomy. In order to prevent hepatobiliary
complications such as stasis stones, cholangitis, or
secondary biliary cirrhosis, these strictures should
be managed surgically even in anicteric and otherwise asymptomatic patients. Synchronous biliary
and pancreatic ductal drainage into the same jejunal
limb has several theoretical disadvantages, including an increased risk of peptic ulceration due to
diversion of bile and pancreatic juice away from
the stomach and the possibility of a combined pancreaticobiliary fistula should the anastomoses break
down. The authors' experience suggests that synchronous decompression of the main pancreatic
duct, the common bile duct, or a coexisting pseudocyst can be accomplished with no increase in
morbidity or mortality.

PANCREATIC RESECTION

Lateral pancreaticojejunostomy is not appropriate
for relieving pain in patients with "small-duct" disease and leads to an unacceptably high failure rate.

In this setting, pancreatic resection yields improved results, but the risks of insulin-requiring diabetes and exocrine insufficiency increase appreciably. The choice of proximal or distal pancreatectomy and the magnitude of the resection are determined primarily by the location and extent of chronic pancreatitis. Although the reported operative risks for pancreatic resection and duct drainage are comparable, extended pancreatic resection is technically formidable and associated with significant metabolic sequelae.

Near-total distal pancreatectomy (NTP) has generally been reserved for management of patients with small-duct disease or recurrent pain following previous duct drainage or more limited pancreatic resection. This procedure removes 80% to 95% of the distal pancreas, leaving in situ a small rim of tissue along the C-loop of the duodenum. One must be careful to identify the intrapancreatic course of the common bile duct to avoid inadvertent bile duct injury. In addition, either the superior or inferior pancreaticoduodenal vessels must be identified and carefully preserved to ensure viability of the duodenum and the remaining pancreas. The authors' experience with 87 patients who underwent NTP for relief of pain associated with chronic pancreatitis indicates an acceptable mortality rate of 2% and a 60% to 75% incidence of postoperative insulin-requiring diabetes. Control of diabetes is acceptable in most patients. However, diabetic complications can adversely affect long-term survival, especially among alcoholic patients. In the authors' series the incidence of late deaths related directly to continued alcohol consumption or diabetes in alcoholic patients was nearly twice that observed in nonalcoholic patients.

Pancreaticoduodenectomy (Whipple resection) has been advocated for treatment of chronic pancreatitis involving primarily the head of the pancreas. Despite the technical difficulty of this procedure and the added complexity of re-establishing biliary, gastric, pancreatic, and intestinal continuity, a Whipple resection can be performed with mortality and morbidity rates of less than 5% and 25% to 30%, respectively. The indications for pancreaticoduodenectomy are summarized in Table 36-4. Preservation of islet tissue in the body and tail of the pancreas usually prevents severe endocrine insufficiency. The 35% incidence of postoperative in-

Table 36-4. Indications for Pancreaticoduodenectomy in Patients with Chronic Pancreatitis

Extensive disease localized to the head of the pancreas with relative sparing of the distal gland

Failure of an earlier duct drainage procedure

Multiple small pseudocysts localized to the head and/or uncinate portions of the pancreas

Symptomatic gastric or biliary obstruction associated with multiple pseudocysts or extensive fibrosis

Hemorrhage from inflammatory aneurysms involving major peripancreatic vessels

Source: Frey CF. Role of subtotal pancreatectomy and pancreaticojejunostomy in chronic pancreatitis. *J Surg Res* 1981; 31:361–371. Used with permission.

sulin-requiring diabetes after a Whipple resection is significantly less than that observed after NTP.

Pancreatic exocrine insufficiency also contributes to early and late morbidity after extensive pancreatic resection and may lead to severe nutritional deficiencies. The severity of postpancreatectomy steatorrhea correlates with the extent of pancreatic resection and may be worsened by associated procedures such as pyloric ablation or distal gastrectomy that alter upper gastrointestinal tract physiology. Steatorrhea after a traditional Whipple resection can usually be controlled with pancreatic exocrine supplements, but postgastrectomy complications such as dumping, diarrhea, and alkaline reflux gastritis or esophagitis are unavoidable. More recently, Traverso and Longmire modified the pancreaticoduodenectomy to include preservation of the pylorus (Fig. 36-7). This procedure is especially appropriate for a benign process such as chronic pancreatitis, since extending the margins and thereby the magnitude of the resection is not necessary. If performed for appropriate indications and in properly selected patients, pancreaticoduodenectomy will yield excellent pain relief in 70% to 80% of patients.

Late failures, defined by recurrence or persistence of pancreatitis and pain, are more common after duct drainage than after resection. Late failures after duct drainage may occur despite radiological evidence of a widely patent pancreaticojejunal anastomosis and usually indicate incomplete drainage of the head or uncinate regions of the pancreas with foci of smoldering pancreatitis. Several alternatives have been proposed to correct this shortcoming,

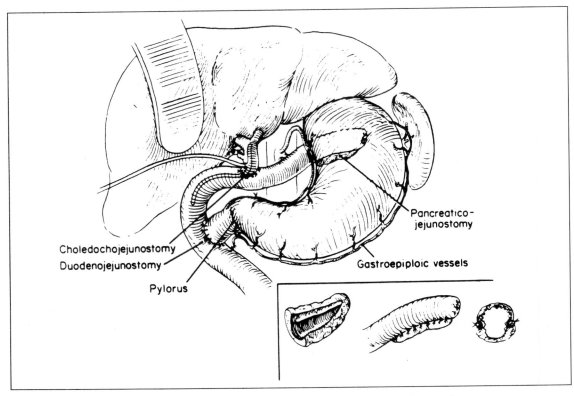

Figure 36-7. Reconstruction of gastrointestinal, biliary and pancreatic continuity after a pylorus-sparing Whipple's resection. (From Traverso LW, Longmire WP. Preservation of the pylorus in pancreatico-duodenectomy: A follow-up evaluation: *Ann Surg* 1980; 192:307. Used with permission.)

including nonanatomical resection of the pancreatic head, leaving the posterior pancreatic capsule and a rim of intact pancreatic tissue along the inner aspect of the duodenal C-loop (Fig. 36-8). The main pancreatic duct and the cored-out head of the pancreas are then drained synchronously into a defunctionalized Roux-en-Y limb of jejunum. Advocates of this "hybrid" procedure anticipate better long-term pain relief than conventional duct drainage and decreased late mortality and morbidity compared to pancreatic resection. To date, limited but promising experience has been reported with this procedure. Pain relief is reported in the majority of patients, but the follow-up period is short, and limited information is available concerning postoperative pancreatic function.

PANCREATIC DENERVATION

Interest in chemical or surgical denervation of the pancreas to control the pain associated with chronic

pancreatitis was originally stimulated by histologic evidence of neuropathology in these patients, but until recently received limited attention. In one neuroanatomical study of the pancreas in patients with chronic pancreatitis, Bockman et al. reported perineural inflammation and destruction of the protective sheath or perineureum that surrounds nerves and protects against potentially noxious agents. This approach is particularly appealing because the disruption of nerve fibers that mediate pancreatic pain should ameliorate symptoms without incurring irreversible changes in pancreatic function.

Anatomical studies of pancreatic innervation indicate that fibers which mediate pain interconnect only through the celiac and superior mesenteric plexuses. Although early reports of surgical splanchnicectomy and celiac ganglionectomy from France were enthusiastic, follow-up studies among patients with diffuse pancreatic fibrosis and no discernible extrapancreatic pathology indicated a 30% late fail-

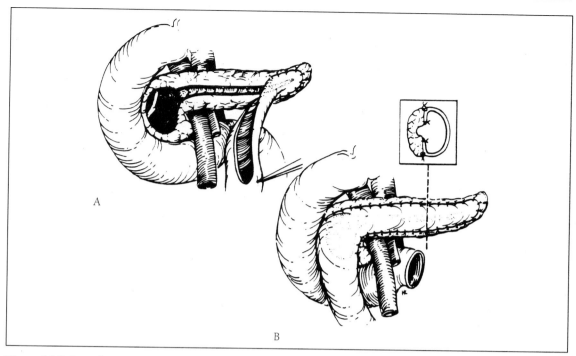

Figure 36-8. Lateral pancreaticojejunostomy with coring out of the pancreatic head. The posterior pancreatic capsule is left intact and care is taken to preserve the intrapancreatic portion of the common bile duct. (From Frey CF, Smith GJ. Description and rationale of a new operation for chronic pancreatitis. *Pancreas* 1987; 2:701–707. Used with permission.)

ure rate. Subsequent efforts to more fully denervate the pancreas have included complete mobilization of the pancreas with resection of all postganglionic nerve plexuses, including those surrounding the splenic and hepatic arteries, and creation of a denervated splenopancreatic "flap" (Fig. 36-9). These procedures are innovative and intriguing in design. Although preliminary results are encouraging, follow-up is short, and the numbers of patients studied are too small to draw any firm conclusions.

ISLET CELL AND SEGMENTAL PANCREATIC AUTOTRANSPLANTATION

Subtotal or total pancreatectomy successfully relieves pain in the majority of patients with chronic pancreatitis, but clinically troublesome insulin-requiring diabetes develops in a significant percentage of patients. Intraportal autotransplantation of islet tissue into the liver has been attempted in selected patients with varying results. Through 1982, 71 patients with chronic pancreatitis who had undergone subtotal pancreatectomy with intraportal islet

cell transplantation were reported to the Human Pancreas and Islet Transplant Registry. Of this group, 33 patients (46%) reportedly had remained insulin-independent indefinitely or for an extended time.

The main obstacles to successful islet cell autotransplantation include insufficient functioning islet cell mass to maintain euglycemia, imperfect methods for isolating and purifying islet cells, and ongoing controversy regarding the most appropriate site and route of islet cell implantation. Fasting normoglycemia is not a good indicator of beta cell reserve, and glucose tolerance testing should be performed to unmask subtle abnormalities in glucose homeostasis. Previous beliefs that islet cell purification was necessary to ensure successful islet cell engraftment have been called into question by experimental evidence in large animals that dispersed autologous pancreatic tissue injected into the spleen or portal vein can prevent the development of diabetes. Limited clinical studies of intraportal autotransplantation of dispersed pancreatic tissue following

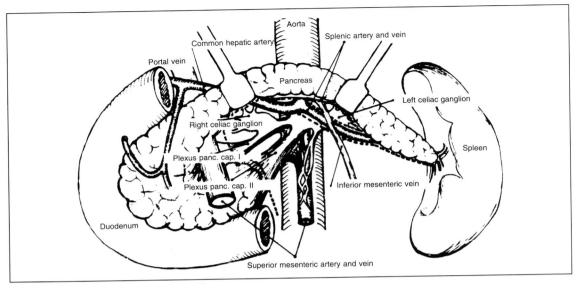

Figure 36-9. General anatomy and plan of operative procedure to extensively denervate the pancreas. The dotted line denotes the limits of the dissection. (From Hiraoka T, et al. A new surgical approach for control of pain in chronic pancreatitis. *Am J Surg* 1986; 152:550. Used with permission.)

pylorus-sparing pancreaticoduodenectomy have demonstrated insulin independence in those individuals receiving more than 100,000 islet cells. These studies show unequivocally that gross exocrine contamination of islet cells does not jeopardize engraftment when the dispersed tissue is distributed into a large, well-vascularized space such as the portal circulation.

Successful segmental autotransplantation of the body and tail of the pancreas was described nearly 15 years ago. Initial trials were complicated by a 20% operative failure rate attributed to in situ vascular thrombosis of the autograft. Other complications related to control of exocrine secretions. Management of the transected pancreas became the subject of considerable controversy because pancreatic fistulas developed in nearly 60% of the reported autotransplant recipients. Efforts to control pancreatic exocrine secretion have included duct ligation, occlusion of the pancreatic duct with synthetic polymers such as neoprene and prolamine (Ethibloc), and internal drainage of the transected pancreas into a defunctionalized Roux-en-Y limb of jejunum. Enteral drainage is physiologically more appealing than the other alternatives, but the number of patients studied is insufficient to draw any

firm conclusions. Prospective, comparative studies of segmental autotransplantation versus intraportal islet cell autotransplantation will be needed to determine which approach is most beneficial for abrogating the long-term endocrine effects of pancreatic resection for chronic pancreatitis.

RECURRENT PAIN AFTER PREVIOUS SURGERY

The patient with chronic pancreatitis who presents with persistent or recurrent pain following a previous operation constitutes one of the most distressing and difficult problems in clinical practice. A comprehensive history should be obtained to determine if the quality and intensity of pain are similar to the quality and intensity experienced prior to the initial surgery. If the nature of the pain has changed significantly, one must consider the possibility of biliary or gastroduodenal pathology and schedule the appropriate diagnostic tests. Prior medical records, including the operative report, should be reviewed whenever possible to determine whether the first operation was "logical" and performed in a technically satisfactory manner and whether the patient had developed a postoperative complication (pancreatic fistula or abscess) that might have compromised the outcome.

One must also consider the possibility of a coexisting carcinoma of the pancreas, especially if the patient presents with recurrent pain and new-onset diabetes. Serological markers such as CA 19-9 are generally too insensitive to reliably discriminate between cancer and chronic pancreatitis, and radiological evidence of pancreatic calcification by no means excludes cancer. Imaging with ultrasound or CT may fail to demonstrate a focus of cancer in a background of chronic pancreatitis. However, a percutaneous pancreatic biopsy may be warranted if imaging studies demonstrate a mass lesion that was absent on previous examinations. The major problem with pancreatic biopsy in this setting is not false-positive findings but false-negative results produced by sampling error. In many cases, extended patient follow-up may be the only reliable method of establishing the correct diagnosis.

In patients with mild to moderate pain that does not require narcotic analgesics, a trial of pancreatic extract therapy is warranted. Reasonable evidence now exists in selected patients with moderate pancreatic insufficiency (no gross steatorrhea) that administration of pancreatic enzyme preparations may decrease abdominal pain by inhibiting exocrine secretion. The presence of abnormal fecal fat excretion may be a good prognostic indicator, since patients with frank steatorrhea do not generally respond to this form of therapy.

Endoscopic retrograde pancreatography (ERP) should be obtained whenever feasible to define pancreatic ductal anatomy. ERP may be difficult or impossible in a patient who has previously undergone anastomosis of the pancreas to a defunctionalized loop of intestine, but the potential benefits justify the added difficulty and risk. If stenosis of a previous pancreaticojejunostomy can be demonstrated, revision may be possible with good results. Disease progression with formation of intraductal calculi or strictures may be amenable to endoscopic therapy alone or combined with extracorporeal shock wave lithotripsy. Unfortunately, patency of a pancreaticojejunal anastomosis does not always ensure long-term pain relief. In one small series, Warshaw documented a 20% incidence of persistent or recurrent pain and progression of pancreatic insufficiency after duct drainage despite ERP evidence of anastomotic patency. This result is not entirely unexpected, since the pathogenesis of pain in chronic pancreatitis is multifactorial.

The most significant dilemma arises in the patient who has undergone previous resection and presents with no radiological evidence of duct dilatation. Limited re-resection is unlikely to be beneficial except for patients with very focal pancreatitis, and near-total (NTP) or total pancreatectomy (TP) is usually necessary in most cases. NTP (80% to 95% distal pancreatectomy) can be performed with a mortality rate of less than 4%, but up to 15% of patients remain narcotic-dependent after the operation and nearly 10% later require completion pancreatectomy for complications of persistent pancreatitis. More importantly, 50% of patients who undergo NTP develop insulin-requiring diabetes, and 40% of late deaths following NTP are directly related to complications related to pancreatic insufficiency or persistent alcoholism.

Total pancreatectomy can also be performed with low mortality following previous surgery for chronic pancreatitis, but severe metabolic sequelae, including malabsorption, diabetes, accelerated fatty infiltration of the liver, and osteopenia, may be difficult to manage. The duodenum and pylorus should be conserved whenever possible to minimize postgastrectomy symptoms and steatorrhea. Pancreatogenic diabetes is characteristically unstable because both of the glucoregulatory hormones insulin and glucagon are absent and because it is associated with frequent episodes of hypoglycemia. Although successful relief of pain is achieved in 50% to 70% of patients, approximately 30% of patients complain of persistent pain and therefore must be classified as "treatment failures." These patients are particularly difficult to manage because the metabolic consequences of total pancreatectomy are irreversible.

Other surgical options should be weighed before recommending near-total or total pancreatectomy. If one is an advocate of resection for "small-duct" disease, intraportal islet cell autotransplantation or segmental pancreatic transplantation should be considered. Intraportal injection of dispersed autologous pancreatic tissue has been performed in a limited number of patients ($n = 27$) at the University of Minnesota since 1977. Eight of the 27 patients (30%) underwent simultaneous pylorus-sparing total pancreatectomy, and of these 8 patients, all 5 who received more than 100,000 islet cells remained insulin-independent. Recent data show that impure islet preparations are capable of successful engraftment as long as a large, well-vascularized space such as the portal circulation is available. Successful islet autotransplantation in chronic pancreatitis will be limited by the volume of functioning islet tissue that can be isolated from glands that are largely replaced with scar tissue.

Similar limitations apply to the use of segmental pancreatic autotransplantation in chronic pancreatitis. This technique consists of removing the body and tail of the pancreas, transplanting it to the upper thigh or retroperitoneum, and anastomosing the splenic artery and vein to either the femoral or iliac artery and vein. The pancreatic duct can be managed either by occlusion with some type of polymer or anastomosis to a defunctionalized loop of intestine. From a technical standpoint, this procedure can now be performed successfully in approximately 80% of patients. Long-term insulin independence for 24 to 54 months has been demonstrated, but the number of patients studied is insufficient to justify drawing any firm conclusions.

Surgical denervation of the pancreas has theoretical appeal since the metabolic consequences of extensive pancreatic resection can be avoided. The results of pancreatic denervation are variable and partly reflect the fact that no single standardized procedure has been described. Limited neurectomy is not likely to provide long-term benefit because the fibers that mediate pain accompany sympathetic fibers which are distributed to multiple plexuses surrounding the hepatic, splenic, and superior mesenteric arteries and their various branches. An extensive neurectomy procedure described by Hiraoko and colleagues (see Fig. 36-9) has been performed successfully in two patients, but the long-term results are not known. Percutaneous celiac ganglion block with phenol or alcohol has been used successfully to treat pain in pancreatic cancer but provides unsatisfactory pain control in chronic pancreatitis. Despite its clinical limitations, celiac ganglion block may be useful in predicting the outcome after surgical neurectomy.

Conclusions

The treatment of chronic pancreatitis must be highly individualized, and no single form of therapy is uniformly appropriate for all patients. Therapeutic decisions should be based on objective information regarding pancreatic function and ductal anatomy and should be tempered by awareness of the potential metabolic consequences of specific interventions. Figure 36-10 is a suggested plan for pain management in chronic pancreatitis. Patients presenting with pain and mild to moderate disease should be treated initially with pancreatic extracts, possibly octreotide and nonnarcotic analgesics. Patients presenting with pain and evidence of pancreatic calcification or steatorrhea have more advanced disease but also warrant a trial of medical therapy. Imaging studies including CT and ERCP should be obtained to define the pancreatic ductal anatomy and to thereby determine whether endoscopic or surgical intervention is feasible. In selected patients with obstructive pancreatitis, endoscopic treatment including sphincterotomy alone or combined with stone extraction, stricture dilation, and temporary stenting should be considered. On occasion, extracorporeal shock wave lithotripsy may be useful in patients with impacted pancreatic ductal stones that prove resistant to conventional extraction techniques.

Patients with extensive large-duct disease, failed attempts at previous endoscopic therapy, and small-duct disease should be considered for surgery. Patients with ERP evidence of large-duct disease should initially undergo duct drainage rather than pancreatic resection to relieve pain and to possibly delay irreversible impairment of pancreatic function. Whipple resection may be indicated in selected patients with disease localized primarily in the head of the pancreas and complicated by biliary or gastric outlet obstruction.

Small-duct disease is a particularly difficult problem. Segmental pancreatic resection may be useful for the occasional patient with focal pancreatitis, but in general more extensive resection is necessary to achieve satisfactory pain relief. The metabolic consequences of near-total or total pancreatectomy are significant and perhaps even prohibitive in patients with alcoholic pancreatitis, in whom continued alcohol intake is associated with increased late mortality. Consequently, this approach should be limited to referral centers with established expertise in segmental pancreatic autotransplantation or intraportal islet autotransplantation done to delay or prevent the onset of diabetes.

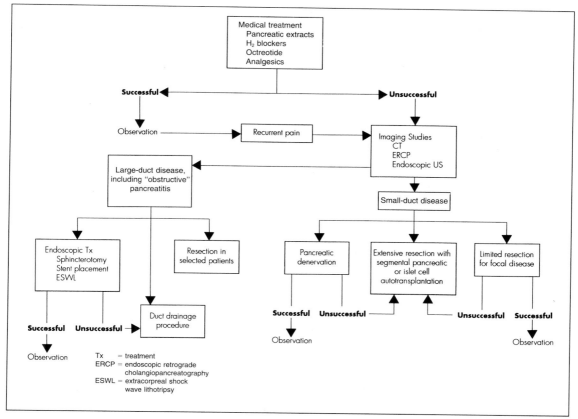

Figure 36-10. Schematic for management of chronic pancreatitis and pain refractory to medical treatment.

Surgical denervation of the pancreas by extensive local neurectomy or transhiatal bilateral splanchnicotomy is appealing because it preserves functioning pancreatic tissue. This option may be especially logical in patients with small-duct disease and continued alcohol intake. However, before this approach is unequivocally embraced, additional work will be necessary to develop a standardized procedure that is technically feasible, effective long-term, and safe. Percutaneous celiac ganglion block yields only short-term relief but may help predict the outcome of neurectomy.

Successful management of chronic pancreatitis requires a comprehensive understanding of pancreatic physiology and anatomy and a willingness to provide extended patient care. Collaboration between gastroenterologists, radiologists, and surgeons interested in this disease is also essential to ensure optimal results. Treatment should never be dictated by a single medical, endoscopic, or surgical strategy but rather should be individualized on the basis of general medical considerations, pancreatic ductal anatomy, functional pancreatic reserve, and the presence of comorbid conditions (e.g., alcoholism) that might adversely influence long-term results.

Selected Readings

Bockman DE, et al. Analysis of nerves in chronic pancreatitis. *Gastroenterology* 1988; 94:1459–1465.

Delhaye M, et al. Extracorporeal shock-wave lithotripsy of pancreatic calculi. *Gastroenterology* 1992; 102: 610–620.

Ebbehoj N, et al. Comparison of regional pancreatic tissue pressure and endoscopic retrograde pancreatographic morphology in chronic pancreatitis. *Scand J Gastroenterol* 1991; 25:756–760.

Eckhauser FE, et al. Near total pancreatectomy for chronic pancreatitis. *Surgery* 1984; 96:599–606.

Farney AC, et al. Autotransplantation of dispersed pancreatic islet tissue combined with total or near-total pancreatectomy for treatment of chronic pancreatitis. *Surgery* 1991; 110:427–439.

Hiraoka T, et al. A new surgical approach for control of pain in chronic pancreatitis. *Am J Surg* 1986; 152: 550–553.

Nealon WH, Thompson JC. Progressive loss of pancreatic function in chronic pancreatitis is delayed by main pancreatic duct decompression. *Ann Surg* 1993; 217:458–468.

Owyang C, Lowie DA, Tatum D. Feedback regulation of pancreatic enzyme secretion: Suppression of CCK release by trypsin. *J Clin Invest* 1986; 77: 2042–2047.

Sarles H, et al. Renaming pancreatic stone protein as "lithostatine." *Gastroenterology* 1990; 99:990–905.

Singh S, Reber HA. The pathology of chronic pancreatitis. *World J Surg* 1990; 14:2–10.

37

Pancreatic Fistulas

Richard A. Kozarek
L. William Traverso

Etiology and Pathogenesis

Etiologically, pancreatic fistulas are the consequence of pancreatic duct disruption and have classically been divided into internal and external fistulas (Table 37-1). Internal fistulas may be intra-abdominal and present most commonly as pseudocysts (discussed in detail in Chapter 31) and occasionally as pancreatic ascites or pancreaticoenteric fistulas. Alternatively, they may present as a mediastinal pseudocyst or pancreaticopleural communication. The latter is most commonly associated with chronic and often massive pleural effusion and occasionally with a pancreaticobronchial fistula. External fistulas, in turn, by definition communicate with the skin and as such are almost invariably iatrogenic or associated with penetrating trauma.

The pathogenesis of internal fistulas is usually felt to be inflammatory. This inflammation often involves a primary duct radical with consequent proximal duct stricture and obstruction, distal duct hypertension, and subsequent rupture, which releases pancreatic juice and enzymes into pancreatic and peripancreatic tissue. When pancreatic juice ruptures anteriorly, it does so at the junction of the body and head (genu) or at the tail of the gland. A direct communication can occur with contiguous bowel, resulting in a pancreaticoenteric fistula. More commonly, free rupture into the lesser sac occurs, forming a pseudocyst. If the lesser sac does not contain the fluid, pancreatic ascites results. Rupture into the retroperitoneal space, in turn, may track through the aortic or esophageal hiatus and, if contained, is associated with a mediastinal pseu-

docyst. Often, however, secretions rupture into one or both pleural cavities, causing chronic pleural effusions or an occasional pancreaticobronchial fistula. In several series, many of the patients who develop thoracic manifestations of internal fistulas have a history of previous or active pulmonary tuberculosis, suggesting that pre-existing lung disease may increase the risk of pancreaticopleural communication. External fistulas, in turn, have been associated with penetrating injury to the pancreas, including that caused by percutaneous biopsy. More frequently, external fistulas are the consequence of gastric or pancreaticobiliary surgery, and an incidence approaching 20% has been claimed with extensive pancreatic resection. Alternatively, external fistulas may be the consequence of percutaneous drainage procedures, especially in the setting of infected necrosis or ongoing ductal obstruction associated with a pseudocyst. Table 37-2 outlines the various etiologies that have been associated with internal and external pancreatic fistulas.

Diagnosis

An external pancreatic fistula is not difficult to diagnose (Fig. 37-1). Occurring in the setting of recent pancreatic surgery or percutaneous drainage of a pseudocyst, or following abdominal trauma, these fistulas usually have an amylase concentration in the thousands and put out a variable volume contingent on the site and presence of upstream obstruction. Approximately one third of these patients have concomitant infectious complications of their fistu-

Table 37-1. Types of Pancreatic Fistulas

Internal
    Abdominal: Pseudocyst
                  Pancreatic ascites
                  Pancreaticoenteric communication
    Thoracic: Pseudocyst
                Pleural effusion
                Pancreaticobronchial communication
External
    Pancreaticocutaneous

Table 37-2. Etiology of Pancreatic Fistulas

Internal
    Chronic pancreatitis (usually alcoholic)
    Trauma
        Blunt
        Surgical
        Needle aspiration of pancreas
    Neoplasm
    Acute pancreatitis
    Miscellaneous
        Papillary stenosis
        Duplication cyst
External
    Trauma
        Surgical resection
        Penetrating injury
        Percutaneous drainage of pancreatic fluid collections

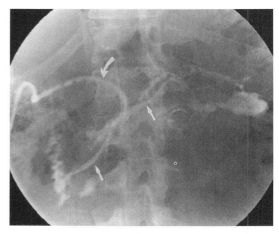

Figure 37-1. Large arrow depicts percutaneous tube communicating with pancreatic duct (small arrows). Note filling of irregular cystic cavity.

Table 37-3. Symptoms and Signs of Pancreatic Fistulas

Internal
    Subdiaphragmatic
        Weight loss
        Increased girth (ascites)
        Abdominal pain
    Supradiaphragmatic
        Cough
        Shortness of breath (pleural effusion)
        Pleuritic pain
        Recurrent pneumonitis
External
    High-amylase fistual ± fistulous tract infection/bleeding

Table 37-4. Diagnostic Modalities for Pancreatic Fistulas

Internal
    Abdominal
        CT/US: pseudocyst, dilated pancreatic duct, ductal calculi
        ERCP: ductal disruption site, ductal obstruction
        Ascites analysis: high amylase, albumin > 3 g/dl
    Chest
        CT: pseudocyst, pleural effusion
        ERCP: ductal disruption, pseudocyst, obstruction
        Thoracentesis: high amylase

las which may be clinically manifested as fever, tachycardia, and progressive abdominal pain and ileus.

Internal pancreatic fistulas, in turn, can be subtle, and signs and symptoms are contingent on presentation above or below the diaphragm (Table 37-3). In the largest series to date, Lipsett and Cameron reviewed 50 internal pancreatic fistula patients seen at Johns Hopkins from 1963 to 1990. Thirty-four presented with pancreatic ascites, 9 with pancreatic pleural effusion, and 7 with both. Patients with ascites complained of abdominal distention, discomfort, and weight loss. Approximately one half had a previous history of pancreatitis, and a small subset had extremity lesions resembling erythema nodosum. Patients with pancreaticopleural fistulas, in turn, had variable degrees of cough, chest pain, and dyspnea.

The diagnosis of an internal fistula presupposes a high amylase content in ascitic or pleural fluid (Table 37-4). The level of serum amylase is often elevated as well, and is usually related to enzyme diffusion across the peritoneal or pleural surface. Ascitic fluid albumin is usually more than 3 g/dl, a feature that helps to distinguish pancreatic from cirrhotic ascites.

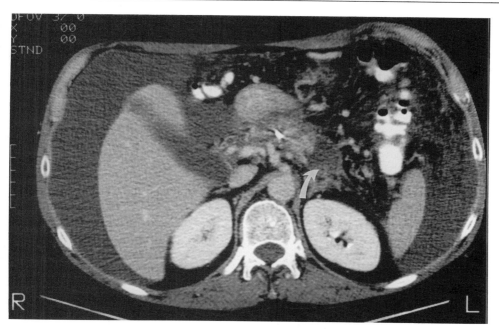

Figure 37-2. Arrow depicts leaking pseudocyst in patient with pancreatic ascites. Note perihepatic and perisplenic fluid accumulation.

Radiographic studies may show nonspecific changes such as the ground glass appearance of ascites or unilateral or bilateral pleural effusions. The latter can be massive. Abdominal imaging modalities are often nonspecific (see Table 37-4). Abdominal ultrasound or CT (Fig. 37-2) may not demonstrate the site of disruption but may demonstrate ductal dilatation, pseudocyst, or calcifications in up to 80% of patients. Endoscopic retrograde cholangiopancreatography (ERCP) is essential in both diagnosing and managing pancreatic fistulas. Findings may include delineation of the site of duct disruption (usually the main pancreatic duct), as well as factors precluding response to conservative therapy, such as obstructing proximal calculi, strictures, or frank ductal discontinuity.

Internal pancreaticoenteric fistulas, in contrast, are often a natural consequence of spontaneous pseudocyst decompression or the result of a percutaneously placed tube eroding into a contiguous loop of bowel. One may help the latter resolve simply by removing the catheter or switching to a smaller diameter, more compliant tubing.

Management

Options

The management of pancreatic fistulas is contingent not only on whether the fistula is internal or external but also on the site of ductal disruption and whether proximal ductal obstruction is present. Classical treatment depends on proper diagnosis and minimization of pancreatic secretion. This goal has been achieved by restricting the patient to clear liquids or nothing orally (NPO) in conjunction with total parenteral hyperalimentation (TPN) (Table 37-5). In addition, attempts to appose leaking mucosa (serosal apposition) have been recommended, and such therapy may include multiple paracenteses or thoracenteses or even placement of an indwelling chest tube. Historically, attempts to further minimize pancreatic secretion have included the use of atropine or acetazolamide (Diamox), but more recent studies have used somatostatin analogs such as octreotide (Sandostatin). Those who fail medical therapy have conventionally undergone surgery, including pancreatic re-

Table 37-5. Management of Pancreatic Fistulas

Reduction of pancreatic secretion
   NPO or clear liquids
   Hyperalimentation
   Octreotide
Correction of ductal disruption
   Endoscopic prosthesis
   Surgery
      Resection
      Pancreaticoenteric anastomosis
Treatment of complications
   Bleeding
   Infection

section, bypass therapy, or Roux-en-Y cystojejunostomy.

Controversies

In contrast to the conventional approach, the physicians at Virginia Mason Medical Center have become increasingly convinced that the placement of transpapillary endoprostheses can speed fistula closure, precluding the need for surgery in a patient subset or converting an urgent surgical situation into an elective one. Internal endoprostheses may function simply to bypass a proximal stricture or stone and can occasionally "plug" a main ductal disruption. More likely, however, they work by bypassing the pancreatic component of the sphincter of Oddi, thereby converting the pancreatic duct into a low-pressure system. They are of little use in frank ductal transection or in the "discontinuous" pancreas occasionally seen with a long-standing pseudocyst.

Preferred Method

INTERNAL FISTULA

The approach to internal pancreatic fistulas depends on making an accurate diagnosis and on delineating pancreatic ductal anatomy. For pancreatic ascites and chronic pleural effusions, the diagnosis requires a high amylase concentration in aspirated fluid and abdominal and/or chest CT imaging to determine the presence or absence of an associated pseudocyst.

Once a diagnosis has been confirmed, pancreatic secretion should be minimized. The patient may be put on a low-fat diet in conjunction with high-dose pancreatic enzyme replacement, on clear liquids, or on NPO in conjunction with hyperalimentation and possibly octreotide. Traditionally, medical therapy has usually been continued for 2 to 3 weeks before surgical intervention is felt to be warranted. Traditional therapy in the authors' institution, however, has evolved into early diagnostic pancreatography following antibiotic coverage, both to delineate ductal anatomy and to define an anatomy amenable to a conservative or endoscopic approach. Patients with an intact duct and a defined site of ductal rupture undergo transpapillary stent placement to bridge the site of ductal disruption (Fig. 37-3), a single large-volume paracentesis or thoracentesis, and, if there is a significant pseudocyst present, subsequent percutaneous drainage of the latter. Patients are rapidly refed (within 48 hours) contingent upon their reaccumulation of fluid as determined by chest x-ray, ultrasound, abdominal girth measurements, percutaneous catheter output, or a combination of the foregoing.

ERCP has the ability not only to diagnose and treat patients with an amenable anatomy but also to identify patients who are unlikely to respond to conservative management. Individuals with complete ductal occlusion or transection (Fig. 37-4), as well as those with the occasional malignant internal fistula, are unlikely to respond to a reduction in pancreatic stimulation and to heal their fistulas spontaneously. Hyperalimentation in this group should be limited to improving nutrition for early operative intervention. This intervention may include distal or proximal gland resection contingent on the site of the leak, cystogastrostomy, or Roux-en-Y cystoenterostomy if a mature pseudocyst is present.

Internal pancreaticoenteric fistulas into the stomach, duodenum, or jejunum, may require no intervention and are the mechanism by which pseudocysts "spontaneously" resolve. Pancreaticoenteric fistulas following percutaneous drainage of fluid collections seem to be primarily a consequence of tube erosion into contiguous gut, particularly in the setting of peripancreatic necrosis. Treatment may require conversion to a smaller diameter, more pliable catheter, catheter removal, transpapillary endoprosthesis placement (Fig. 37-5), or surgical debridement and resection. Pancreaticocolic fistulas

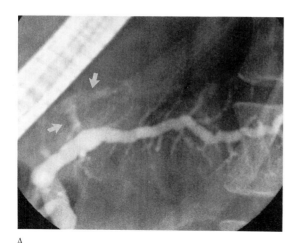

A

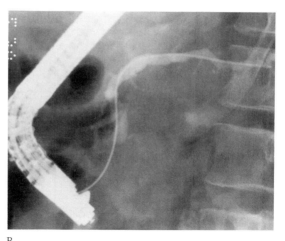

B

Figure 37-3. A. Arrows depict site of ductal disruption at endoscopic pancreatography in patient with pancreatic ascites. B. Guidewire placement to midbody of pancreatic duct. C. 7 French pancreatic duct stent inserted beyond site of ductal disruption.

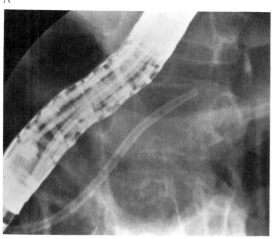

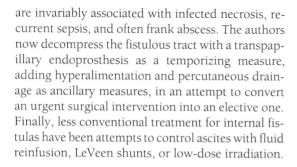

C

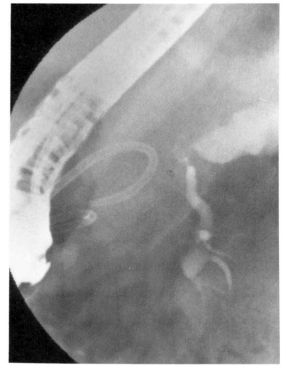

are invariably associated with infected necrosis, recurrent sepsis, and often frank abscess. The authors now decompress the fistulous tract with a transpapillary endoprosthesis as a temporizing measure, adding hyperalimentation and percutaneous drainage as ancillary measures, in an attempt to convert an urgent surgical intervention into an elective one. Finally, less conventional treatment for internal fistulas have been attempts to control ascites with fluid reinfusion, LeVeen shunts, or low-dose irradiation.

EXTERNAL FISTULA

Most external fistulas are the consequence of surgery or percutaneous pseudocyst drainage and less commonly the result of trauma or neoplasia (percu-

Figure 37-4. ERCP depicting complete ductal disruption with pseudocyst. Pigtail catheters are noted in additional fluid collections.

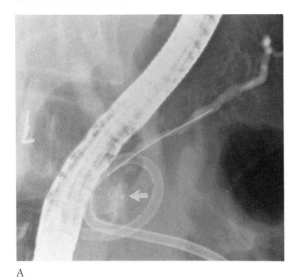

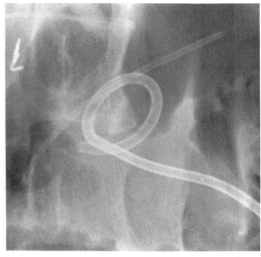

A   B

Figure 37-5. A. ERCP depicting nitinol wire in pancreatic duct in patient with chronic fistula resulting from pseudocyst drainage. Note pigtail catheter and extravasation (arrow) from head of pancreas. B. A 7 French pancreatic duct stent allowed for removal of the percutaneous catheter within 1 week.

taneous needle biopsy). Treatment is contingent on a number of factors, including the volume of output, the presence of ductal discontinuity, or a proximal obstruction related to a stricture or stone, and on whether bacterial tissue necrosis supervenes. Most low-volume fistulas that are unassociated with obstruction or infection heal spontaneously even if the patient is fed (low-fat diet and high-dose pancreatic enzyme supplementation). Treatment consists of replacing a large-diameter pigtail catheter with a soft, straight catheter of 8 to 10 French diameter. Most of these fistulas will spontaneously close, and the catheters can be retrieved when only 10 to 15 ml of fluid are drained daily and ultrasound confirms no residual pseudocyst cavity. The absence of ongoing ductal communication radiographically or a low amylase content in the drain output is reassuring, but these signs do not preclude fistula closure if the ductal anatomy is normal.

Patients with a high-volume fistula usually have ductal transection or proximal obstruction. Traditionally, such patients have been placed NPO and hyperalimented; more recently, they have received variable doses of octreotide (50–300 mcg SQ q8h) in an attempt to decrease pancreatic stimulation and allow healing. Whereas the latter treatment methods are still considered the treatments of choice for most postoperative and many post-traumatic fistulas, transpapillary stenting may shorten the treatment time dramatically in those patients with proximal stenoses. Moreover, direct pancreatography, either percutaneously or by means of ERCP, may select patients who are unlikely to respond to medical treatment and should then be considered for early surgical intervention.

Results

Internal Fistula

Bowel rest and hyperalimentation. in conjunction with repeated thoracenteses or paracenteses have been associated with successful therapy in approximately one half of patients with internal fistulas. For instance, in the Hopkins series, 34 patients had ascites, 9 had pleural effusion, and 7 had both. Conservative management was successful in 21 of 42 patients, and 71% (15 of 21) were discharged within 2 weeks of admission. Five deaths occurred in the medically managed group, all in patients managed conservatively for more than 3 weeks. Uchigama et al. compiled 37 cases of pancreatic ascites from the Japanese literature. Twelve were healed with conservative measures alone, and 18 required surgery. Seven poor-risk patients were treated with external drainage alone.

The recent addition of octreotide to the therapeutic armamentarium may improve the percentage of patients responding to medical management as well as accelerate healing in selected patients. For instance, Parekh and Segal defined 23 patients with pancreatic ascites or effusions, 10 of whom healed with medical therapy after a mean of 30 ± 2 days. Five additional patients (3 ascites, 2 effusion) subsequently responded to octreotide. These authors correlated healing with ductal anatomy as delineated by ERCP. Whereas 9 of 11 patients with mild to moderate chronic pancreatitis responded to conservative therapy, only 1 of 10 patients with severe chronic pancreatitis responded. In the present authors' experience, octreotide has been invariably unsuccessful when treating patients with end pancreatic fistulas or those in whom necrosis has resulted in isolated pancreatic segments.

Traditionally, surgical therapy has been limited to patients who have failed several weeks of medical therapy. Using bypass or resective therapy, Lipsett and Cameron operated on 24 of 50 patients with internal fistulas. One surgical failure and 2 deaths (8.3%) occurred in this series. These authors as well as others feel strongly that the type and timing of surgery should be dictated by pancreatography, and recurrence rates of up to 50% have been noted when surgery has been undertaken without ERCP or operative pancreatography. Recurrence rates of 15% have been reported with or without surgery, and mortality rates for both medical and surgical management of internal fistulas range from 15% to 25%.

Because of these facts and because of previous experience in draining pseudocysts by means of transpapillary endoprostheses, it was logical to attempt similar therapy in pancreatic ascites and effusions. To date, the authors have stented disrupted ducts in four patients with pancreatic ascites and in two with effusions. Transpapillary stents were placed in all patients and pleural effusions and ascites were percutaneously drained under ultrasound control. All patients were fed a low-fat diet within 3 days, were discharged within a week, and resolved their fluid accumulations without compli-

cation. Stents were retrieved at a mean of 4 weeks, and ascites and effusion had not recurred at a mean follow-up of 14 months. Likewise, treatment of internal pancreaticoenteric fistulas may require transpapillary stenting. For instance, of eight patients with pancreaticoduodenal (five) or pancreaticocolonic fistulas (three), three healed following the removal of a percutaneous drainage catheter, three healed following transpapillary endoprosthesis placement, and two required surgery.

External Fistula

PREVENTION

Since a 12% external fistula rate has been claimed by some authors following a Whipple's resection, and since a higher fistula rate has been noted by others after acute surgery for penetrating pancreatic trauma, many surgeons feel that measures to prevent fistulas may be more important than steps to treat a fistula once it has developed. Most surgeons concur with the need for Jackson-Pratt drainage after a major pancreatic resection. Others use a modified pancreaticojejunal anastomosis, fibrin glue, or octreotide. In a recent randomized, double-blind, placebo-controlled trial of 246 German patients undergoing major pancreatic resection, patients received either placebo or 100 mcg of octreotide SQ three times daily for 7 days perioperatively. The complication rate was 32% in patients receiving octreotide and 55% in placebo-treated patients, primarily as a result of decreased anastomotic leak in high-risk patients.

TREATMENT

The conventional medical therapy for external fistulas depends in large part on the etiology of the fistula, the output of the fistula, and the presence or absence of bacterial infection. For instance, using TPN and NPO status, Martin and her colleagues attempted the medical management of 35 patients with pancreatic fistulas (external 26, internal 9). All but 5 patients required surgical intervention. An overall operative success rate of 83% was noted, with 1 postoperative death (3%). In contrast, Saari et al. reported on 19 patients with external fistulas. Fourteen of these patients had necrotizing or chronic pancreatitis, and all were treated with hyperalimentation and constant infusion with octreotide. Sixty-eight percent of the patients (13 of 19) closed their fistula in a median treatment time of 7 days (range 2–14 days). Only 1 of 6 patients with an obstructed duct healed, but all patients without bacterial contamination of the tract were successfully managed with medical therapy. In addition to parenteral hyperalimentation and octreotide, some evidence suggests that high-dose pancreatic enzyme supplementation may further speed the healing of external pancreatic fistulas. For instance, Garcia-Pugés et al. have reported 5 patients with external pancreatic fistulas in whom fistula flow and trypsin output were dramatically reduced after enzyme initiation. All fistulas closed between 1 and 12 days.

Conclusions

Internal and external pancreatic fistulas presuppose a ductal disruption as a consequence of acute or chronic pancreatitis, penetrating or surgical trauma, or rarely, obstructing neoplasm. Treatment results and the need for eventual surgical intervention are contingent upon the etiology, the site of ductal disruption (main duct vs. side branch), the presence of duct discontinuity or proximal obstruction, and the presence or absence of bacterial contamination or infection. Whereas the surgical bypass or resective approaches to pancreatic fistulas have remained defined over the years, octreotide,

percutaneous drainage techniques, and transpapillary stents or drains have dramatically changed the medical approaches to these problems.

Selected Readings

Büchler M, et al. Role of octreotide in the prevention of postoperative complications following pancreatic resection. *Am J Surg* 1992;163:125–131.

Eckhauser F, et al. Surgical management of pancreatic ascites, and pancreaticopleural fistulas. *Pancreas* 1991;6:S66–S75.

Garcia-Pugés AM, et al. Oral pancreatic enzymes accelerate closure of external pancreatic fistulas. *Br J Surg* 1988;75:824–825.

Kozarek RA, et al. Endoscopic transpapillary therapy for disrupted pancreatic duct and peripancreatic fluid collections. *Gastroenterology* 1991;100:1362–1370.

Lansden FT, Adams DB, Anderson MC. Treatment of external pancreatic fistulas with somatostatin. *Am Surg* 1989;55:695–698.

Lipsett PA, Cameron JL. Internal pancreatic fistulas. *Am J Surg* 1992;163:216–220.

Maki HS, Kolts RL, Kuehner ME. Prevention of pancreatic fistula by modified pancreaticojejunal anastomosis. *Am J Surg* 1990;160:533–534.

Parekh D, Segal I. Pancreatic ascites and effusion. Risk factors for failure of conservative therapy and the role of octreotide. *Arch Surg* 1992;127:707–712.

Szentes MJ, et al. Invasive treatment of pancreatic fluid collections with surgical and nonsurgical methods. *Am J Surg* 1991;161:600–605.

Torres AJ, et al. Somatostatin in the management of gastrointestinal fistulas. *Arch Surg* 1992;127:97–100.

38

Pancreatic Trauma

Jake Krige
Philippus C. Bornman
Steven J. Beningfield
Ivor C. Funnell

Pancreatic injuries are best managed by early diagnosis and an accurate definition of the nature and extent of injury. Both are necessary for planning the optimal surgical strategy. Failure to accomplish these fundamental goals may result in serious sequelae if the injury is underestimated or inappropriately treated. The management of combined injuries to the pancreas and duodenum may be complex, especially if there is devitalized tissue and associated damage to contiguous to vital structures such as the bile duct, portal vein, vena cava, aorta, and colon. Major complications, including pancreatic fistula, pseudocyst, abscess, or hemorrhage, develop in one third of surviving patients. The gravity of major pancreatic injuries and the potentially serious complications necessitate a comprehensive and multidisciplinary approach.

Etiology and Classification

Trauma to the pancreas is uncommon, accounting for 1% to 4% of severe abdominal injuries. Recent data, however, indicate an increasing incidence of pancreatic trauma as a result of more frequent high-speed automobile accidents and an escalation in civil violence associated with increasingly dangerous weapons. Not surprisingly, these injuries occur predominantly to young men. In North American cities, penetrating abdominal injuries from gunshot wounds are the most common cause of pancreatic trauma, whereas in Western Europe and the United Kingdom the cause is usually road traffic accidents. This geographical difference in etiology results in considerable variation in the reported incidence and severity of pancreatic injury.

Associated Injuries

Isolated injuries to the pancreas are infrequent, with the incidence of associated injuries ranging from 50% to 90%. The mean number of organs injured in the same patient is 3.5. These associated injuries cause most of the morbidity and mortality linked with pancreatic trauma. The organs most commonly injured are the liver (42%), stomach (40%), major vessels (35%), thorax (31%), colon and small bowel (29%), central nervous system, skeleton, and extremities (25%), and duodenum (18%). Colonic injuries are more common after penetrating than blunt trauma and are associated with an increased incidence of postoperative sepsis. Penetrating injuries also result in damage to retroperitoneal vessels in one third of all cases.

Mechanism of Injury

The unique anatomic features of the pancreas influence the site and type of injury. The proximity to major vascular structures and surrounding viscera adds to the complexity of the injuries. The leakage of pancreatic exocrine secretions with duct disruption exacerbates the mechanical effects of pancreatic injury, causing surrounding edema and tissue necrosis.

Damage to the pancreas is caused by either penetrating or blunt trauma. The nature and consequence of penetrating injuries depend on the type and kinetic energy of the wounding force. Simple lacerations of the pancreas are usually the result of stab wounds, which also often injure surrounding vessels or bowel. Penetrating injuries with adjacent contusions occur in single-fragment missile wounds, and severe fragmentation occurs with shotgun wounds. High-velocity missiles produce devastating and often lethal abdominal injuries.

Blunt trauma to the pancreas and duodenum is usually the result of a direct blow to the upper abdomen caused by assault, pedestrian road traffic accidents, or torso deceleration against unyielding surfaces or steering wheels, as occurs with unrestrained drivers or passengers without seat belts.

Handlebars may inflict similar injuries to motorcyclists. In children, blunt traumas due to bicycle handlebars, falls, and car accidents are most commonly encountered.

The mechanism of injury in blunt trauma relates to the direction of the impact force and the retroperitoneal location of the pancreas closely applied to the lumbar spine. Blunt upper abdominal midline trauma results in posterior compression of the anterior abdominal wall against the spine, with injury to the pancreas over or to the left of the portal vein and superior mesenteric vessels (Fig. 38-1). Impact forces concentrated to the right produce crush injuries of the pancreatic head and duodenum against the spine. Serious associated injuries, include liver lacerations and avulsions of the common bile duct and gastroduodenal, right, and middle colic vessels, compounding the effect of the pancreatic trauma. Blunt injury to the left of the vertebrae results in damage to the pancreatic tail and spleen. In view of the difficulties in clinical diagnosis, a high index of suspicion is essential when a history of these forms of injury is obtained.

Classification of Injuries

Comparisons between various forms of treatment are often difficult to interpret because isolated pancreatic injuries are infrequent, experience in most centers is limited, and no universally acceptable injury classification system is available. Several classifications have been applied to pancreatic injuries.

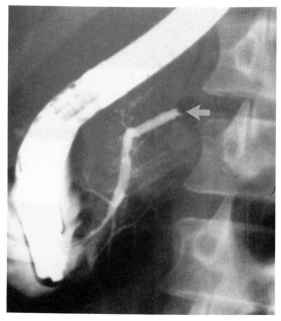

Figure 38-1. ERCP showing pancreatic duct cutoff (arrow) in the neck after blunt trauma.

The system proposed by Lucas is the most widely used (Fig. 38-2):

Class I. Simple superficial contusion or peripheral laceration with minimal parenchymal damage. Any portion of the pancreas can be affected, but the main pancreatic duct is intact.

Class II. Deep laceration, perforation, or transection of the neck, body, or tail of the pancreas with or without pancreatic duct injury.

Class III. Severe crush, perforation, or transection of the head of the pancreas with or without duct injury.

Class IV. Combined pancreaticoduodenal injuries, subdivided into the following:
a. Minor pancreatic injury
b. Severe pancreatic injury and duct disruption.

Diagnosis

The retroperitoneal location of the pancreas contributes to the delay in diagnosis because clinical signs may be subtle and late in onset. Blunt trauma to the pancreas may be clinically occult, and parenchymal

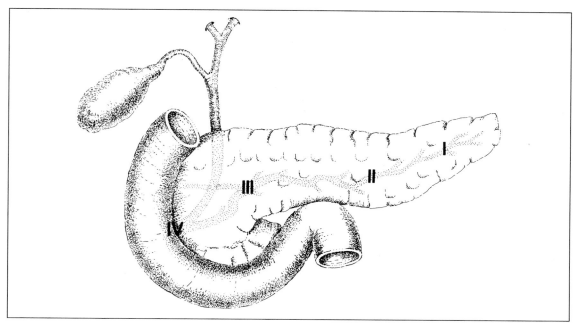

Figure 38-2. Site and severity classification of pancreatic injuries. Class I: contusion, peripheral laceration, intact duct; II: distal laceration, transection, possible ductal disruption, no duodenal injury; III: proximal laceration, transection, suspected ductal injury, no duodenal injury; IV: severe combined pancreaticoduodenal injury. (Reprinted with permission from Lucas CE. Diagnosis and treatment of pancreatic and duodenal injury. *Surg Clin North Am* 1977; 57:49.)

and duct injury may go unrecognized during the initial evaluation or during surgery. Awareness of these factors and recognition of the mechanism of injury should lead to a high index of suspicion. Delay in diagnosis and intervention is the most important cause of increased morbidity and mortality. Where there is concern over the stable patient without clinical signs of intra-abdominal bleeding or peritoneal irritation, careful repeated clinical evaluation, measurement of serum amylase levels, and early imaging of the pancreas are necessary.

Amylase

Serum amylase levels correlate poorly with the presence or absence of pancreatic trauma. Amylase levels may be normal in severe pancreatic damage or may be elevated when no demonstrable injury to the gland has occurred. Measuring serum isoamylase levels has also yielded disappointing results. The incidence of hyperamylasemia in patients with proven blunt pancreatic trauma ranges from 25% to 75%. In patients with hyperamylasemia after blunt abdominal trauma, the pancreas has been found to be injured in 10% to 90% of patients.

Serum amylase levels are equally unhelpful in penetrating injury to the pancreas. Any perforation of the duodenum or upper gastrointestinal tract may produce an elevated serum amylase concentration due to absorption of intraluminal amylase following leakage into the peritoneal cavity. Increased levels of amylase in diagnostic peritoneal lavage fluid has been suggested as a measure for evaluating pancreatic injury. Current data indicate that levels of amylase in lavage fluid over 100 IU/liter correlate with the presence of abdominal injury but are not specific for pancreatic injury. Therefore, although an elevated amylase level is not a reliable indicator of pancreatic injury, it should initiate further investigations.

Imaging

PLAIN RADIOGRAPH

A plain radiograph of the abdomen may raise the suspicion of pancreatic trauma, especially when associated with duodenal trauma. Gas bubbles in the retroperitoneum, adjacent to the right psoas muscle, around the kidneys, or anterior to the upper lumbar vertebrae seen on frontal or cross-table radiographs may indicate duodenal injury. Free intraperitoneal gas may also be seen. Fractures of the transverse processes of the lumbar vertebrae are evidence of forceful retroperitoneal trauma. Other indirect signs of pancreatic injury are displacement of the stomach or transverse colon and a general "ground glass" appearance. A meglumine diatrizoate (Gastrografin) meal may demonstrate a duodenal leak with or without distortion of the duodenal C-loop.

COMPUTERIZED TOMOGRAPHY

Computerized tomography (CT) is uniquely suited to the evaluation of pancreatic trauma. The main indications for CT are in hemodynamically stable patients with abdominal pain or tenderness after trauma who have suspected pancreatic injury (Fig. 38-3) and in those with late complications of pancreatic trauma. Dynamic incremental bolus CT provides the optimal contrast enhancement of the pancreas necessary to identify subtle fractures. Pancreatic injuries are diagnosed on the basis of pancreatic lacerations or on evidence of posttraumatic pancreatitis. Pancreatic lacerations may be

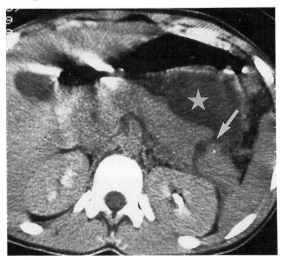

Figure 38-3. CT showing pancreatic fracture (arrow) through the tail with an anterior fluid collection (star).

seen as linear, wedge-shaped, or irregular low-density areas traversing the gland.

Important limitations and difficulties exist with the CT evaluation of pancreatic injuries. Pancreatic lacerations may be too small or poorly demonstrated to detect. Complete pancreatic transection may misleadingly appear as minimal separation on CT. The timing of CT scanning in pancreatic trauma is important. False-negative scans are more likely if performed within 12 hours of trauma. Early blunt pancreatic injury may be overlooked because lacerations and fractures of the pancreas may initially only have minor changes in density with minimal separation of parenchyma at the site of the injury. The hematoma may mask the injury by obscuring lacerations or may appear as a focal high-density mass.

Pancreatic injuries may be simulated by fluid in the lesser sac, by peripancreatic hematoma secondary to splenic or renal injury, or by unopacified bowel loops. Normal variations in pancreatic morphology may also be misleading. Pancreatic injuries may be difficult to identify because of motion or streak artifacts. Gastric decompression, adequate patient sedation, the use of dilute oral meglumine diatrizoate, and the withdrawal of the nasogastric tube into the lower esophagus may prevent these artifacts. Faster scanning is also helpful in reducing artifact. If any question exists regarding the diagnosis of a pancreatic laceration, further scans with either additional oral or intravenous contrast in different patient positions should be obtained.

The CT features of pancreatitis after blunt abdominal trauma are indirect evidence of a pancreatic injury and in some patients may be the only clue. The CT findings of posttraumatic pancreatitis are also time-dependent and may not be evident on scans performed immediately after an injury. The features of posttraumatic pancreatitis are edema and infiltration of the peripancreatic soft tissues, thickening of the anterior pararenal fascia, and focal or diffuse pancreatic enlargement. Subtle areas of heterogeneous density may occur within the gland. In some patients, traumatic edema and contusion result in diffuse low attenuation of the pancreas. Additional information, including injuries or lacerations of adjacent viscera, may be evident on CT. A high index of suspicion must be maintained for pancreatic injury in all patients with a history of severe blunt injury to the epigastrium despite a negative CT.

ULTRASOUND

Ultrasound (US) is less sensitive than CT in the diagnosis of acute pancreatic injuries. US is useful, however, in the follow-up of patients with posttraumatic pancreatic fluid collections, pseudocysts, or other complications. US may be more useful in children and thin patients in identifying the status of the pancreatic duct.

ENDOSCOPIC RETROGRADE
CHOLANGIOPANCREATOGRAPHY

Endoscopic retrograde cholangiopancreatography (ERCP) is the most accurate method of detecting pancreatic duct injury, and its use in acute abdominal trauma is supported by a small group of enthusiasts. Preoperative endoscopic pancreatography is appealing because it obviates opening the duodenum and performing difficult operative cannulation of the papilla during laparotomy when a pancreatic duct injury is suspected. However, even in centers with the necessary expertise, the often impractical logistics involved in arranging ERCP tend to outweigh the potential benefits. ERCP is seldom feasible in patients with pancreatic trauma because most require urgent laparotomy for bleeding or associated injuries. ERCP after blunt trauma to the pancreatic head or neck may also be technically difficult because of distortion of recognizable landmarks, including the papilla, in the medial wall of the duodenum caused by intramural hematoma or surrounding peripancreatic edema. In addition, the patient's supine position, the need for high-quality x-ray facilities, and the necessity for complete visualization of the pancreatic duct add to the technical difficulties.

Because of these difficulties, the authors have used ERCP infrequently as a preoperative diagnostic procedure in the acute situation. In the unusual event of an elevated serum amylase level or a CT abnormality in a stable patient without acute abdominal signs, the demonstration of an intact main pancreatic duct or leakage from a peripheral duct may enable one to avoid an operation (Fig. 38-4). The real merit of ERCP is in evaluating late complications of pancreatic trauma such as fistulas, stric-

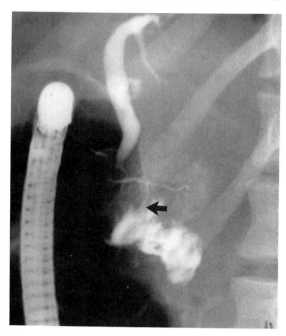

Figure 38-4. ERCP showing localized contrast extravasation (arrow) from a side duct in the uncinate process.

tures, and pseudocysts (Fig. 38-5), where it is valuable in defining the ductal injury.

Management

The initial management of the patient with pancreatic trauma is similar to that of any patient with severe abdominal injury. The priorities of primary management include maintenance of a clear airway, urgent resuscitation, and ventilatory and circulatory support. The mechanism and type of injury are determined while physical examination and resuscitation are in progress. One should rapidly obtain the following information: venous access, volume replacement, hemoglobin concentration, white blood cell count, packed blood cell volume, blood grouping and cross-match, urea and creatinine levels, electrolyte analysis, and blood gas estimation. A nasogastric tube and urinary catheter are essential.

The criteria for performing a laparotomy in patients with abdominal trauma differ from center to center. Urgent laparotomy is required in all patients with evidence of major intraperitoneal bleed-

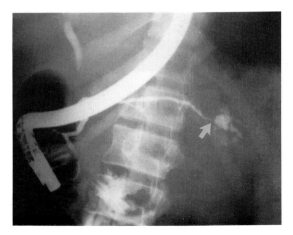

Figure 38-5. Pancreatic duct fistula in the tail with site of duct injury (arrow).

ing, associated visceral trauma, or clinical findings suggesting peritonitis. In patients who are stable and have no obvious clinical signs of intraperitoneal injury, management differs in various institutions. Some advocate mandatory laparotomy in all patients who have injuries that penetrate the peritoneum. The authors practice a policy of careful observation and repeated clinical abdominal examination with selective exploration if signs deteriorate. Blunt trauma to the upper abdomen in the stable patient is evaluated by careful clinical examination and special investigations when necessary.

If a laparotomy is indicated, a long midline incision is used. In the presence of shock and a hemoperitoneum, the first priority is to identify the source of bleeding. Immediate survival is dependent upon successful control and repair of major vascular injuries. The inaccessible retropancreatic position of the superior mesenteric, splenic, and portal veins makes proximal and distal clamping or circumferential control of individual vessels impractical during massive bleeding. Rapid initial control is best obtained by surgical packing or digital pressure. Early duodenal mobilization and bimanual compression of the bleeding site are helpful if an injury to a major portal or superior mesenteric vein is suspected. Vigorous resuscitation with blood and blood components should continue until bleeding has been staunched and normovolemia is achieved. The application of soft bowel clamps is a useful

temporary method of limiting gross peritoneal contamination from disrupted bowel before definitive repair. Attention is directed to other priority visceral injuries before the pancreatic trauma is dealt with.

Intraoperative Evaluation

In most patients, the diagnosis of pancreatic injury is made at laparotomy. Determining the presence and extent of a pancreatic injury intraoperatively requires recognizing the features that indicate a potential pancreatic injury, adequately exposing the pancreas, defining the integrity of the pancreatic parenchyma, and determining the status of the major pancreatic duct. This process may be complicated by the extent and severity of associated injuries. Gross inspection and palpation of the pancreas alone can be misleading because retroperitoneal or subcapsular hematoma, as well as peripancreatic edema, may mask major parenchymal and duct injuries. Clues suggesting pancreatic injury include retroperitoneal bile staining or hematoma at the base of the transverse mesocolon or visible through the gastrohepatic ligament. Metastatic fat necrosis may be present if there has been undue delay before laparotomy. With such findings, complete visualization of the gland and accurate determination of the duct status are crucial. Failure to recognize a major pancreatic duct injury is the principal cause of pancreatic injury–related postoperative morbidity.

The lesser sac is entered through the gastrocolic omentum just outside the gastroepiploic arcade. By retracting the transverse colon downward and the stomach upward, one exposes the anterior surface and the superior and inferior borders of the body and tail of the pancreas (Fig. 38-6). If the posterior surface of the pancreas requires exposure, the pancreas should be mobilized upward by dividing the inferior avascular peritoneal attachments. Surrounding hematoma may complicate adequate assessment of the tail, and further detailed evaluation may require division of the lateral peritoneal attachments. The spleen and the tail and body of the pancreas are reflected forward and medially by developing a plane between the kidney and the pancreas. This maneuver permits full exposure and bimanual palpation of the tail and body of the pancreas. For full inspection of the pancreatic head and

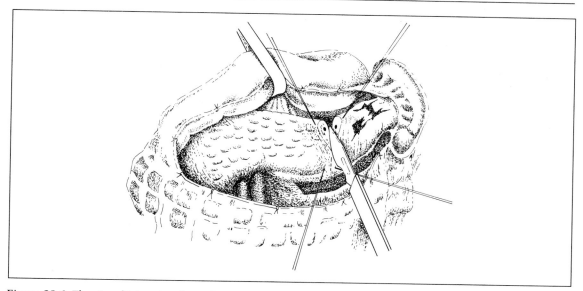

Figure 38-6. The site of injury involving the body and tail of the pancreas is exposed through the lesser sac. Distal resection is the favored treatment for ductal injuries of the body and tail.

uncinate process, the Kocher maneuver is necessary to mobilize the second part of the duodenum medially toward the superior mesenteric vessels. The dissection and downward reflection of the hepatic flexure of the colon and the mesocolon further improve exposure of the second portion of the duodenum and uncinate process. All penetrating wounds should be traced through their entire intraabdominal course to exclude pancreatic or other visceral injury.

Blunt trauma to the pancreas can result in transection of the major duct with or without transection of the gland. Minor contusions or lacerations of the pancreatic substance do not usually require further definitive treatment, but this decision can only be made after careful local exploration to rule out a major duct injury.

Operative Pancreatography

Several radiological methods of intraoperative pancreatography to delineate the pancreatic duct have been recommended. The easiest and simplest method is to inject contrast medium into the gallbladder to obtain a cholecystocholangiogram. An alternative method is to perform a cholangiogram by directly puncturing the common bile duct with a 23-gauge needle. Small incremental volumes of contrast are injected to obtain a cholangiogram. The objective is to define the distal and intrapancreatic bile duct as well as the integrity of the ampulla. Unfortunately, in this situation no absolute reliance can be placed on the findings because there may be only partial filling of the pancreatic duct even if there is obvious reflux of contrast via a common channel. In the presence of an open duodenal injury, the papilla may be conveniently accessible and should be located. A firm squeeze on the gallbladder helps to identify the papillary opening by producing bile in the lumen. A fine lacrimal probe passed through the papilla into the pancreatic duct may provide sufficient information by demonstrating the position of an intact duct beyond the site of the injury (Fig. 38-7). Should a duodenotomy and papillary cannulation be required, a Fogarty catheter or Bakes' dilator passed through a small incision in the supraduodenal bile duct is useful to indicate the position of the papilla after trauma to the head of the pancreas (Fig. 38-8). Previously advised techniques suggesting distal pancreatic resection and cannulation of the duct through the tail are of historical interest. A skilled endoscopist may be of assistance in performing an intraoperative ERCP if logistics permit.

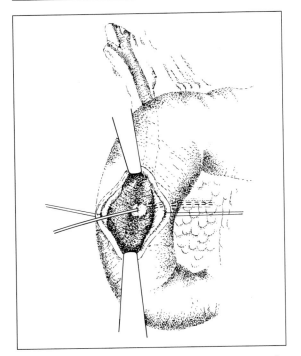

Figure 38-7. After a longitudinal duodenotomy, small right-angle retractors are used to expose the papilla of Vater. A probe in the pancreatic duct indicates the position of the pancreatic duct.

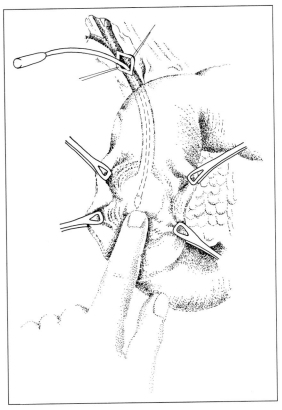

Figure 38-8. The exact level of the ampulla can be determined by palpating a small Bakes' dilator passed down the bile duct.

Class I: Contusions and Lacerations Without Duct Injury

Seventy percent of pancreatic injuries are minor, consisting of contusions, hematomas, and superficial capsular lacerations without any underlying major duct injury. Control of bleeding and simple external drainage without repair of capsular lacerations are sufficient treatment. If the laceration is deeper and concern exists about division of larger side ducts, oversewing the laceration may reduce leakage from these minor ducts. However, meticulous care must be taken to avoid an iatrogenic injury to the main pancreatic duct by a suture inadvertently placed too deep. Either a Penrose drain or a soft closed suction or sump drain is used. The closed suction drain is preferred because pancreatic secretions are more effectively controlled, skin excoriation at the drain exit site is reduced, and bacte-

rial colonization is less than when sump or gravity drains are used.

Premature extraction of drains may result in peripancreatic collections, increasing the risk of sepsis. Drains should therefore be removed only when drainage ceases or when a well-established tract has formed. If the drainage volume is large and the amylase concentration elevated, the drain should be left in place until the nature, location, and extent of the pancreatic fistula are defined. Sinography is the simplest radiological modality and may demonstrate a communication with the main pancreatic duct. However, the interpretation can be misleading because extensions of the tract may simulate ductal structures. An ERCP is indicated when there is a persistent leak for more than 10 days.

Class II: Distal Injury With Duct Disruption

Injury to the neck, body, or tail of the pancreas with major lacerations or transection and associated duct disruption is best treated by distal pancreatectomy. A splenectomy is usually necessary. Distal pancreatic resection with preservation of the spleen prolongs operative time and is contraindicated in an unstable patient with multiple injuries. Although splenectomy in the adult may increase the potential risk of sepsis, the incidence is small and does not justify the extra time necessary to salvage the spleen in the critically injured patient. Splenic preservation is a safe and reasonable course of action in isolated pancreatic injuries or when associated injuries are not life-threatening.

The optimal management of the divided pancreatic duct and the resection margin after distal pancreatectomy is controversial. Some surgeons have advocated the use of a Roux-en-Y pancreatojejunostomy to incorporate and drain the resection margin in order to prevent the development of a pancreatic fistula. In patients with multiple injuries, incurring the added risk of an anastomotic leak is not warranted, and this procedure is not recommended. Oversewing or stapling the transected end of the pancreas and using simple methods to buttress or seal the cut margin are adequate measures and have not led to increased fistula formation.

A visible pancreatic duct should be ligated using a nonabsorbable suture. Although individual ligation of the pancreatic duct has been stressed in the past, identification of the cut end may be difficult, especially after blunt trauma with surrounding edema and hematoma. Routine ligation of the duct is probably not essential, and omitting this specific step has not resulted in an increase in postoperative fistulas. The resection margin of the pancreas should be fashioned in a central "V" pattern to resemble a fish mouth so that the cut end of the pancreas can be oversewn to allow closure without tension (Fig. 38-9A). Mattress sutures placed through the full thickness of the pancreas ensure hemostasis along the resection margin and minimize leakage from the transected parenchyma

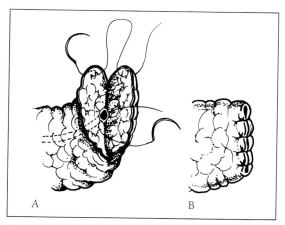

Figure 38-9. The proximal resection margin of the pancreas is fashioned into a "fish mouth," and after duct ligation (A), is closed with interrupted mattress sutures (B).

(see Fig. 38-9B). Fish-mouthing should not be attempted if the cut end of the pancreas is edematous because sutures are under tension and tend to cut out. Several operative techniques have been devised to further minimize a fistula from the resection margin. A small omental patch may be used to bolster the cut surface, or the closed pancreatic stump can be positioned against the retroperitoneum or buttressed against the mesocolon. A drain is placed near the closed end.

Although anecdotal reports of successful primary pancreatic duct repair have been published, most surgeons advise against this maneuver because of complications such as fistula, stricture formation, and pancreatitis. The time required for duct repair also adds an unacceptable risk to patients with pancreatic trauma and major associated injuries. In addition, salvaging the distal pancreas by duct repair has little to offer, because even major pancreatic resections seldom produce functional impairment.

Class III: Proximal Injury With Probable Duct Disruption

It is important to exclude a pancreatic duct injury in trauma to the head of the pancreas. The specific technique used to identify or exclude a pancreatic duct injury is controversial. Some authorities feel that pancreatography should be used whenever the possibility of duct injury in the head of the pancreas exists, whereas others use direct local exploration and evaluation with selective transduodenal intra-operative pancreatography. The risk of pancreatography involves the potential complications of a duodenotomy in an acute multitrauma situation. Those surgeons with preference for intraoperative pancreatography argue that the procedure is generally safe and reliable, and that the advantage of accurate ductal definition outweighs any potential disadvantage if there is uncertainty about the status of the pancreatic duct. The more conservative groups, however, express reservations regarding the use of a duodenotomy to perform pancreatography, and favor careful local inspection and exploration of the defect to define the integrity of the duct.

Injuries to the head of the pancreas that do not involve the main pancreatic duct are best managed by simple external drainage. Even if there is a suspected isolated duct injury (as with a localized sharp penetrating injury) and a distal resection is not justified, external drainage of the injured area is often the safest option. A controlled fistula thus created either settles spontaneously or may later require elective internal drainage after the exact site of duct leakage is defined. Techniques describing onlay Roux-en-Y loop anastomoses to incorporate injured areas in the head of the pancreas are not advisable because of the difficulty of ensuring the integrity of the anastomosis in the acute event.

Distal pancreatectomy may be feasible even if the pancreatic duct is injured to the right of the portal vein, as long as the ampulla and duodenum are uninvolved. In most patients, resection of the pancreas distal to the neck has no permanent functional sequelae unless, as on rare occasions, pre-existing chronic pancreatitis exists. If concern exists that the residual pancreatic tissue is insufficient to sustain adequate endocrine and exocrine function, preservation of the body and tail using Roux-en-Y pancreaticojejunostomy is a reasonable option. This choice, however, is inappropriate when the magnitude of other injuries demands an abbreviated procedure.

Class IV: Combined Major Pancreaticoduodenal Injuries

Severe combined pancreatic head and duodenal injuries are uncommon, and usually result from gunshot wounds or blunt trauma with other associated intra-abdominal injuries. In determining the best option for patients with combined injuries, it is crucial to define the integrity of the common bile duct, pancreatic duct, and ampulla and the viability of the duodenum. If the existing injury is in the second part of the duodenum, careful retraction of the edges of the wound or extension of the laceration in the direction of the papilla may provide adequate exposure of the papilla. Gentle passage of a probe through the ampulla up the bile duct is generally sufficient to exclude injury to the bile duct and ampulla. Alternatively, a cholangiogram performed through the gallbladder or bile duct may provide the same information. If there is obstructed flow of contrast into the duodenum without extravasation, it can be assumed that the common bile duct and ampulla are intact. The presence of bile staining in the retroperitoneum or around the lower bile duct in the hepatoduodenal ligament is confirmation of bile duct injury or ampullary avulsion. If the duodenal injury involves the third or fourth part which is remote from the ampulla, and concern exists about ductal integrity, a duodenotomy opposite the papilla is helpful to adequately evaluate the ductal system.

If the common bile duct and ampulla are shown to be intact, the duodenal laceration is repaired, and the pancreatic injury is treated according to the site of the injury. As with class III injuries, division or damage to the main pancreatic duct and parenchyma near the junction of the head and neck is optimally managed by resection of the neck, body, and tail. Penetrating injury in the pancreatic head without devitalization is best treated by careful drainage of the area. Localized ischemia at the site of the duodenal injury should be debrided before primary duodenal closure; if there is concern about the integrity of the duodenum, decompression using a carefully placed nasogastric tube is useful. Where there is loss of tissue, a controlled fistula via a lateral or side duodenostomy using a T tube or a small Foley catheter with an inflated bulb has been recommended to reduce tension at the suture line.

With severe injury to the duodenum in association with a lesser pancreatic head injury, some authors advise diversion of gastric and biliary contents away from the duodenal repair. Several complex and innovative techniques have been described to deal with this situation. Diversion can be accomplished by a duodenal "diverticulization" procedure which employs primary closure of the duodenal wound, a vagotomy, an antrectomy with an end-to-side gastrojejunostomy, T tube common bile duct drainage, and a tube duodenostomy (Fig. 38-10A). The aim is to convert a potentially uncontrolled lateral duodenal fistula into a controlled end-fistula by diverting gastric and biliary contents away from the duodenal injury, while making provision for early enteral nutrition via a gastrojejunostomy.

An alternative option that avoids a vagotomy and antrectomy is the "pyloric exclusion" procedure. The pylorus is closed with an absorbable suture performed through a gastrotomy, and a side-to-side gastrojejunostomy provides temporary diversion of gastric flow away from the duodenum while the duodenal and pancreatic injuries heal (see Fig. 38-10B). The pylorus opens when the sutures dissolve 3 or 4 weeks later, or the sutures can be removed endoscopically after an intact duodenum has been confirmed. In selected patients, pyloric exclusion has proved useful in managing severe duodenal injuries combined with pancreatic head

injuries in which a Whipple's procedure is not justified. The authors believe that the same objectives can be achieved by less complex procedures, and in this situation they use primary duodenal closure, external catheter drainage near the site of the repair, a diverting gastrojejunostomy without closure of the pylorus, polymeric silicone and a fine-bore (Silastic) nasojejunal feeding tube.

Reconstruction may not be possible in combined injuries of the proximal duodenum and head of the pancreas with devitalization, complete disruption of the ampulla involving the proximal pancreatic duct and distal common bile duct, or avulsion of the duodenum from the pancreas. In these situations, the only rational option is resection. Pancreaticoduodenectomy may be necessary in 1% to 2% of pancreatic injuries and in up to 5% of combined pancreaticoduodenal injuries. The mortality of a Whipple's procedure for trauma has been reported to be between 30% and 50%, suggesting that this procedure should be reserved as a last resort. The need for resection is usually obvious when there is massive destruction with gross devitalization, or when there is pancreatobiliary, duodenal, and ampullary disruption requiring debridement that results in a near-complete pancreaticoduodenectomy.

Five patients in the authors' recent experience have undergone a pylorus-preserving Whipple's resection for trauma without mortality. Technical problems arise in the reconstruction of pancreatic

Figure 38-10. Duodenal diverticulization (A) and pyloric exclusion (B) procedures.

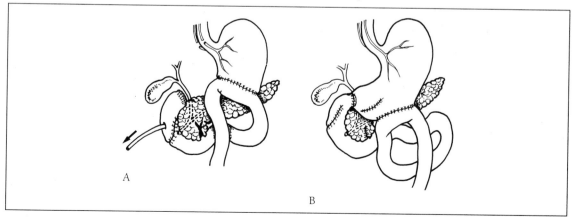

A

B

and biliary anastomoses because of the small size of the ducts (Fig. 38-11). For the pancreatic anastomosis, invagination of the end of the pancreas into a Roux-en-Y jejunal loop is the most widely used technique. The authors have also used a pancreaticogastrostomy in this situation with minimal morbidity. Biliary-enteric continuity is usually restored by a side-to-side choledochojejunostomy or hepaticojejunostomy using a high bile duct reconstruction technique with preplaced sutures. If the small size of the common bile duct precludes a safe choledochojejunal anastomosis, a side-to-side cholecystojejunostomy with ligation of the common bile duct can be used as an alternative in the unstable patient as a rapid means of achieving biliary continuity. However, this procedure is a suboptimal biliary drainage procedure which may require revision in the long term.

Since major vascular injuries are frequent, massive blood loss, coagulopathy, and hypothermia are often present by the time the pancreatic repair is undertaken. Gross bowel edema and localized pancreatitis may aggravate the technical aspects of the pancreaticoduodenectomy and jeopardize the anastomosis. In unstable patients with serious associated injuries, simple controlled drainage and delayed reconstruction may be the most judicious and appropriate procedure.

Figure 38-11. Ultrasound demonstrating pancreatic fracture with separation of the pancreatic head (H) from the body (B) with an interposed fluid collection (star). The pancreatic duct (PD) is clearly seen

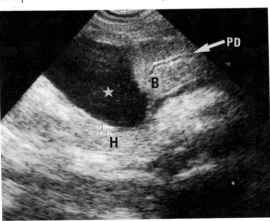

Postoperative Care

The principles of postoperative care in patients with pancreatic injuries are similar to those in patients with other major abdominal injuries. Attention must be paid to ventilatory status, fluid balance, renal function, intestinal ileus, and nasogastric tube losses. Meticulous charting of drain content and volume is important. Prolonged ileus and pancreatic complications may preclude normal oral intake in severely injured patients. The standard composition of regular tube feeds increases pancreatic secretion. The low-fat and higher pH (4.5) formulation of an elemental diet is less stimulating to the pancreas, and should be tried before instituting parenteral nutrition. A catheter jejunostomy using a submucosal needle technique or a fine-bore polymeric silicone nasogastric tube with a weighted tip placed at the initial operation in all complex pancreatic injuries allows the option of early postoperative enteral feeding rather than total parenteral nutrition. The enteral route is more efficient for nitrogen utilization and may be more effective in restoring immune competence. In addition, the morbidity and cost of enteral nutrition are considerably less than for parenteral nutrition.

Results and Complications

Fistulas

Fistula is the most common complication, and 10% to 20% of major injuries to the pancreas result in a pancreatic fistula. The majority of fistulas are minor and resolve spontaneously within 1 or 2 weeks of the injury, provided that adequate external drainage has been established. High-output fistulas (> 700 ml/d) usually indicate major pancreatic duct disruption and are less likely to close spontaneously. An ERCP is then indicated to establish the cause and site of the fistula as well as to plan further therapy if a high-output fistula fails to progressively decrease in volume or persists more than 10 days. Nutritional support should be provided throughout this period. Somatostatin has been used in this situation with variable results. Persistent fistulas without evidence of obvious downstream duct narrowing may require internal drainage into a Roux-en-Y jejunal loop, or resection if they are near the tail.

Pseudocysts

Pseudocysts may be a late presentation of isolated pancreatic trauma in up to 10% of patients and should be suspected when a palpable mass is noted in the epigastrium or left upper quadrant or when the level of serum amylase is persistently elevated. Nonoperative treatment options include percutaneous ultrasound-guided aspiration or catheter drainage and endoscopic drainage. Endoscopic pancreatography is useful in planning the management strategy and in identifying the site and extent of duct disruption (Fig. 38-12). Posttraumatic pancreatic pseudocysts can be treated by percutaneous aspiration or catheter drainage provided no major duct injury, stricture, or demonstrable communication with the main pancreatic duct is present on ERCP.

In the authors' experience, endoscopic drainage of selected traumatic pseudocysts is technically feasible and safe. As with surgical drainage, success relies on the close proximity and intimate juxtaposition of the cyst to the bowel wall. Ultrasound and CT are helpful in assessing this relationship (Fig. 38-13). The final decision and choice of the drainage site are best made by endoscopic demonstration of an obvious intraluminal bulge. The addition of

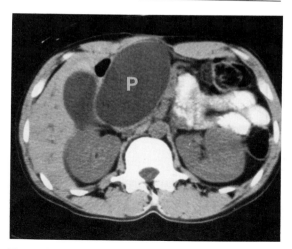

Figure 38-13. CT scan showing a posttraumatic pseudocyst (P) arising from the head of the pancreas.

endoscopic ultrasound increases the efficacy of this technique. A tendency exists for posttraumatic pseudocysts to recur if there is main pancreatic duct disruption. Surgery remains the definitive treatment and may become necessary if conservative methods fail. The site, size, and maturity of the cyst dictate the surgical options, although the ultimate decision is made at operation. In general, mature proximal cysts are best drained internally into adjacent stomach or bowel, whereas small distal cysts with duct strictures in the body or the tail are better handled by distal resection.

Abscesses

Peripancreatic, subhepatic, and subphrenic fluid collections are commonly seen on US or CT after pancreatic trauma. Clinical evidence of intra-abdominal sepsis mandates guided aspiration to obtain fluid for bacteriology and amylase content. In contrast, pancreatic abscesses are uncommon and usually result from inadequate debridement of devitalized pancreatic tissue or ineffective drainage of the lesser sac and pancreatic bed in the presence of ongoing duct leakage. An abscess should be suspected in any patient who develops an elevated temperature, raised white blood cell count, prolonged ileus, or unexplained upper abdominal tenderness in the postoperative period. US or CT scan is necessary to confirm the diagnosis.

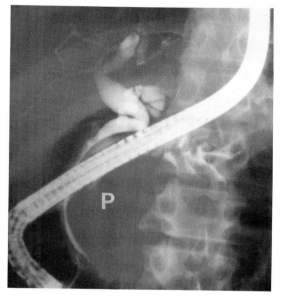

Figure 38-12. ERCP demonstrating displacement of the bile duct by a pseudocyst (P) in the head of the pancreas.

Pancreatic abscesses require prompt drainage. Empiric broad-spectrum parenteral antibiotic therapy should be instituted to cover the full bacterial spectrum until definitive culture results become available. Percutaneous aspiration or catheter drainage is usually effective in patients with accessible unilocular collections and no evidence of pancreatic necrosis. The presence of necrotic pancreatic tissue generally mandates surgery with debridement of nonviable tissue and generous external catheter drainage, although the percutaneous insertion of large-bore drainage catheters may be beneficial in selected cases. Secondary hemorrhage from the pancreatic bed or surrounding vessels as a consequence of infected devitalized tissue and retroperitoneal autodigestion from uncontrolled pancreatic drainage is an uncommon but formidable complication after pancreatic trauma. Failing control by angiographic embolization, operative exposure and packing with abdominal swabs may be life-saving.

A rare but frequently lethal complication is hemorrhagic necrotizing pancreatitis. The first indication of this problem may be abdominal pain, blood-stained pancreatic drainage, shock, or a fall in hemoglobin concentration in a rapidly deteriorating and severely ill patient. As with secondary bleeding in pancreatic sepsis, full intensive care support, operative control of bleeding, and debridement are necessary.

Conclusions

Injuries to the pancreas are uncommon but may result in considerable morbidity and mortality because of the magnitude of the associated trauma and a delay in diagnosis. Early diagnosis of isolated blunt pancreatic injury is hampered by the retroperitoneal location, which may conceal the clinical features. Prognosis is determined by the cause of injury, the extent of blood loss and the presence or absence of shock, the rapidity of resuscitation, the magnitude of associated injuries, and the nature and site of the pancreatic injury. Early mortality is due to uncontrolled or massive bleeding from associated vascular or visceral injuries. Late mortality is a consequence of infection and multiple organ failure. The priority during laparotomy is to control

bleeding and bowel contamination. Surrounding hematoma and edema may mask an injury, and unless they are carefully evaluated at operation, a serious pancreatic injury may be overlooked. Neglect of major duct injury may lead to life-threatening complications, including pancreatitis, pseudocyst, fistula, sepsis, and hemorrhage.

Most pancreatic injuries are minor and can be treated by external drainage. The most common major injury is a prevertebral fracture of the body or neck of the pancreas, which requires a distal pancreatectomy. Major fractures to the right of the portal vein with an intact bile duct are similarly best treated by distal resection. Persistent pancreatic exocrine or endocrine insufficiency seldom occurs after major resections. Duodenal diversion is an option for combined pancreatic and duodenal injuries. Pancreaticoduodenectomy is reserved for maximal injuries to the head of pancreas and duodenum in which salvage is not feasible. All procedures should include effective drainage of the pancreatic injury. The extent of the late complications of pancreatic trauma in stable patients is best evaluated by US or CT and ERCP. The trend to increasingly conservative surgery for most pancreatic injuries represents a simplification of past methods and allows for preservation of pancreatic tissue without increasing morbidity. With careful assessment of the injury by inspection and judicious use of pancreatography, pancreatic complications can be reduced without the need for complex resections, enteric diversions, and pancreaticoenteric anastomoses.

Selected Readings

Feliciano DV, et al. Management of combined pancreatoduodenal injuries. *Ann Surg* 1987; 205:673–680.

Frey CF, Wardell JW. Injuries to the pancreas. In Trede M, Carter DC (eds), *Surgery of the Pancreas*. Edinburgh: Churchill Livingstone, 1993.

Funnell IC, et al. Endoscopic drainage of traumatic pancreatic pseudocysts. *Br J Surg* 1994; 81 (in press).

Glancy KE. Review of pancreatic trauma. *West J Med* 1989; 151:45–51.

Jurkovich GJ, Carrico CJ. Pancreatic trauma. *Surg Clin North Am* 1990; 70:575–593.

Lewis G, et al. Traumatic pancreatic pseudocysts. *Br J Surg* 1993; 80:89–93.

Lucas CE. Diagnosis and treatment of pancreatic and duodenal injury. *Surg Clin North Am* 1977; 57: 49–65.

Smego DR, Richardson JD, Flint LM. Determinants of outcome in pancreatic trauma. *J Trauma* 1985; 25:771–776.

Wilson RH, Moorehead RJ. Current management of trauma to the pancreas. *Br J Surg* 1991; 78: 1196–1202.

Wisner DH, Wold RL, Frey CF. Diagnosis and treatment of pancreatic injuries: An analysis of management principles. *Arch Surg* 1990; 125:1109–1113.

39

Islet Cell Tumors

BRUCE E. STABILE
LIN CHANG

Etiology and Pathogenesis

The islets of Langerhans are organized collections of cells within the pancreas belonging to the diffuse neuroendocrine system. Normal islets are populated by highly differentiated peptide-secreting cells with varied and specific endocrine and paracrine functions. These cells are commonly referred to as APUD cells because they share the properties of amine precursor uptake and decarboxylation. Tumors arising from the pancreatic islets are thus termed apudomas, a group of neoplasms that also includes the peptide-producing endocrine tumors of the gastrointestinal tract and the pituitary, thyroid, and parathyroid glands and the adrenal medulla.

Tumors arising from pancreatic islets are considered *entopic* when they produce hormones normally secreted by islet cells such as insulin, glucagon, somatostatin and pancreatic polypeptide. Tumors are referred to as *ectopic* if they produce nonpancreatic hormones such as gastrin, vasoactive intestinal polypeptide (VIP), growth hormone–releasing factor (GRF), adrenocorticotropic hormone (ACTH), or parathyroid hormone (PTH)–like peptides.

With the exception of insulinoma, pancreatic islet cell tumors are more often malignant than benign. They metastasize to regional lymph nodes, to the liver, and occasionally to other distant sites such as lung or bone. Whereas insulinomas of the pancreas are typically small (< 2 cm) and gastrinomas of either the pancreas or duodenum may be truly minute (< 5 mm), most of the other islet tumors are large (> 3 cm) and easily localized. Even when benign, gastrinomas are often multiple. Multiplicity is the rule when islet cell tumors are part of the multiple endocrine neoplasia–type I (MEN-I) syndrome. In addition to islet cell tumors of the pancreas and duodenum, patients with MEN-I syndrome also have parathyroid gland hyperplasia and adenomas of the pituitary. Gastrinoma is the most common functional pancreatic endocrine tumor found in MEN-I patients, followed by insulinoma, glucagonoma, and vipoma. Although large islet cell tumors have a greater likelihood of being malignant, even minute duodenal gastrinomas may metastasize to regional lymph nodes. Little correlation exists between tumor size and plasma hormone concentrations or the severity of clinical symptoms.

The clinical syndromes of hormonal excess caused by islet cell tumors typically are the manifestations of a single peptide. However, most if not all of the tumors produce multiple hormones. These hormones are readily detectable by immunohistochemical staining of tumor tissue, and elevated plasma levels are measurable by individual highly specific radioimmunoassays.

The etiology of the MEN-I syndrome, as well as some proportion of sporadic islet cell tumors, appears to be a specific gene deletion on the long arm of chromosome 11. In cases of MEN-I this defect is inherited as an autosomal dominant trait. Although the mechanisms of pathogenesis remain to be elucidated, apparently all cells within the islet population are capable of neoplastic change, albeit with markedly different frequencies and malignant potentials.

Table 39-1. Islet Cell Tumor Characteristics

	Pancreatic Primary (%)	Duodenal Primary (%)	Multiple Primaries (%)	Malignant Tumor (%)	MEN-I Syndrome (%)
Insulinoma	99	—	12	5	8
Gastrinoma	50	40	40	55	24
Glucagonoma	99	—	4	70	2
Vipoma	80	15	15	40	6
Somatostatinoma	50	50	10	75	—
PPoma	99	—	60	30	50
GRFoma	40	5	50	35	40
ACTHoma	100	—	—	100	—
PTH-like-oma	100	—	—	100	—
Neurotensinoma	100	—	—	90	—

Islet cell tumors exert their morbidity and mortality both through their devastating syndromes of hormonal excess and as a consequence of malignant growth. Since early diagnosis is now much more frequent and effective medical therapies are available, most deaths are due to advanced metastatic disease. This situation is exclusively the case for nonfunctioning islet cell tumors. Regardless of the hormonal products produced by malignant islet cell tumors, their malignant behavior is profoundly less aggressive than that of adenocarcinoma of the exocrine pancreas. Some important characteristics of the various islet cell tumors are presented in Table 39-1.

Clinical Features and Diagnosis

Insulinoma

Insulinomas are the most common islet cell tumor. The average age of patients at the time of presentation is between 40 and 50 years. About 60% of reported cases have been in females. The clinical features reflect the hypoglycemia that occurs from excessive insulin secretion by the tumor. Hypoglycemia induces a range of symptoms, reflecting cerebral dysfunction and activation of the autonomic nervous system with release of catecholamines. The symptoms of adrenergic excess that occur in response to hypoglycemia include sweating, weakness, tremulousness, palpitations, irritability, and hunger. The neuroglycopenic symptoms consist of headache, visual disturbances, dizziness, lightheadedness, and confusion and may progress to seizures, coma, and death. Symptoms usually occur during fasting or a few hours postprandially and are relieved by carbohydrate ingestion. When long delays occur in establishing the diagnosis, patients typically develop obesity because of increased oral intake in response to the hypoglycemic symptoms.

The diagnosis of insulinoma can be difficult because hypoglycemia in the presence of an elevated plasma insulin concentration may be present in a variety of other conditions. The differential diagnosis includes B cell hyperplasia or nesidioblastosis, factitious hypoglycemia due to surreptitious administration of excessive insulin or oral hypoglycemic agents, and autoantibodies against insulin or the insulin receptor. The diagnosis of insulinoma is based on the presence of three elements: (1) the recognition that the symptoms may be due to hypoglycemia secondary to insulinoma; (2) the presence of Whipple's triad (hypoglycemic symptoms associated with fasting, documented hypoglycemia during symptoms, and relief of symptoms following glucose ingestion); and (3) the demonstration that the plasma insulin concentration is inappropriately elevated relative to the plasma glucose level.

Almost all patients with insulinoma develop symptoms due to hypoglycemia during a 72-hour fast, and this fact provides a reliable diagnostic test. Approximately 90% will have symptoms within 48 hours of fasting, 80% within 24 hours, and 40% within 2 hours. The plasma glucose level during symptomatic hypoglycemia is usually less than

40 mg/dl, and the insulin level is greater than 5 uU/ml. The ratio of plasma immunoreactive insulin to plasma glucose is considered to be diagnostically more accurate than absolute levels of insulin and glucose. An insulin (uU/ml) to glucose (mg/dl) ratio greater than 0.4 reliably identifies an insulinoma. In addition, elevated plasma concentrations of proinsulin and C-peptide, and the absence of antibodies to insulin and of detectable sulfonylurea in the serum or urine can be helpful in differentiating insulinoma from other conditions. Very rarely, provocative testing is needed when the diagnosis of insulinoma is not secure. Most of these tests, such as the insulin suppression test, have relatively low diagnostic accuracy and are potentially dangerous.

Gastrinoma (Zollinger-Ellison Syndrome)

Gastrinoma has an estimated incidence of 0.1 to 0.4 per million people per year. Approximately 1 in 750 patients with peptic ulcer disease has a gastrinoma. The age range of affected individuals is 7 to 90 years, but the majority are between 30 and 50 years old. The predominance of males to females is in the order of 2:1 to 3:2.

The diagnosis of Zollinger-Ellison (ZE) syndrome rests on the findings of an elevated plasma gastrin level and gastric acid hypersecretion in the appropriate clinical setting. Peptic ulcer disease is the most common clinical presentation and is seen in more than 90% of patients. Patients typically are found to have a solitary ulcer in the first portion of the duodenum. Less common ulcer sites are the more distal duodenum and the proximal jejunum. The ulcer symptoms are more refractory to standard therapy than in common peptic ulcer disease. In addition, up to two thirds of patients with gastrinoma have gastroesophageal reflux disease.

Diarrhea is the second most common symptom of ZE syndrome and is present in roughly one half of patients. The diarrhea is usually watery and voluminous and persists with fasting. The etiology of the diarrhea is multifactorial, though acid hypersecretion appears largely responsible. The voluminous acid load causes intestinal mucosal damage and inactivates pancreatic enzymes, resulting in malabsorption and steatorrhea.

An elevated plasma gastrin level of over 1000 pg/ml (normal < 100 pg/ml) in a patient with gastric acid hypersecretion and the appropriate symptoms and signs is virtually diagnostic of ZE syndrome. However, the finding of hypergastrinemia can be associated with other conditions. These include a Billroth II gastrectomy with a retained gastric antrum, hypochlorhydria or achlorhydria with or without pernicious anemia, antral G cell hyperplasia, renal insufficiency, massive small bowel resection, gastric outlet obstruction, and the use of antisecretory drugs such as H_2 receptor antagonists or omeprazole. Measurement of the gastric basal acid output is very useful in differentiating gastrinoma from these other conditions. A basal acid output of 15 meq/hr or greater (or 5 meq/hr after an acid-reducing operation) is highly suggestive of a gastrinoma.

Several provocative tests are available that can confirm the diagnosis of gastrinoma and exclude other conditions associated with hypergastrinemia. The secretin stimulation test is the most safe and reliable. In the setting of a gastrinoma, secretin injection (2 U/kg) causes a paradoxical rise in the plasma gastrin level of 200 pg/ml or greater above the basal level (Fig. 39-1). The level remains unchanged in other conditions.

Glucagonoma

The diagnosis of glucagonoma is based on the finding of an elevated plasma glucagon level in the clinical setting of glucose intolerance, dermatitis, hypoaminoacidemia, weight loss, and anemia. The usual age of patients with glucagonoma is between 40 and 60 years. More than three fourths present with a characteristic dermatitis known as necrolytic migratory erythema that is believed to be a consequence of hypoaminoacidemia. The rash is found on the extremities and in the intertriginous and periorificial areas. The lesions initially appear erythematous and scaly, progress to bullous, and finally become encrusted. Atrophic glossitis, cheilitis, nail dystrophy, and hair thinning are associated features. Thromboembolic events can occur in patients with glucagonoma and may be fatal. The cause of the hypercoagulable state is not known.

An elevated glucagon level of over 1000 pg/ml (normal < 100 pg/ml) is strongly suggestive of glucagonoma. Other conditions associated with hyperglucagonemia include hepatic failure, renal failure,

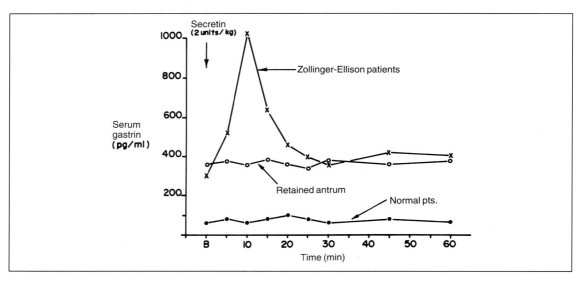

Figure 39-1. Serum gastrin responses to secretin injection in patients with Zollinger-Ellison syndrome, in patients with retained antrum after Billroth II gastrectomy, and in normal controls.

exercise, prolonged fasting, and infection. In general, glucagon concentrations over 500 pg/ml are not seen in these other clinical settings. However, unlike gastrinoma, glucagonoma cannot be differentiated from the other conditions by provocative testing.

Vipoma

The vipoma syndrome is characterized by an elevated VIP concentration in association with a high-volume secretory diarrhea, hypokalemia, and hypochlorhydria. Other common names for the vipoma syndrome are Verner-Morrison syndrome, pancreatic cholera, and the WDHA syndrome (watery diarrhea, hypokalemia, and achlorhydria).

The most common clinical feature is the secretory diarrhea seen in virtually all patients, which is watery and voluminous (> 1 liter/d) and persists with fasting. A net chloride and sodium secretion into the small intestine occurs with no osmotic gap. Associated symptoms include abdominal cramps and weakness, and flushing is present in a minority of patients. Electrolyte disturbances are common. The diagnosis of vipoma is based on the finding of an elevated plasma VIP level in the setting of a secretory diarrhea. The fasting VIP level should be obtained when the diarrhea is present since VIP values can be normal between periods of diarrhea in some patients.

Somatostatinoma

Somatostatinomas are very rare tumors that not only secrete excessive amounts of somatostatin but may also produce VIP, pancreatic polypeptide, gastrin, calcitonin, or other peptide hormones. A range of clinical features may be present in the somatostatinoma syndrome because the hormone inhibits the release of virtually all of the other gut hormones and has additional direct effects on various gastrointestinal functions. The clinical syndrome classically includes mild diabetes mellitus, cholelithiasis, diarrhea, steatorrhea, hypochlorhydria, and weight loss. Abdominal pain associated with gallstone disease is quite common and is presumably due to gallbladder stasis induced by somatostatin. Although the tumor may arise from the pancreas or the duodenum, the typical clinical features of somatostatinoma are more frequently associated with the pancreatic lesions.

Because the clinical presentation of somatostatinoma is often nonspecific, the tumor is usually found unexpectedly at the time of surgical exploration for gallstone disease, during upper endoscopy, or on abdominal imaging studies. A reliable radio-immunoassay to detect increased plasma concentrations of somatostatinlike immunoreactivity (SLI) is available.

Pancreatic Polypeptide Tumor and Nonfunctioning Islet Cell Tumors

Pancreatic endocrine tumors exclusively secreting pancreatic polypeptide (PPomas) and nonfunctioning islet cell tumors are both uncommon and are not accompanied by any identifiable clinical syndrome. These tumors are usually diagnosed when the patients complain of symptoms attributable to a large tumor mass that is often metastatic at time of presentation. Patients typically are found to have weight loss, hepatomegaly, jaundice, and abdominal pain due to advanced disease. In a very small number of cases, PPomas have been associated with diarrhea and a pruritic skin rash.

Elevated plasma levels of pancreatic polypeptide have been detected in patients with various other islet cell tumors of the pancreas and with carcinoid tumors. High levels of the hormone have also been noted in the elderly and in those with renal failure, diabetes mellitus, and certain inflammatory diseases. It has been suggested that plasma pancreatic polypeptide levels are clinically useful in PPoma patients to monitor the response of the tumor to treatment.

Very Rare Islet Cell Tumors

GRF-omas are islet cell tumors that secrete excessive amounts of growth hormone–releasing factor (GRF). Most of the patients present with acromegaly. Because 40% of patients with GRF-oma have an associated gastrinoma, they may also have significant abdominal complaints. ACTH-omas are tumors that are manifested by Cushing's syndrome because of excessive production of adrenocorticotropic hormone (ACTH). These tumors have been associated with gastrinoma and MEN-I and less commonly with sporadic gastrinoma. Rarely, tumors secreting PTH-like peptide hormone or tumors secreting the vasoactive peptide neurotensin have been reported.

Management

Medical Options

SYMPTOMATIC TREATMENT

In general, medical therapy should not be given to asymptomatic patients, even with advanced islet cell tumors, unless the tumor exhibits an aggressive biologic behavior. For symptomatic patients, medical therapy should be administered. General supportive management is necessary to restore biochemical and hemodynamic stability in severe cases. The pharmacologic options are of two types: medications for treating the clinical syndrome of hormonal excess and medications for treating the tumoral process.

Initial supportive medical management is needed in all patients with functioning tumors, especially those with insulinoma, vipoma, or glucagonoma. Instituting a dietary regimen consisting of small frequent meals can alleviate symptoms in patients with insulinoma. In extreme cases, 10% dextrose may be required to treat profound refractory hypoglycemia. In patients with vipoma, fluid and electrolyte repletion is essential to correct the hypokalemia and metabolic acidosis. Those patients with severe necrolytic migratory erythema due to glucagonoma may benefit from parenteral amino acids to correct the hypoaminoacidemia.

Beneficial pharmacologic therapies can be used to treat patients with insulinoma. Approximately 60% of patients improve on diazoxide because it attenuates hypoglycemia by inhibiting insulin release and by enhancing glycogenolysis. Patients not responding to diazoxide may respond to the calcium channel antagonist verapamil or to phenytoin.

Efficacious pharmacotherapy is also available for ZE syndrome patients in the form of the histamine H_2 receptor antagonists and, more recently, omeprazole. The most important factor for long-term success with these medications is adequate dosing in order to lower the basal gastric acid output to less than 10 meq/hr. Long-term treatment with H_2 antagonists can effectively control gastric acid hypersecretion in patients with gastrinoma for many years; however, tachyphylaxis is common, and many patients require yearly dosage increases. Omeprazole, the first of the substituted benzimidazoles, has important advantages that make it the drug of choice for gastrinoma patients. Omeprazole irreversibly inactivates the hydrogen-potassium adenosine triphosphatase (H^+K^+-ATPase) that is responsible for the generation of hydrogen ion by the parietal cell. Compared to the H_2 receptor antagonists, the drug has a longer duration of action (> 24 hours) requiring less frequent dosing (once or twice daily), greater potency (median dose 60 mg/d), fewer and milder side effects, greater efficacy (complete symptomatic relief in 80% and partial relief in an additional 10%), and far less tachyphylaxis (only 10% of patients need increases in dosage).

Several medications have been reported to decrease the diarrhea associated with vipoma. With the exception of a few specific antidiarrheal agents such as loperamide, these medications are no longer used. Octreotide acetate, the long-acting synthetic analog of somatostatin, is now the principal pharmacologic therapy used in the treatment of the clinical syndromes of both vipoma and glucagonoma. Octreotide reduces plasma concentrations of circulating peptides, inhibits gastric and pancreatic secretions, decreases gallbladder contractility, and alters gut motility. Because the reduction of clinical symptoms induced by octreotide is infrequently associated with a comparable reduction in the level of the index peptide, octreotide appears also to depress somatostatin receptor sensitivity. Although octreotide has been found to be very useful in achieving symptomatic relief in patients with and without metastatic disease, its antitumor effects appear to be very limited.

Octreotide has great efficacy in patients with vipoma and is considered first-line medical therapy. Approximately 80% to 85% of patients with vipoma have a symptomatic response with octreotide. Most experience a dramatic reduction in diarrhea volume within 12 to 24 hours after starting therapy. However, many patients initially responsive to octreotide eventually develop tachyphylaxis and require increased dosages to control symptoms.

In patients with glucagonoma, octreotide reliably improves the rash, minimizes weight loss, and decreases diarrhea and abdominal cramping, but it does not appear to control the diabetes mellitus, probably because of a reduction in plasma insulin along with glucagon that is caused by the drug. The beneficial effects of octreotide last longer than 6 months in 75% of patients. The intravenous administration of amino acids and zinc also reportedly improves the troublesome rash.

Because 90% of insulinomas are benign and are treated by surgical resection, octreotide has been used largely for symptomatic relief in patients with metastatic disease. In preoperative patients octreotide has been relatively unreliable in maintaining normal blood glucose levels. In the presence of metastatic disease, octreotide controls hypoglycemia in the majority of patients, but approximately 30% experience recurrent symptoms, only some of which respond to increased dosages of the drug.

Octreotide also has been used in some patients with gastrinoma because of its inhibitory effects on plasma gastrin and gastric acid secretion. However, since octreotide is currently available only in injectable form, it is not generally indicated because of the excellent symptomatic control afforded by oral omeprazole or H_2 antagonist therapy.

The long-term use of octreotide is often complicated by the need to increase dosage. With higher doses, up to 50% of patients experience side effects, including abdominal pain, nausea, vomiting, diarrhea or constipation, and pain at the injection site. Most symptoms are not severe enough to necessitate discontinuing the medication. Other less common untoward effects are steatorrhea, development of cholelithiasis or gallbladder sludge, and a rebound effect after discontinuation of the drug.

NONSURGICAL TREATMENT OF METASTATIC DISEASE

Medical treatments used for metastatic disease include chemotherapy, interferon, octreotide, and hepatic artery embolization. About 60% of patients with noninsulinoma islet cell tumors have malignant disease. With the more recently available treatments for the hormonal syndromes, patients' long-term mortality has become less dependent on the complications of hormonal excess and more related to tumor growth.

The studies that have sought to assess the efficacy of chemotherapy for islet cell carcinomas have grouped the various tumors together because of their rarity. Streptozotocin, a glycosamine nitrosourea compound used alone or in combination, has been the most extensively studied agent. Approximately one third of patients with malignant islet cell tumors obtain an objective response (greater than 50% reduction in tumor mass) with streptozotocin alone. A significantly higher overall response rate (40% to 60%) and median duration of response occur with the use of combination chemotherapy. Effective combinations include streptozotocin plus 5-fluorouracil and streptozotocin plus doxorubicin. Chlorozotocin alone has recently been shown to have an efficacy similar to streptozotocin plus fluorouracil and was attended by fewer gastrointestinal side effects.

Human leukocyte interferon may be useful in some patients with metastatic islet cell tumors who have failed chemotherapy. Interferon administration can induce objective reductions in tumor mass and in tumor hormone marker levels. Adverse reactions are less severe than with chemotherapy and include flulike symptoms, leukopenia, and anemia. Octreotide typically reduces the levels of circulating peptides and symptoms in patients with metastatic islet cell tumors but rarely decreases objective tumor size (50% minimum reduction).

Hepatic artery occlusion has been used for many years to treat liver metastases in patients with islet cell carcinoma. Angiographic transcatheter hepatic artery embolization with or without postocclusion intra-arterial chemotherapy (chemoembolization) has been shown to decrease tumor mass, improve symptoms, and reduce tumor hormone levels in some cases. The combined chemoembolization technique appears to be more effective than either embolization or chemotherapy alone.

Surgical Options

Appropriate surgical management of an islet cell tumor is predicated on (1) a thorough knowledge of the nature and severity of the clinical syndrome caused by the hormonal excess, (2) a prediction of the natural history of the disease based on the results of preoperative staging, (3) the adequacy of medical control of the hormonal syndrome, (4) the potential morbidities, mortalities, and expected benefits of the various surgical options, (5) the availability of additional nonsurgical treatments, and (6) the fitness of the patient to withstand a major operative intervention. Since all islet cell tumors are potentially malignant and operative removal represents the only proven curative therapy, all symptomatic patients should have institution of medical treatment at the outset to control the clini-

cal syndrome. This treatment is followed by operative intervention with the intention to remove all tumor to achieve cure. The only exception would be those patients with diffuse metastatic disease.

Intraoperative surgical decision making depends on the results of preoperative tumor localization studies, the knowledge of whether the patient has sporadic or familial (MEN-I) disease, and the results of surgical exploration. For the management of primary tumors, the surgical options include simple enucleation and formal resection. Enucleation is appropriate for small tumors that are judged to be well encapsulated and noninvasive. This procedure is most particularly applicable to insulinomas and benign gastrinomas of the head and uncinate process of the pancreas. Resection is more appropriate for locally invasive and large tumors of the body and tail of the pancreas. Distal pancreatectomy with splenectomy is the standard operation in such cases. For large or invasive tumors of the head of the gland, a Whipple pancreatoduodenectomy is required. In most instances a pylorus-preserving operation can be used without compromising the curative potential of the resection. Pancreatic resection is also applied when involvement or proximity of the tumor to the main pancreatic duct renders enucleation unsafe. Small duodenal wall gastrinomas are treated by full-thickness elliptical excision. Large or invasive tumors of the duodenum are treated by a Whipple's resection. Removal of enlarged or suspicious regional lymph nodes is indicated in all cases. Even when no nodal involvement is suspected, a sampling of normal lymph node tissue and frozen-section examination are recommended to rule out occult metastatic disease. When liver metastases are present but small and relatively few in number, simple wedge excisions may be performed. Formal lobectomy may be considered for solitary large or multiple unilobar hepatic tumors if cure is a reasonable expectation or palliative debulking is required to control symptoms.

Controversies

PREOPERATIVE TUMOR LOCALIZATION

Accurate preoperative tumor localization represents the ideal if tumor-directed surgical therapy is to achieve maximal curative potential while avoiding unnecessary negative abdominal explorations and blind pancreatic resections with their attendant morbidity and mortality. Imaging studies that define a specific tumor mass are localization techniques, whereas those that provide only an inferential tumor presence based on hormone levels from multiple venous samplings are regionalization studies. In the latter studies, the tumor can only be assumed to be present within a particular region of the pancreas or duodenum.

Abdominal computed tomography (CT) is the most widely applied localization technique but has good sensitivity only for hepatic metastases and the larger (> 1.5 cm) pancreatic tumors (Fig. 39-2). This also appears to be the case for magnetic resonance imaging (MRI) scans (Fig. 39-3). Small tumors and particularly those in the duodenal wall and lymph nodes are poorly visualized by CT, MRI, or abdominal ultrasonography. The same limitations apply to visceral angiography. Selective angiography with injection of secretin (for gastrinoma) or calcium (for insulinoma) appears to enhance the characteristic blush of some islet cell tumors (Fig. 39-4). Endoscopic ultrasonography appears to be useful in identifying tumors in the head and uncinate process of the pancreas but is less sensitive for tumors of the distal body and tail of the gland. The recently introduced ^{111}In-labeled octreotide scan appears to hold promise for defining occult tumors in any anatomic location (Fig. 39-5). Transhepatic portal venous sampling with multiple hormone measurements was the first regionalization technique introduced and is predicated on the finding of a gradient of hormone level that allows one to identify the region from which the hypersecretion of hormone derives. A new technique that involves selective intra-arterial injection of secretin or calcium followed by hepatic vein sampling for hormone levels provides a similar regionalization of tumors.

Because most of the localization and regionalization techniques for islet cell tumors are invasive and expensive, their limited accuracy and questionable impact on clinical outcome have brought their usefulness into question. A number of criticisms regarding their widespread use have been enunciated. (1) All of the tests have had demonstrated false-positive as well as false-negative results. (2) A true positive finding does not exclude the possibility of additional nonvisualized tumors, and thus complete surgical exploration is still required. (3) The localization potential of the tests is very poor out-

Figure 39-2. CT scan showing a large glucagonoma of the body of the pancreas.

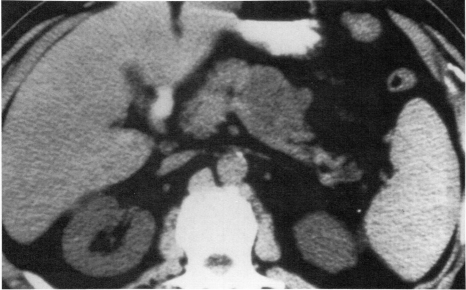

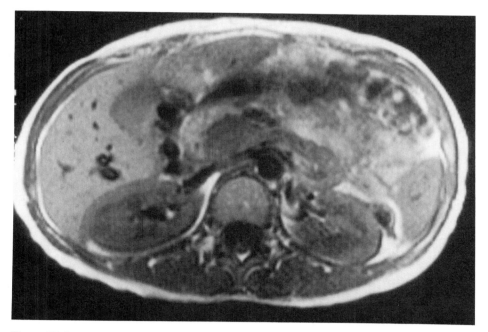

Figure 39-3. MRI scan showing a nonfunctioning islet cell tumor in the uncinate process of the pancreas.

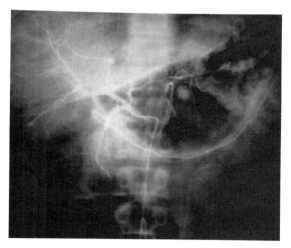

Figure 39-4. Hepatic artery angiogram with calcium injection demonstrating an insulinoma of the body of the pancreas deriving its blood supply from the dorsal pancreatic artery.

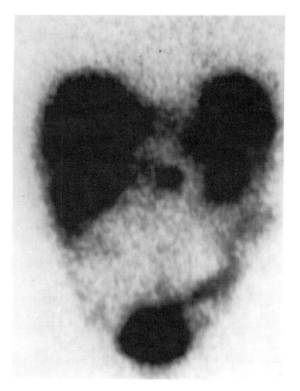

Figure 39-5. ^{111}In-labeled octreotide scan demonstrating a gastrinoma in the neck of the pancreas that appears as a "hot spot" in the midline upper abdomen.

side of the liver and pancreas. (4) The regionaliza-tion studies which measure hormone levels are use-ful only for occult insulinomas because the vast majority of occult gastrinomas are located in the gastrinoma triangle encompassing the head of the pancreas and duodenum (Fig. 39-6). Virtually all other islet cell tumors are large and readily visual-ized by CT. (5) Thorough surgical exploration by palpation plus intraoperative ultrasonography, en-doscopic transduodenal illumination, duodenot-omy, and extensive lymph node sampling appears to be more accurate than preoperative localization techniques when tumors are small or in unusual locations. (6) The techniques have little efficacy in MEN-I patients because clinical benefit is derived only from the removal of large and readily apparent tumors. Thus, it may be argued that extensive pre-operative localization and regionalization attempts should be confined almost exclusively to patients with sporadic insulinomas that are not visualized by abdominal CT or endoscopic ultrasonography.

ADVISABILITY OF OPERATION

The role of surgery for patients with insulinoma is both well defined and well accepted. The cure rates are very high (> 90%), and morbidity and mortality low. Most tumors are single and benign, and amen-able to simple enucleation. In contrast, the other islet cell tumors that are typically malignant require more extensive operative procedures and are diffi-cult to cure. In addition, newer medical therapies can control the lethal sequelae of hormonal excess in most patients. The role of surgery in noninsu-linoma islet cell tumors is thus the subject of contin-uing controversy.

Because of its relative frequency, the variability of its natural history, and the introduction of nu-merous drugs capable of controlling its clinical se-quelae, gastrinoma has been the most controversial of the islet cell tumors. Before the introduction of the histamine H_2 receptor antagonist drugs, virtu-ally all patients with gastrinomas required total gas-trectomy for the control of acid hypersecretion and its complications of ulcer bleeding and perforation. With the availability of the H_2 antagonists and omep-razole, operation is now recommended primarily for cure of the tumoral process rather than for con-trol of acid hypersecretion. Total gastrectomy is almost never required unless the patient is non-compliant with the medical regimen.

Whereas the early experience with treatment of the tumoral process in gastrinoma patients was poor, modern effective medical therapy has made possible a systematic and thorough preoperative evaluation directed toward a controlled elective exploration intended to eradicate all tumor. With

Figure 39-6. The gastrinoma triangle in which most gastrinomas, and virtually all occult gastrinomas, are found.

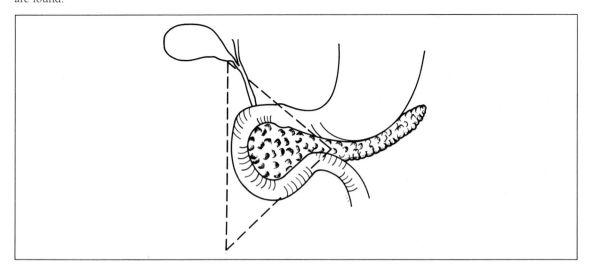

better understanding of the nature and location of occult gastrinomas, curative excisions have been increasing. The intraoperative discovery rate is now approximately 90%, and cures have been obtained even when the disease is found to be metastatic to regional lymph nodes. Thus an aggressive approach to patients without MEN-I or extensive hepatic metastases is indicated. Even when occult tumor remains undiscovered at exploration, the prognosis is very good, because these minute tumors tend to follow a benign clinical course. Only patients with tumor spread to the liver have limited longevity (Fig. 39-7).

METHOD OF TUMOR EXCISION

Although formerly a subject of considerable disagreement, the method of islet cell tumor excision is now fairly standardized. With the exception of insulinoma, most islet cell tumors of the body and tail of the pancreas are relatively large and invasive. Thus distal pancreatectomy with splenectomy is the most appropriate option. A Whipple resection is performed for bulky or invasive tumors of the pancreatic head or duodenum. Enucleation is appropriate for virtually all small benign gastrinomas and insulinomas unless the main pancreatic duct is jeopardized. When multiple tumors are present throughout the gland, distal resection is performed,

and the remaining tumors in the head are enucleated if possible.

OPERATIVE MANAGEMENT OF METASTATIC DISEASE

Because of the relatively indolent nature of malignant neuroendocrine tumors, the management of metastases to lymph nodes and liver has been a controversial subject. Unlike with adenocarcinoma, the successful removal of metastatic islet cell tumor deposits in lymph nodes portends a good prognosis, thus arguing for an aggressive approach. En bloc or anatomic lymph node dissection does not appear to confer any benefit beyond simple excision. This observation is most pertinent to patients with small duodenal gastrinomas, in whom adjacent lymph node deposits are surprisingly common. A number of investigators also have documented the occurrence of tumors that appear to be primary in lymph nodes, and these patients have had excellent long-term results following lymph node excision alone.

In contrast to the surgical results with lymphatic metastases, the results with resection of liver deposits have not been particularly gratifying. Although apparent long-term cures have occurred after resection of solitary liver metastases, an aggressive approach to multiple metastases is infrequently indicated except for palliation of inadequately controlled hormonal manifestations. Recent

Figure 39-7. Survival curves for gastrinoma patients showing comparable longevity among those with no tumor found, those with tumor confined to the pancreas or duodenum, and those with lymph node involvement. Hepatic metastases are associated with a limited survival.

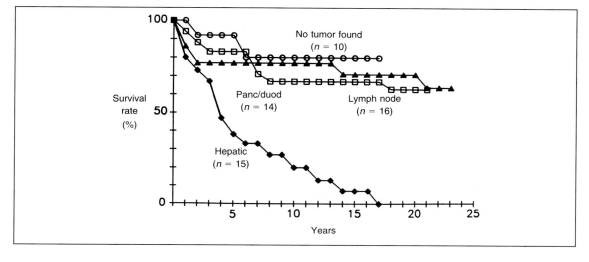

experience with chemoembolization of multiple liver metastases suggests that comparable palliation may be achieved with this much less invasive technique.

TREATMENT OF ISLET CELL TUMORS IN MEN-I SYNDROME

In patients with gastrinoma or insulinoma and MEN-I syndrome, the tumors tend to be multiple, diffuse, and difficult or impossible to cure. Because only a relatively small number of such patients have been adequately studied, their management remains problematic.

In patients with gastrinoma and MEN-I, the hypercalcemia attending hyperparathyroidism exacerbates hypergastrinemia and gastric acid hypersecretion. Therefore, parathyroidectomy is often performed because it facilitates medical management. A number of authorities advocate surgical exploration of the abdomen if a single, dominate pancreatic or duodenal gastrinoma is localized preoperatively. In patients with no anatomic tumor localization, nonoperative management is generally preferred. In this setting, symptomatic control with antisecretory therapy is usually sufficient.

Insulinoma differs from gastrinoma in the setting of MEN-I syndrome because malignancy is far less frequent and extrapancreatic insulinomas are extremely rare. However, in almost 50% of patients with hyperinsulinemia and MEN-I syndrome, no tumor can be localized by CT or selective angiography. In such instances, a regionalization study such as a selective intra-arterial calcium injection with hepatic vein sampling or transhepatic portal venous sampling for insulin should be employed. If preoperative localization or regionalization attempts are successful, surgical resection is usually recommended, especially for patients who are poorly controlled on medical therapy. When all preoperative localization and regionalization attempts fail to identify the source of insulin hypersecretion, some investigators advocate surgical exploration and the use of intraoperative ultrasonography to facilitate tumor discovery. Others recommend simply continuing medical therapy and obtaining periodic CT scans of the abdomen. Surgical intervention is then recommended for those patients who develop a demonstrable tumor.

Conclusions

Because of the complexities inherent in the diagnosis, localization, and management of islet cell tumors, a multidisciplinary approach is absolutely essential. Appropriate consultation and input from the gastroenterologist, endocrinologist, radiologist, surgeon, and medical oncologist are required if patients are to receive a treatment that maximizes both the length and quality of their lives. Clearly, recognition of the various clinical syndromes manifested by patients with islet cell tumors requires a thorough knowledge of their classic presentations as well as their more subtle variations. With a proper index of suspicion, diagnosis is readily afforded by radioimmunoassay of the appropriate hormone. In all instances of confirmed islet cell tumors, additional investigations for the presence of hyperparathyroidism and pituitary lesions should be pursued. If the MEN-I syndrome is discovered or strongly suspected, screening of first-order family members is also appropriate.

Once the diagnosis of an islet cell tumor is confirmed, medical therapy should be instituted immediately. For insulinoma, diazoxide is still the most useful drug for control of hypoglycemia, but octreotide may be used adjunctively. For gastrinoma, omeprazole is uniformly effective, but acid secretory levels should be monitored to ensure a safe level of suppression (< 10 meq/hr). For glucagonoma, octreotide is highly effective in controlling the troublesome necrolytic migratory erythema and in reversing the severe catabolic effects of glucagon excess. In many instances, institution of intravenous hyperalimentation rapidly accelerates the correction of severe hypoaminoacidemia and its sequelae. Patients with vipoma require intravenous volume and electrolyte repletion and octreotide to control the massive secretory diarrhea. Patients with the other very rare functioning islet cell tumors generally benefit from octreotide, with the notable exception of those with somatostatinoma.

The preoperative localization efforts must be tailored to the individual patient, the patient's fitness for major surgical intervention, and the type of tumor diagnosed. All patients should undergo CT of the abdomen and endoscopic ultrasonography, if available. These tests alone will locate most islet cell tumors except for small gastrinomas and insulinomas. In the latter case, an aggressive preoperative localization effort is justifiable to eliminate the need for blind pancreatic resection and its high failure rate. If all of the localization techniques fail, then a regionalization technique such as selective arteriography with calcium stimulation and hepatic vein sampling for insulin levels should be done. This examination will maximize the likelihood that an appropriate resection can be accomplished if intraoperative localization techniques also fail to demonstrate the occult insulinoma.

For gastrinomas not apparent on CT and endoscopic ultrasonography, additional invasive localization techniques are probably superfluous. However, the ^{111}In octreotide scan may prove to be useful in demonstrating multiple tumors and those in ectopic locations. Since most occult gastrinomas are found in the gastrinoma triangle, the most important localization maneuvers are performed intraoperatively. These include ultrasonography, transduodenal illumination, and duodenotomy with bidigital palpation of the duodenal wall. Extensive lymph node sampling will also detect the occasional ectopic tumor and the frequent occult lymph node metastasis. Patients with glucagonoma, vipoma, and the other islet cell tumors generally have single primary tumors that are readily visualized by noninvasive preoperative imaging techniques. When preoperative localization is not possible, intraoperative ultrasonography is a useful adjunct that should be routinely employed.

Surgical intervention should be offered to all patients who are fit and do not have widely metastatic disease or MEN-I syndrome without a preoperatively imaged dominant tumor. In addition, patients with poor medical control on maximal therapy should be considered for debulking procedures or chemoembolization therapy. An aggressive surgical approach should be taken in all insulinoma patients because of the high lethality and devastating morbidity attending uncontrolled hypoglycemia. Gastrinoma patients without hepatic metastases or MEN-I syndrome should all be explored to maximize the chance for permanent cure of the tumoral process, which is malignant in more than 50% of cases. Patients with vipoma and glucagonoma generally require injection therapy with octreotide for control of symptoms. Even though vipomas and glucagonomas are often malignant, cure remains possible with aggressive resection. Failing complete extirpation of tumor, significant palliation can be afforded by medical therapy.

At operation it is the surgeon's responsibility to identify, stage, and excise all tumor to the extent that is safe and possible. Enucleation is preferred for benign tumors, particularly those in the head of the pancreas. Resection is applied without hesitation for disease that is bulky and locally invasive, and when enucleation would jeopardize the integrity of the pancreatic duct. Small duodenal tumors are managed by elliptical full-thickness excisions in most instances. Aggressive excision of regional lymph nodes is performed in all patients other than those with apparently benign insulinomas. Easily accessible and resectable liver metastases are removed if they are few in number and particularly when medical control of the hormonal syndrome is suboptimal. Chemoembolization can be a useful adjunct in patients with unresectable symptomatic hepatic metastases. In most patients with surgically incurable islet cell tumors the hormonal syndromes can be controlled with medical therapy. Chemotherapy with cytotoxic drugs or interferon provides useful palliation in some cases.

Selected Readings

Doherty GM, et al. Results of a prospective strategy to diagnose, localize and resect insulinoma. *Surgery* 1991; 110:989–997.

Howard TJ, et al. Biologic behavior of sporadic gastrinoma located to the right and the left of the superior mesenteric artery. *Am J Surg* 1993; 165: 101–105.

Maton P. Use of octreotide acetate for control of symptoms in patients with islet cell tumors. *World J Surg* 1993; 17:504–510.

Moertel CG, et al. Streptozotocin-doxorubicin, streptozotocin-fluorouracil, or chlorozotocin in the treatment of advanced islet cell carcinoma. *N Engl J Med* 1992; 326:519–523.

Norton JA. Neuroendocrine tumors of the pancreas and duodenum. *Curr Probl Surg* 1994; 31:77–164.

Norton JA, Doppman JL, Jensen RT. Curative resection in Zollinger-Ellison syndrome: Results of a 10 year prospective study. *Ann Surg* 1992; 215:8–18.

Solcia E, et al. The gastroenteropancreatic endocrine system and related tumors. *Gastroenterol Clin North Am* 1989; 18:671–693.

Stabile BE, Morrow DJ, Passaro E Jr. The gastrinoma triangle: Operative implications. *Am J Surg* 1984; 147:25–31.

Thompson GB, et al. Islet cell carcinomas of the pancreas: A twenty-year experience. *Surgery* 1988; 104:1011–1017.

Van Eyck CHJ, et al. Use of isotope-labelled somatostatin analog for visualization of islet cell tumors. *World J Surg* 1993; 17:444–447.

40

Cystic Neoplasms

Mark A. Talamini
Elliot K. Fishman
Ralph H. Hruban
Henry A. Pitt

A cyst is defined as an abnormal sac containing fluid, air, or a semisolid material. The most common cyst associated with the pancreas is the pseudocyst. The difference between pseudocysts and true cysts is that pseudocysts are not lined with epithelium. The second most common pancreatic cysts are neoplastic cysts. Cystic tumors of the pancreas are an interesting group of lesions both from a diagnostic and a biologic point of view. Considerable controversy persists regarding their classification. Most authorities agree that serous and mucinous cystadenomas and cystadenocarcinomas should be classified as cystic neoplasms of the pancreas. However, the proper classification of cystic neuroendocrine tumors, papillary and cystic (Hamoudi) tumors, mucinous duct ectasia, and adenocarcinomas that produce large amounts of extracellular mucin remains a matter of debate.

Etiology and Classification

Cystic neoplasms of the pancreas may be either benign or malignant, and they are easily confused with simple cysts or pseudocysts. Further confusion arises from the fact that an adenocarcioma of the pancreas is capable of producing mucin in sufficient quantities to create a cystic structure or duct ectasia. Adenocarcinoma of the pancreas can also cause pancreatitis from pancreatic duct obstruction, which can evolve into a pseudocyst. Thus the presentation of a cyst within the pancreas gives rise to a spectrum of possibilities which can be difficult to precisely differentiate preoperatively. In the operating room an accurate diagnosis can be difficult even with the gross specimen in hand.

In a recent review of 50 patients with cystic neoplasms of the pancreas from The Johns Hopkins Hospital between 1984 and 1991, the authors classified these lesions into three broad categories (Table 40-1): group 1, benign cystadenomas; group 2, cystadenocarcinomas; and group 3, adenocarcinomas masquerading as cystadenocarcinomas. Groups 1 and 3 were further subdivided: 1a, serous cystadenomas; 1b, mucinous cystadenomas; 3a, mucin-producing carcinomas presenting as cysts; and 3b, adenocarcinomas with an associated pseudocyst or simple cyst. This classification system includes the "true" cystic neoplasms and those lesions most likely to be confused with them on both a clinical and pathologic basis.

Group 1 includes the benign cystic neoplasms of the pancreas. Serous cystadenomas (group 1a) are benign neoplasms that have also been referred to as microcystic adenomas or glycogen-rich cystadenomas. Grossly, these lesions contain serous fluid and are made up of numerous small cysts, which give these tumors a honeycomb or sponge-like appearance (Fig. 40-1A). The fibrous septa are hypervascular, which causes enhancement on a CT scan with intravenous contrast, and they often develop central calcification. At the microscopic level, serous cystadenomas are lined by a cuboidal epithelium containing large amounts of intracellular glycogen (see Fig. 40-1B). The cells show little to

Table 40-1. Classification of Cystic Neoplasms

Group 1:	Cystadenoma
	1a. Serous cystadenoma
	1b. Mucinous cystadenoma
Group 2:	Cystadenocarcinoma
Group 3:	Adenocarcinoma
	3a. Producing mucin and creating a cyst
	3b. Associated with a pseudocyst or simple cyst

no pleomorphism, and serous cystadenomas are generally believed not to have malignant potential. However, the literature does contain isolated reports of serous cystadenocarcinoma of the pancreas. The majority of serous cystadenomas are identified by pain, an abdominal mass, or by incidental finding on a computerized tomography (CT) scan.

Mucinous cystadenomas (group 1b) are quite different in that the cystic elements are considerably larger (Fig. 40-2A). These lesions have malignant

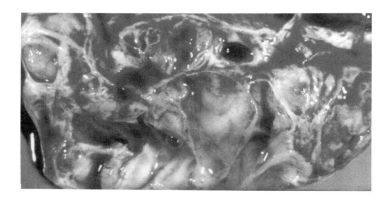

A

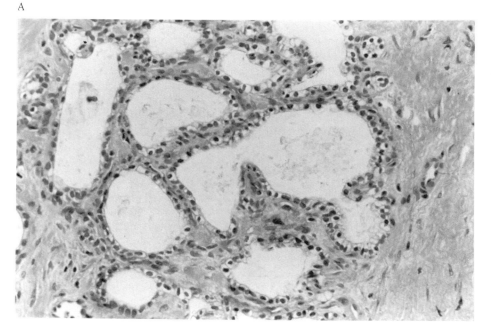

B

Figure 40-1. A. Gross appearance of a serous (microcystic) cystadenoma of the pancreas. B. Microscopic pathology of a serous cystadenoma. Note the single layer of cuboidal epithelium.

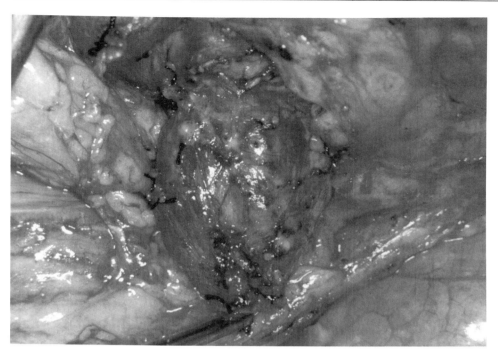

A

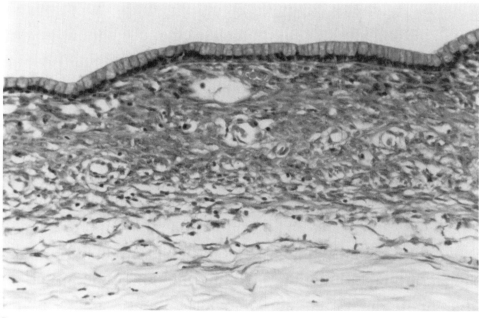

B

Figure 40-2. A. Gross appearance of a mucinous cystadenoma being enucleated from the uncinate. B. Microscopic pathology of a mucinous cystadenoma. Note the ovarian stroma.

potential and with time may develop into a cystadenocarcinoma. On cut section the cysts are filled
with tenacious mucous secretions. Histologically,
mucinous cystadenomas are lined with columnar
epithelium containing intracellular mucin. Cellular pleomorphism can occur sporadically in the
epithelium in such a way that atypia can exist in
one area and carcinoma in another. Thus, in order to rule out malignant degeneration, the pathologist must examine the entire lesion by light
microscopy. In addition, some mucinous cystadenomas, particularly those in women, may have
an "ovarian stroma"–like cellular subepithelial
stroma similar to that seen in mucinous cystic tumors of other organs (see Fig. 40-2B). Mucinous
cystadenomas are more common in the body and
tail of the pancreas, whereas microcystic serous
adenomas are evenly distributed throughout the
pancreas. The etiology of these two lesions is
obscure.

Mucinous cystadenocarcinomas (group 2)
probably arise from malignant degeneration of
long-standing mucinous cystadenomas. Mucinous
cystadenocarcinomas present as single macrocystic
masses which generally have less than six cysts,
each of which is usually greater than 2 cm (Fig.
40-3A). Although cystadenocarcinomas may be
unilocular, the epithelial lining will often have papillary invaginations and may have solid components
(see Fig. 40-3B). As was true for mucinous cystadenoma, on cut section the cysts are filled with tenacious mucus. Some cystadenocarcinomas stain for
serotonin and somatostatin, suggesting that they
arise from ectodermal stem cells. As with cystadenomas, cystadenocarcinomas have little or no peri-
cystic inflammatory reaction. Cystadenocarcinomas
may be adherent to but rarely invade adjacent organs. Although they are less aggressive than the
more common infiltrating adenocarcinoma of the
pancreas, these lesions are malignant, and they can
metastasize to the peritoneum, liver, and distant
sites.

Considerable confusion can arise when a
garden-variety adenocarcinoma of the pancreas
is accompanied by a cyst. This clinical situation
can have two possible causes. First, a mucin-
producing adenocarcinoma can create mucin to
such an extent that a mucinous cyst is created

(group 3a). Second, a pancreatic adenocarcinoma
can obstruct the pancreatic duct, causing accompanying pancreatitis with pseudocyst formation
(group 3b).

Another potentially confusing situation is mucinous ductal ectasia. This lesion also occurs as
the result of mucin overproduction and papillary
hyperplasia, which causes dilatation of the pancreatic duct. Mucinous ductal ectasia may be a premalignant lesion. A similar situation can occur, however, with long-standing duct obstruction, as with
pancreas divisum. These confusing entities can only
be differentiated from true cystic neoplasms in the
pathology laboratory when the entire specimen has
been examined.

A potentially more dangerous situation exists
in differentiating a cystadenoma or cystadenocarcinoma from a pseudocyst. Relying on clinical findings, a surgeon may drain what appears to be a
pseudocyst. In some instances, this cystic structure
may actually be a mucinous cystadenoma. The only
sure way to differentiate a pseudocyst from a cystic
neoplasm is through pathologic evaluation of an
excised piece of the cyst's wall. This confusion is
further enhanced by the fact that a long-standing
pseudocyst can become epithelialized by progressive growth of pancreatic ductal epithelium along
the wall of the pseudocyst. Nevertheless, if a piece
of cyst wall demonstrates a continuous epithelium,
the surgeon must assume that the lesion is a cystic
neoplasm, and must alter the plan from cyst drainage to cyst excision.

True cysts of the pancreas are extremely rare
lesions. Pancreatic cysts may also be rarely observed
in patients with polycystic disease of the kidneys
or liver and in the Von Hipple-Lindau syndrome.
Lymphoepithelial cysts of the pancreas have also
been reported. The presentation and radiologic
picture of these cysts may be identical to that of
cystic pancreatic neoplasms. However, each of
these lesions has a distinctive histologic picture that
differentiates it from cystic neoplasms. Similarly,
cystic islet cell tumors, papillary and cystic (Hamoudi) tumors, and other rare neoplasms may have
a clinical and radiologic picture that can mimic
cystic neoplasms of the pancreas. However, each
of these lesions also has a distinct histologic appearance.

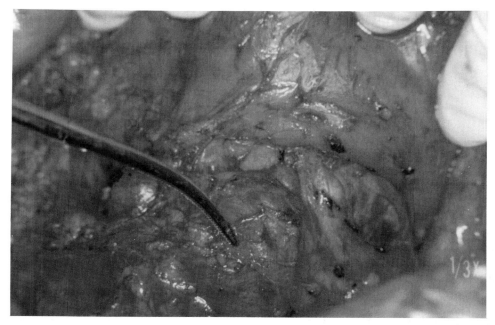

A

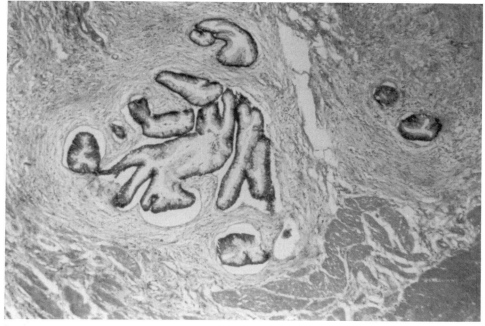

B

Figure 40-3. A. Gross appearance of a mucinous cystadenocarcinoma of the pancreatic head.
B. Microscopic pathology of a mucinous cystadenocarcinoma.

Table 40-2. Presentation of Cystic Neoplasms

	Group 1 Cystadenoma (%)	Group 2 Cystadenocarcinoma (%)	Group 3 Adenocarcinoma (%)
Pain	61	67	73
Anorexia	26	42	47
Weight loss	17	50	33
Jaundice	4*	25	33
Asymptomatic	26*	0	7

*$P < 0.05$ vs. groups 2 and 3.
Source: Adapted from Talamini MA, et al. The spectrum of cystic tumors of the pancreas. *Am J Surg* 1992; 163:117–124.

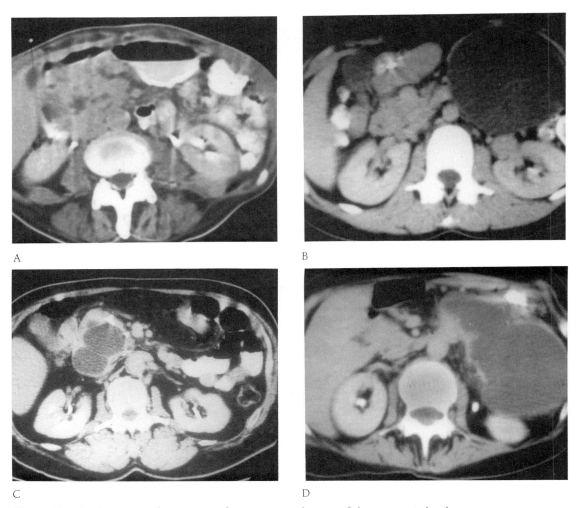

A

B

C

D

Figure 40-4. A. Computerized tomogram of a serous cystadenoma of the pancreatic head.
B. Computerized tomogram of a mucinous cystadenoma of the pancreatic tail. C. Computerized
tomogram of a cystadenocarcinoma of the pancreatic head. D. Computerized tomogram of a mucin-
producing adenocarcinoma of the pancreatic tail.

Diagnosis

Clinical Presentation

The majority of cystic neoplasms present with pain (Table 40-2). However, this symptom cannot be used to classify these patients because pain is common for group 1 (cystadenoma), group 2 (cystadenocarcinoma), and group 3 (adenocarcinoma) patients. Nonspecific symptoms such as nausea, vomiting, anorexia, and weight loss are also common and cannot differentiate among the cystic neoplasms. Jaundice is present more commonly in group 2 and 3 patients with malignant cystic tumors. However, a rare group 1 patient with a cystadenoma may also present with obstructive jaundice. Malignant cystic tumors are rarely asymptomatic, whereas approximately one quarter of cystadenomas will be discovered incidentally during workup or surgery for another abdominal problem.

Radiologic Evaluation

The widespread use of CT scanning has led to both an understanding of the radiographic characteristics and an increase in the incidental finding of these tumors. Microcystic adenomas exhibit a honeycomb cystic structure which enhances on CT scan with intravenous contrast because of hypervascularity (Fig. 40-4A). These lesions may also have central calcification. The presence of septations on CT is a reasonably reliable sign differentiating a cystic lesion from a pseudocyst. However, some pseudocysts may be multilocular, especially when they become infected. Unfortunately, unless a mass is observed near the lesion or hepatic metastases are present, CT is not effective in differentiating a mucinous cystadenoma (see Fig. 40-4B), a cystadenocarcinoma (see Fig. 40-4C), or an adenocarcinoma producing large amounts of mucin (see Fig. 40-4D). Spiral CT, however, may be useful in detecting vascular encasement or invasion, a finding consistent with a malignant process. In differentiating among these lesions, sonography may play a role because it can also detect septations within a large lesion, suggesting that a neoplasm exists rather than a pseudocyst.

The gastroenterologist may also participate in the diagnostic process. Pancreatography often reveals duct displacement rather than occlusion, suggesting a benign lesion. Endoscopic retrograde cholangiopancreatography (ERCP) is also vital to the diagnosis of duct ectasia (Fig. 40-5). In these rare patients the pancreatic duct is ectatic, and large amounts of mucin extrude from the ampulla at the time of the examination. In addition to the pancreatogram, the cholangiogram may provide useful information for the surgeon when bile duct obstruction is present, usually with malignant lesions.

The interventional radiologist can provide two examinations, transhepatic cholangiography and angiography, both of which are often helpful in the workup of cystic tumors of the pancreas. Transhepatic cholangiography provides useful information regarding the invasive nature of the lesion by demonstrating occlusion of the common bile duct in the head of the pancreas. This finding is usually observed with malignant cystic tumors. Bowing of the duct, on the other hand, suggests a benign lesion as opposed to a sharp cutoff occlusion, which suggests invasion of the duct by a malignancy. Arteriography can demonstrate encasement or occlusion, strongly suggesting malignancy. However, very large benign tumors may also cause venous narrowing. Lesions in the body or tail of the pancreas can also cause splenic vein thrombosis.

Fluid Analysis

Several groups have suggested that pseudocysts, serous cystadenomas, mucinous cystadenomas, and cystadenocarcinomas can be differentiated by an analysis of cyst fluid. Fluid viscosity, amylase or

Figure 40-5. ERCP demonstrating pancreatic duct ectasia.

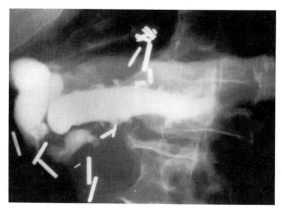

lipase enzyme levels, and cytology have been analyzed (Table 40-3). However, none of these parameters are specific enough to differentiate among benign, potentially malignant, and malignant lesions.
For example, cystic neoplasms may communicate
with the pancreatic duct and may have high amylase
levels. In addition, potentially malignant mucinous
cystadenomas will often have negative cytology.

More recently, carcinoembryonic antigen
(CEA), carbohydrate antigen (CA) 15.3, and CA
72-4 have also been suggested as tools to differentiate among the lesions in the differential diagnosis
(see Table 40-3). CA 15.3 levels are usually less
than 30 U/ml in pseudocysts and cystadenomas
and greater than 30 U/ml in cystadenocarcinomas.
CA 72-4 levels, on the other hand, are low in pseudocysts and serous cystadenomas, intermediate in
mucinous cystadenomas, and high in cystadenocarcinomas. More data are necessary, however, to
determine whether this test will accurately differentiate between pseudocysts and mucinous cystadenomas. Moreover, the advisability of aspirating cystadenocarcinomas must also be questioned because
of concerns about spilling malignant cells into the
peritoneal cavity.

Thus diagnostic uncertainty remains, despite a
wide variety of means to investigate these lesions.
Differentiation between mucinous cystadenoma and
cystadenocarcinoma is particularly difficult. The
pathologist must fully examine the entire specimen
to be certain that no area contains epithelium consistent with cancer. Differentiation between pseudocysts and mucinous cystadenomas is also important. In the Johns Hopkins series, five patients
eventually found to have cystic tumors of the pan-

creas had been previously explored. Four of these
patients had been previously classified as having
pancreatic pseudocysts. Thus, despite the plethora
of possible preoperative studies, operative resection
remains the safest and most reliable means of definitive diagnosis and therapy.

Management

The optimal management of a patient suspected of
having a cystic neoplasm of the pancreas remains
surgical resection. Of the 50 patients recently observed at The Johns Hopkins Hospital, 74% underwent resection. Thirty-six percent underwent
pancreaticoduodenectomy, 32% had a distal pancreatectomy, 14% underwent a palliative bypass,
and 12% were only biopsied. Total pancreatectomy was necessary in 4% of patients, and 2%
underwent enucleation of the lesion. The benign
lesions, serous cystadenomas and mucinous cystadenomas (group 1), were resected in 91% of the
23 patients. Eight of the 12 patients (67%) with
cystadenocarcinomas (group 2) had the lesion resected. In comparison, only 53% of the 15 patients
with adenocarcinomas masquerading as cystic lesions (group 3) could be resected.

A surgical exploration is also important when
attempting to differentiate a pseudocyst from a mucinous cystadenoma or cystadenocarcinoma. During any operative procedure for a pseudocyst, a
piece of the wall must be sent to the pathologist
for examination. If the specimen reveals a simple
columnar cell lining, the patient has a mucinous
cystic neoplasm, and the lesion should be entirely
resected. Similarly, if the biopsy demonstrates signs

Table 40-3. Fluid Analysis of Cystic Lesions

	Pseudocyst	Serous Cystadenoma	Mucinous Cystadenoma	Cystadeno- carcinoma
Viscosity	Low	Low	Usually high	High
Amylase	High	Variable	Variable	Variable
Cytology	Negative	50% positive	Usually positive	Usually positive
CEA[a] (ng/ml)	Low < 25	Low < 25	High > 25	High > 25
CA[b] 15.3 (U/ml)	Low < 30	Low < 30	Low < 30	High > 30
CA 72-4 (U/ml)	Low < 10	Low < 10	10–250	High > 700

[a]CEA = carcinoembryonic antigen.
[b]CA = carbohydrate antigen.
Source: Adapted from Alles AJ, et al. Expression of CA 72-4 (TA6-72) in the fluid contents of pancreatic cysts: A new marker to distinguish malignant pancreatic cystic tumors from benign neoplasms and pseudocysts. *Am Surg* 1994; 219:131–134.

of cystadenocarcinoma, a neuroendocrine tumor, or another rare tumor, resection should be undertaken.

Options and Controversies

Several options are available for the diagnosis and management of cystic neoplasms. When alternatives exist, controversies abound. For example, these lesions may be diagnosed by CT scan, ultrasound, magnetic resonance imaging, or endoscopic ultrasound. CT scan is presently the diagnostic procedure of choice even though this modality may not differentiate among the various cystic tumors. Lesions other than cystic neoplasms that appear with low density on CT may also cause confusion. Most importantly, with contrast enhancement a typical adenocarcinoma may appear cystic because of low blood flow. Papillary and cystic neoplasms (Hamoudi tumors) (Fig. 40-6), some cystic islet cell tumors, and, of course, pseudocysts may also be confused with true cystic neoplasms.

The CT appearance of a serous cystadenoma is usually quite characteristic. Thus, when a patient presents with a honeycomb cystic lesion of the pancreas which enhances with intravenous contrast, the temptation is to observe rather than resect. The literature suggests that almost all of these lesions are benign. However, such patients should be explored, for two reasons. First, four patients with malignant serous cystadenocarcinoma have been reported.

Figure 40-6. Computerized tomogram of a papillary and cystic (Hamoudi) tumor of the head of the pancreas.

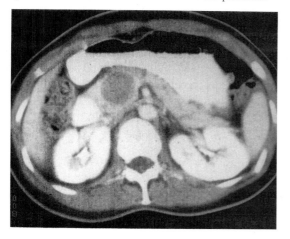

Second, diagnostic uncertainty is always present with cystic tumors of the pancreas, and some lesions may not fall clearly into one category or another. Given such uncertainty, surgical exploration is the safest course.

Mucinous cystadenomas may cause minimal or no symptoms and may be confused with pseudocysts. A clear move toward percutaneous drainage of pseudocysts has taken place over the last decade. Randomized studies are now under way to determine whether percutaneous or surgical drainage is preferable for pseudocysts. Even during an open operation, a cystic neoplasm of the pancreas may be confused with a pseudocyst. At laparotomy a lesion assumed to be a pseudocyst may actually be a cystic tumor of the pancreas. This potential confusion can be clarified by biopsy of the cyst wall. However, the distinction between a mucinous cystic neoplasm and a pseudocyst may be difficult with a percutaneous biopsy. The recent reports which examine CA 15.3 and CA 72-4 levels as well as characteristics of cyst fluid may improve the precision of percutaneous aspiration. However, initial reports need to be confirmed, and concerns about the spread of tumor cells may prevent the widespread employment of this option.

Another area of potential controversy is the management of the rare patient with duct ectasia. Whether these lesions are true cystic neoplasms or are acquired as the result of sphincter stenosis has yet to be clearly defined. If the ectatic duct is acquired and the patient presents with pain or pancreatitis, lateral pancreatojejunostomy may be adequate therapy. However, if the ectatic duct indicates that the lesion is a cystic neoplasm, resection should be undertaken. Since these lesions may involve the entire pancreas, however, resection would mean that total pancreatectomy would be required to remove the abnormal epithelium. Whether such a radical operation is indicated in these patients remains unclear, since reports with a reasonable number of patients with long-term follow-up have yet to be published.

Preferred Approach

The preferred approach to a cystic neoplasm of the pancreas is surgical exploration and, when possible, resection. A careful history and physical examination should give important clues to the differential diagnosis of pseudocysts versus cystic tumors of the pancreas. A prior history of pancreatitis, alcohol ingestion, or gallstone pancreatitis suggests pancreatitis as the origin of the cyst. The CT scan may also help to differentiate a pseudocyst from a cystic tumor by the presence or absence of inflammation. If uncertainty persists, an ERCP may discriminate between a pseudocyst and a cystic tumor of the pancreas by the presence or absence of inflammatory ductal changes.

If a pseudocyst is unlikely, the location of the lesion would dictate the next step in the workup. A cystic lesion in the head of the pancreas should be treated as any other mass in this region. Transhepatic or endoscopic cholangiography should be performed if the patient is jaundiced. The placement of a percutaneous drainage catheter or endoscopic endoprosthesis should be done on a case-by-case basis. If a standard CT scan raises the possibility of vascular encasement, arteriography or a spiral CT should be performed and should include the hepatic or superior mesenteric venous phase. Encasement of the portal or superior mesenteric veins or the hepatic or superior mesenteric arteries makes resection for cure unlikely. In addition, anatomic variants discovered in the preoperative arteriogram are more easily dealt with in the operating room. If the lesion is in the body or tail of the pancreas, ERCP may be helpful in providing a pancreatogram. However, the usefulness of this information can be debated, and this test may be avoided in selected patients. Similarly, arteriography with venous phase studies will reveal the state of the splenic vein and the possible presence of left-sided portal hypertension. However, this information may also be available from a spiral CT scan which is coupled with a properly timed contrast injection.

At the time of operative exploration, a complete and thorough laparotomy must be performed to seek evidence of metastatic disease in the form of peritoneal studding, hepatic metastasis, or mesenteric lymph node metastases. If the lesion is found to be unresectable, the patient should undergo biopsy for a definitive tissue diagnosis, and biliary and/or gastric bypass as necessary. Patients presenting with back pain should also receive a celiac block with absolute ethanol diluted to 50%

with saline. Patients whose tumors appear resectable should undergo a pancreatic resection for attempted cure. Resection may require pancreatoduodenectomy, distal pancreatectomy, or, rarely, total pancreatectomy. Enucleation or local resection of cystadenomas may be acceptable in carefully selected patients.

The role of radiation and chemotherapy in patients with cystic neoplasms has yet to be clearly defined. In general, the authors have recommended radiation with 5-fluorouracil as a radiosensitizer for patients with unresectable but localized tumors. Although the data are anecdotal, some of these patients have survived for long periods of time. Similarly, chemotherapy may be considered in patients with metastatic disease. The choice of agents should probably be similar to that employed for other adenocarcinomas. Response rates of 20% to 30% should be expected, and the decision to continue therapy should be based on response and toxicity.

Results

As expected, patients with benign cystadenoma have an excellent survival. In the Johns Hopkins series, only one death occurred in this group from an unrelated cause (Fig. 40-7). In patients with cystadenocarcinoma, the 1-, 3-, and 5-year survival rates were 90%, 72%, and 72%, respectively. In patients with infiltrating adenocarcinoma masquerading as a cystic lesion, survival was worse, with 1-, 3-, and 5-year survival rates of 41%, 14%, and 14%, respectively. Thus patients with true cystadenocarcinoma have a survival rate that is significantly better than those with adenocarcinoma of the pancreas. On the other hand, adenocarcinomas that produce large amounts of mucin or that present with pancreatitis and pseudocyst formation may have a slightly worse prognosis than the typical adenocarcinoma.

A recent preliminary report has correlated DNA cytometry with survival. In the group with cystadenocarcinoma of the pancreas, those patients with diploid low S-phase tumors had the longest survival but still succumbed to the disease within 10 years. The authors concluded that DNA cytometry may help to identify patients with aggressive tumors who

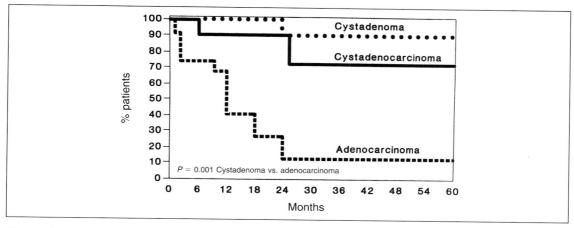

Figure 40-7. Actuarial 5-year survival for patients with cystadenoma, cystadenocarcinoma, and adenocarcinoma masquerading as a cystic neoplasm. (Reprinted with permission from Talamini MA, et al. The spectrum of cystic tumors of the pancreas. *Am J Surg* 1992; 163:117–124.)

could most benefit from adjuvant chemoradiation therapy.

Conclusions

The differential diagnosis of patients with cystic lesions of the pancreas is large. This chapter has focused on cystadenomas, cystadenocarcinomas, and adenocarcinomas producing mucin or causing nonneoplastic cysts and therefore masquerading as cystadenocarcinomas. In the evaluation of these patients, even with sophisticated CT scans, diagnostic uncertainty remains. Although percutaneous aspiration and cyst fluid analysis have been recommended by some authorities, these techniques may not accurately differentiate among cystic pancreatic lesions and may cause the spillage of tumor cells. In addition, differentiation among the possible tumor types may be difficult even in the operating room. Moreover, the correct diagnosis can often not be established until the cyst has been resected and completely examined histologically. With the good long-term survival rates for cystadenomas and cystadenocarcinomas, an aggressive surgical approach is prudent.

Selected Readings

Albores-Saavedra J, et al. Cystic tumors of the pancreas. *Pathol Ann* 1990; 25:19–50.

Alles AJ, et al. Expression of CA 72-4 (TA6-72) in the fluid contents of pancreatic cysts: A new marker to distinguish malignant pancreatic cystic tumors from benign neoplasms and pseudocysts. *Ann Surg* 1994; 219:131–134.

Furukawat T, et al. The mucus-hypersecreting tumor of the pancreas. *Cancer* 1992; 70:1505–1513.

Iselin CE, et al. Computed tomography and fine-needle aspiration cytology for preoperative evaluation of cystic tumors of the pancreas. *Br J Surg* 1993; 80: 1166–1169.

Pyke CM, et al. The spectrum of serous cystadenoma of the pancreas. *Ann Surg* 1992; 215:132–139.

Satoh K, et al. An immunohistochemical study of the c-erbB-2 oncogene product in intraductal mucin-hypersecreting neoplasms and in ductal cell carcinomas of the pancreas. *Cancer* 1993; 72:51–56.

Talamini MA, et al. The spectrum of cystic tumors of the pancreas. *Am J Surg* 1992; 163:117–124.

Warshaw AL, et al. Cystic tumors of the pancreas: New clinical, radiologic, and pathologic observations in 67 patients. *Ann Surg* 1990; 212:432–445.

Yeo CJ, Sarr MG. Cystic and pseudocystic disease of the pancreas. *Curr Probl Surg* 1994; 31:165–252.

Zinner MJ, Sharbaji MS, Cameron JL. Solid and papillary epithelial neoplasms of the pancreas. *Surgery* 1990; 108:475–480.

41

Ampullary Carcinoma

Andrew J. Oishi
Michel M. Murr
Bret T. Petersen
Michael G. Sarr

Etiology and Pathogenesis

The ampulla of Vater is located in an anatomically complex and busy physiologic region comprising the interface of the pancreas, duodenum, and pancreatobiliary ductal system. An inordinately high incidence of malignancy arises in this area, possibly because of the local production of carcinogens through the combined interaction of pancreatic exocrine enzymes, bile salts, and duodenal content. Neoplasms presenting clinically as periampullary masses may arise from the pancreas, the duodenum, the distal bile duct, or the ampulla itself, all potentially masquerading as an ampullary cancer. Most periampullary neoplasms (90%) are adenocarcinomas of pancreatic ductal origin, yet when one examines the subgroup of surgically resectable periampullary malignances, ampullary cancer accounts for a much larger percentage of the total (approximately 20%–30%).

Historically, attempts to preoperatively differentiate ampullary cancers from other periampullary malignancies were not necessary because diagnostic approaches were limited and treatment options were similar, regardless of the site of origin. Currently, however, it has become very important to classify periampullary neoplasms according to the histologic cell of origin because of the now-appreciated differences in the prognosis, survival, and biologic behavior associated with each site of origin. This differentiation requires a team approach involving the gastroenterologist, the radiologist, and the surgeon. Thus, whenever possible, periampullary neoplasms should be subclassified as primary ampullary tumors, periampullary duodenal neoplasms, or periampullary neoplasms involving or infiltrating the ampulla. This differentiation is important because the treatment approach and surgical aggressiveness vary significantly with the site of origin.

Although any epithelial or submucosal cell type of the ampulla may undergo malignant transformation, adenocarcinoma is by far the most common malignant ampullary neoplasm. Carcinoid tumors, neuroendocrine neoplasms, and sarcomas may arise from the ampulla, but these are exceedingly rare. More common are benign neoplasms such as villous adenomas. As in the colon, ampullary and periampullary carcinomas are now thought to evolve through an adenoma-carcinoma sequence. Potentially premalignant adenomas, therefore, require ablative therapy. This treatment is often accomplished in a less aggressive manner than for carcinoma. The remainder of this chapter will concentrate on ampullary cancer, discussing periampullary benign neoplasms when appropriate.

Diagnosis

Clinical Presentation

Most patients present in the sixth and seventh decades of life with jaundice and/or complaints of nonspecific constitutional symptoms. Malaise, anorexia, weight loss, or abdominal pain of several weeks or months in duration are common symptoms. The jaundice is usually progressive but in a small percentage may be intermittent and associated with cholangitis. This clinical presentation of intermittent jaundice appears to be related to repeated necrosis and sloughing of the obstructing tumor mass, which allows for temporary resolution of the jaundice and cholangitis. Hematemesis or melena is rare, although anemia due to occult gastrointestinal bleeding from the ulcerated tumor may be seen in up to a third of patients. The triad of intermittent painless jaundice, anemia, and a palpably enlarged gallbladder has been considered relatively specific for ampullary cancer; however, this triad is seen in less than 10% of patients. In rare cases, patients may complain of gray or "silver-colored" stool which occurs as the result of acholic stool combined with melena and is considered virtually pathognomonic of periampullary neoplasms. Infrequently, ampullary carcinoma may present as pancreatitis.

Patients with the genetic syndrome familial adenomatous polyposis (FAP) are predisposed to the development of ampullary and periampullary adenomas with subsequent malignant transformation. Periampullary cancers in such patients tend to present 10 to 15 years later than the associated colon cancers, that is, in the 40s and 50s.

Laboratory Tests

The majority of patients have some abnormality in serum liver function tests. The earliest and often the only abnormality is an increase in alkaline phosphatase, a sensitive marker of cholestasis. As the ampullary cancer progresses, jaundice and hyperbilirubinemia occur; later, as biliary obstruction progresses, increases in serum aminotransaminases may be found as well. A smaller percentage (about 30%) of patients may have a microcytic, hypochromic anemia due to chronic gastrointestinal bleeding from the tumor surface. The prothrombin time may be increased as a result of cholestasis-induced malabsorption of fat-soluble vitamins, including vitamin K. Although a number of tumor markers such as carcinoembryonic antigen (CEA) and carbohydrate antigen (CA) 19-9 have been studied, most have been directed toward pancreatic adenocarci-

noma; currently, no reliable serum marker exists for the diagnosis of primary ampullary carcinoma.

Radiologic Imaging

Transabdominal ultrasonography is often used in the initial evaluation of those patients with abdominal pain or suspected extrahepatic biliary obstruction. This simple, noninvasive test is particularly useful in diagnosing biliary dilatation and in identifying liver metastases. The presence of gallstones in the gallbladder does not exclude ampullary malignancy, since they may coexist in as many as 30% of patients. Ultrasound may demonstrate simultaneous common bile and pancreatic duct dilatation (the "double-duct sign"), suggesting a periampullary obstruction of both the pancreatic and bile duct. Visualization of the ampullary tumor mass is often difficult, but as many as 80% of these tumors appear as an ill-defined mass between the duodenum and the common bile duct. The presence of ascites in the absence of known cirrhosis suggests advanced unresectable disease and mandates further investigation. Although the accuracy of ultrasonography in detecting ampullary and periampullary tumors is operator-dependent, in experienced hands it has a sensitivity and specificity approaching 90%.

Computed tomography (CT) with both intravenous and oral contrast is usually used for staging rather than diagnosis; however, because CT is an essential imaging procedure in the evaluation of ampullary tumors, the authors believe it should be the first imaging modality (thus supplanting ultrasonography) for the older patient presenting with painless jaundice and a clinical picture of malignancy. As with ultrasound, CT can demonstrate biliary and pancreatic ductal dilatation, a mass lesion at the ampulla, and the presence of ascites. With periampullary carcinoma, the most important finding is that of a distal obstruction, that is, with dilatation of the retroduodenal and intrapancreatic portions of the common bile duct. The presence of a dilated intrapancreatic common bile duct tends to differentiate ampullary tumors from most cancers of the head of the pancreas, especially if there is no recognizable mass in the head or uncinate process of the pancreas (Fig. 41-1).

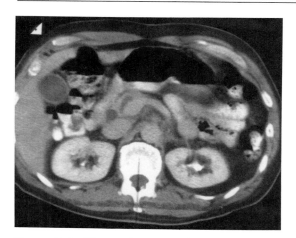

Figure 41-1. CT scan of patient with ampullary cancer. Note presence of dilated intrapancreatic portion of common bile duct, indicative of a very distal obstruction.

CT is superior to ultrasound in its ability to demonstrate local metastatic disease as well as other evidence of unresectability such as encasement of the superior mesenteric vessels, local tumor extension, and regional lymphadenopathy. The limitations of CT are its inability to reliably detect hepatic metastases less than 1 to 2 cm in diameter or small lymphatic, omental, or peritoneal metastases (less than 1 to 2 mm), resulting in an overestimation of resectability. When endoscopic approaches fail, CT-guided percutaneous biopsy may be useful in confirming the diagnosis of cancer in a patient who is being considered for nonoperative management. A negative biopsy, however, does not exclude the presence of carcinoma, because false-negative results occur in about 10% to 30% of patients. Magnetic resonance imaging currently offers no additional benefit over CT and therefore has a limited role in the evaluation of patients with ampullary carcinoma.

Upper gastrointestinal (GI) barium studies or hypotonic duodenography may demonstrate a large ampullary mass causing an indentation of the duodenal lumen, producing the characteristic "inverted 3" sign. A GI series is no longer a commonly used diagnostic test in the evaluation of ampullary neoplasms because of its low sensitivity. Typically, many ampullary tumors are not large enough to be recognized reliably on contrast examination and are difficult to differentiate from a normal ampulla, resulting in a false-negative examination in as many as 40% of cases.

The use of mesenteric angiography in the preoperative evaluation of a large ampullary carcinoma is controversial. The purported benefit of angiography is to demonstrate vascular involvement. When it is combined with CT, the accurate assessment of unresectability of periampullary malignancies may exceed that achieved with either modality alone. Other potential benefits of angiography include the demonstration of major arterial anomalies (which can occur in up to 34% of patients) as well as the ability to evaluate atherosclerotic changes in the celiac or superior mesenteric artery which, in theory, might alter the technique of attempted surgical resection. Conversely, other studies have shown that angiography offers little added benefit to CT in demonstrating unresectability or in changing the surgical approach, and that it places the patient at risk for procedure-related complications. Recent advances in endoscopic ultrasonography may allow for an accurate assessment of major vascular involvement in a less invasive manner than angiography (see below). The authors do not routinely utilize angiography in the evaluation of ampullary cancer.

Cholangiography usually demonstrates a combination of proximal dilatation of the biliary tree and an obstructing, irregular filling defect of the very distal common bile duct. The choice of either an endoscopic retrograde cholangiopancreatographic (ERCP) or percutaneous transhepatic (PTC) route depends on the apparent level of obstruction, the upper gut anatomy, the presence or absence of coagulopathy, and local expertise. Both cholangiographic approaches have similar sensitivity and specificity, and both allow for the placement of indwelling biliary stents for preoperative or palliative drainage of the biliary tree. Endoscopic cholangiography has the added advantages of (1) direct visualization of the ampulla and surrounding duodenum by the endoscopists; (2) access for biopsy confirmation of malignancy; (3) the ability to definitively treat alternative diagnoses (e.g., choledocholithiasis); and (4) less discomfort and fewer potential complications from percutaneous puncture of the hepatic parenchyma. In addition, demonstration of a normal pancreatic duct at ERCP virtually excludes ductal carcinoma of the pancreas as the site of origin. Similarly, an obvious mass on CT or ultrasonography with an endoscopically (visually) normal ampulla essentially excludes ampullary cancer.

Percutaneous transhepatic cholangiography may provide better imaging of the proximal biliary tree and may be necessary when a tumor extends proximally to involve the bifurcation of the right and left main hepatic duct or when endoscopic cholangiography cannot be performed for technical reasons. The authors' practice is to perform endoscopic cholangiography when an ampullary mass is suspected and to proceed to percutaneous transhepatic cholangiography only if the proximal extent of the tumor cannot be evaluated adequately by ERCP, ultrasonography, or CT.

Endoscopy

Fiberoptic endoscopy revolutionized the diagnosis and preoperative evaluation of ampullary and periampullary neoplasms and is the diagnostic procedure of choice in most situations. Using the standard side-viewing "duodenoscope," the ampulla can be visualized (Fig. 41-2), biopsied, and cannulated for cholangiography or biliary decompression.

Figure 41-2. Endoscopic photography of an ampullary carcinoma.

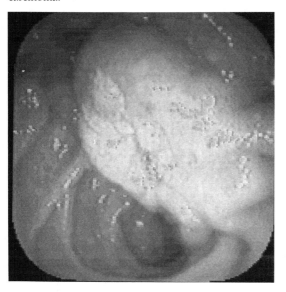

End-viewing endoscopes are not adequate for either surveillance or diagnostic examinations of the ampulla or periampullary region. The endoscopic appearance of ampullary cancer varies widely. Small intra-ampullary lesions may cause almost imperceptible changes to the ampulla. Whereas intraduodenal lesions may appear polypoid (and potentially benign); infiltrating or ulcerated lesions are clearly malignant. This spectrum of change may make the preoperative diagnosis of carcinoma difficult. Biopsy of the tumor surface or brush cytology may be negative in up to 30% of carcinomas; therefore, a negative biopsy does not exclude invasive cancer. Many biopsies demonstrate adenomatous tissue while underestimating the true degree of dysplasia or invasiveness. Although a greater risk of bleeding exists with endoscopic snare biopsy, its use for polypoid or papillary lesions may reduce the incidence of false negatives and thus aid in the diagnosis of cancer.

When common bile duct dilatation exists without an obvious ampullary tumor, the judicious use of sphincterotomy with biopsy of the interior of the ampulla can establish the diagnosis in up to 40% of such occult presentations of ampullary cancer. Biopsy sensitivity is improved by resampling 7 to 10 days after sphincterotomy to allow for resolution of cautery artifact and inflammation.

Endoscopic ultrasonography (EUS) has recently been reported to be an accurate and reliable modality for diagnosing and staging ampullary carcinomas. In several studies, the accuracy of EUS in staging and in determining resectability has averaged over 90%. Furthermore, EUS may be superior to angiography or CT in demonstrating involvement of the superior mesenteric or portal vein by tumor, although it is less reliable for detecting celiac or superior mesenteric arterial involvement. The actual role for EUS in the evaluation of the patient with a periampullary neoplasm is yet to be defined.

For patients with familial adenomatous polyposis, endoscopic surveillance with a side-viewing duodenoscope is advised every 3 to 5 years beginning at the time of diagnosis. Minor adenomatous foci can be ablated with cold biopsy, cautery, or laser with subsequent intensified follow-up. Extensive adenomatous change should prompt aggressive laser ablation or local surgical excision. Endoscopic sphincterotomy should be performed prior to ag-

gressive therapy to prevent pancreatitis or cholangitis.

Management

Staging

The proper management of patients with ampullary
cancer requires a multidisciplinary team approach.
The diagnostic and interventional radiologist,
endoscopist, and surgeon all contribute to management decisions and are essential for the proper
selection of patients for resectional or palliative surgery or nonoperative therapy. A suggested plan for
evaluation and appropriate treatment is shown in
Fig. 41-3.

The primary staging system for ampullary cancer used currently in the United States is the 1987
TNM system (Table 41-1). Regardless of the staging
system used, ampullary carcinoma is classified according to the extent of local invasion, the presence
or absence of regional lymph node metastases, and
the presence or absence of distant metastatic disease—the factors influencing resectability and,
hence, prognosis. Patients who do not have preoperative evidence of unresectability and who are good
operative risks should undergo surgical exploration. Conversely, when preoperative evaluation reveals local metastases or when a patient is not an
operative candidate because of serious medical conditions, nonoperative palliation with a biliary endoprosthesis and palliative radiation therapy should

Figure 41-3. Management of patients with ampullary cancer.

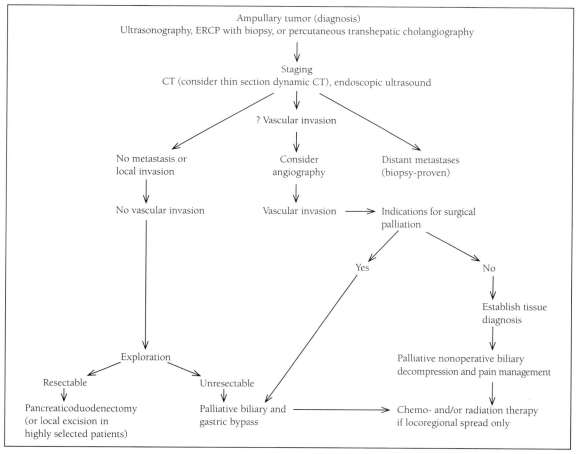

Table 41-1. TNM Staging of Ampullary Carcinoma

		Group Staging Criteria			
T1	Tumor limited to the ampulla of Vater	Stage I	T1–T2	N0[a]	M0[b]
T2	Tumor invades duodenal wall	Stage II	T3	N0	M0
T3	Tumor invades < 2 cm into pancreas	Stage III	any T	N1[a]	M0
T4	Tumor invades > 2 cm into pancreas and/or adjacent organs	Stage IV	any T	any N	M1[d]

[a]N0 = no regional lymph node metastases.
[b]M0 = no distant metastases.
[c]N1 = regional lymph node metastases.
[d]M1 = distant metastases.

be considered. Preoperative endoscopic or percutaneous biopsy is useful in this latter situation because malignancy must be confirmed before appropriate palliative chemotherapy or radiotherapy will be initiated.

After cholangiography, patients with obstructive jaundice may undergo preoperative biliary drainage by placement of a nasobiliary drain or an indwelling stent (endoprosthesis). However, the routine use of preoperative biliary drainage is controversial. Preoperative biliary drainage has been claimed to improve hepatic function and to reduce the incidence of postoperative complications, yet it is difficult to show objective improvements in operative morbidity or mortality. The resolution of the deleterious effects of jaundice (e.g., immunosuppression) may require 4 to 6 weeks of decompression, which is impractical.

Pancreaticoduodenectomy

In 1935, Whipple, Parsons, and Mullins reported on three patients managed successfully with a two-stage pancreaticoduodenectomy as a cure for ampullary carcinoma. Since this pioneering report, radical pancreaticoduodenectomy has gone through a number of technical modifications. Although universal acceptance of this procedure was limited by a high complication rate and an operative mortality rate of up to 25%, recent advancements in surgical technique, anesthesia, and pre- and postoperative care have resulted in a decrease in the morbidity rate (though it still remains about 40%) and, more importantly, a decrease in the mortality rate to less

than 5% in most experienced centers. Radical pancreaticoduodenectomy is the curative procedure of choice for patients with ampullary cancer.

The operation is initially carried out via an upper midline or limited right subcostal incision. A diligent search for evidence of unresectability is carried out before any attempt at resection is initiated. The entire abdominal cavity is examined for evidence of peritoneal or hepatic metastases. If no peritoneal metastases are found, the incision is extended, and the exploration is continued. The duodenum and pancreatic head are widely mobilized and lifted off the vena cava and aorta (Kocher maneuver). The celiac and superior mesenteric artery are palpated for evidence of tumor involvement. Nodal groups in the hepatoduodenal ligament and the superior pancreatic and celiac axis regions are biopsied routinely. The plane between the neck of the pancreas and the anterior surface of the superior mesenteric vein is developed.

If there is no evidence of tumor outside the anticipated resection margins and if the diagnosis of cancer has not been established preoperatively, consideration is given to intraoperative biopsy. This step is easily accomplished by transduodenal core-needle biopsy or by fine-needle aspiration cytology. Because a negative biopsy does not rule out the possibility that the mass is malignant, repeated attempts at biopsy to establish the diagnosis are not indicated. Once resectability is established, pancreaticoduodenectomy is carried out. This procedure involves en bloc resection of the distal stomach, the duodenum, the gallbladder, and the distal common bile duct and pancreatic head. Gastrointestinal continuity is restored with a pancreaticojejunostomy (or pancreaticogastrostomy), a hepaticojejunostomy, and a gastrojejunostomy. Recently, a pylorus-preserving pancreaticoduodenectomy, as reported by Traverso and Longmire in 1978, has gained popularity. Its proposed advantages include improved postoperative gastrointestinal function, less dumping, and reduced jejunal anastomotic ulceration. Although these postoperative benefits have not been shown conclusively, advantages exist in decreased operative time and reduced intraoperative blood loss. In a very small minority of cases, total pancreatectomy is required because technical reasons preclude performing a safe pancreaticojejunal anastomosis; this possibility should always be discussed with the patient preoperatively.

Regardless of the type of pancreaticoduodenectomy performed (standard vs. pylorus-preserving vs. total pancreatectomy), the incidence of postoperative complications remains high and ranges from 25% to 50%. Delayed gastric emptying and anastomotic leak from the pancreaticojejunostomy are the most common, significant postoperative morbidities. Perioperative treatment with both octreotide (a somatostatin analog) and erythromycin (a motilin agonist) in an attempt to decrease pancreatic exocrine secretion and to increase gastric emptying, respectively, may decrease the incidence of these complications. Intra-abdominal sepsis, bile leak, gastrointestinal bleeding, and intra-abdominal hemorrhage occur less frequently; together they account for only a quarter of the complications but are responsible for over 80% of the operative mortalities. Potential late complications include weight loss, dumping, and pancreatic exocrine and endocrine insufficiency.

Local Excision

In 1899, Halstead reported the first local excision of an ampullary carcinoma with reimplantation of the pancreatic and bile ducts. Because of the potential for local recurrence and the recent improved results with pancreaticoduodenectomy, local resection is rarely performed. Recent reports suggest that patients undergoing local excision may be at high risk for local recurrence. Nevertheless, local excision for ampullary cancer can be performed with curative intent in either selected, high-risk patients with small tumors in whom medical conditions preclude radical resection or in patients likely to have benign tumors. Periampullary resection as opposed to pancreaticoduodenectomy may be the procedure of choice in ampullary villous adenomas with histologic evidence of dysplasia or carcinoma in situ. Local excision may also be indicated as palliation in patients with unresectable disease and with an ulcerated, bleeding tumor surface that is causing anemia or life-threatening hemorrhage.

The operation is performed via an upper midline or right subcostal incision. As with radical resection, a careful exploration to rule out metastatic disease or other evidence of resectability is imperative. A Kocher maneuver allows for complete inspection of the duodenum and pancreatic head. If the tumor is resectable, a longitudinal duodenotomy is made that is centered over the ampulla. (Passage of a biliary Fogarty catheter through the cystic duct into the common duct and out into the duodenum may aid in the placement of the duodenotomy.) One then excises the tumor completely, taking a full thickness of the duodenal wall and including segments of the bile and pancreatic ducts (Fig. 41-4). If necessary, the two ducts are sutured together to form a common septum, and then the posterior wall of the duodenum is approximated to the joined pancreatic and common duct openings (see Fig. 41-4). If there is concern about restoration of biliary or pancreatic drainage, the common and pancreatic ducts may be stented or a T tube choledochostomy may be placed.

Palliation

Although the resectability rate of ampullary cancer is much greater than that for periampullary cancers arising from the pancreas, 20% to 35% of patients are not candidates for curative resection. These patients present challenging management problems because optimal palliation of their symptoms is often difficult. Obstructive jaundice, duodenal obstruction, and abdominal or back pain are the most frequent symptoms requiring intervention. Regardless of whether palliation is performed operatively or nonoperatively, relief of these symptoms is the primary goal.

OPERATIVE PALLIATION

Surgical options include biliary-enteric drainage, gastrojejunostomy, and intraoperative chemical splanchnicectomy (celiac plexus block). The procedure of choice for biliary drainage is a hepaticojejunostomy; however, a cholecystojejunostomy may be constructed if technical considerations preclude a common duct-enteric anastomosis. Gastrojejunostomy should be considered in conjunction with biliary-enteric bypass even if duodenal obstruction has not developed or does not appear "impending." The addition of a gastroenterostomy to a biliary enteric bypass may slightly increase the duration

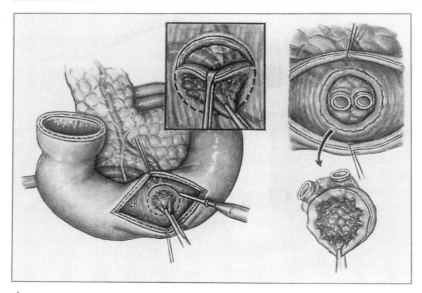

A

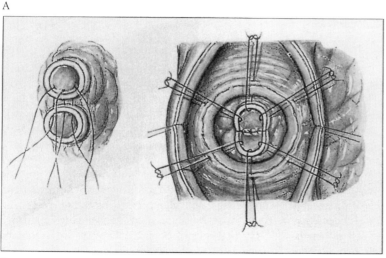

B

Figure 41-4. Transduodenal resection of an ampullary cancer. A. Duodenotomy and transmural resection of periampullary mass; note separate openings of intrapancreatic common bile duct and pancreatic duct. B. Anastomosis of common bile duct with pancreatic duct. C. Mucosa-to-mucosa anastomosis of common bile duct/pancreatic duct to duodenal mucosa. (Asbun HJ, Rossi RL, Munson JL. Local resection for ampullary tumors. *Arch Surg* 128:515–520. Copyright 1993 American Medical Association.)

of postoperative hospitalization but will prevent reoperation for subsequent duodenal obstruction, which occurs in as many as 15% of patients with periampullary cancer in which a gastrojejunostomy has not been performed. A randomized trial of chemical splanchnicectomy with 50% alcohol in-

jected into the para-aortic and celiac ganglia showed a significant reduction of pain associated with pancreatic cancer and no increase in morbidity. No similar studies comparing the efficacy of operative chemical splanchnicectomy for the relief of pain associated with periampullary cancer exist, but it

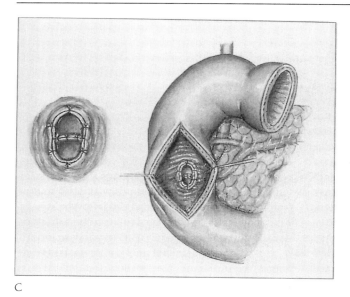

C

Figure 41-4. (continued)

NONOPERATIVE PALLIATION

is reasonable to expect similar benefits, and this simple procedure should be considered in patients with unresectable lesions.

The most common technique of palliating jaundice involves placing a biliary endoprosthesis through the area of obstruction, thus providing for biliary decompression while maintaining internal drainage of bile into the duodenum. Endoscopic placement of these stents is preferred over a percutaneous route because it avoids transhepatic puncture and the attendant risks of hemorrhage, hemobilia, and bile leak. A combined approach involving endoscopic stenting over a percutaneously passed wire may be helpful when the tumor obscures the papillary os or prevents wire access below. Percutaneous placement is normally reserved for situations when biliary decompression cannot be established endoscopically. Depending on tumor anatomy, endoscopic sphincterotomy without stent placement may provide adequate palliation; however, with this form of management there is a risk of recurrent tumor obstruction. Although generally not indicated, palliative laser therapy of unresectable lesions may be useful for control of persistent bleeding.

Patients who later develop duodenal obstruction and are not candidates for surgical gastroenterostomy may be treated with percutaneous endoscopic tube gastrostomy (PEG) for gastric decompression. Although PEG does not allow a patient to be fed orally, it is effective in relieving symptoms relatd to gastric outlet obstruction. A separate tube can be advanced distal to the obstruction endoscopically for enteral hydration and nutrition, thus avoiding the need for parenteral hyperalimentation. However, many believe this means of "palliation" is inappropriate because, although it may prolong survival, the quality of life is poor except in patients with a good performance status and realistic expectations.

Percutaneous chemical splanchnicectomy with injections of 50% ethanol or 6% phenol should be used liberally for the nonoperative treatment of back pain associated with ampullary cancer. Satisfactory reduction of pain can be expected in most patients.

Several randomized studies have shown comparable survival rates when nonoperative stent placement is compared to surgical bypass for relief of malignant biliary obstruction. Nonoperative palliation is associated with fewer procedure-related complications, a shorter initial period of hospitalization, and possibly a decreased mortality rate when compared to surgical bypass. The principal limitation to palliative stenting is the tendency of the stent (whether the original plastic stents or the newer metal expandable stents) to occlude from biliary sludge and debris, resulting in the recurrence of jaundice or cholangitis, which often requires rehospitalization. To avoid this complication, routine changes of the plastic stents have been suggested at intervals of 3 to 6 months. Recent trials with self-expanding metal stents have demonstrated improved patency and decreased incidence of recurrent jaundice and cholangitis. Most metal stents, however, are permanent once placed, and delayed or late occlusion may still occur as a result of tumor ingrowth. It is anticipated that newer sheathed metal stents will overcome this problem. Because of the problems with duodenal obstruction and stent occlusion, the quality of life may be better with operative palliation in selected patients with unresectable malignancies who at the time of presentation have a good performance level and are expected to live longer than 6 months.

Radiotherapy and Chemotherapy

The role of chemotherapy and radiotherapy, either as adjuvant treatment in surgically resected cases or as palliative therapy, is undefined for ampullary carcinoma. Combined modality therapy with chemotherapy (5-fluorouracil) with radiation has been shown to improve survival in patients with resectable periampullary and pancreatic carcinomas, and similar results have been extrapolated (albeit without data) to ampullary carcinoma. Combination chemotherapy with 5-fluorouracil, adriamycin, and mitomycin-C (FAM) showed no improvement in survival when compared to surgical resection alone; this therapeutic protocol was poorly tolerated.

The benefits of chemotherapy and radiotherapy in the palliative treatment of unresectable ampullary carcinoma have not been proven. Few studies have examined palliative chemotherapy and radiation therapy specifically for ampullary cancer. Most studies include periampullary or pancreatic cancers, making interpretation of the results difficult. Good evidence exists, however, that combina-

tion chemotherapy and radiation prolong survival and improve the quality of life in patients with unresectable pancreatic ductal adenocarcinoma. The subjective improvement in patient outlook with the use of palliative methods of treatment should also not be overlooked.

Figure 41-5. Survival of patients with ampullary carcinoma undergoing curative resection. A. Overall survival. B. Survival according to histologic differentiation/grade. C. Survival according to nodal status. (Monson JR, et al. Radical resection for carcinoma of the ampulla of Vater. *Arch Surg* 126:353–357. Copyright 1991 American Medical Association.)

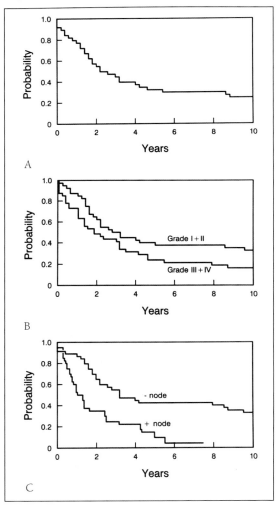

Results

The hospital mortality rate following either resection or operative palliation ranges from 1% to 5%. Operative mortality is similar regardless of whether pancreaticoduodenectomy, local excision, or palliative biliary and gastric bypass is performed. This observation is not surprising because it likely reflects the appropriate bias toward selecting better operative candidates for radical surgery and poorer candidates for less radical procedures.

The overall 5-year survival rates for patients with ampullary cancer undergoing radical resection range from 25% to 55% (Fig. 41-5). Favorable prognostic indicators include tumors confined to the ampulla or duodenum, a well-differentiated histology, the absence of regional nodal metastases, and negative resection margins. Survival data for local excision of ampullary carcinoma are difficult to interpret because most published series are small and include patients with periampullary carcinomas as well as benign ampullary adenomas. In a collective review of 86 patients who underwent local excision for an ampullary tumor, 5-year survival rates ranged from 0% to 50%, and the results of many series often approached results obtained with radical resection. Survival for patients with unresectable carcinoma is dismal. The mean survival following palliative intervention is less than 10 months, with few (if any) patients surviving beyond 5 years.

Conclusions

It is important to differentiate among various periampullary neoplasms because biologic behavior differs with each site of origin. Most patients with ampullary carcinoma present with jaundice, which may be intermittent. CT and endoscopy with biopsy are the diagnostic tests of choice. Cholangiography and pancreatography help to define anatomy, but the need for angiography or preoperative biliary drainage is controversial. Pancreaticoduodenectomy is the treatment of choice, whereas local excision should be reserved for carefully selected high-risk patients with small tumors. Palliative therapy may be performed either operatively or nonoperatively. The benefits of radiotherapy and chemotherapy have not been proven in patients with ampullary carcinoma, partly because of the relative rarity of this disease. Five-year survival rates in resected cases range from 25% to 55% and are affected by tumor differentiation and nodal status.

Selected Readings

Asbun HJ, Rossi RL, Munson JL. Local resection for ampullary tumors. *Arch Surg* 1993; 128:515–520.

Buck JL, Elsayed AM. Ampullary tumors: Radiologic-pathologic correlation. *Radiographics* 1993; 13: 193–212.

Hyoty MK, Nordback IH. Biliary stent or surgical bypass in unresectable pancreatic cancer with obstructive jaundice. *Acta Chir Scand* 1990; 156:391–396.

Lambert R, et al. Laser treatment of tumors of the papilla of vater. *Endoscopy* 1988; 20:227–231.

Lillemoe KD, et al. Current status of surgical palliation of periampullary carcinoma. *Surg Gynecol Obstet* 1993; 176:1–10.

Miedema BW, et al. Complications following pancreaticoduodenectomy. *Arch Surg* 1992; 127:945–950.

Monson JR, et al. Radical resection for carcinoma of the ampulla of Vater. *Arch Surg* 1991; 126:353–357.

Ponchon T, et al. Contribution of endoscopy to diagnosis and treatment of tumors of the ampulla of Vater. *Cancer* 1989; 64:161–167.

Rosch T, et al. Staging of pancreatic and ampullary carcinoma by endoscopic ultrasonography. *Gastroenterology* 1992; 102:188–199.

Willett CG, et al. Patterns of failure after pancreaticoduodenectomy for ampullary carcinoma. *Surg Gynecol Obstet* 1993; 176:33–38.

42

Pancreatic Cancer

JOHN L. CAMERON
LOUISE B. GROCHOW
FRANCIS D. MILLIGAN
ANTHONY C. VENBRUX

Carcinoma of the pancreas has increased significantly in incidence over the past several decades. Between 25,000 and 30,000 new cases of pancreatic cancer are diagnosed each year in the United States, and it is now the fifth most common cause of cancer death. In the past pancreatic cancer was a particularly frustrating disease to manage; by the time most patients were diagnosed, they were inoperable because of disseminated disease. Among that smaller group of patients who were operable, most were unresectable. Prior to the past decade, that small group of patients that was resectable incurred a hospital mortality rate of 25%. The remaining small number that were successfully resected and left the hospital generally died a painful death during the next 12 months. The other patients who were inoperable or unresectable had a mean survival of less than 6 months, and usually had inadequate palliation of pain.

Over the past decade the management of pancreatic cancer has improved substantially. Preoperative diagnosis can be made with great accuracy, patient selection and preoperative staging are much more precise, and the resectability rate of those patients undergoing surgery has increased remarkably. The hospital mortality rate for surgical resection has dropped below 5% in virtually all age groups, effective adjuvant therapy has been developed, and up to one quarter of patients undergoing pancreaticoduodenectomy are now surviving 5 years.

Etiology and Pathogenesis

As with most malignancies, the exact etiology of pancreatic cancer is unknown. A number of potential risk factors have been studied, but convincing data have only been established for smoking as a causative factor. Coffee and alcohol have also been studied, but current data do not support an association between excess intake of these liquids and pancreatic cancer. Nitrosamine intake can cause pancreatic cancers in animals, but an association between excess ingestion of nitrosamines and human pancreatic cancer has not been established. Both chronic pancreatitis and diabetes have also been suggested as possible risk factors. Recent data suggest that patients with chronic pancreatitis are at increased risk for developing pancreatic cancer, whereas long-standing diabetics are not at increased risk. However, elderly patients with new-onset diabetes are more likely than the general population to be harboring a pancreatic cancer.

Recent studies have demonstrated that the majority of pancreatic cancers have point mutations at codon 12 of the K-*ras* oncogene and that an association exists between this tumor marker and smoking. As with other gastrointestinal tumors, many patients with pancreatic cancer also have a defect in the p53 suppressor gene. Considerable work is ongoing in the genetics of pancreatic cancer, and future studies of rare patients with hereditary

475

tumors may help to unravel the pathogenesis of these tumors.

Diagnosis

Clinical Presentation

In the majority of patients with adenocarcinoma of the pancreas the lesion originates in the head of the gland, and these patients will be the focus of this discussion. The less frequent lesions that arise in the body and tail of the gland will not be discussed. Most patients with cancer of the head of the pancreas do not present until they develop obstructive jaundice. Even though this is often at a relatively late stage, even the newer diagnostic tools have not allowed for an earlier diagnosis. Pancreatic cancer generally arises at the "knee" of the main pancreatic duct and remains asymptomatic until it obstructs the adjacent common bile duct at its "knee." Thus the stage of pancreatic tumor seen today is identical to that seen two decades ago, as determined by diameter of tumor and incidence of positive lymph nodes. A substantial number of patients have abdominal pain, and the adage that patients usually have painless jaundice is generally not true. Many patients have back pain as well, and weight loss is a common feature. Occasional patients in whom the lesion develops in the uncinate process, or at the junction of the head and neck of the pancreas, do not have jaundice but rather abdominal pain and weight loss. Nausea and vomiting are seen less frequently.

Radiologic Tests

When a patient presents with obstructive jaundice and is suspected of having a periampullary carcinoma, the first study ordered after the initial diagnostic blood tests should be a computerized tomographic (CT) scan. This study will not only allow one to confirm the diagnosis of biliary obstruction by imaging dilated bile ducts but will also demonstrate a mass in the head of the pancreas. Furthermore, by determining the site at which the dilated bile duct is obstructed, one can usually differentiate pancreatic cancer from the more distally obstructing malignant lesions (distal bile duct, ampullary, and duodenal cancer). In addition to providing diagnostic accuracy, a CT scan also allows one to stage

the patient by determining whether or not liver metastases are present and whether or not the major vessels are encased or occluded (Fig. 42-1). The authors prefer CT scan to ultrasound because of its improved imaging of the pancreas, particularly in the presence of bowel gas. The accuracy of CT in detecting liver metastases is also superior to that of sonography. Some have suggested that for staging pancreatic cancer magnetic resonance imaging (MRI) is superior to the CT scan. In some instances MRI provides more accurate imaging of the vessels; in general, however, CT is to be preferred.

In many institutions endoscopic retrograde cholangiopancreatography (ERCP) plays a major role in the initial management of a patient with a suspected periampullary cancer. In a patient with obstructive jaundice secondary to a periampullary tumor, endoscopy allows one to differentiate duodenal and ampullary tumors from distal bile duct and pancreatic neoplasms and to confirm them by biopsy. In addition, pancreatic cancers can generally be differentiated from distal bile duct tumors through the demonstration of an obstructed pancreatic duct (Fig. 42-2). Finally, some potential benefit exists with ERCP if the patient is deeply jaundiced and there is a potential delay in surgical decompression. The biliary obstruction can be decompressed by the insertion of an endoprosthesis.

In other institutions percutaneous transhepatic cholangiography (PTC), with the insertion of a per-

Figure 42-1. Spiral CT scan demonstrating a low-density adenocarcinoma in the uncinate encasing the superior mesenteric artery.

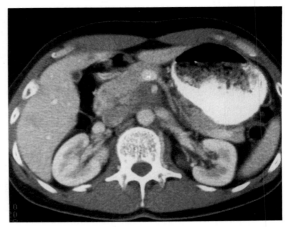

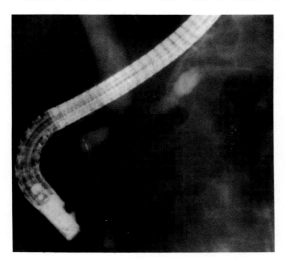

Figure 42-2. ERCP demonstrating a "double-duct" sign with occlusion of the pancreatic and bile ducts.

cutaneous biliary stent, is preferred over ERCP in patients presenting with periampullary tumors. The success of PTC and stent placement is close to 100% in such patients. In addition, the biliary tree above the obstructing lesion is well visualized, and this information can be of great benefit to the surgeon. The stent can also be of technical aid at the time of surgery, particularly if the patient has recently undergone a right upper quadrant procedure. Finally, the percutaneously placed stent can be used to decompress the biliary anastomosis following surgery, and obviates the use of a T tube.

Staging

As already mentioned, the CT scan is a useful tool not only in diagnosing carcinoma of the head of the pancreas but also in staging the extent of the disease. Liver metastases down to 1 cm in diameter can generally be visualized. In addition, encasement or occlusion of the portal, superior mesenteric, and splenic veins can often be imaged. Encasement or occlusion of the hepatic, splenic, and superior mesenteric arteries can also be seen. MRI can provide the same staging function, and some studies have suggested that vascular involvement can be diagnosed with greater accuracy by MRI.

Many institutions, including the authors', consider selective visceral angiography to be of substan-

tial benefit in staging patients with carcinoma of the head of the pancreas (Fig. 42-3). In a prospective study carried out at The Johns Hopkins Hospital, 90 consecutive patients with periampullary cancer were studied. All patients had CT scans which suggested a periampullary cancer, with no evidence of unresectability. Although patients with other tumors were included, the majority of patients (78 patients) had carcinoma of the head of the pancreas. Among the 90 patients, 48 had normal visceral angiograms. At the time of surgery, 77% of the 48 patients successfully underwent a pancreaticoduodenectomy. In 17 patients vessel encasement was demonstrated. Of these 17 patients, 35% were successfully resected. In some instances the encased vessel was resected and reconstructed, and in others it was felt that the angiogram was falsely positive. In 11 patients major vessel occlusion was found, and in none of these patients was resection possible. The study showed that the combination of CT scan and angiography results in a high degree of staging accuracy in patients with carcinoma of the head of the pancreas.

Others have suggested that CT scan and laparoscopy are effective in staging patients with carcinoma of the pancreas. At the Massachusetts General Hospital preoperative laparoscopy in combination with biopsy and peritoneal cytology has been advocated by Warshaw and colleagues. This routine has also proved to be highly accurate and has resulted in a resectability rate virtually identical to that of the combination of CT scan and angiography. The disadvantage of laparoscopy with cytology is that it requires an additional general anesthetic for the laparoscopy and a delay of several days to wait for cytology. Each technique—CT and angiography, and CT and laparoscopy—determines resectability via different criteria. However, the results are virtually identical.

Management

Surgical Resection

All patients with pancreatic cancer who are acceptable anesthetic risks and via staging are demonstrated to be potentially resectable for cure should be explored. The operative procedure of choice is a pylorus-preserving pancreaticoduodenectomy.

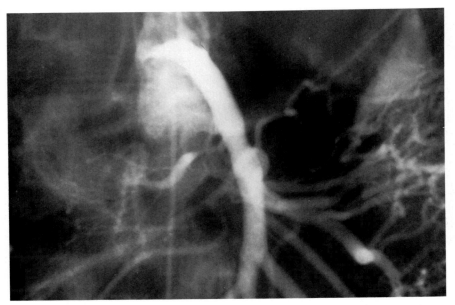

Figure 42-3. Superior mesenteric artery angiogram of same patient as in Fig. 42-1 demonstrating encasement of the artery.

Current evidence suggests that the smaller margins obtained with pylorus preservation do not decrease long-term survival over the more classic Whipple's operation, which includes a hemigastrectomy. In addition, most data suggest that a partial pancreatectomy which removes only the uncinate process, head, and neck of the gland achieves the same prolongation of survival as does total pancreatectomy, with less postoperative morbidity because of the absence of insulin dependency.

Until 1980 throughout the country, pancreaticoduodenectomy carried a hospital mortality rate of 25%. This rate has dropped substantially, and now many institutions are reporting hospital mortality rates for pancreaticoduodenectomy of less than 5%. During one 3-year period at The Johns Hopkins Hospital, 145 consecutive patients underwent pancreaticoduodenectomy without hospital mortality. Four of these patients were in their 80s, and 36 were over age 70. During the past 10 years, the authors have performed pancreaticoduodenectomies in 20 patients over age 80, and in one patient over age 90. Only one death occurred in this group. Thus, with reasonable patient selection pancreaticoduodenectomy can now be performed in virtually

any age group with an acceptably low hospital mortality.

The reason for the substantial drop in hospital mortality is not entirely clear. Undoubtedly, better anesthesia, better intensive care units, more sophisticated support for organ failure, and better anticipation and management of postoperative complications all play a role. However, in addition, in the authors' institution improved experience with the procedure has also played a major role. Before 1980 at The Johns Hopkins Hospital, generally fewer than 10 pancreaticoduodenectomies for periampullary cancer were performed annually. The hospital mortality rate was 24%. Since 1980, the number of Whipple's operations performed each year has increased substantially, and now between 60 and 80 procedures are performed each year (Fig. 42-4). Prior to 1980, a large number of surgeons were performing 1 or 2 Whipple's operations every several years. Now, a small number of surgeons who do virtually nothing but pancreatic, biliary, and liver surgery are performing all of the pancreaticoduodenectomies. This change has resulted in an increased familiarity with anatomy, a substantial decrease in operative time and blood loss, and better

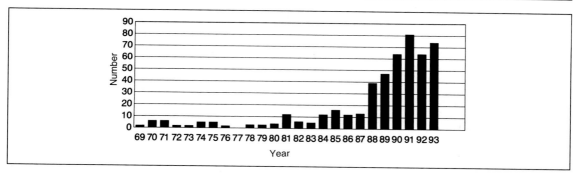

Figure 42-4. Number of pancreaticoduodenectomies per year at The Johns Hopkins Hospital, 1969–1993.

anticipation and management of postoperative complications, and probably is the main reason for the marked drop in mortality in the authors' institution.

Morbidity continues to be substantial following pancreaticoduodenectomy, but in most instances postoperative complications are not life-threatening. The two most common postoperative complications are delayed gastric emptying and pancreatic cutaneous fistula. The incidence of delayed gastric emptying is approximately 30%. This problem is defined as the need to reinsert a nasogastric tube 10 or more days following pancreaticoduodenectomy. Delayed gastric emptying is not a life-threatening complication and always resolves, but it keeps the patient in the hospital for an additional week to 10 days. A study carried out by Yeo and associates at The Johns Hopkins Hospital suggests that delayed gastric emptying following pancreaticoduodenectomy is secondary, at least in part, to the loss of the prokinetic hormone motilin. Motilin is produced primarily in the duodenum, which is removed during a Whipple's operation. The antibiotic erythromycin is a motilin agonist that in other clinical situations has improved gastric emptying. In a prospective randomized study carried out at The Johns Hopkins Hospital, the administration of erythromycin intravenously decreased the incidence of delayed gastric emptying and made the reinsertion of a nasogastric tube unnecessary in a significant percentage of patients following pancreaticoduodenectomy.

The second most common complication following the Whipple's procedure is the development of a pancreatic-cutaneous fistula. This problem occurs with an incidence of between 10% and 20%. The standard reconstruction following pancreaticoduodenectomy is an end-to-end pancreaticojejunostomy, an end-to-side hepaticojejunostomy, and then a duodeno- or gastrojejunostomy. Multiple small series and case reports suggest that the incidence of pancreatic-cutaneous fistulas might be decreased following a Whipple's procedure if the pancreas is anastomosed to the back wall of the stomach instead of to the jejunum. A prospective randomized study is being carried out at The Johns Hopkins Hospital comparing these two types of anastomoses. Recent European studies have also suggested that the prophylactic administration of the somatostatin analog octreotide can decrease the incidence of pancreatic-cutaneous fistula following pancreaticoduodenectomy. Even though this approach has theoretic appeal, available data do not prove the efficacy of octreotide for this purpose.

POSTOPERATIVE SURVIVAL

Before 1980, most institutions reported a 5-year survival rate for patients with carcinoma of the head of the pancreas of less than 5% following pancreaticoduodenectomy. Over the past decade, this situation has changed. In a series of 50 patients reported from The Johns Hopkins Hospital in 1987, the 5-year survival rate was approximately 20%. In a more recent update from the Hopkins series, now with 195 patients, the 5-year survival rate was 26% (Fig. 42-5). In a series of 128 patients from the Memorial Sloan-Kettering Institute, Brennan and colleagues have reported a 21% 5-year survival rate following

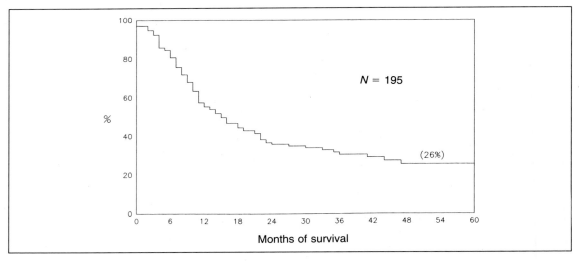

Figure 42-5. Actuarial 5-year survival rates of 195 patients with pancreatic cancer at The Johns Hopkins Hospital.

pancreaticoduodenectomy. Trede et al. from the Mannheim Clinic in Germany have also reported a 25% 5-year survival rate following pancreaticoduodenectomy in a series of 130 patients.

The reasons for the improvement in 5-year survival are not clear. A variety of parameters allow one to predict long-term survival, such as size of the primary tumor, blood vessel invasion, and lymph node involvement. These factors do not appear to have changed in prevalence over the past several decades, however, and thus do not explain why patients are surviving longer now than in the past. In a series of 81 patients from The Johns Hopkins Hospital, data suggest that fewer blood transfusions during surgery is an independent predictor of long-term survival. Thus patients with the same tumor stage who receive less blood at the time of surgery have a better chance of surviving long-term. In the Hopkins series, if a patient received more than 2 units of blood during surgery, the 5-year survival rate was 8%. With less than 2 units, the survival rate was 30% (Fig. 42-6). In virtually all institutions the amount of blood loss and the number of units of blood transfused have decreased for pancreaticoduodenectomy over the last two decades. This factor could, in large part, explain the improvement in survival. The teleologic explanation for this phenomenon is that blood transfusions

are immunosuppressive, and that if blood is given while the tumor is being manipulated and tumor cells are being shed into the blood, a metastasis is more likely to occur.

ADJUVANT THERAPY

Data from the Gastrointestinal Tumor Study Group's prospective randomized study published several years ago demonstrated that adjuvant radiation and chemotherapy can prolong survival following pancreaticoduodenectomy for carcinoma of the head of the pancreas. Forty-three patients were prospectively randomized. One-half received no adjuvant therapy, and the second half received 4000 rads of external beam radiotherapy to the pancreatic bed and low-dose weekly intravenous 5-fluorouracil (5-FU) for 24 months. Mean survival was doubled in the group that received adjuvant therapy. Most oncologists presently judge this adjuvant regimen to be inadequate, and hope persists that adjuvant therapy will improve over the next decade.

The limited activity of available adjuvant treatments (5-fluorouracil and radiation therapy) is a motivation for research into new drugs and alternative cytotoxic approaches. Ongoing multimodality studies at Johns Hopkins are evaluating more intensive chemotherapy with continuous infusion of 5-FU and leucovorin with concurrent radiation to

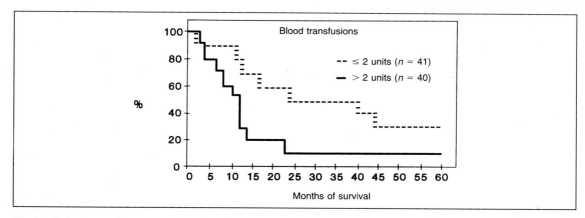

Figure 42-6. Actuarial 5-year survival rates for patients with pancreatic cancer receiving 2 or fewer units of blood during pancreaticoduodenectomy. (Reprinted with permission of Cameron JL, et al. Factors influencing survival following pancreaticoduodenectomy for pancreatic cancer. *Am J Surg* 1991; 161:120.)

the pancreatic bed and the liver. Other approaches include preoperative chemotherapy and radiation to reduce the viability of cells shed at surgery, immunomodulatory regimens, and studies of new drugs.

Palliation

Many patients with carcinoma of the head of the pancreas who present with obstructive jaundice are not candidates for resection. At the time of diagnosis they may have evidence of tumor dissemination in the form of liver metastases, or serosal or distant spread. In addition, some patients will not be resectable because of major vessel involvement. Unless such patients have duodenal obstruction, they probably do not benefit substantially from operative palliation. Their jaundice may be palliated either endoscopically with an endoprosthesis, or percutaneously and transhepatically with a percutaneously placed stent or endoprosthesis. The palliation of pain in a patient who is unresectable can be managed with celiac axis blocks with 50% alcohol. This procedure can be performed percutaneously under fluoroscopy and can be very effective in palliating pain.

ENDOSCOPIC PALLIATION

Biliary endoprostheses can be placed in patients with obstructive jaundice secondary to malignancy,

such as pancreatic cancer, with a success rate of between 85% and 95%. Tumor involvement of the duodenal wall and papilla sometimes makes successful placement of a biliary endoprosthesis impossible. However, if a cannula and guidewire can be passed into the biliary tree, an endoprosthesis can be positioned within the bile duct and manipulated through the area of obstruction.

Plastic stents between 7 French and 11.5 French in diameter are available in various lengths and shapes and can be placed through most obstructing lesions in the biliary tree between the papilla of Vater and the bifurcation of the left and right intrahepatic ducts. Successful placement results in the rapid drainage of bile and the prompt relief of pruritis, fever, and cholangitis so that the patient can live more comfortably even though the pancreatic cancer may be enlarging in size. However, plastic stents may occlude anywhere between 1 week to several months after insertion, and symptoms of fever, abdominal pain, and jaundice may recur. On rare occasions, the tumor may occlude the stent, but usually a clogging phenomenon occurs, the mechanism of which is not entirely understood. A deposition of calcium bilirubinate and other organic materials as well as bacteria develops within the lumen of the stent, which can result in occlusion. The endoprosthesis can be changed easily as soon as obstruction occurs, but it is best to change the stents at 3- to 4-month intervals prophylactically even though the patient is free of symptoms.

To decrease the likelihood of possible stent occlusion and to make a larger passage through the obstructing lesion, metallic mesh stents have been developed. However, metallic stents are more expensive, and once in place cannot be removed. The most frequently used metallic stent at this time is the Wallstent, which can be delivered through an 8 French tube but which can expand to approximately 30 French. Proper placement of the stent is essential and requires some skill. Stent blockage may occur, especially from growth of tumor, either through the mesh of the stent or at the stent margins. Blockage can be overcome either by placement of a conventional stent through the Wallstent or by recanalization with a diathermy probe or cautery. At the present time, multicenter studies are in progress to assess the associated complications and long-term performance of the Wallstent, as well as to evaluate the success and complication rates of the Wallstent versus the conventional biliary stent. Newer metallic stents of various types are also being tested in the hope that they will be less susceptible to occlusion.

PERCUTANEOUS TRANSHEPATIC PALLIATION

The technique of decompressing obstructed bile ducts by transhepatic catheter placement was first reported by Molnar and Stokum in 1974. Since that time, percutaneous techniques have improved considerably. Percutaneous transhepatic cholangiography (PTC) and percutaneous biliary drainage (PBD) are well-established nonsurgical procedures which may be used preoperatively to decompress the biliary system or to palliate the patient with malignant obstructive jaundice who is not an appropriate surgical candidate. At the authors' institution, many patients with malignant obstruction due to pancreatic carcinoma undergo preoperative biliary decompression (Fig. 42-7). After a diagnostic PTC, access into the biliary system is gained using a coaxial system of steerable guidewires and catheters, which is followed by placement of an 8.3 Ring biliary drainage catheter (Cook, Inc., Bloomington, Ind.). This catheter not only decompresses the obstructed biliary system but frequently serves as an intraoperative marker during pancreaticoduodenectomy.

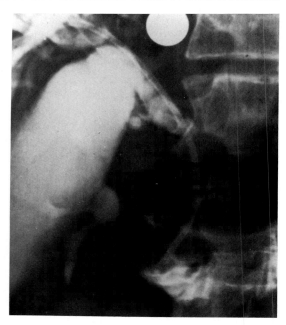

Figure 42-7. Percutaneous transhepatic biliary drainage in a patient with pancreatic cancer.

If the patient presents with obstructive jaundice due to pancreatic malignancy and is felt to be unresectable based on (1) clinical evaluation, (2) cross-sectional imaging by CT, MRI, or ultrasound (US), or (3) angiography, transhepatic palliation is an option. The 8.3 Ring catheter placed initially is stiff and uncomfortable for the patient and is therefore exchanged for a softer, more comfortable tube approximately 24 to 48 hours after PBD. The stent is then exchanged approximately every 2 to 3 months. Cholangiography and biliary catheter exchange procedures are generally performed on an outpatient basis. Antibiotics are administered intravenously prior to the cholangiogram and biliary catheter exchange.

Percutaneous biliary drainage in patients with malignancies may be associated with a significant morbidity and mortality. Previously reported studies on PBD have reported major complications in 5% to 25% and procedure-related deaths in 0% to 5%. Many of the patients reported in the literature have malignant biliary obstruction. A review by Ye and Ho combining the results of six groups of investigators (702 patients) reports major complications of 8% and death in 2%. In this retrospective review, 609 of the 702 patients (87%) had malignant biliary obstructions. The high complication rate is generally attributed to the fact that these patients are more debilitated than those presenting with biliary obstruction due to benign causes.

Another option in those patients who are not appropriate surgical candidates because of underlying cardiac, pulmonary, or other medical conditions, or in those patients who are found to be unresectable on CT, angiography, or laparoscopy, is transhepatic palliation using a biliary endoprosthesis. This treatment option has recently received greater clinical acceptance. Such devices should be used only in patients with a limited life expectancy, such as 6 months or less. Biliary endoprostheses are placed either endoscopically or transhepatically. In the setting of preoperative biliary decompression through PTC and PBD, transhepatic access is already available and conversion to an endoprosthesis is feasible.

Biliary endoprostheses are constructed of plastic or metal and are fluoroscopically advanced across the obstruction. Recent improvements in materials have reduced the incidence of premature closure of such devices. Plastic endoprostheses are generally larger and are constructed in such a fashion that a "mushroom" configuration at one end or a subcutaneous "anchoring" button is necessary to prevent migration. Metal endoprostheses, approved for biliary applications by the U.S. Food and Drug Administration (FDA), consist of three designs: (1) the Wallstent (Schneider [USA] Inc., Minneapolis, Minn.), (2) the Gianturco Z-stent (Cook, Inc., Bloomington, Ind.), and (3) the Palmaz stent (Johnson & Johnson Interventional Systems Co., Warren, NJ). The first two endoprostheses are self-expanding metallic stents, whereas the Palmaz stent is a balloon-expandable metallic stent.

The metallic endoprostheses are significantly more expensive (approximately ten times the cost of a plastic endoprosthesis). The metallic Wallstent requires only a 7 French transhepatic tract for placement, compared with the 10 to 13 French tract size required for placement of the plastic endoprostheses. Because of the reduced size of the transhepatic tract required for the Wallstent, this endoprosthesis may be placed in a single step (i.e., immediately after PTC/PBD if there is no significant hemobilia),

thus offsetting the increased cost. In general, percutaneous transhepatic placement of plastic endoprostheses requires more than one step (i.e., PTC/PBD), tube tract maturation, tract dilation, and endoprosthesis placement.

The advantages of an endoprosthesis include (1) restoration of bile flow into the duodenum and (2) conversion of an internal and external biliary drainage catheter (stent) into a device which is completely intrahepatic, thus eliminating the care required for a conventional biliary drainage catheter (i.e., dressing changes, flushing of the tube twice daily, leakage at the skin entry site, complications such as cholangitis, and drain and routine catheter [stent] exchanges).

The disadvantages of an endoprosthesis include (1) premature occlusion with its associated complications, (2) possible dislodgement, and (3) increased cost for the metallic endoprosthesis. Once an endoprosthesis is placed, transhepatic access is generally eliminated. Thus, if the patient survives beyond 6 months, the plastic endoprosthesis must be endoscopically exchanged. Metallic endoprostheses cannot be exchanged either endoscopically or by a transhepatic approach, and in most series the patency rates of metallic endoprostheses are similar to those of the plastic devices. Should premature occlusion occur, percutaneous transhepatic intervention to relieve jaundice (i.e., PBD) is necessary if endoscopic treatment fails.

Clinical results using percutaneously placed transhepatic biliary endoprostheses as palliation for malignant obstruction have varied considerably. In a large series of 334 patients published by Lammer et al., the results since 1982 of transhepatic placement of endoprostheses are reported. Of the 334 patients, 320 had malignant biliary obstruction. Plastic endoprostheses were placed transhepatically in 297 patients, and metallic endoprostheses in 37 patients. Of the 297 patients receiving plastic endoprostheses, malignancy was the cause of obstruction in 289 patients. Premature occlusion of plastic endoprostheses was noted in 25 of 297 patients (8.4%).

In this series, 31 of 37 patients receiving metallic endoprostheses had malignancy as the cause of biliary obstruction. Overall stent failure (occlusion, dislocation, etc.) occurred in 12% of the 37 patients receiving metallic endoprostheses. Specifically, reocclusions occurred in 4 of the 31 patients (13%) with·malignant biliary obstruction treated with the metallic endoprostheses.

In a series published by Gordon et al., 50 consecutive patients with malignant biliary obstruction were treated with the Wallstent endoprostheses. Follow-up ranged between 9 and 22 months. Patient survival rates in this group were 7.5 months. The overall endoprosthesis patency rate was 5.8 months. Stent occlusion requiring a second intervention occurred in 24% of patients.

The complications associated with plastic or metallic biliary endoprosthesis placement used to palliate patients include bleeding; bile peritonitis; biliary pleural effusion; intrahepatic, subphrenic, and subhepatic abscesses; cholangitis; ascites; fistula; and, rarely, duodenal perforation. These complications have also been observed in patients undergoing PTC/PBD procedures. In most series, the long-term patency of plastic and metal endoprostheses is similar. Thus, unless a patient has a limited life expectancy, routine biliary catheter exchanges are, in the authors' opinion, the best means of percutaneous transhepatic palliation of jaundice.

SURGICAL PALLIATION

For patients who are staged preoperatively and thought to be resectable, and then at the time of surgery are found to be unresectable, surgical palliation is appropriate. In addition, patients who preoperatively are known to be unresectable but who present with duodenal obstruction with or without jaundice are also candidates for surgical palliation. In the past, many series reporting the results of surgical palliation for carcinoma of the head of the pancreas reported mortality rates in the range of 15% to 20%. These results were in the era, however, when pancreaticoduodenectomy carried a mortality rate of 25%. Today surgical palliation can be carried out effectively with a low hospital mortality. In a series of 118 patients who were explored at The Johns Hopkins Hospital with the hope of performing a curative resection and at the time of surgery were found to be unresectable, all were palliated effectively, with a hospital mortality rate of 2.5%.

The authors' choice for biliary bypass is to perform a hepaticojejunostomy rather than a cholecystojejunostomy. This procedure was performed in the majority of the 118 patients in this series. In addition, the authors have felt that all patients should undergo a palliative gastrojejunostomy. Previously, many surgeons were reluctant to perform this procedure routinely because of the delayed gastric emptying that often would result, even in patients who had no emptying problems preoperatively. The authors have eliminated this incidence of delayed gastric emptying by routinely performing retrocolic gastrojejunostomies. In addition, as a third procedure at the time of palliation, the authors perform a chemical splanchnicectomy by injecting 20 cc of 50% alcohol on either side of the aorta at the level of the celiac axis.

Late gastric outlet obstruction occurred in only 4 patients (3%) in this series. Recurrent jaundice occurred in only 2 patients (2%), and both patients were managed with percutaneous transhepatic stents. The celiac plexus blocks were effective in controlling pain. This was documented by a prospective randomized study comparing alcohol injection into the celiac axis at the time of palliative bypass to the injection of saline into the celiac axis. This study demonstrated clearly that effective pain palliation can be achieved by chemical splanchnicectomy (Fig. 42-8). This study was carried out by Lillemoe and his colleagues at Johns Hopkins, and included these 118 patients plus 19 other patients. These 137 patients were prospectively randomized, and the study clearly demonstrated effective pain

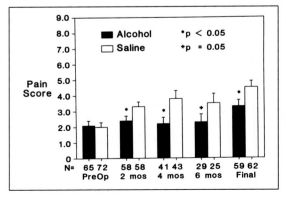

Figure 42-8. Mean pain scores for patients with unresectable pancreatic cancer receiving alcohol chemical splanchnicectomy and saline controls. (Reprinted with permission of Lillemoe KD, et al. Chemical splanchnicectomy in patients with unresectable pancreatic cancer: A prospective randomized trial. *Ann Surg* 1993; 217:447.)

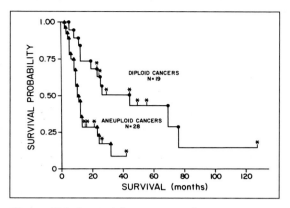

Figure 42-9. Survival for patients with pancreatic cancer after pancreaticoduodenectomy with diploid or aneuploid tumors. (Reprinted with permission of Allison DC, et al. Pancreatic cancer cell DNA content correlates with long-term survival after pancreaticoduodenectomy. *Ann Surg* 1991; 214:648.)

palliation from the procedure. Thus, in the vast majority of patients with unresectable pancreatic cancer, pain can be effectively palliated, late gastric outlet obstruction can be prevented, and jaundice can be permanently palliated.

RADIOTHERAPY AND CHEMOTHERAPY

Very few regimens have been demonstrated to have any effect in terms of prolonging survival or improving the quality of life in the patient with unresectable carcinoma of the pancreas. Shrinkage of measurable masses occurs in only 10% to 20% of patients with metastatic pancreatic carcinoma treated with 5-fluorouracil as a single agent, and the tumor response is generally brief. The addition of other agents (doxorubicin, mitomycin-C) increases toxicity but has not been shown to improve the response rate or survival time. Trials of drugs with novel cytotoxic mechanisms are suitable for such patients. Patients with localized unresectable pancreatic cancer are treated at Johns Hopkins and many other institutions with palliative external beam radiation, which may decrease analgesic requirements and improve survival.

Conclusions and New Approaches

Substantial progress has been made in the management of carcinoma of the head of the pancreas over the past decade. Patients can be diagnosed and

staged rapidly and with great accuracy. When patients are candidates for pancreaticoduodenectomy, this procedure can be carried out with a very low hospital mortality. Morbidity remains substantial but is not life-threatening and is virtually all self-limited. Adjuvant therapy has been demonstrated to be of benefit. Survival can clearly be prolonged by surgery. Patients with carcinoma of the head of the pancreas who undergo pancreaticoduodenectomy are clearly surviving longer today than a decade or more ago.

Potential new approaches for the future include the preoperative staging of patients by image cytometry. Using small specimens obtained from aspiration biopsy, the DNA status of tumors can be documented via image cytometry. If a tumor is diploid, the 5-year survival rate is in the range of 50% (Fig. 42-9). The authors have not had a long-term survival in a patient with an aneuploid tumor. This approach could make it possible to stage patients biologically with aspiration biopsies. If a 40-year-old male had involvement of the portal vein such that pancreaticoduodenectomy would require portal vein resection and reconstruction and the tumor was demonstrated to be diploid by preoperative aspiration biopsy, the procedure should probably be performed. In contrast, if the tumor was demonstrated to be aneuploid, such an extended pancreaticoduodenectomy would probably be unwarranted.

Molecular studies have demonstrated a high prevalence of point mutations at codon 12 of the K-*ras* oncogene in pancreatic cancer. In the authors' series from The Johns Hopkins Hospital, this point mutation is present in over 90% of the patients studied. In addition, the mutation is more prevalent in patients who are cigarette smokers. This mutation may be one of the mechanisms by which cigarette smoking predisposes to carcinoma of the pancreas. Attempts are now under way to screen for patients who may have alimentary tract neoplasms, including pancreatic cancer, by looking for evidence of this point mutation in the stool.

Screening tools are needed to improve long-term survival for carcinoma of the head of the pancreas. If a Whipple's procedure is done prior to nodal spread, the 5-year survival rate can be as high as 50%. Currently, most patients who are resectable with carcinoma of the head of the pancreas already have nodal spread. Some means of demonstrating a tumor marker in the blood or stool, which would allow one to identify a pancreatic neoplasm before obstructive jaundice develops, might well lead to a substantial improvement in long-term survival. In addition, new and improved adjuvant regimens need to be developed. The current regimen demonstrated to be effective by the Gastrointestinal Tumor Study Group is clearly not an ideal regimen, and every expectation exists that better regimens will be developed over the next decade.

Selected Readings

Allison DC, et al. Pancreatic cancer cell DNA content correlates with long-term survival after pancreaticoduodenectomy. *Ann Surg* 1991; 214:648.

Cameron JL, et al. Factors influencing survival following pancreaticoduodenectomy for pancreatic cancer. *Am J Surg* 1991; 161:120.

Cameron JL, et al. One hundred and forty-five consecutive pancreaticoduodenectomies without mortality. *Ann Surg* 1993; 217:430.

Crist DW, Sitzmann JV, Cameron JL. Improved hospital morbidity, mortality and survival following the Whipple procedure. *Ann Surg* 1987; 206:358.

Davids PHP, et al. Randomized trial of self-expanding metal stents versus polyethylene stents for distal malignant biliary obstruction. *Lancet* 1992; 340:1488.

Gastrointestinal Tumor Study Group. Further evidence of effective adjuvant combined radiation and chemotherapy following curative resection of pancreatic cancer. *Cancer* 1987; 59:2006.

Gordon RL, et al. Malignant biliary obstruction: Treatment with expandable metallic stents—Follow-up and reintervention in patients with hilar and nonhilar obstruction. *Radiology* 1992; 182:697.

Klassen DJ, et al. Treatment of locally unresectable cancer of the stomach and pancreas: A randomized comparison of 5-fluorouracil alone or with radiation plus concurrent and maintenance 5-fluorouracil. An ECOG study. *J Clin Oncol* 1985; 3:373.

Lillemoe KD, et al. Chemical splanchnicectomy in patients with unresectable pancreatic cancer: A prospective randomized trial. *Ann Surg* 1993; 217:447.

Yeo CJ, et al. Erythromycin accelerates gastric emptying after pancreaticoduodenectomy: A prospective, randomized placebo controlled trial. *Ann Surg* 1993; 218:229.

Index

① at what point is Jim at w/ the disease?
(Ranges from Asymptomatic to patients w/ secondary
    biliary disease) Primary to secondary

② Treatment?
        Medical treatment doesn't seem to have an
        effect on the progressiveness of the disease — —
Are any of   A. Interventional Radiology
these an   B. ~~~~ Endoscopic therapy
option?   C. Surgical therapy
Is there a
by-pass type
surgery?
~~~~~~~~~~~~~~~

③ Jim also has ulcerative colitis (which is common)
    says that it should raise the ~~stm~~ suspicion of
    " Concomitant biliary disease" - what is that?

④